Evidence-Based Endocrine Surgery

Rajeev Parameswaran • Amit Agarwal
Editors

Evidence-Based Endocrine Surgery

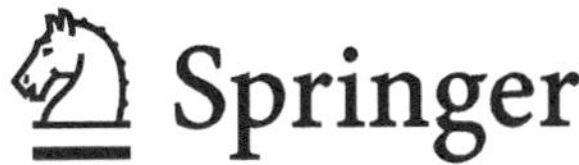

Springer

Editors
Rajeev Parameswaran
Division of Endocrine Surgery
National University Hospital
Singapore

Amit Agarwal
Department of Endocrine Surgery
SGPGI Hospital
Lucknow
India

ISBN 978-981-13-3818-2 ISBN 978-981-10-1124-5 (eBook)
https://doi.org/10.1007/978-981-10-1124-5

This Springer imprint is published by the registered company Springer Nature Singapore Pte Ltd.
The registered company address is: 152 Beach Road, #21-01/04 Gateway East, Singapore 189721, Singapore

Acknowledgements

To those most dear to us

My wife Chithra Rajeev and my children Reshma and Pranav for their constant support and encouragement, without which this project would not have been possible

To my parents and Almighty God

To my mentors, colleagues, fellows and medical students for enriching my academic life

To all my colleague authors, who are also my dear friends for their contributions to the textbook

To the publishers for supporting this project

Rajeev Parameswaran

My parents for their love, my wife Vijaya Mohan for her support, my sons Arpit and Vedanta for their understanding and my colleagues, students and well-wishers for their admiration and encouragement

Amit Agarwal

Contents

Part I

Thyroid

1 Evidence-Based Surgery

Rajeev Parameswaran and Amit Agarwal

Surgery has always been learnt via the apprenticeship model with the teachers showing the way to perform based on their experience. This model of learning was not ideal, as it meant that learning was dependent on the mistakes made by oneself or others. The appearance of the concept of evidence-based medicine in the late twentieth century in a document published from McMaster University changed the way clinicians practice effective and efficient clinical care today [1]. Evidence-based surgery incorporates integration of best available evidence from research, clinical circumstances, and patient and clinical experience to treat patients effectively [2].

Evidence-based medicine has four main components [2], known as 1-2-3-4; one goal, two fundamental principles, three components, and four steps. The goal of evidence-based practice is to improve the health-related quality of life through decisions in relation to clinical and healthcare policies. The two fundamental principles include *hierarchy of evidence* and *insufficiency of evidence alone* in decision-making. The three components include *evidence*, *expertise*, and *expectations of patients*. The four steps are *ask*, *acquire*, *access*, and *apply*. In relation to surgery, evidence-based practice can be divided into two categories [3]:

- Evidence-based surgical decision-making
- Evidence-based surgical guidelines

The knowledge to practice evidence-based surgery is obtained from data obtained through research, measuring evidence through statistics and clinical experience and practice.

Hierarchy of Evidence

The results of the research designs are not all equal in terms of the risk, error, and bias, with some research providing better evidence than others. The validity of results obtained from research is therefore based on the type of studies, with randomized controlled trials providing the most reliable evidence [2, 4]. Once the studies have been selected, it is important to identify those studies that carry a higher methodological weight. Hierarchies of evidence allow for research-based recommendations to be graded and reflect the susceptibility of bias observed in the various types of study. The simplest hierarchical tool that is commonly used is Sackett's levels of evidence (Table 1.1).

R. Parameswaran (✉)
Division of Endocrine Surgery, National University Hospital, Singapore, Singapore
e-mail: rajeev_parameswaran@nuhs.edu.sg

A. Agarwal
Sanjay Gandhi Post Graduate Institute of Medical Sciences (SGPGIMS), Lucknow, Uttar Pradesh, India

R. Parameswaran, A. Agarwal (eds.), *Evidence-Based Endocrine Surgery*,
https://doi.org/10.1007/978-981-10-1124-5_1

Table 1.1 Sackett's level of evidence

Level	Type of evidence
I	Large RCT with clear results
II	Small RCT with not so clear results
II	Cohort and control cases studies
IV	Historical cohorts or control cases studies
V	Series of cases, studies with no controls

RCT randomized clinical trials

Randomized Controlled Trials

The randomized controlled trial (RCT) is one of the simplest, most powerful, and revolutionary tools of research [5, 6] and offers the maximum protection against bias [7] [8]. RCT is a study in which individuals are allocated randomly to receive one of several interventions, with the control group receiving an accepted treatment or no treatment at all (Fig. 1.1). The outcomes from RCT's can be described as continuous or discrete [9]. The problem is that RCTs in surgery are less performed when compared with medical interventions, and this may be due to problems such as standardization of interventions, issues with recruitment, and blinding of subjects and investigators [10, 11]. Similarly, trials may have to be discontinued earlier than planned [12], and this can have a significant scientific, ethical, and economic impact [13, 14].

A meta-analysis is a systematic review of randomized controlled trials where the outcomes of the studies are pooled. The advantage of meta-analyses is that it effectively increases the sample size, with the Cochrane collaborators calling the results of meta-analyses the "pinnacle of scientific knowledge" as it improves the statistical power of the evidence given by a single RCT [2]. However, the problem with pooling of data is that the outcomes are dependent on the quality of the RCT's. Even meta-analyses are not without their pitfalls and commonly include *publication, bias, heterogeneity*, and *robustness of studies.*

Observational Studies: Case-Control and Cohort Studies

Case-control studies are those where the subjects meet the definition of a "case" and subjects that are not cases. These are typically retrospective studies as they look back in time to identify causable factors and have a longitudinal aspect to the data. An outline of the study design is shown in Fig. 1.2. These studies can be used for study of common diseases and useful for studying etiologies of rare disease as well. However, these studies are not without bias—*incidence bias*, *selection bias*, and *"healthy volunteer" effect.* The biases in case-control studies may be minimized by the following criteria: *appropriate case selection* (representative of all patients with the disease), *appropriate controls* from the healthy population, and *information from cases and controls are collected the same way*. An example of such a study in thyroidology is that of metabolic and cardiovascular risk in patients with a history of thyroid cancer from Italy [15].

Cohort studies unlike case-control studies are truly not retrospective but prospective in the sense that the risk factor is collected first and then the disease outcomes are collected downstream, after a period of follow-up. These studies are useful to make observations or study associations between a risk factor and subsequent development of a disease. A flow chart of such a study is shown in Fig. 1.3. Cohort studies can be of many types:

- Nonconcurrent, historical, or retrospective cohort studies
- Concurrent or prospective cohort studies
- Nested cohort studies

The advantages of cohort studies are that the cases diagnosed are incident, rather than prevalence obtained from case-control studies; provide information about the natural history of the disease and estimates of risk, less risk of bias; and study multiple outcomes. Unlike case-control studies where rare disease can be studied, prospective cohort studies help study a rare exposure. The disadvantages of cohort studies are that the study durations are generally very long, follow-up can be expensive, and large study populations are required. An example of a cohort study in endocrine surgery is that of a Korean study considering the benefits and risks of prophylactic central neck dissection for papillary thyroid cancer [16].

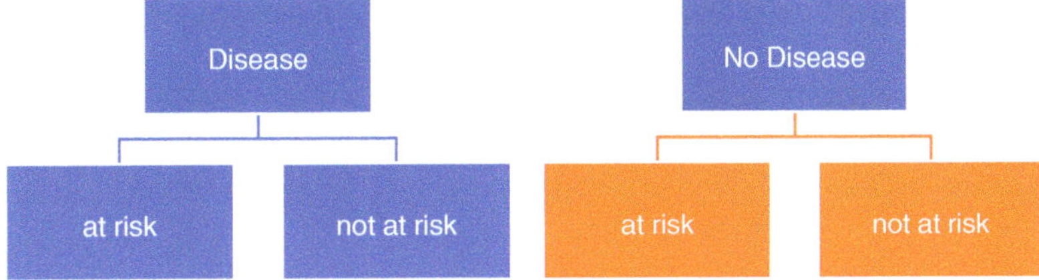

Fig. 1.1 Layout of a case-control study with patients with or without disease identified at the start of the study, and information is collected retrospectively

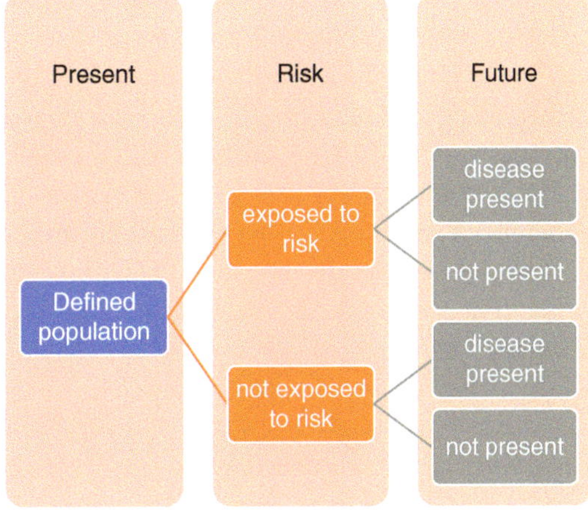

Fig. 1.2 Layout of a prospective cohort study, which may be longitudinal concurrent or nonconcurrent historical [1]

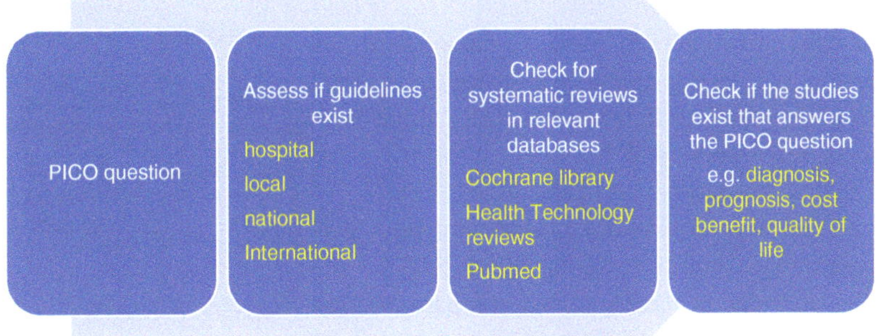

Fig. 1.3 Finding evidence in surgery based on McCulloch and Badenoch

Case Reports and Series

Case report describes a single case and series describes similar cases, with both describing clinical characteristics about individual patients. Case reports represent the lowest evidence of published clinical evidence and are generally uncontrolled descriptive studies of outcomes related to a type of intervention [17]. Retrospective case series are the most common evidence in surgical literature and makes causal inferences about the relationships between outcomes and risk factors [17]. Case series have inherent biases and are usually based on single center or surgeon's experience which cannot be generalized to the population. Despite its drawbacks, case series can be used for hypothesis generation and providing information on rare diseases [18].

Identifying the Evidence

Identifying the best evidence can be challenging but is an essential skill required for surgeons in their day-to-day practice. Various methods have been employed to perform a search on a research topic, but the most widely used is the PICO (Population/problem, Intervention/exposure, Comparison, and Outcome) tool developed by the McMaster University (Table 1.2). PICO enables researchers to frame research questions and search terms, enabling a systematic search strategy [19, 20]. It is the best tool adopted by most researchers and has been adopted by the Cochrane collaboration [21].

Other tools besides PICO that have been proposed for qualitative research include SPICE (setting, population, intervention, comparison, and evaluation) [22], ECLIPSE (expectation, client group, location, impact, professionals, service) [23], and CIMO (context–intervention–mechanism–outcome) [24]. None of the abovementioned tools are suitable for use with qualitative research questions. Once the appropriate tool has been selected, the next step is to work through finding the sequence of evidence (as shown in Fig. 1.3) [25].

Sources of Evidence

There are wide range of sources for collection of data for research, with each of them having advantages and disadvantages (Table 1.3). No matter whatever the source, this should be appraised critically before it is applied to the patient.

The first option of getting an evidence in surgical practice is mainly from senior colleagues or a peer with significant experience. This source of evidence is sought mainly by inexperienced professionals and turn to colleagues for help and advice when faced with clinical uncertainties as shown in a study on dental practitioners [26]. Similarly, one may seek the opinion of an expert, an advanced practitioner in his or her specialty. In terms of evidence, these sources are considered as low level, and other problem is that it is not uncommon to see disagreements between experts. Similarly, books though are a good source of information, the time it takes to research and publish a book is quite long, and the information may be out of date after a few years.

The *Internet* has changed the world, in terms of how people work and obtain information, with

Table 1.2 Outline of PICO

PICO	
P: patient population	Group for which you need evidence
I: intervention	Operation or treatment whose effect you need to study
C: comparison	What is the evidence that the proposed intervention produces better or worse results than no intervention or a different type of intervention?
O: outcomes	What are the effects and end points of the intervention?

Table 1.3 Examples of the various sources of evidence available for the surgeon

Colleagues
Books
The Internet
Journals
Electronic databases
Specialist organizations
Guidelines

an estimated 52% using the Internet globally. One can practically obtain information on any subject from anywhere, with relatively easy access. The information that can be accessed from the Internet include research evidence, clinical guidelines, and patient information and resources [27]. The disadvantage with the Internet is that not all information obtained from the Internet may be accurate and can be time-consuming. A search on Google retrieved a total of 52,200 sites using the search words evidence-based endocrine surgery, but of these many might be factually inaccurate or useless. Criteria to help individuals assess the quality of health-related websites have been published by many organizations [28].

Journal reading is most common method of keeping up to date in surgery, and there are many journals published in surgery and their subspecialties (both with low and high impact factor). Journals unlike books contain more recent information on various topics, which are available in print form or electronic version (e-version). There are over 1000 journals published worldwide, and to read articles of interest in one's specialty is a big task. Ways of keeping pace with research articles in journals are the following: decide which specialist journal is most relevant to your clinical practice and review contents regularly, host journal clubs, and use evidence-based supplements.

Electronic databases are specialized bibliographic databases that are available electronically and focusing on a subspecialty. The most commonly used database for medical-related information is MEDLINE, compiled by the US National Library of Medicine (NLM). It is freely available on the Internet and can be searched by the free search engine PubMed. Currently the database contains over 25 million records from 5633 publications to date. Over 80% of the published articles are in English, and the most common topic published is cancer.

Specialist organizations like Cochrane collaboration (www.cochrane.org) provide high-quality information to make health decisions and maintain a database of systematic reviews, meta-analyses, and randomized controlled trials. Two similar organizations are the NHS Centre for Reviews and Dissemination (CRD) based in UK and the National Library for Health (NeLH).

Clinical Practice Guidelines

Clinical practice guidelines were developed to support clinicians in decision-making along with their knowledge and experience. However, clinical practice guidelines are now being used for broader purposes: as institutional policy, to inform insurance coverage, for deriving quality of care criteria, and for medicolegal liability standards [29]. However clinical guidelines are not without problems in terms of bias and misguidance [30], and despite this many clinicians follow this. Some of the examples of clinical guidelines in endocrine surgery are shown in Table 1.4.

Table 1.4 Examples of guidelines available for clinicians involved in the management of thyroid disease

2017	European Thyroid Association Guidelines regarding thyroid nodule molecular fine-needle aspiration cytology diagnostics [31]
2017	Radioactive iodine therapy, molecular imaging, and serum biomarkers for differentiated thyroid cancer: 2017 guidelines of the French Societies of Nuclear Medicine, Endocrinology, Pathology, Biology, Endocrine Surgery and Head and Neck Surgery [32]
2017	2017 Guidelines of the American Thyroid Association for the Diagnosis and Management of Thyroid Disease During Pregnancy and the Postpartum [33]
2016	2015 American Thyroid Association Management Guidelines for Adult Patients with Thyroid Nodules and Differentiated Thyroid Cancer: The American Thyroid Association Guidelines Task Force on Thyroid Nodules and Differentiated Thyroid Cancer [34]

Why Evidence-Based Surgery?

Practicing evidence-based surgery is challenging, and applying it to surgical practice is a four-step process: creating evidence, summarizing evidence, disseminating evidence, and implementing evidence into practice [1, 35]. Evidence-based practice is more evident in the field of general medicine than in surgery as high-quality surgical research is very difficult [36, 37]. In 1996 only about 7% of the papers published in surgery was from RCTs [38] compared to 24% of surgery in 2009 [39], much lesser than the 50% of RCTs in general medicine [40]. Clinicians are now recognizing this shortfall [11, 41] and pushing for evidence-based practice in surgery [41, 42].

Currently there is a lot of discrepancy between our knowledge and the way we practice [43], and this gap can be bridged with evidence-based practice. So many our clinical practices are guided by what is taught during the apprenticeship of surgical training, and one example of this is the use of drains in thyroid surgery. Surgical practices are also dependent on policies dictated by the needs of the population in a country, and healthcare policies. A lot of these policies and practices are aimed at reducing the cost of health, rather than actual value to the patient. Value-based surgery focuses on patient outcomes, quality of life, and cost using evidence-based practice [44].

Besides the benefits to the patients and healthcare industry by the practice of evidence-based surgery, the benefits are also to the surgeon in the form of improved teamwork, decision-making, enhanced research, and improvements in training and satisfaction [45]. The benefits of evidence-based surgery are summarized in Fig. 1.4. To promote improved outcomes and benefits, there is a concerted effort by national, regional, and international societies and organizations to use evidence-based surgery [46].

National surgical organizations have increasingly focused on using EBM to enhance the practice and outcome of surgical care. The ACS are exemplary in this process but are not alone. Efforts are occurring in all surgical specialties through national and regional societies and organizations.

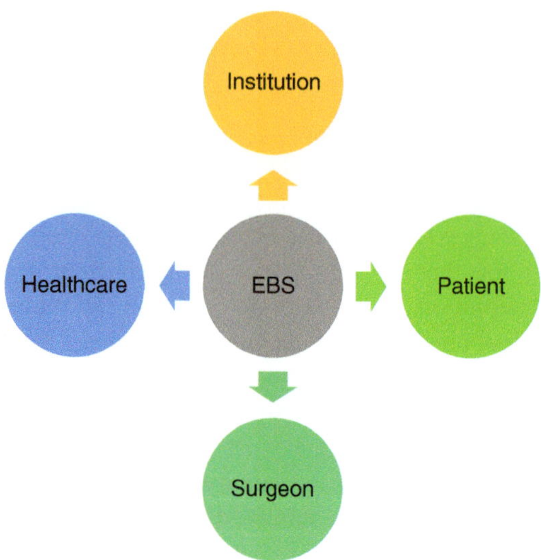

Fig. 1.4 Benefits of Evidence Based Surgery (adapted from Athanasiou T, Debas HT, Darzi A. Key topics in surgical research and methodology)

Conclusion

Evidence-based surgery is not just about doing randomized controlled trials but for the global benefit of patients and healthcare. The principle of evidence-based practice is obtained from best available evidence and requires a change in mentality at all levels of healthcare. As surgeons, one should move away from the old-fashioned approach to surgery and embrace the change of evidence-based practice. To do surgeons must gather, analyze, and collate data to derive best practice and outcomes for the benefit of patients ultimately. For the next generation of surgeons, surgery should not be about intuitions but based on best evidence. As Ubbink and Legemate put in their editorial article in *British Journal of Surgery, evidence-based surgery is not a passing creed—it is a lasting need.*

References

1. Evidence-Based Medicine Working Group. Evidence-based medicine. A new approach to teaching the practice of medicine. JAMA. 1992;268(17):2420–5.
2. Sackett DL. Evidence-based medicine: how to practice and teach EBM. 2nd ed. Edinburgh: Churchill Livingstone; 2000.

3. Eddy DM. Evidence-based medicine: a unified approach. Health Aff (Millwood). 2005;24(1):9–17.
4. Mulrow CD. The medical review article: state of the science. Ann Intern Med. 1987;106:485–8.
5. Jadad AR, Rennie D. The randomized controlled trial gets a middle-aged checkup. JAMA. 1998;279(4):319–20.
6. Silverman WA, Iain C. Sir Austin Bradford Hill: an appreciation. Control Clin Trials. 1992;13(2):100–5.
7. Miller JN, Colditz GA, Mosteller F. How study design affects outcomes in comparisons of therapy. II: surgical. Stat Med. 1989;8(4):455–66.
8. Colditz GA, Miller JN, Mosteller F. How study design affects outcomes in comparisons of therapy. I: medical. Stat Med. 1989;8(4):441–54.
9. Sprague S, McKay P, Thoma A. Study design and hierarchy of evidence for surgical decision making. Clin Plast Surg. 2008;35(2):195–205.
10. Solomon MJ, McLeod RS. Should we be performing more randomized controlled trials evaluating surgical operations? Surgery. 1995;118(3):459–67.
11. McCulloch P, Taylor I, Sasako M, Lovett B, Griffin D. Randomised trials in surgery: problems and possible solutions. BMJ. 2002;324(7351):1448–51.
12. Goodman SN. Stopping trials for efficacy: an almost unbiased view. Clin Trials. 2009;6(2):133–5.
13. Iltis AS. Stopping trials early for commercial reasons: the risk-benefit relationship as a moral compass. J Med Ethics. 2005;31(7):410–4.
14. Kasenda B, von Elm E, You J, Blümle A, Tomonaga Y, Saccilotto R, et al. Prevalence, characteristics, and publication of discontinued randomized trials. JAMA. 2014;311(10):1045–52.
15. Giusti M, Mortara L, Degrandi R, Cecoli F, Mussap M, Rodriguez G, et al. Metabolic and cardiovascular risk in patients with a history of differentiated thyroid carcinoma: a case-controlled cohort study. Thyroid Res. 2008;1(1):2.
16. Lee DY, Cho J-G, Oh KH, Woo J-S, Jung K-Y, Baek S-K, et al. The benefits and risks of prophylactic central neck dissection for papillary thyroid carcinoma: prospective cohort study. Int J Endocrinol. 2015;2015:1–6.
17. Brighton B, Bhandari M, Tornetta P 3rd, Felson DT. Hierarchy of evidence: from case reports to randomized controlled trials. Clin Orthop Relat Res. 2003;413(413):19–24.
18. Urschel JD, Goldsmith CH, Tandan VR, Miller JD. Users' guide to evidence-based surgery: how to use an article evaluating surgical interventions. Can J Surg. 2001;44(2):95.
19. Booth A, O'Rourke AJ, Ford NJ. Structuring the presearch reference interview: a useful technique for handling clinical questions. Bull Med Libr Assoc. 2000;88(3):239–46.
20. Schardt C, Adams MB, Owens T, Keitz S, Fontelo P. Utilization of the PICO framework to improve searching PubMed for clinical questions. BMC Med Inform Decis Mak. 2007;7(1):16.
21. Higgins J, Green SP, Cochrane C, Wiley I. Cochrane handbook for systematic reviews of interventions. Hoboken, NJ; Chichester: Wiley-Blackwell; 2008.
22. Booth A. Clear and present questions: formulating questions for evidence based practice. Library Hi Tech. 2006;24(3):355–68.
23. Wildridge V, Bell L. How CLIP became ECLIPSE: a mnemonic to assist in searching for health policy/management information. Health Inf Libr J. 2002;19(2):113–5.
24. Denyer D, Tranfield D, Aken vJEJ. Developing design propositions through research synthesis. Organ Stud. 2008;29(3):393–413.
25. McCulloch P, Badenoch D. Finding and appraising evidence. Surg Clin North Am. 2006;86(1):41–57. viii
26. Glenny AM, Iqbal A. General dental practitioners' knowledge of and attitudes towards evidence based practice. Br Dent J. 2002;193(10):587–91.
27. John J. Sources of evidence. Evid Based Dent. 2003;4(2):37–9.
28. Kim P, Eng TR, Deering MJ, Maxfield A. Published criteria for evaluating health related web sites: review. BMJ. 1999;318(7184):647–9.
29. Fervers B, Carretier J, Bataillard A. Clinical practice guidelines. J Visc Surg. 2010;147(6):e341–9.
30. Lenzer J. Evidence Based Medicine. Why we can't trust clinical guidelines. BMJ. 2013;346:f3830.
31. Paschke R, Cantara S, Crescenzi A, Jarzab B, Musholt TJ, Sobrinho Simoes M. European Thyroid Association Guidelines regarding thyroid nodule molecular fine-needle aspiration cytology diagnostics. Eur Thyroid J. 2017;6(3):115–29.
32. Zerdoud S, Giraudet AL, Leboulleux S, Leenhardt L, Bardet S, Clerc J, et al. Radioactive iodine therapy, molecular imaging and serum biomarkers for differentiated thyroid cancer: 2017 guidelines of the French Societies of Nuclear Medicine, Endocrinology, Pathology, Biology, Endocrine Surgery and Head and Neck Surgery. Ann Endocrinol (Paris). 2017;78(3):162–75.
33. Alexander EK, Pearce EN, Brent GA, Brown RS, Chen H, Dosiou C, et al. 2017 Guidelines of the American Thyroid Association for the diagnosis and management of thyroid disease during pregnancy and the postpartum. Thyroid. 2017;27(3):315–89.
34. Haugen BR, Alexander EK, Bible KC, Doherty GM, Mandel SJ, Nikiforov YE, et al. 2015 American Thyroid Association management guidelines for adult patients with thyroid nodules and differentiated thyroid cancer: The American Thyroid Association Guidelines Task Force on Thyroid Nodules and Differentiated Thyroid Cancer. Thyroid. 2016;26(1):1–133.
35. Cook DJ, Sibbald WJ, Vincent JL, Cerra FB. Evidence based critical care medicine; what is it and what can it do for us? Evidence Based Medicine in Critical Care Group. Crit Care Med. 1996;24(2):334–7.
36. McLeod RS, Wright JG, Solomon MJ, Hu X, Walters BC, Lossing A. Randomized controlled

trials in surgery: issues and problems. Surgery. 1996;119(5):483–6.
37. Lilford R, Braunholtz D, Harris J, Gill T. Trials in surgery. Br J Surg. 2004;91(1):6–16.
38. Horton R. Surgical research or comic opera: questions, but few answers. Lancet. 1996;347(9007):984–5.
39. Ubbink DT, Legemate DA. Evidence-based surgery. Br J Surg. 2004;91(9):1091–2.
40. Howes N, Chagla L, Thorpe M, McCulloch P. Surgical practice is evidence based. Br J Surg. 1997;84(9):1220–3.
41. Jenkins TR. It's time to challenge surgical dogma with evidence-based data. Am J Obstet Gynecol. 2003;189(2):423–7.
42. TR R. What is the future of surgery? Arch Surg. 2003;138(8):825–31.
43. Pang T, Gray M, Evans T. A 15th grand challenge for global public health. Lancet. 2006;367(9507):284–6.
44. Porter ME, Teisberg EO. How physicians can change the future of health care. JAMA. 2007;297(10):1103–11.
45. Athanasiou T, Debas HT, Darzi A. Key topics in surgical research and methodology. Heidelberg: Springer; 2010.
46. Maier RV. What the surgeon of tomorrow needs to know about evidence-based surgery. Arch Surg. 2006;141(3):317–23.

Graves' Disease

2

Chiaw-Ling Chng

Introduction

Graves' disease (GD) is an autoimmune disease with a myriad of clinical manifestations and exerts a profound effect on the metabolism of the individual affected [1]. It is the most common cause of hyperthyroidism in areas of sufficient iodine intake, with annual incidence of 21 cases per 100,000 per year [2]. The disease shows female predominance, with female-to-male ratio between 5:1 and 10:1 [3]. Although the onset of GD can occur at any age, it is most common between 40 and 60 years of age [4]. In this review, pathogenesis, diagnosis, and treatment, including recent advances in the understanding of this disease, will be discussed.

Etiology

The pathogenesis of this autoimmune disease is thought to be multifactorial, with the primary trigger being loss of immunotolerance and development of autoantibodies that stimulate thyroid follicular cells by binding to TSH receptor. These antibodies result in continuous and unregulated thyroid stimulation, resulting in excess production of thyroid hormones and thyroid gland enlargement. A genetic predisposition, coupled with environmental stressors, underlies the pathogenesis of this disease. A higher concordance rate of the condition is found in monozygotic twins than dizygotic twins [5]. Several disease susceptibility loci have been identified for GD, including specific polymorphisms of HLA [6], CTLA-4 [7, 8], CD40 [9], protein tyrosine phosphatase-22 [10], thyroglobulin [6], and TSH receptor [6, 7]. Among these, HLA is the major genetic factor in the susceptibility to GD [6]. Environmental factors postulated to contribute to this condition include psychosocial stress [11], smoking [12], and childbirth [13]. In particular, a positive family history of thyroid disease, especially in maternal relatives, is associated with an increased incidence of the disease at a younger age of onset [14]. The interaction between these predisposing factors in the pathogenesis of GD is likely to be complex, and further studies are required to elucidate the precise roles of these factors in the cause of this condition.

Presentations, Investigations, and Treatment Options

Clinical Presentation

The clinical presentation of overt hyperthyroidism due to GD is characterized by a variety of signs and symptoms related to the widespread

C.-L. Chng
Department of Endocrinology, Singapore General Hospital, Singapore, Singapore
e-mail: chng.chiaw.ling@singhealth.com.sg

R. Parameswaran, A. Agarwal (eds.), *Evidence-Based Endocrine Surgery*,
https://doi.org/10.1007/978-981-10-1124-5_2

Table 2.1 Symptoms and signs of overt hyperthyroidism

System	Symptoms	Signs
Metabolic/ thermoregulatory	Increased appetite Weight loss Heat intolerance Increased perspiration and polydipsia	Warm moist skin
Cardiovascular	Palpitations	Tachycardia Increased systolic blood pressure atrial fibrillation Congestive cardiac failure
Respiratory	Dyspnea	Tachypnea
Gastrointestinal	Increased bowel movement	
Reproductive	Irregular menses oligomenorrhea Reduced libido and reduced fertility	Gynecomastia (in males)
Neuromuscular	Tremor of extremities Muscle weakness	Fine hand tremors Proximal myopathy Hyperreflexia
Dermatological	Hair loss Pruritus	Palmar erythema
Psychiatric	Anxiety and irritability Insomnia Altered mood	Altered mood, e.g., mania or depression

actions of thyroid hormones (Table 2.1). The most common presenting symptoms are weight loss (61%), heat intolerance (55%), and tremulousness (54%), and the most common physical finding is a palpable diffuse goiter (69%) [15].

Older patients are less likely to have tachycardia and tremor, and they more often present with weight loss or depression, a clinical entity referred to as apathetic hyperthyroidism [13, 16]. Atrial fibrillation and congestive cardiac failure are also more common presenting problems in patients over age of 50 years old [16]. It is important to note that these signs and symptoms of overt hyperthyroidism are not specific to GD and can be found in patients with hyperthyroidism from other causes such as toxic nodular goiter or hyperthyroid phase of thyroiditis. However, GD is uniquely characterized by extra-thyroidal manifestations, including Graves' orbitopathy (GO), thyroid dermopathy and thyroid acropachy, and thyrotoxic periodic paralysis.

Graves' Orbitopathy

GO is the main extra-thyroidal manifestation of GD, affecting 25% of patients at diagnosis. Majority of the presentation is mild, with moderate to severe form affecting 5% of cases, which can progress to sight-threatening disease. The disease is autoimmune in etiology and is characterized by inflammation and extensive remodeling of the soft tissues surrounding the eyes [17]. Proliferation of subpopulations of orbital fibroblasts plays a crucial role in the pathogenesis of this condition, leading to expansion of retro-orbital fat and enlargement of extraocular muscles [18]. Disease manifestations include redness and swelling of the conjunctivae and lids, forward protrusion of the globes (proptosis), ocular pain, debilitating double vision, and even sight loss due to compressive optic neuropathy or breakdown of the cornea [19]. There is some evidence to suggest Asian patients with GO may manifest milder phenotypic features, with less proptosis, extraocular muscle involvement, and restriction, although dysthyroid optic neuropathy may occur more readily [20]. Patients with GO are more likely to be women by a 2:1 ratio, while men with GD appear to be at higher risk for the development of more severe disease [21]. Smoking is the most important risk factor for the occurrence and progression of GO. Other risk factors for developing or worsening GO include thyroid dysfunction (both hyperthyroidism and hypothyroidism), radioiodine therapy, and higher level of TSH receptor antibodies (TRAB) [22]. Apart from smoking cessation, current treatment options for GO include supportive measures, high-dose intravenous steroids, or other immunosuppressive therapy such as cyclosporine, methotrexate, or azathioprine. Radiotherapy or orbital decompression surgery may be recommended depending on the severity and activity of the disease [23].

Thyroid Dermopathy and Acropachy

Both thyroid dermopathy and acropachy are rare extra-thyroidal manifestation of GD. Thyroid dermopathy is characterized by slightly pigmented thickened skin, primarily involving the pretibial area (hence the term "pretibial myxedema"), although involvement of the upper body, particularly sites of repeated trauma and surgical scars, can occur [24]. Thyroid dermopathy is present in about 0.5–4.3% of patients with GD and 13% those with severe GO [25, 26] . One quarter of these patients have acral changes called thyroid acropachy, of which the most common manifestation is clubbing of the fingernails [24, 27]. Almost all patients with dermopathy have significant GO, and both conditions are characterized by an accumulation of glycosaminoglycans (GAGs) in either the dermis and subcutaneous tissues (thyroid dermopathy) or retro-orbital space (GO) [24, 28]. The onset of thyroid dermopathy typically follows GO and on the average occurs 12–24 months after the diagnosis of thyrotoxicosis, although this interval may be longer in some cases [24]. Thyroid acropachy almost always occurs in association with GO and thyroid dermopathy [29]. It is usually asymptomatic but can occasionally be painful due to the associated periostitis [27]. Similar to GO, normalization of thyroid function should be the first goal in the treatment of these extra-thyroidal manifestations. Smoking is associated with severity of thyroid dermopathy and acropachy; hence patients should be strongly advised to stop smoking [30]. Most patients with mild asymptomatic skin changes may not require intervention. The lesions may partially or completely resolve over time, spontaneously, or as a result of systemic corticosteroid therapy given for the associated GO [24, 31]. Specific treatment for the skin lesions include topical steroid therapy, intralesional steroid injection, complete decompress physiotherapy, and surgical excision [30]. No specific treatment is available for thyroid acropachy although pain management with anti-inflammatory agents may be needed in cases with painful periostitis of acropachy [29].

Thyrotoxic Periodic Paralysis

Thyrotoxic periodic paralysis (TPP) is a potentially lethal complication of hyperthyroidism characterized by hypokalemia and muscle paralysis affecting mainly males of Asian descent [32]. The clinical presentation of TPP is characterized by the classic triad of flaccid paralysis, signs of thyrotoxicosis, and hypokalemia due to intracellular potassium shifts during the paralytic episode. The paralytic attack is characterized by recurrent, transient episodes of muscle weakness that range from mild weakness to complete flaccid paralysis, affecting the proximal muscles more than the distal muscles [32]. Electrocardiographic changes resulting from hypokalemia leading to life-threatening ventricular arrhythmias were previously reported [33, 34]. Triggering factors for these attacks include carbohydrate-rich meals, strenuous exercise, trauma, infection, and emotional stress [35, 36]. The exact pathogenesis of this condition remains unknown, although it has been hypothesized that hormonal modulators (such as excessive levels of T_3 and testosterone), carbohydrate-rich meals (with resultant hyperinsulinemia), and rest following exercise could alter ion channel dynamics in the cell membranes of neuromuscular junctions in genetically susceptible individuals harboring ion channel mutations (e.g., Kir2.6 mutations) [36]. Treatment of TPP should include control of the underlying hyperthyroidism, use of β-adrenergic blockers, and judicious replacement of potassium to avoid rebound hyperkalemia during recovery of the paralysis when the potassium is shifted back into the intravascular compartment [32, 37]. In general, definitive therapy, i.e., RAI or thyroidectomy, is recommended for treatment of hyperthyroidism in patients with TPP in view of the potential lethal consequences of this condition.

Investigations

Thyroid function testing in GD typically reveals overt hyperthyroidism, with elevated free T_4 and/or T_3 coupled with suppressed TSH. In mild hyperthyroidism, only serum T_3 may be raised and associated with subnormal TSH, while serum T_4 can be normal. This is known as "T_3-toxicosis" and may reflect early stages of hyperthyroidism [38]. The ratio of total T_3/total T_4 is also helpful in differentiating hyperthyroidism caused by GD or toxic nodular goiter from painless or postpartum thyroiditis [39]. This ratio is typically >20 in hyperthyroidism from GD or toxic nodular goiter due to increased T_3 production compared to T_4 by the hyperactive gland, whereas T_4 is more elevated than T_3 in thyroiditis [40]. The latest American Thyroid Association (ATA) Guidelines for Diagnosis and Management of Hyperthyroidism and other causes of thyrotoxicosis recommend measurement of TSH receptor antibodies (TRAB), determination of the radioactive iodine uptake (RAIU), or measurement of thyroidal blood flow on ultrasound if the diagnosis is not apparent based on initial clinical and biochemical evaluation, depending on the available local expertise and resources [41].

There are two currently available methods of measuring TRAB. The first are competition-based assays that detect TRAB in patient's sera by their ability to compete for binding of TSH receptor (TSHR) with a known TSHR ligand (TSH or monoclonal anti-TSHR antibody). These assays cannot differentiate between stimulating or non-stimulating TRAB (inhibitory or neutral) but are widely available commercially for clinical use. The second are assays that detect cyclic adenosine monophosphate (cAMP) production in cells incubated with patients' sera, also known as bioassays. These assays can measure the ability of TRAB to stimulate or inhibit TSHR activity (thyroid-stimulating or thyroid-blocking antibodies). However, bioassays are seldom utilized in the management of GD since the presence of TRAB in a thyrotoxic patient is usually adequate to diagnose a patient with the condition. Interestingly, it has been found that the more specific thyroid-stimulating antibodies correlated better with GO, whereas TRAB tend to be associated with hyperthyroidism in Asian patients with GD [42]. The utility of TRAB is not limited to diagnosis of GD but also in the prognosis of disease remission with medical treatment [43, 44] and in the assessment of the risk of fetal/neonatal hyperthyroidism in maternal Graves' disease [45].

The two most commonly used agents for imaging the thyroid are technetium pertechnetate (Tc-99m) and iodine-123 (I-123). A radioiodine uptake scintigraphy measures the percentage of administered radioiodine (I-123) that is concentrated into the thyroid gland after a fixed interval, usually 24 h. Unlike I-123, which is both concentrated and organified within the thyroid, technetium pertechnetate is only concentrated in the thyroid. A technetium uptake scintigraphy measures the percentage of administered technetium that is trapped in the thyroid after a fixed interval, usually 20 min. Technetium pertechnetate is readily available and associated with less total body radiation, thus more widely used than I-123 [46]. Diffuse increased uptake of Tc-99m or I-123 is suggestive of GD, whereas a diffuse reduced uptake is seen in subacute, painless, or postpartum thyroiditis [47]. The use of isotope uptake tests in the diagnosis of GD has declined considerably over the past 20 years [48], presumably due to advent of third generation TRAB assays with excellent sensitivity and specificity [49] and the associated high cost and inconvenience of isotope scans [50].

Thyroid ultrasonography with color flow Doppler was first employed in 1988 in the diagnosis of GD, where the term "thyroid inferno," referring to the pulsatile blood flow pattern in GD (Fig. 2.1), was obvious in all 16 patients with GD compared to controls in the study by Ralls et al. The role of ultrasound with color Doppler evaluation was further confirmed by a larger prospective study, with high sensitivity and specificity in the diagnosis of GD [51]. Quantitative Doppler evaluation which measures the peak systolic velocity of the inferior thyroid artery was recently proposed as a potential quantitative tool to supplement the qualitative tool of tissue vascularity in the diagnosis of GD [52].

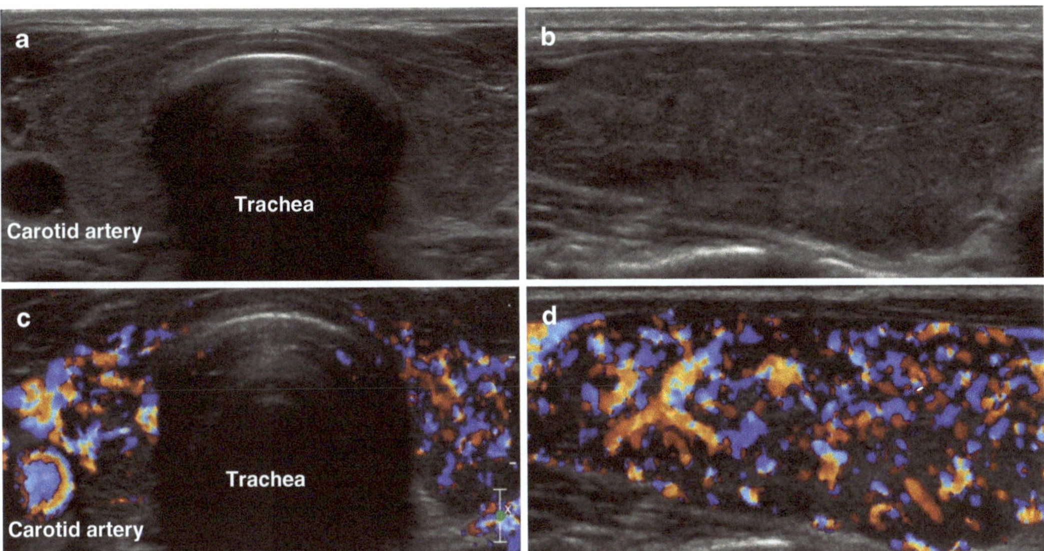

Fig. 2.1 Thyroid ultrasound appearance in Graves' disease. (**a**) Transverse image of the thyroid gland and (**b**) longitudinal image of the right thyroid lobe showing heterogenous thyroid echotexture. (**c**) Transverse image of the thyroid gland and (**d**) longitudinal image of the right thyroid lobe with color flow Doppler demonstrating increased vascularity (thyroid inferno)

Treatment

The three treatment options for GD are antithyroid drugs (ATDs), radioactive iodine ablation (RAI), and thyroidectomy. The choice of therapy depends on patient preference and several clinical factors as outlined in Table 2.2.

Antithyroid Drugs (ATD)

The thioamide compounds, methimazole (MMI), its prodrug derivative, carbimazole (CMZ), and propylthiouracil (PTU), are the mainstay of medical management of GD. The main mode of action of thioamides is to inhibit thyroid hormone synthesis by interfering with thyroid peroxidase-mediated and coupling of tyrosine residues [53]. PTU, at larger doses, also inhibits peripheral conversion of T_4 to T_3 via inhibition of type 1 deiodinase [53]. The choice of ATDs as the first-line treatment is largely driven by practical considerations and regional preferences. ATDs are more favored in Asia and Europe compared to the United States, which tend to prefer RAI as the first-line treatment [54, 55]. Two widely used ATD regimes for GD treatment are the "titration" regime, which involves a titrating dose of ATD over 12–18 months of treatment period and the "block and replace" regime, which entails a fixed high dose of ATD combined with levothyroxine over 6 months. Recent studies have not found superiority of one regime over the other in terms of long-term efficacy or maintaining stable thyroid function [56, 57]. However, the "block and replace" regime is generally less favored in clinical practice due to the higher pill load, more drug-related adverse effects, and potential patient non-compliance issues [53, 58]. This regime is also contraindicated in the management of GD in pregnancy due to the risk of fetal hypothyroidism and goiter. Treatment with ATDs should be considered in patients with clinical characteristics that may predict remission with medical treatment: women, mild hyperthyroidism, small goiter, and low TRAB levels at diagnosis [41, 59]. A typical initial adult dose of ATD will comprise of 30–40 mg of CMZ (equivalent to 20–30 mg MMI or 300-400 mg PTU) followed by gradual titration to maintenance dose (generally 5–10 mg CMZ) depending on the severity of hyperthyroidism at diagnosis and response to the ATD treatment. In addition, β-adrenergic blockers (e.g., propranolol) are typically prescribed in the initial management of these patients for relief of symptoms caused by increased sympathetic action

Table 2.2 Factors favoring, advantages, and disadvantages of the three treatment modalities for Graves' disease

Factors that favor ATDs	*Factors that favor RAI*	*Factors that favor thyroidectomy*
Patient preference	Patient preference	Patient preference
Facilities for surgery or radioiodine are not available	Relapsed GD	Relapsed GD
Patients unable to adhere to radiation safety rules, e.g., parents of young children and nursing home residents	Persistent thyrotoxicosis in patients with previous operated or irradiated necks	Concomitant suspicious nodules or thyroid cancer
Patients with contraindications to RAI, e.g., pregnancy and severe GO	High surgical risk	Concomitant moderate to severe GO
Persistent thyrotoxicosis in patients with previous operated or irradiated necks	Patients with contraindications or serious adverse effects to ATD	Symptomatic and large goiters
High surgical risk	Patients with thyrotoxic periodic paralysis	May be preferred in women considering pregnancy in less than 6 months who wants to avoid potential risk of ATD-related birth defects
Patients with characteristics that favor remission with ATD, e.g., women, small goiter, mild hyperthyroidism, low TRAB levels		Concomitant primary hyperparathyroidism requiring surgery
		Patients with contraindications or serious adverse effects to ATD
		Patients with thyrotoxic periodic paralysis
Advantages of ATDs	*Advantages of RAI*	*Advantages of thyroidectomy*
Outpatient treatment	Outpatient treatment	No radiation exposure
Low risk of hypothyroidism	Achievement of desired end point, i.e., hypothyroidism in the majority of patients treated with a single administration of sufficient radiation dose	Low disease recurrence rate after surgery (especially with total thyroidectomy)
No exposure to radioactive material, anesthetic, or surgical risks	No anesthetic or surgical risks	Rapid normalization of thyroid dysfunction
No adverse effects on GO	Reduces goiter size	Definitive histology results
Disadvantages of ATDs	*Disadvantages of RAI*	*Disadvantages of thyroidectomy*
High relapse rate upon withdrawal	Permanent hypothyroidism	Permanent hypothyroidism (especially with total thyroidectomy)
Regular monitoring of thyroid function required	Risk of de novo development of GO or exacerbation of pre-existing mild GO	Permanent scar
Potential serious adverse effects	Requires compliance to radiation safety rules	Potential anesthetic and surgical risk—e.g., recurrent laryngeal nerve palsy and hypoparathyroidism
Risk of carbimazole or methimazole associated birth defects	Conception needs to be delayed (usually 6 months) in women considering pregnancy	High cost
		Require hospitalization

such as sweating, anxiety, palpitations, and tremors. Biochemical monitoring of thyroid function should be performed every 4 to 6 weeks in the first 3–6 months of therapy, followed by three monthly intervals when biochemical euthyroidism is achieved. The use of thioamides is associated with uncommon adverse effects. Minor side effects include pruritus, urticaria, and rash, which occur in 3–6% of patients on ATDs [60]. These can be generally managed with concurrent antihistamines in mild cases. Switching to another ATD or consideration for other treatment modalities such as RAI or surgery may be required if the side effect is persistent. Major side effects associated with ATD usage include agranulocytosis, hepatotoxicity, and antineutrophil cytoplasmic antibody (ANCA)-positive vasculitis. Agranulocytosis (defined as absolute neutrophil count or ANC <500) occurs in approximately 0.1–0.3% of treated patients and tends to manifest in the first 90 days of drug initiation [53, 61, 62]. CMZ-/MMI-induced hepatotoxicity is often cholestatic, whereas PTU is associated with hepatocellular damage, including fatal fulminant hepatic necrosis [63]. The incidence of ATD-associated hepatotoxicity is between 0.03 and 0.07% and most often occurs in the first 3 months of therapy [64, 65]. PTU is associated with higher reported rates of liver failure compared to CMZ/MMI [64, 66]. The US Food and Drugs Administration, the European Medicines Agency, and the UK Medicines and Healthcare Regulatory agency have all issued warnings on the risk of liver failure with PTU [67]. Hence, the current ATA guidelines recommend that CMZ/MMI should be used in all patients (including children) selected for treatment with ATDs, except during first trimester of pregnancy, in the treatment of thyroid storm, and in patients who have minor adverse effects with CMZ/MMI who refused RAI or surgery [41]. All patients should be counselled on these potential side effects prior to initiation of ATD, and baseline full blood count and liver function should be considered prior to initiating ATDs [41]. Although low white cell count and elevated liver enzymes may be encountered in newly diagnosed GD patients, it is recommended that initiation of ATDs must be seriously reconsidered if the neurotrophil count is <1000/mm^3 or liver transaminase levels are more than fivefold upper limit of normal [41]. ANCA-positive vasculitis is an uncommon adverse effect associated with ATD. It has been more commonly reported in children, patients of Asian ethnicity, and PTU usage and its risk increase with duration of therapy [68, 69]. Other rare adverse effects of CMZ/MMI have also been reported [70, 71], including higher risk of congenital birth defects such as aplasia cutis and choanal atresia when used in the first trimester of pregnancy [72]. The main disadvantage of ATDs is the high relapse rate after discontinuation of therapy, which is estimated to be 50–55% [56]. The risk of relapse is highest in the first 6 months after withdrawal of ATD. In particular, patients who are male, young, smokers, has large goiter, high TRAB levels at diagnosis or persistently positive TRAB levels prior to stopping the drug are more likely to have disease recurrence [73, 74]. Patients who have relapse after ATD discontinuation will typically be advised to consider definitive treatment with RAI or thyroidectomy, although recent growing evidence suggest long-term low-dose ATD may be considered in selected groups [75, 76].

Radioactive Iodine Ablation (RAI)

In the treatment of GD with RAI, the radioactive form of iodine (I-131) is taken up by iodide transporter of the thyroid the same way as natural iodine and is similarly processed. The beta particles released result in ionizing damage to the thyroid follicular cells and gradual destruction of the gland, leading to volume reduction and control of the thyrotoxicosis. Radioiodine is given orally as a single dose of I-131 labelled sodium iodide in liquid or capsule form. The goal of RAI therapy is to render the patient hypothyroid, which can be achieved in 80% of patients after one administration of sufficient radiation dose [77]. The optimal method for determining iodine-131 treatment doses remains controversial. Radioiodine can be administered in fixed amounts or calculated doses based on the estimated thyroid gland size (either clinically or from imaging) and the 24 h radioiodine uptake. The current literature does not support the superiority of one method over the other [77, 78]. Absolute contraindications to radioiodine treatment are pregnancy, lactation, and inability to comply with radiation safety rules. Pretreatment with ATD prior to RAI is generally not required, except in older patients and in patients with coexisting ischemic heart disease due to potential increased risk of complications due to short-term worsening of hyperthyroidism following administration of RAI. Radioiodine treatment may result in de novo development of GO or exacerbation of pre-existing mild GO, particularly in smokers, in severe hyperthyroidism (high free thyroid hormone levels and/or TSH receptor autoantibodies), and hyperthyroidism of recent onset [79, 80]. The current European Thyroid Association/European Group on Graves' Orbitopathy Guidelines recommend that oral prednisone prophylaxis be given in radioiodine-treated patients at high risk of progression or de novo development of GO [80].

Thyroidectomy

Thyroidectomy is the least often used treatment modality of GD but may be preferred in selected cases, such as presence of large goiter and concomitant suspicious thyroid nodules or thyroid cancer and in patients who prefer rapid and definitive treatment for their disease. Patients treated with surgery or medication showed a gradual fall in serum TRAB levels with disappearance of TRAB in 50–60% of patients after 1 year, whereas increasing TRAB levels was found in those treated with RAI [81]. This surge in TRAB levels during the 1st year after RAI is associated with a risk of developing or worsening of GO [82]. Current literature suggest GO remain stable or even improve in some patients after thyroidectomy [83, 84]. Hence, thyroidectomy instead of RAI is the recommended definitive treatment for patients with moderate to severe GO whose hyperthyroidism cannot be adequately controlled with ATDs. Near-total or total thyroidectomy is the recommended procedure of choice in view of virtually 0% risk of recurrence, whereas subtotal thyroidectomy may have an 8% chance of persistence or recurrence of hyperthyroidism at 5 years [85]. Notably, more recent data support the safety of total thyroidectomy for benign thyroid disease if the surgery is performed at a high-volume center, keeping the risk of permanent morbidity at <2% [86]. In a recent meta-analysis of 23 studies comparing these two surgical approaches, total thyroidectomy was associated with a decrease in recurrent hyperthyroidism but with only a small increase in both temporary and permanent hypoparathyroidism [87]. Progression of GO and incidence of permanent recurrent laryngeal nerve palsy were similar between these two groups [87]. The rates of complications of thyroid surgery are inversely correlated with surgeon's experience and annual volume of thyroidectomies. In a study of 166,954 patients who underwent total thyroidectomy for thyroid disease, it was demonstrated that the likelihood of experiencing a postoperative complication decreased with increasing surgeon work volume in a dose-dependent fashion up to 26 (95% CI 22–32) total thyroidectomies per year [88]. Based on the results of this study, the authors identified a surgeon volume threshold of more than 25 total thyroidectomies per year to define a high-volume thyroid surgeon [88]. The risk of permanent hypoparathyroidism has been determined to be <2%, permanent recurrent laryngeal nerve palsy to be <1%, and frequency of bleeding necessitating reoperation to be between 0.3 and 0.7% following thyroidectomy by high-volume surgeons [89, 90].

Perioperative Management of GD for Thyroid and Non-thyroid Surgery

Patients with GD should be as close as possible to clinical and biochemical euthyroidism using ATDs before going to surgery. Elective surgeries should be postponed until this is achieved. This is rarely an issue in patients undergoing thyroidectomy for treatment of their GD since surgery is considered a second-line treatment. Surgery in patients with poorly controlled thyrotoxicosis can potentially precipitate thyroid storm—a life-threatening condition caused by the exaggeration of clinical manifestations of thyrotoxicosis associated with significant risk of mortality [91]. However, it is common for TSH values to remain suppressed in prolonged hyperthyroidism in patients who otherwise have normalized their T_4 and T_3 on ATDs and should not be considered a contraindication to surgery.

In the unusual circumstances where urgent non-thyroid surgery or urgent thyroidectomy is required in an overtly hyperthyroid patient with GD, rapid preoperative preparation using several drugs is employed. The same multimodality approach targeting at different steps in the production and metabolism of thyroid hormones is also used in the management of thyroid storm. Since there is insufficient time to render the patient completely euthyroid before the surgery, the aim of rapid preoperative preparation is to normalize T_4 and T_3 levels, with greater emphasis on normalizing T_3 levels, since T_3 is three to five times more active than T_4. Thioamides (MMI, CMZ, or PTU) mainly inhibit thyroid hormone synthesis and may take several weeks to render the patient euthyroid. Hence, other drugs are usually required in this situation, which include iodine, β-adrenergic blockers, steroids, oral cholecystographic agent (iopanic acid), and cholestyramine (Table 2.3). Potassium iodide in the form of Lugol's iodine or saturated solution of potassium iodide (SSKI) decreases thyroidal iodide uptake and release of thyroid hormones via the Wolff-Chaikoff effect. This effect can be seen within 24 h of administration and is maximal at approximately 10 days of treatment. In patients undergoing thyroidectomy, it has been shown to decrease thyroid gland vascularity and blood loss as well [92]. However, iodine is generally not recommended to be given in the absence of pretreatment with thioamides in view of potential iodine-induced thyrotoxicosis via the Jod-Basedow effect. Metabolism of iopanic acid results in release of iodine. In addition, iopanic acid is also a potent inhibitor of the peripheral conversion of T_4 to T_3. Hence, iopanic acid is more effective than potassium iodide in inhibiting thyroid hormone secretion and metabolism and can be used in patients who cannot tolerate thioamides in the expectation that definitive surgical cure will occur before the delivered iodine acts as a substrate for increased thyroid hormone synthesis [93]. However, this drug is no longer widely available as its production is currently restricted. Steroids (hydrocortisone, betamethasone, or dexamethasone) in high doses also inhibit peripheral conversion of T_4 to T_3. Cholestyramine, which inhibits enterohepatic circulation of thyroid hormones, contributed to more rapid and complete decline in thyroid hormones when combined with ATDs and β-adrenergic blocker, is a useful adjunctive treat-

Table 2.3 Drugs used in rapid preoperative preparation of thyrotoxic patients for surgery

Drug class	Mechanism of action	Comment
Thioamides (e.g., propylthiouracil 200 mg 6–8 h)	Inhibit new thyroid hormone synthesis PTU at larger doses, also inhibit peripheral conversion of T_4 to T_3	PTU can be administered through nasogastric tube or rectally via an enema
Iodine (e.g., SSKI 1 drop thrice daily (35–50 mg iodide per drop) or Lugol's iodine three to five drops thrice daily (8 mg iodine per drop))	Decreases thyroidal iodide uptake and release of thyroid hormones	Should not be used until thioamides are on board
Steroids (e.g., intravenous hydrocortisone 100 mg 8 h)	Vasomotor stability inhibits peripheral conversion of T_4 to T_3	
Oral cholecystographic agent (e.g., iopanic acid 500 mg twice daily)	Inhibits thyroid hormone release Inhibits peripheral conversion of T_4 to T_3	No longer widely available
Cholestyramine	Inhibits enterohepatic circulation of thyroid hormones	Common gastrointestinal side effects include constipation and abdominal discomfort
β-adrenergic blockers (e.g., propranolol 40–80 mg 8 h)	Improve thyrotoxic symptoms Inhibits peripheral conversion of T_4 to T_3 at higher doses	Precaution should be used in patients with history of moderate to severe heart failure and reactive airway disease

ment in patients with GD [94]. In cases where the use of ATDs is contraindicated, e.g., drug allergy, various combinations of the other classes of drugs presented in Table 2.3 have been proposed in the literature [93, 95, 96]. In the postoperative period, ATDs, iodine, and cholestyramine should be stopped after thyroidectomy, while β-adrenergic blockers and steroids should be tapered off gradually. Thyroxine should be started at a daily dose appropriate for the patient's weight (1.6 μg/kg for adults or lower at 1.0 μg/kg in elderly patients), with monitoring of the patient's thyroid function 6–8 weeks later. In the postoperative period after non-thyroid surgery in a thyrotoxic patient, ATDs and β-adrenergic blockers should be continued while the other agents could be stopped or gradually weaned off.

Preoperative parathyroid hormone and vitamin D levels and early postoperative changes in calcium levels have been found to be useful predictors of post-thyroidectomy hypocalcemia [97]. Recent studies suggest optimization of calcium and vitamin D levels preoperatively reduce the risk of transient postoperative hypocalcemia related to parathyroid injury or increased bone turnover [98, 99]. In addition, early postoperative monitoring of calcium and parathyroid hormone levels and routine supplementation with calcium and calcitriol are recommended to reduce the development of hypocalcemic symptoms [41].

Surgery or RAI Ablation in Patients with Large Grave's Goiter

The management of patients with large Graves' goiters represents a unique challenge to physicians. Larger goiter size at the onset of disease is associated with higher relapse rate following ATD therapy [100]. Thus, these patients will generally be advised to consider early definitive treatment with RAI or thyroidectomy. Both treatments are effective in reducing goiter size, although direct comparison between these two modes of treatment for this subset of patients is currently lacking. In a randomized prospective study by Peters et al., the relative reduction in thyroid size by RAI was just as marked in patients with larger goiters as in those with small glands [101]. However, whether larger goiter size is associated with higher treatment failure with RAI remains controversial, since thyroid volume is also associated with other disease factors that may adversely impact the outcome of RAI therapy, such as disease severity and immunoreactivity [102].

A pertinent concern with prescribing RAI therapy for Graves' disease patients with large goiters is the occurrence of radiation thyroiditis following RAI therapy. Although mostly asymptomatic, the acute inflammation may lead to transient thyroid swelling and potential airway compromise in these patients. Other factors contributing to this rare complication are the topo-anatomical relationship between the goiter and trachea, compression of the recurrent laryngeal nerve by the thyroid swelling, and possible allergic reaction to radioiodine [103]. Therefore, in the case of significant tracheal compression (i.e., smallest cross-sectional tracheal area < 60 mm^2), prophylactic glucocorticoids are advocated during RAI to prevent radiation-induced swelling of the goiter and potential respiratory deterioration [104]. The current guidelines recommend surgery for large Graves' goiter, especially if symptomatic compression is present [41]. However, in those with asymptomatic large Graves' goiter, other patient and disease factors as outlined in Table 2.2 in this Chapter should also be taken into consideration before recommending the optimal treatment for these patients.

Conclusion

Graves' disease is a complex autoimmune disease with a wide range of clinical manifestations. The three treatment modalities currently are antithyroid drugs, radioiodine ablation, and thyroidectomy. Each treatment modality has its own advantages and disadvantages, and the choice of therapy depends on both patient preference and clinical factors that may favor one treatment modality over the other. However, there is no treatment to date that specifically targets the pathogenic culprit—TSH receptor antibodies. Current ongoing research on the use of TSH receptor blocking monoclonal antibodies and small molecule antagonists with high affinity for the TSH receptor (SMANTAGs) may represent novel approaches to treatment of this disease in the future [105].

Clinical Pearls

1. Graves' disease (GD) is an autoimmune thyroid disease characterized by signs and symptoms of thyrotoxicosis, coupled with unique extra-thyroidal manifestations.
2. Measurement of TSH receptor antibodies titer, determination of the radioactive iodine uptake, or measurement of thyroidal blood flow on ultrasound can be employed if the diagnosis of GD is not apparent based on initial clinical and biochemical evaluation, depending on the available local expertise and resources.
3. The current treatment modalities for GD are antithyroid drugs, radioiodine ablation, and thyroidectomy. The main disadvantage of antithyroid drug treatment is the high disease relapse rate upon drug withdrawal, whereas ablative/surgical treatments induce permanent hypothyroidism.
4. Thyroidectomy may be preferred in selected cases, such as presence of large symptomatic goiter and concomitant suspicious thyroid nodules or thyroid cancer and in patients who prefer rapid and definitive treatment for their disease.

References

1. Chng C-L, Lim AYY, Tan HC, et al. Physiological and metabolic changes during the transition from hyperthyroidism to euthyroidism in Graves' disease. Thyroid. 2016;26:1422–30.
2. Nyström HF, Jansson S, Berg G. Incidence rate and clinical features of hyperthyroidism in a long-term iodine sufficient area of Sweden (Gothenburg) 2003–2005. Clin Endocrinol (Oxf). 2013;78:768–76.
3. Brent GA. Graves' disease. N Engl J Med. 2008;358:2594–605.
4. Weetman A. Graves' disease. N Engl J Med. 2000;343:1236–48.
5. Brix TH, Kyvik KO, Hegedüs L. What is the evidence of genetic factors in the etiology of Graves' disease? A brief review. Thyroid. 1998;8:727–34.
6. Lee HJ, Li CW, Hammerstad SS, Stefan M, Tomer Y. Immunogenetics of autoimmune thyroid diseases: a comprehensive review. J Autoimmun. 2015;64:82–90.
7. Akamizu T, Sale MM, Rich SS, et al. Association of autoimmune thyroid disease with microsatellite markers for the thyrotropin receptor gene and CTLA-4 in Japanese patients. Thyroid. 2000;10:851–8.
8. Yanagawa T, Hidaka Y, Guimaraes V, Soliman M, DeGroot LJ. CTLA-4 gene polymorphism associated with Graves' disease in a Caucasian population. J Clin Endocrinol Metab. 1995;80:41–5.
9. Kurylowicz A, Kula D, Ploski R, et al. Association of CD40 gene polymorphism (C-1T) with susceptibility and phenotype of Graves' disease. Thyroid. 2005;15:1119–24.
10. Heward JM, Brand OJ, Barrett JC, Carr-Smith JD, Franklyn JA, Gough SC. Association of PTPN22 haplotypes with Graves' disease. J Clin Endocrinol Metab. 2007;92:685–90.
11. Winsa B, Adami H-O, Bergström R, Gamstedt A, Dahlberg PA, Adamson U, Jansson R, Karlsson A. Stressful life events and Graves' disease. Lancet. 1991;338:1475–9.
12. Wiersinga WM. Smoking and thyroid. Clin Endocrinol. 2013;79:145–51.
13. Cooper DS. Hyperthyroidism. Lancet. 2003;362:459–68.
14. Manji N, Carr-Smith JD, Boelaert K, et al. Influences of age, gender, smoking, and family history on autoimmune thyroid disease phenotype. J Clin Endocrinol Metab. 2006;91:4873–80.
15. Muldoon BT, Mai VQ, Burch HB. Management of Graves' disease: An overview and comparison of clinical practice guidelines with actual practice trends. Endocrinol Metab Clin North Am. 2014;43:495–516.
16. Klein I, Ojamaa K. Hormone action. N Engl J Med. 2001;344:501–9.
17. Bahn RS. Graves' ophthalmopathy. N Engl J Med. 2010;362:726–38.
18. Bahn RS. Current insights into the pathogenesis of graves' ophthalmopathy. Horm Metab Res. 2015;47:773–8.
19. Wiersinga WM. Management of Graves' ophthalmopathy. Nat Clin Pract Endocrinol Metab. 2007;3:396–404.
20. Chng C-L, Seah LL, Khoo DHC. Ethnic differences in the clinical presentation of Graves' ophthalmopathy. Best Pract Res Clin Endocrinol Metab. 2012;26:249–58.
21. Burch HB, Wartofsky L. Graves' ophthalmopathy: current concepts regarding pathogenesis and management. Endocr Rev. 1993;14:747–93.
22. Bartalena L. Prevention of Graves' ophthalmopathy. Best Pract Res Clin Endocrinol Metab. 2012;26:371–9.
23. Bartalena L. Graves' orbitopathy: imperfect treatments for a rare disease. Eur Thyroid J. 2013;2:259–69.

24. Schwartz KM, Fatourechi V, Ahmed DDF, Pond GR. Extensive personal experience: dermopathy of Graves' disease (pretibial myxedema): long-term outcome. J Clin Endocrinol Metab. 2002;87:438–46.
25. Fatourechi V, Garrity JA, Bartley GB, Bergstralh EJ, Gorman CA. Orbital decompression in Graves' ophthalmopathy associated with pretibial myxedema. J Endocrinol Investig. 1993;16:433–7.
26. Bartley GB, Fatourechi V, Kadrmas EF, Jacobsen SJ, Ilstrup DM, Garrity JA, Gorman CA. The incidence of Graves' ophthalmopathy in Olmsted County, Minnesota. Am J Ophthalmol. 1995;120:511–7.
27. Fatourechi V, Ahmed DDF, Schwartz KM. Thyroid acropachy: report of 40 patients treated at a single institution in a 26-year period. J Clin Endocrinol Metab. 2002;87:5435–41.
28. Fatourechi V, Bartley GB, Eghbali-Fatourechi GZ, Powell CC, Ahmed DDF, Garrity JA. Graves' dermopathy and acropachy are markers of severe Graves' ophthalmopathy. Thyroid. 2003;13:1141–4.
29. Bartalena L, Fatourechi V. Extrathyroidal manifestations of Graves' disease: a 2014 update. J Endocrinol Investig. 2014;37:691–700.
30. Fatourechi V. Thyroid dermopathy and acropachy. Best Pract Res Clin Endocrinol Metab. 2012;26:553–65.
31. Fatourechi V. Thyroid dermopathy and acropachy. Expert Rev Dermatol. 2011;6:75–90.
32. Kung AWC. Clinical review: thyrotoxic periodic paralysis: a diagnostic challenge. J Clin Endocrinol Metab. 2006;91:2490–5.
33. Bernard E, Med M, Cheah JS. Electrocardiographic changes in thyrotoxic periodic paralysis. J Electrocardiol. 1979;12:263–70.
34. Loh KC, Pinheiro L, Ng KS. Thyrotoxic periodic paralysis complicated by near-fatal ventricular arrhythmias. Singap Med J. 2005;46:88–9.
35. Chang CC, Cheng CJ, Sung CC, Chiueh TS, Lee CH, Chau T, Lin SH. A 10-year analysis of thyrotoxic periodic paralysis in 135 patients: focus on symptomatology and precipitants. Eur J Endocrinol. 2013;169:529–36.
36. Maciel RMB, Lindsey SC, Dias MR, Silva D, Maciel RMB, Lindsey SC, Dias MR. Novel etiopathophysiological aspects of thyrotoxic periodic paralysis. Nat Rev Endocrinol. 2011;7:657–67.
37. Vijayakumar A, Ashwath G, Thimmappa D. Thyrotoxic periodic paralysis: clinical challenges. J Thyroid Res. 2014;2014:649502.
38. Woeber KA. Triiodothyronine production in Graves' hyperthyroidism. Thyroid. 2006;16:687–90.
39. Carlé A, Knudsen N, Pedersen IB, Perrild H, Ovesen L, Rasmussen LB, Laurberg P. Determinants of serum T4 and T3 at the time of diagnosis in nosological types of thyrotoxicosis: a population-based study. Eur J Endocrinol. 2013;169:537–45.
40. Shigemasa C, Abe K, Taniguchi SI, Mitani Y, Ueda Y, Adachi T, Urabe K, Tanaka T, Yoshida A, Mashiba H. Lower serum free thyroxine (T4) levels in painless thyroiditis compared with Graves' disease despite similar serum total T4 levels. J Clin Endocrinol Metab. 1987;65:359–63.
41. Ross DS, Burch HB, Cooper DS, et al. 2016 American Thyroid Association Guidelines for diagnosis and management of hyperthyroidism and other causes of thyrotoxicosis. Thyroid. 2016;26:1343–421.
42. Goh SY, Ho SC, Seah LL, Fong KS, Khoo DHC. Thyroid autoantibody profiles in ophthalmic dominant and thyroid dominant Grave's disease differ and suggest ophthalmopathy is a multiantigenic disease. Clin Endocrinol. 2004;60:600–7.
43. Feldt-Rasmussen U, Schleusener H, Carayon P. Meta-analysis evaluation of the impact of thyrotropin receptor antibodies on long term remission after medical therapy of Graves' disease. J Clin Endocrinol Metab. 1994;78:98–102.
44. Carella C, Mazziotti G, Sorvillo F, Piscopo M, Cioffi M, Pilla P, Nersita R, Iorio S, Amato G, Braverman LE, Roti E. Serum thyrotropin receptor antibodies concentrations in patients with Graves' disease before, at the end of methimazole treatment, and after drug withdrawal: evidence that the activity of thyrotropin receptor antibody and/or thyroid response modify during. Thyroid. 2006;16:295–302.
45. Abeillon-Du Payrat J, Chikh K, Bossard N, et al. Predictive value of maternal second-generation thyroid-binding inhibitory immunoglobulin assay for neonatal autoimmune hyperthyroidism. Eur J Endocrinol. 2014;171:451–60.
46. Czepczyński R. Nuclear medicine in the diagnosis of benign thyroid diseases. Nucl Med Rev Cent East Eur. 2012;15:113–9.
47. Smith JR, Oates E. Radionuclide imaging of the thyroid gland: patterns, pearls, and pitfalls. Clin Nucl Med. 2004;29:181–93.
48. Bartalena L. Diagnosis and management of graves disease: a global overview. Nat Rev Endocrinol. 2013;9:724–34.
49. Tozzoli R, Bagnasco M, Giavarina D, Bizzaro N. TSH receptor autoantibody immunoassay in patients with Graves' disease: improvement of diagnostic accuracy over different generations of methods. Systematic review and meta-analysis. Autoimmun Rev. 2012;12:107–13.
50. Franklyn JA. What is the role of radioiodine uptake measurement and thyroid scintigraphy in the diagnosis and management of hyperthyroidism? Clin Endocrinol (Oxf). 2010;72:11–2.
51. Cappelli C, Pirola I, De Martino E, Agosti B, Delbarba A, Castellano M, Rosei EA. The role of imaging in Graves' disease: a cost-effectiveness analysis. Eur J Radiol. 2008;65:99–103.
52. Hari Kumar KVS, Pasupuleti V, Jayaraman M, Abhyuday V, Rayudu BR, Modi KD. Role of thyroid Doppler in differential diagnosis of thyrotoxicosis. Endocr Pract. 2009;15:6–9.
53. Cooper DS. Antithyroid drugs. N Engl J Med. 2005;352:905–17.
54. Wartofsky L, Glinoer D, Solomon B, Nagataki S, Lagasse R, Nagayama Y, Izumi M. Differences and

similarities in the diagnosis and treatment of graves' disease in Europe, Japan, and the United States. Thyroid. 1991;1:129–35.
55. Vaidya B, Williams GR, Abraham P, Pearce SHS. Radioiodine treatment for benign thyroid disorders: results of a nationwide survey of UK endocrinologists. Clin Endocrinol (Oxf). 2008;68:814–20.
56. Abraham P, Avenell A, McGeoch SC, Clark LF, Bevan JS. Antithyroid drug regimen for treating Graves' hyperthyroidism. Cochrane Database Syst Rev. 2010;1:1–75.
57. Vaidya B, Wright A, Shuttleworth J, Donohoe M, Warren R, Brooke A, Gericke CA, Ukoumunne OC. Block & replace regime versus titration regime of antithyroid drugs for the treatment of Graves' disease: a retrospective observational study. Clin Endocrinol (Oxf). 2014;81:610–3.
58. Abraham P, Avenell A, Park CM, Watson WA, Bevan JS. A systematic review of drug therapy for Graves' hyperthyroidism. Eur J Endocrinol. 2005;153:489–98.
59. Okosieme O, Lazarus J. Current trends in antithyroid drug treatment of Graves' disease. Expert Opin Pharmacother. 2016;17:2005–17.
60. Sundaresh V, Brito JP, Wang Z, Prokop LJ, Stan MN, Murad MH, Bahn RS. Comparative effectiveness of therapies for graves' hyperthyroidism: a systematic review and network meta-analysis. J Clin Endocrinol Metab. 2013;98:3671–7.
61. Nakamura H, Miyauchi A, Miyawaki N, Imagawa J. Analysis of 754 cases of antithyroid drug-induced agranulocytosis over 30 years in Japan. J Clin Endocrinol Metab. 2013;98:4776–83.
62. Watanabe N, Narimatsu H, Noh JY, Yamaguchi T, Kobayashi K, Kami M, Kunii Y, Mukasa K, Ito K, Ito K. Antithyroid drug-induced hematopoietic damage: a retrospective cohort study of agranulocytosis and pancytopenia involving 50,385 patients with Graves' disease. J Clin Endocrinol Metab. 2012. https://doi.org/10.1210/jc.2011-2221.
63. Ruiz JK, Rossi GV, Vallejos HA, Brenet RW, Lopez IB. Fulminant hepatic failure associated with propylthiouracil. Ann Pharmacother. 2003;37:224–8.
64. Wang MT, Lee WJ, Huang TY, Chu CL, Hsieh CH. Antithyroid drug-related hepatotoxicity in hyperthyroidism patients: a population-based cohort study. Br J Clin Pharmacol. 2014;78:619–29.
65. Andersen S, Olsen J, Laurberg P. Antithyroid drug side effects in the population and in pregnancy. J Clin Endocrinol Metab. 2016;101:1606–14.
66. Andersohn F, Konzen C, Garbe E. Systematic review: agranulocytosis induced by nonchemotherapy drugs. Ann Intern Med. 2007;146:657–65.
67. Akmal A, Kung J. Propylthiouracil, and methimazole, and carbimazole-related hepatotoxicity. Expert Opin Drug Saf. 2014;13:1397–406.
68. Rivkees SA, Szarfman A. Dissimilar hepatotoxicity profiles of propylthiouracil and methimazole in children. J Clin Endocrinol Metab. 2010;95: 3260–7.
69. Balavoine A-S, Glinoer D, Dubucquoi S, Wémeau J-L. Antineutrophil cytoplasmic antibody-positive small-vessel vasculitis associated with antithyroid drug therapy: how significant is the clinical problem. Thyroid. 2015;25:1273–81.
70. Lim AY, Kek PC, Soh AW. Carbimazole-induced myositis in the treatment of Graves' disease: a complication in genetically susceptible individuals? Singapore Med J. 2013;54:e133–6.
71. Chng C-L, Kek PC, Khoo DH-C. Carbimazole-induced acute pancreatitis and cholestatic hepatitis. Endocr Pract. 2011;17:960–1.
72. Taylor PN, Vaidya B. Side effects of anti-thyroid drugs and their impact on the choice of treatment for thyrotoxicosis in pregnancy. Eur Thyroid J. 2012;1:176–85.
73. Allahabadia A, Daykin J, Holder RL, Sheppard MC, Gough SCL, Franklyn JA. Age and gender predict the outcome of treatment for Graves' hyperthyroidism. J Clin Endocrinol Metab. 2000;85:1038–42.
74. Nedrebo BG, Holm PI, Uhlving S, Sorheim JI, Skeie S, Eide GE, Husebye ES, E a L, Aanderud S. Predictors of outcome and comparison of different drug regimens for the prevention of relapse in patients with Graves' disease. Eur J Endocrinol. 2002;147:583–9.
75. Azizi F, Ataie L, Hedayati M, Mehrabi Y, Sheikholeslami F. Effect of long-term continuous methimazole treatment of hyperthyroidism: comparison with radioiodine. Eur J Endocrinol. 2005;152:695–701.
76. Villagelin D, Romaldini JH, Santos RB, Milkos AB, Ward LS. Outcomes in relapsed Graves' disease patients following radioiodine or prolonged low dose of methimazole treatment. Thyroid. 2015;25:1282–90.
77. Leslie WD, Ward L, Salamon EA, Ludwig S, Rowe RC, Cowden EA. A randomized comparison of radioiodine doses in Graves' hyperthyroidism. J Clin Endocrinol Metab. 2003;88:978–83.
78. De Rooij A, Vandenbroucke JP, Smit JWA, Stokkel MPM, Dekkers OM. Clinical outcomes after estimated versus calculated activity of radioiodine for the treatment of hyperthyroidism: systematic review and meta-analysis. Eur J Endocrinol. 2009;161:771–7.
79. Acharya SH, Avenell A, Philip S, Burr J, Bevan JS, Abraham P. Radioiodine therapy (RAI) for Graves' disease (GD) and the effect on ophthalmopathy: a systematic review. Clin Endocrinol. 2008;69:943–50.
80. Bartalena L, Baldeschi L, Boboridis K, Eckstein A, Kahaly GJ, Marcocci C, Perros P, Salvi M, Wiersinga WM. The 2016 European Thyroid Association/European Group on Graves' Orbitopathy Guidelines for the Management of Graves' Orbitopathy. Eur Thyroid J. 2016;55:9–269.
81. Laurberg P, Wallin G, Tallstedt L, Abraham-Nordling M, Lundell G, Törring O. TSH-receptor autoimmunity in Graves' disease after therapy with

anti-thyroid drugs, surgery, or radioiodine: a 5-year prospective randomized study. Eur J Endocrinol. 2008;158:69–75.
82. Wiersinga WM, Bartalena L. Epidemiology and prevention of Graves' ophthalmopathy. Thyroid. 2002;12:855–60.
83. Järhult J, Rudberg C, Larsson E, Selvander H, Sjövall K, Winsa B, Rastad J, F a K. Graves' disease with moderate-severe endocrine ophthalmopathy-long term results of a prospective, randomized study of total or subtotal thyroid resection. Thyroid. 2005;15:1157–64.
84. De Bellis A, Conzo G, Cennamo G, et al. Time course of Graves' ophthalmopathy after total thyroidectomy alone or followed by radioiodine therapy: a 2-year longitudinal study. Endocrine. 2012;41:320–6.
85. Palit TK, Miller CC, Miltenburg DM. The efficacy of thyroidectomy for Graves' disease: a meta-analysis. J Surg Res. 2000;90:161–5.
86. Barczyński M, Konturek A, Stopa M, Cichoń S, Richter P, Nowak W. Total thyroidectomy for benign thyroid disease: is it really worthwhile? Ann Surg. 2011;254:724–9. discussion 729–30
87. Feroci F, Rettori M, Borrelli A, Coppola A, Castagnoli A, Perigli G, Cianchi F, Scatizzi M. A systematic review and meta-analysis of total thyroidectomy versus bilateral subtotal thyroidectomy for Graves' disease. Surgery. 2014;155:529–40.
88. Adam MA, Thomas S, Youngwirth L, Hyslop T, Reed SD, Scheri RP, Roman SA, Sosa JA. Is there a minimum number of thyroidectomies a surgeon should perform to optimize patient outcomes? Ann Surg. 2017;265:402–7.
89. Röher HD, Goretzki PE, Hellmann P, Witte J. Complications in thyroid surgery. Incidence and therapy. Chirurg. 1999;70:999–1010.
90. Abbas G, Dubner S, Heller KS. Re-operation for bleeding after thyroidectomy and parathyroidectomy. Head Neck. 2001;23:544–6.
91. Swee DS, Chng CL, Lim A. Clinical characteristics and outcome of thyroid storm: a case series and review of neuropsychiatric derangements in thyrotoxicosis. Endocr Pract. 2015;21:182–9.
92. Erbil Y, Ozluk Y, Giriş M, Salmaslioglu A, Issever H, Barbaros U, Kapran Y, Ozarmağan S, Tezelman S. Effect of lugol solution on thyroid gland blood flow and microvessel density in the patients with Graves' disease. J Clin Endocrinol Metab. 2007;92:2182–9.
93. Langley RW, Burch HB. Perioperative management of the thyrotoxic patient. Endocrinol Metab Clin N Am. 2003;32:519–34.
94. Tsai WC, Pei D, Wang TF, Wu DA, Li JC, Wei CL, Lee CH, Chen SP, Kuo SW. The effect of combination therapy with propylthiouracil and cholestyramine in the treatment of Graves' hyperthyroidism. Clin Endocrinol (Oxf). 2005;62:521–4.
95. Panzer C, Beazley R, Braverman L. Rapid preoperative preparation for severe hyperthyroid Graves' disease. J Clin Endocrinol Metab. 2004;89:2142–4.
96. Pagsisihan D, Andag-Silva A, Piores-Roderos O, Escobin MA. Rapid preoperative preparation for thyroidectomy of a severely hyperthyroid patient with graves' disease who developed agranulocytosis. J ASEAN Fed Endocr Soc. 2015;30:48–52.
97. Edafe O, Antakia R, Laskar N, Uttley L, Balasubramanian SP. Systematic review and meta-analysis of predictors of post-thyroidectomy hypocalcaemia. Br J Surg. 2014;101:307–20.
98. Oltmann SC, Brekke AV, Schneider DF, Schaefer SC, Chen H, Sippel RS. Preventing postoperative hypocalcemia in patients with Graves disease: a prospective study. Ann Surg Oncol. 2015;22:952–8.
99. Genser L, Trésallet C, Godiris-Petit G, Li Sun Fui S, Salepcioglu H, Royer C, Menegaux F. Randomized controlled trial of alfacalcidol supplementation for the reduction of hypocalcemia after total thyroidectomy. Am J Surg. 2014;207:39–45.
100. Laurberg P, Buchholtz Hansen PE, Iversen E, Eskjaer Jensen S, Weeke J. Goitre size and outcome of medical treatment of Graves' disease. Acta Endocrinol. 1986. https://doi.org/10.1530/acta.0.1110039.
101. Peters H, Fischer C, Bogner U, Reiners C, Schleusener H. Reduction in thyroid volume after radioiodine therapy of Graves' hyperthyroidism: results of a prospective, randomized, multicentre study. Eur J Clin Investig. 1996;26:59–63.
102. Bonnema SJ, Hegedüs L. Radioiodine therapy in benign thyroid diseases: effects, side effects, and factors affecting therapeutic outcome. Endocr Rev. 2012;33:920–80.
103. Kinuya S, Yoneyama T, Michigishi T. Airway complication occurring during radioiodine treatment for Graves' disease. Ann Nucl Med. 2007;21:367–9.
104. Hegedüs L, Bonnema SJ. Approach to management of the patient with primary or secondary intrathoracic goiter. J Clin Endocrinol Metab. 2010;95:5155–62.
105. Neumann S, Place RF, Krieger CC, Gershengorn MC. Future prospects for the treatment of Graves' hyperthyroidism and eye disease. Horm Metab Res. 2015;47:789–96.

3 Nodular Goitre

Ranil Fernando

Introduction

Goitre or enlargement of the thyroid gland is still a common problem. It has been estimated by the WHO that about 15.8% of the world population have goitres. Nodular goitre is the commonest endocrine surgical disorder encountered world over. The prevalence of nodular disease in the population varies based on the clinical methods used for detection: with palpation around 4% [1], with ultrasound scan studies 10–35% [2] and in post-mortem studies up to 49–57% [3].

There are several causes for nodularity of the thyroid. The nodular enlargement may or may not be accompanied by alteration in the function of the thyroid gland. The decisions relating to the clinical significance and the management strategies of thyroid nodules must be based on current knowledge and best available evidence, as there are several areas which are contentious. The nodular goitres can be classified broadly into those with hormone dysfunction (mainly toxic) and those without (euthyroid) (Table 3.1). Hypothyroidism associated with thyroid nodules is encountered only rarely in surgical practice (except in Hashimoto's thyroiditis), hence not included in this classification.

R. Fernando
Faculty of Medicine, Department of Surgery, University of Kelaniya, Kelaniya, Sri Lanka
e-mail: ranilfern@sltnet.lk

Pathogenesis

Multinodular Goitre

Multinodular enlargement is one of the commonest disorders of the thyroid and usually arises from repeated hyperplasia and degeneration of the gland. The process is generally triggered by iodine deficiency leading to DNA damage and an increase of the spontaneous mutation rate [4]. Multinodular goitre (MNG) has higher replication rates than normal thyroid tissue and this increases the mutagenic load to MNG by preventing DNA repair after the mutation [5].

It is now generally accepted that thyroid cells are heterogeneous genetically and would respond to stimuli differently [6, 7], and the various stimuli include genetics, stress, radiation, excess iodine, goitrogens, smoking, certain drugs like amiodarone and infections. The heterogeneity would explain why certain areas of the thyroid grow and become nodular in response to the various stimuli. The main mechanisms of growth are the cAMP-dependent TSH or EGF pathways [7]. The exact role various factors play varies from patient to patient, community to community and country to country. Iodine deficiency still remains a key factor in the pathogenesis of nodular goitre in certain parts of the world, especially some regions in the Asian subcontinent and sub-Saharan Africa [8].

R. Parameswaran, A. Agarwal (eds.), *Evidence-Based Endocrine Surgery*,
https://doi.org/10.1007/978-981-10-1124-5_3

Table 3.1 Classification of goitres

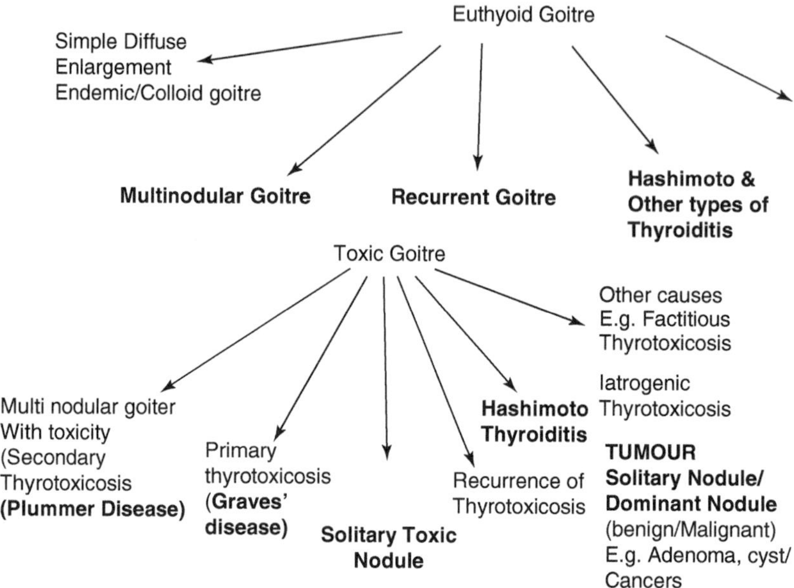

The importance of genetic factors is evident from the clustering of goitre within families and the higher concordance rate for goitre in monozygotic than in dizygotic twins. Studies assessing the role of specific candidate genes or genetic markers in the aetiology of simple goitre have given conflicting data in various families [7]. The possibility that single gene such as (MNG1) on chromosome 14 playing a major role in goitrogenesis within certain families is a postulate that needs to be entertained [7]. Other genes that have been identified as having a possible causative role are thyroglobulin (Tg) gene, the thyroid-stimulating hormone receptor (TSHR) gene, the Na+/I− symporter (NIS) gene and the multinodular goitre marker 1 [7]. Further studies focusing on whole-genome screening in multiplex families as well as large population-based studies should be undertaken that will elucidate the nature of goitrogenesis.

In *toxic multinodular goitre (TMNG)*, autonomously functioning thyroid nodules are seen and usually in long-standing multinodular goitres. TMNG or Plummer's disease was first described by Henry Plummer in 1913 and is the second commonest cause of hyperthyroidism, after Graves' disease. In elderly individuals and in areas of endemic iodine deficiency, TMNG is sometimes the most common cause of hyperthyroidism. As in nodular goitre, there is variable growth of nodules, with some undergoing haemorrhage, degeneration and calcification. Of these some nodules develop autonomous function which is probably the result of somatic mutations of the TSH receptor [9]. The autonomously functioning nodules, usually larger than 2.5 cm in diameter, may cause toxicity in about 10% of patients.

Most causes of recurrent nodular goitre are due to incomplete resection from previous surgery. Goitre recurrence is a difficult issue, as the risk of complications during subsequent surgery is much higher. The other cause of recurrence may be the development of a malignancy in a remnant. Goitres from malignancy and recurrent disease will be discussed in later chapters.

Clinical Presentation

The current consensus appears to be that goitre is diagnosed when a thyroid gland is four to five times enlarged [10]. Goitre is defined as a thyroid gland weighing over 20–25 g or a gland exceeding a volume of over 19 mL in women and 25 mL in men [11]. Nodular enlargement of a thyroid gland is the commonest presentation of a patient

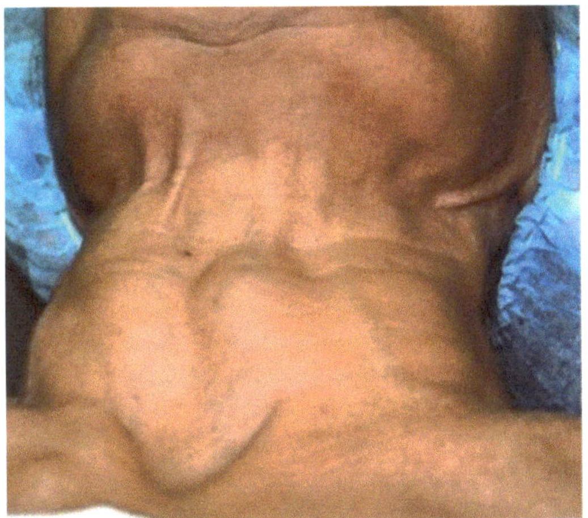

Fig. 3.1 Recurrence of a MNG

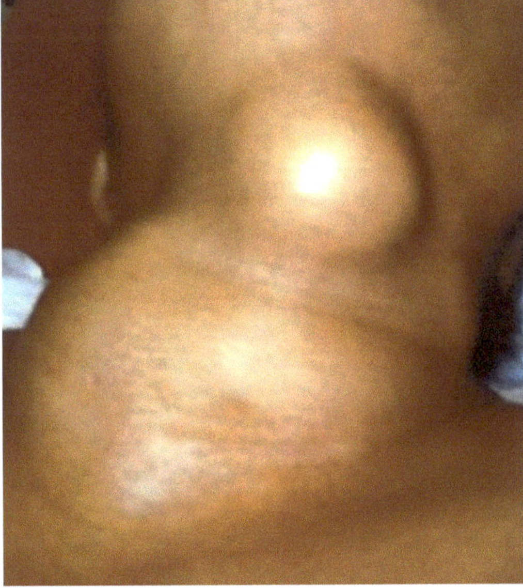

Fig. 3.2

to a surgical unit. Nodular goitres are much commoner in females than males (in a ratio of 3:1), in both endemic and non-endemic regions [12]. Multinodular goitre and other thyroid disorders are common in middle-aged females (fourth and fifth decades of life). However, in current practice one does see a significant number presenting with lumps incidentally on various modalities of imaging like ultrasound neck, CT, MRI, and PET scans (incidentalomas) [13].

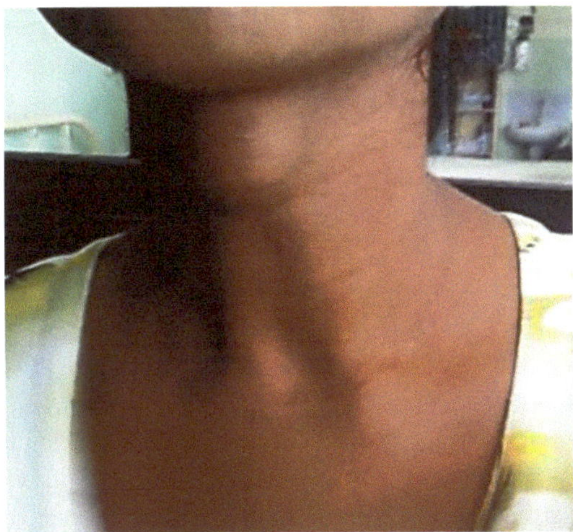

Fig. 3.3

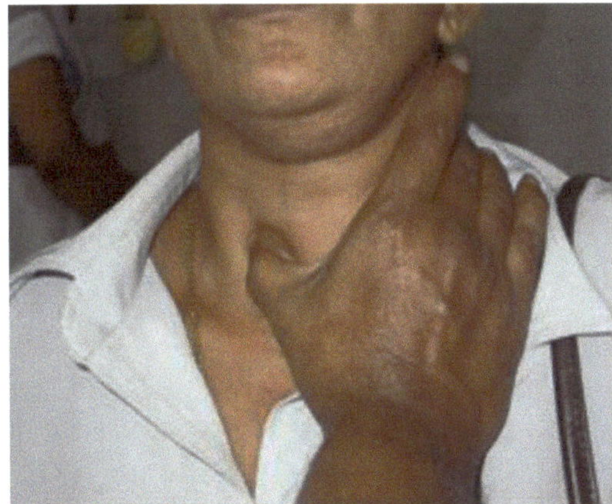

Fig. 3.4 Technique of palpation from the front

The important points to ascertain in clinical evaluation of a nodular goitre, apart from the physical characteristics, are:

1. Thyroid status
2. The position of the trachea
3. The involvement of neck vessels
4. Compressive features (Pemberton's sign)
5. Retrosternal extension
6. Lymph node enlargement

There are rare presentations such as recurrence in an embryological remnant (Figs. 3.1, 3.2, and 3.3). If solitary nodule is the presenting feature, it is very important to ensure that it is truly a solitary nodule and not a dominant nodule in a MNG. Having ascertained that it is a solitary nodule, all features of malignancy including enlargement of lymph nodes must be looked for. If it is a recurrent goitre, the possibility of a malignancy needs to be entertained.

In the examination of a thyroid gland the traditional method of palpating the gland from behind has several disadvantages. **Hence it is critical to examine the thyroid gland BOTH from the front (Fig. 3.4) and from behind**.

In contrast to Graves' disease the presentation of a toxic MNG may be due to the goitre or due to cardiovascular abnormalities such as dyspnoea, atrial fibrillation or cardiac failure. The classical features of sympathetic over activity and eye signs are not commonly seen in toxic MNG. On palpation of goitre in a patient with Hashimoto's thyroiditis, the surface of the gland feels finely granular: micronodular (as opposed to macronodules in a MNG). This is not a fact well described in standard text, but it is a physical sign found in most patients with Hashimoto's thyroiditis.

The final clinical assessment must contain information about the physical characteristics, functional status and possible aetiology of the nodular goitre, e.g. euthyroid benign multinodular goitre with features of compression. This will assist in deciding on the appropriate investigations.

Investigations of Nodular Goitre/ Thyroid Nodule

Morphology of goitre is assessed by clinical examination and ultrasonography. US scan is superior to clinical examination in detecting thyroid nodules as nodules as small as 3 mm can be detected by ultrasonography, using a 5–15 MHz probe, and preferably can be performed by an experienced radiologist or clinician. However, it is not without its limitations. Significant inter-observer and intra-observer variation occurs in sonographic measurements of thyroid volume and therefore proper training and experience are needed before reliance can be placed only on ultrasonography to assess thyroid size and features [14].

In addition, thyroid size differs in different populations. The size of the thyroid is affected by several factors including the iodine status of a population [15]. The differences in thyroid volume (Tvol) between the regions suggest that population-specific references for Tvol in countries with long-standing iodine sufficiency may be more accurate than is a single international reference [15]. The best method of assessing the size of thyroid ultrasonographically is debatable too. The well-known method is based on the three axes of each lobe and a new principle is based on planimetry in two planes. Recently volumetric evaluation of the thyroid gland based on the use of an ellipsoid model is being recommended [16]. The value obtained thus replaces clinical evaluation of volume. With the ellipsoid model, the height, width, and depth of each lobe are measured and multiplied. The obtained result is then multiplied by a correction factor, which is $\pi/6$, or 0.524 [16]. The US Scan findings such as increased vascularity and calcification may indicate the possibility of malignancy [17], but the definitive diagnosis of cancer only comes from histopathology. US scan is also needed to assess lymphadenopathy of the cervical nodes in thyroid disease especially when treating patients with thyroid cancer.

Other Imaging Modalities

CT scan is the best for assessment of retrosternal extension and involvement of surrounding structures such as the carotid artery and the internal jugular vein. PET scan is usually used for assessing recurrence of thyroid cancer. There are many reports of incidental small nodules of thyroid detected during routine PET scans and a positive uptake is suggestive of malignancy, but the PET is not recommended for routine assessment of thyroid nodules and it does not affect the outcome [18]. Plain X-ray of the neck still has a role in assessing the thyroid; it will show tracheal deviation and compression. The management strategies for incidental thyroid lesions/nodules detected by all forms of imaging are currently being debated and the consensus appears to be that detecting lesions less than 1 cm or less is of no value as it does not affect the outcome at all and screening for nodules and thyroid cancer is not recommended [19].

Blood Tests

Functional status is assessed by the thyroid hormone assay—T3, T4 and TSH. These assays are readily available in many countries. If cost constraints do not permit the assay of all three parameters, initial assay of the TSH, which is a very sensitive assay of thyroid pituitary axis, will provide a useful and reliable guide about the thyroid status [20]. The only exception is the very rare possibility of a TSH-secreting lesion in the pituitary. There are other non-thyroidal illnesses that may change the values of thyroid function (non-thyroidal illness syndrome); these must be borne in mind when interpreting thyroid function tests [21].

Other investigations such as thyroid antibodies will assist in diagnosing coexisting Hashimoto's thyroiditis or a Graves' disease and should be done in patients with symptoms of hyperthyroidism, clinical or subclinical. Serum calcitonin measurement is rarely used in the context of nodular goitre unless there is a suspicion of medullary thyroid cancer; however there are proponents of using it in routine thyroid practice [22–24]. **Routine testing of serum antibodies is relatively expensive, particularly in the developing world, and their measurement must be done judiciously, considering the real indication and cost-effectiveness. Serum thyroglobulin level has no role in the diagnosis of a nodular goitre**.

Cyto/Histopathology

Fine-needle aspiration cytology (FNAC) is the cornerstone in the assessment of pathology of the thyroid gland and thyroid nodules. **The British Thyroid Association (BTA)/RCP Thy1–5 system [25] and The Bethesda System for Reporting Thyroid Cytology (TBSRTC)** [26] have made the decision-making in thyroid lesions much more uniform.

In most patients with nodular diseases of the thyroid gland, the diagnosis of the lesion is elucidated on ultrasound and fine-needle cytology, to enable the clinicians to decide on an appropriate management (except cystic lesions). In about 10–20% of the patients the histopathological category causes a management dilemma as the information given in the cytology report is insufficient to decide on the management. In cystic lesions of the thyroid gland with no features to suggest thyroid malignancy, especially where repeated aspirations have not resolved the condition, surgical extirpation may be necessary to provide a histological diagnosis as cytology is generally not very helpful.

Treatment Options

The Natural history of nodular is variable. A nodule may remain dormant for a long period of time or progress rapidly. most nodules progress rather slowly. Rapid progression may indicate a sinsiter cause like a malignancy one the one hand or it may indicate a benign cause like a bleed into a cyst. If there is any change in the pattern of progression such patients will need early reevaluation.

Non-surgical options offer little in terms of treatment for MNG. If the patient does not wish to have sugrey and if the giotre does not have any features of malignancy clinically and cytologically or evidence of toxicity over a long period of time consideration may be given to careful follow up only. Suppressive dose of thyroxine, ethanol injection, radioiodine and recombinant human TSH (rhTSH) have all been tried in small number of selected patients with mixed results [27]. These modalities are not recommended for routine use. In addition, they do not eliminate the underlying pathology.

This leaves surgery as the main option for the definitive management of multinodular goitre. MNGs that need surgical treatment are mainly for the indications listed below *(the 5 Cs)*:

1. Cosmesis
2. Compression (of trachea or superior thoracic aperture)

3. Cancer (fear of it)
4. Comeback (recurrence)
5. Control of toxicity (failed medical therapy in Graves' or toxic MNG)

Though there are few detractors most authors would agree that the best surgical option for MNG is total/near-total thyroidectomy [28, 29]. This is more so in the case of very large goitres, seen in less developed part of the world where other forms of therapy will not be effective. Total thyroidectomy eliminates the need for revision surgery due to recurrence and it would also treat an occult cancer in a MNG. The only proviso is that the total thyroidectomy should be undertaken by an experienced surgeon [29]. The other drawback of total thyroidectomy is the need to have lifelong thyroxine replacement therapy. On balance, there is clear evidence to suggest that total thyroidectomy is the best surgical option for MNG. This is true for newly diagnosed MNGs as well as recurrence but the complication rates of recurrent disease tend to be a little higher [30, 31].

There is no consensus on the best option for a toxic MNG [32]. The treatment options depend on factors that include the age, degree of hyperthyroidism, size of nodule or goitre and patient choice [33]. However, the first aim of treatment is to control the toxicity with anti-thyroid drug therapy and then consider options for dealing with the goitre once the patient is euthyroid as hyperthyroidism recurs following cessation of treatment in about 95% of cases [34]. The available options are to undertake thyroidectomy or suppressive radioiodine therapy.

Surgery offers the only permanent cure in a toxic MNG. Surgery is generally recommended for the presence of compressive symptoms, coexisting thyroid cancer, large goitre, retrosternal extension, need for rapid correction of hyperthyroid state and coexisting hyperparathyroidism [35]. The only drawbacks are the risks involved in a thyroidectomy and the need to be on lifelong thyroxine therapy. In centres where complication rates are around 1% or less, surgery offers the best option of treatment. RAI-suppressive therapy is favourable for elderly patients, presence of comorbidities, previous surgery in the neck and small goitres. The risk of failure of treatment following near-total or total thyroidectomy is less than 1% [33, 36] in comparison to 20% following radioiodine therapy [36, 37].

To summarize, the treatment of Plummer's disease must take into account the goals of therapy, relief of symptoms, durability of cure, risk of malignancy and risk of complications [35].

Recurrent Goitre

Recurrent goitres are a challenging clinical problem (Figs. 3.1 and 3.2), with surgery the only definitive treatment option available, but the risk of complications is much higher in recurrent goitres [30, 38]. Hence the surgery should only be undertaken in units that undertake a large volume of thyroidectomies and the decision to operate must be undertaken with caution. Issues relating to reoperative thyroid surgery are discussed in Chap. 21.

Surgical Technique

The technique of thyroidectomy has evolved a great deal in the last 20 years. The favoured technique now is the capsular dissection with identification and preservation of recurrent laryngeal nerves (RLN), the external branches of the superior laryngeal nerve (EBSLN) and the parathyroids as described by Delbridge et al. [39]. If a parathyroid is accidentally devascularized or removed immediate autotransplantation in the ipsilateral sternocleidomastoid muscle must be undertaken. The other key change is the careful identification of all the embryological remnants. The main embryological remnants are the pyramidal lobe, the tubercle of Zuckerkandl and the thyrothymic remnants. One of the main reasons for recurrent goitres is the subsequent enlargement of the embryological remnants. These are very close to the parathyroids and the nerves and hence the risk of redo surgery is much higher.

Emergence of newer techniques of endoscopic and robotic thyroidectomy has added newer surgical techniques to thyroidectomy and this is further discussed in Chap. 22. The main criticism of the newer techniques is that most of them are not minimally invasive; against all surgical principles the surgeon moves away from the structure and approaches it through a circuitous route. The tissue damage is much more in breast or axillary approaches to the thyroid. In addition, newer complications such as brachial plexus injury have been described in an operation which had a very low complication rate in the open method. Besides this, in most countries the minimally invasive methods, particularly the robotic method, are not cost effective [40, 41].

Thyroidectomy is associated with complications and commonly include superior and recurrent laryngeal nerve palsy, hypoparathyroidism, bleeding, hematoma and seroma. The complications and their management are described in detail in Chap. 20.

Conclusion/Personal Review

Nodular disease of the thyroid is the commonest problem a surgeon is likely to encounter.

In the era of evidence-based medicine, the current available evidence is at best Levels II–VI.

Clinical assessment is invaluable in determining the patient's problems and must contain information about thyroid morphology, hormone status, likely pathology and local effects.

The minimum investigations that are required include thyroid hormone status, ultrasound of the thyroid gland and neck, and fine-needle aspiration cytology. If necessary, additional tests like antibodies or CT for evaluation of retrosternal extension may be needed based on the clinical suspicion.

Treatment is based on the size of goitre and symptoms. Small benign multinodular goitres are usually managed conservatively and observed with regular US scans, FNACs and hormone assays.

If surgery is the preferred option, **the current best evidence is that total thyroidectomy should be the treatment of choice**.

As the late Prof. William Halstead said:

> *The extirpation of the thyroid gland ... typifies, perhaps better than any operation, the supreme triumph of the surgeon's art .... A feat which today can be accomplished by any competent operator without danger of mishap and which was conceived more than one thousand years ago .... There are operations today more delicate and perhaps more difficult .... But is there any operative problem propounded so long ago and attacked by so many ... which has yielded results as bountiful and so adequate?—Dr. William S. Halsted, 1920* (56)

How true especially today!

References

1. Vander JB, Gaston EA, Dawber TR. The significance of nontoxic thyroid nodules. Final report of a 15-year study of the incidence of thyroid malignancy. Ann Intern Med. 1968;69(3):537–40.
2. Bruneton JN, Balu-Maestro C, Marcy PY, Melia P, Mourou MY. Very high frequency (13 MHz) ultrasonographic examination of the normal neck: detection of normal lymph nodes and thyroid nodules. J Ultrasound Med. 1994;13(2):87–90.
3. Wang C, Crapo LM. The epidemiology of thyroid disease and implications for screening. Endocrinol Metab Clin N Am. 1997;26(1):189–218.
4. Paschke R. Molecular pathogenesis of nodular goiter. Langenbeck's Arch Surg. 2011;396(8):1127–36.
5. Krohn K, Fuhrer D, Bayer Y, Eszlinger M, Brauer V, Neumann S, et al. Molecular pathogenesis of euthyroid and toxic multinodular goiter. Endocr Rev. 2005;26(4):504–24.
6. Roger PP, Baptist M, Dumont JE. A mechanism generating heterogeneity in thyroid epithelial cells: suppression of the thyrotropin/cAMP-dependent mitogenic pathway after cell division induced by cAMP-independent factors. J Cell Biol. 1992;117(2):383–93.
7. Brix TH, Hegedus L. Genetic and environmental factors in the aetiology of simple goitre. Ann Med. 2000;32(3):153–6.
8. Okosieme OE. Impact of iodination on thyroid pathology in Africa. J R Soc Med. 2006;99(8):396–401.
9. Palos-Paz F, Perez-Guerra O, Cameselle-Teijeiro J, Rueda-Chimeno C, Barreiro-Morandeira F, Lado-Abeal J, et al. Prevalence of mutations in TSHR, GNAS, PRKAR1A and RAS genes in a large series of toxic thyroid adenomas from Galicia, an iodine-deficient area in NW Spain. Eur J Endocrinol. 2008;159(5):623–31.
10. Delange F. What do we call a goiter? Eur J Endocrinol. 1999;140(6):486–8.
11. Langer P. Minireview: discussion about the limit between normal thyroid goiter. Endocr Regul. 1999;33(1):39–45.

12. Paschke R. Nodulogenesis and goitrogenesis. Ann Endocrinol (Paris). 2011;72(2):117–9.
13. Jin J, McHenry CR. Thyroid incidentaloma. Best Pract Res Clin Endocrinol Metab. 2012;26(1):83–96.
14. Jarlov AE, Nygard B, Hegedus L, Karstrup S, Hansen JM. Observer variation in ultrasound assessment of the thyroid gland. Br J Radiol. 1993;66(787):625–7.
15. Zimmermann MB, Hess SY, Molinari L, De Benoist B, Delange F, Braverman LE, et al. New reference values for thyroid volume by ultrasound in iodine-sufficient schoolchildren: a World Health Organization/Nutrition for Health and Development Iodine Deficiency Study Group Report. Am J Clin Nutr. 2004;79(2):231–7.
16. Shabana W, Peeters E, De Maeseneer M. Measuring thyroid gland volume: should we change the correction factor? Am J Roentgenol. 2006;186(1):234–6.
17. Smith-Bindman R, Lebda P, Feldstein VA, Sellami D, Goldstein RB, Brasic N, et al. Risk of thyroid cancer based on thyroid ultrasound imaging characteristics: results of a population-based study. JAMA Intern Med. 2013;173(19):1788–96.
18. Wong C, Lin M, Chicco A, Benson R. The clinical significance and management of incidental focal FDG uptake in the thyroid gland on positron emission tomography/computed tomography (PET/CT) in patients with non-thyroidal malignancy. Acta Radiol. 2011;52(8):899–904.
19. Ahn HS, Kim HJ, Welch HG. Korea's thyroid-cancer "epidemic"—screening and overdiagnosis. N Engl J Med. 2014;371(19):1765–7.
20. Sheehan MT. Biochemical testing of the thyroid: TSH is the best and, oftentimes, only test needed—a review for primary care. Clin Med Res. 2016;14(2):83–92.
21. Farwell AP. Nonthyroidal illness syndrome. Curr Opin Endocrinol Diabetes Obes. 2013;20(5): 478–84.
22. Elisei R. Routine serum calcitonin measurement in the evaluation of thyroid nodules. Best Pract Res Clin Endocrinol Metab. 2008;22(6):941–53.
23. Dietlein M, Wieler H, Schmidt M, Schwab R, Goretzki PE, Schicha H. Routine measurement of serum calcitonin in patients with nodular thyroid disorders? Nuklearmedizin. 2008;47(2):65–72.
24. Burch HB, Burman KD, Cooper DS, Hennessey JV, Vietor NO. A 2015 survey of clinical practice patterns in the management of thyroid nodules. J Clin Endocrinol Metab. 2016;101(7):2853–62.
25. Perros P, Boelaert K, Colley S, Evans C, Evans RM, Gerrard Ba G, et al. Guidelines for the management of thyroid cancer. Clin Endocrinol (Oxf). 2014;81(Suppl 1):1–122.
26. Cibas ES, Ali SZ, NCI Thyroid FNA State of the Science Conference. The Bethesda system for reporting thyroid cytopathology. Am J Clin Pathol. 2009;132(5):658–65.
27. Fast S, Nielsen VE, Bonnema SJ, Hegedus L. Time to reconsider nonsurgical therapy of benign non-toxic multinodular goitre: focus on recombinant human TSH augmented radioiodine therapy. Eur J Endocrinol. 2009;160(4):517–28.
28. Agarwal G, Aggarwal V. Is total thyroidectomy the surgical procedure of choice for benign multinodular goiter? An evidence-based review. World J Surg. 2008;32(7):1313–24.
29. Vassiliou I, Tympa A, Arkadopoulos N, Nikolakopoulos F, Petropoulou T, Smyrniotis V. Total thyroidectomy as the single surgical option for benign and malignant thyroid disease: a surgical challenge. Arch Med Sci. 2013;9(1):74–8.
30. Rudolph N, Dominguez C, Beaulieu A, De Wailly P, Kraimps JL. The morbidity of reoperative surgery for recurrent benign nodular goitre: impact of previous unilateral thyroid lobectomy versus subtotal thyroidectomy. J Thyroid Res. 2014;2014:231857.
31. Calo PG, Pisano G, Medas F, Tatti A, Tuveri M, Nicolosi A. Risk factors in reoperative thyroid surgery for recurrent goitre: our experience. G Chir. 2012;33(10):335–8.
32. Bhagat MC, Dhaliwal SS, Bonnema SJ, Hegedus L, Walsh JP. Differences between endocrine surgeons and endocrinologists in the management of non-toxic multinodular goitre. Br J Surg. 2003;90(9):1103–12.
33. Erickson D, Gharib H, Li H, van Heerden JA. Treatment of patients with toxic multinodular goiter. Thyroid. 1998;8(4):277–82.
34. van Soestbergen MJ, van der Vijver JC, Graafland AD. Recurrence of hyperthyroidism in multinodular goiter after long-term drug therapy: a comparison with Graves' disease. J Endocrinol Investig. 1992;15(11):797–800.
35. Porterfield JR Jr, Thompson GB, Farley DR, Grant CS, Richards ML. Evidence-based management of toxic multinodular goiter (Plummer's disease). World J Surg. 2008;32(7):1278–84.
36. Kang AS, Grant CS, Thompson GB, van Heerden JA. Current treatment of nodular goiter with hyperthyroidism (Plummer's disease): surgery versus radioiodine. Surgery 2002;132(6):916–923.; discussion 23.
37. Nygaard B, Hegedus L, Ulriksen P, Nielsen KG, Hansen JM. Radioiodine therapy for multinodular toxic goiter. Arch Intern Med. 1999;159(12):1364–8.
38. Muller PE, Jakoby R, Heinert G, Spelsberg F. Surgery for recurrent goitre: its complications and their risk factors. Eur J Surg. 2001;167(11):816–21.
39. Delbridge L, Reeve TS, Khadra M, Poole AG. Total thyroidectomy: the technique of capsular dissection. Aust N Z J Surg. 1992;62(2):96–9.
40. Broome JT, Pomeroy S, Solorzano CC. Expense of robotic thyroidectomy: a cost analysis at a single institution. Arch Surg. 2012;147(12):1102–6.
41. Yoo H, Chae BJ, Park HS, Kim KH, Kim SH, Song BJ, et al. Comparison of surgical outcomes between endoscopic and robotic thyroidectomy. J Surg Oncol. 2012;105(7):705–8.

Epidemiology of Thyroid Cancer

4

Tan Wee Boon and Rajeev Parameswaran

Introduction

In Singapore, thyroid cancer accounted for only the eighth commonest cancer in women, with an annual incidence of 1100 cases per year [1]. The incidence of thyroid cancer has increased over the last few decades in most parts of the world [2–5], and is the fastest growing cancer in women, with it being projected to be the third most common cancer by 2019 [6, 7]. Thyroid cancer is the most common malignancy and the incidence has risen by over 300% in the USA [8] and over 250% in Singapore (unpublished). Most of the increase is in the incidence of small papillary thyroid cancer [9].

The exact cause of the increase in the incidence of thyroid cancer remains a subject of debate. Some of the factors implicated in the rising incidence increased screening [10], and increased diagnostic imaging and pathological detection of small cancers [2, 11]. Population screening with an ultrasound of the thyroid is not recommended in Singapore unlike South Korea. In Korea screening led to an increase from 12.2 cases per 100,000 persons in 1993–1997 to 59.9 cases per 100,000 persons in 2003–2007 amongst people aged 15–79 years [12, 13]. However, it may be the case that the rising incidence is true [14, 15] and may be due to increase in unrecognized carcinogens [16].

Despite the increasing incidence, the mortality of thyroid cancer has remained stable and this may be related to variations in risk factor exposure, improved diagnosis, and early treatment of the disease [2, 17, 18]. The prognosis of almost all types of thyroid cancer has increased except that of anaplastic thyroid cancer. The significant divergence between the increasing incidence and mortality suggests the indolent behavior of thyroid cancers and the effect on mortality is only seen after many years.

Is the Increase Seen for all Thyroid Cancers?

The age-standardized incidence rate (ASR) of thyroid cancer increased by 224% (2.5 per 100,000 in 1974 to 5.6 per 100,000 in 2013) in Singapore. The ASR of males was 1.5 per 100,000 in 1974 vs. 2.7 per 100,000 in 2013 (increased by 180%) while that for female was 3.7 per 100,000 in 1974 versus 8.4 per 100,000 in 2013 (increased by 227%) (Fig. 4.1). The increase is predominantly due to the increase in incidence of papillary subtype (Fig. 4.2). The results are similar to the incidence trends shown in the SEER data and Netherlands Cancer Registry [19–21]. However, a few studies have showed the incidence of follicular cancer to have risen albeit

T. W. Boon · R. Parameswaran (✉)
Division of Endocrine Surgery, National University Hospital, Singapore, Singapore
e-mail: rajeev_parameswaran@nuhs.edu.sg

R. Parameswaran, A. Agarwal (eds.), *Evidence-Based Endocrine Surgery*,
https://doi.org/10.1007/978-981-10-1124-5_4

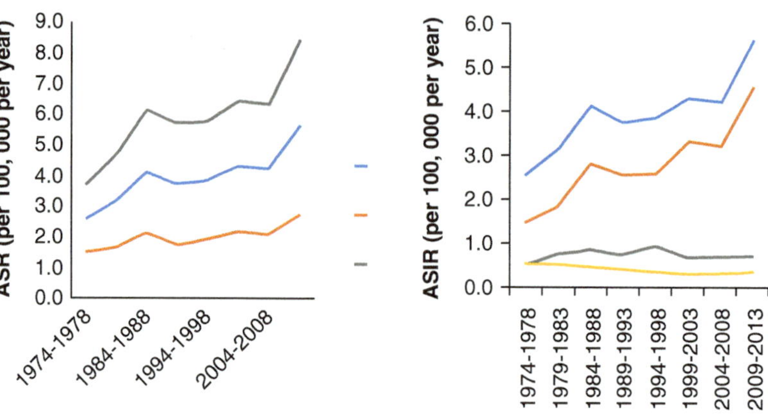

Fig. 4.1 Panel (**a**): The overall age-standardized ratio (ASR) of the cohort based on the histotype. Panel (**b**): ASR of thyroid cancer per gender for the cohort (Singapore National Cancer Registry)

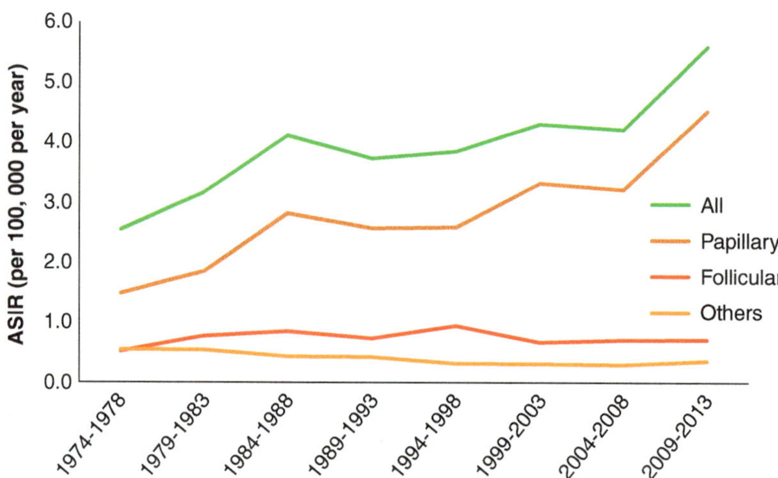

Fig. 4.2 The incidence of different types of thyroid cancer over the last four decades (Singapore National Cancer Registry)

slowly when compared to PTC [22–25]. In relation to medullary thyroid cancer, studies have shown stable and increased rates [22, 24]; ATC has shown a decreasing trend [24].

Is the Increase Seen for all Sizes of Thyroid Cancer?

The increase in incidence has shown a shift towards the detection of small cancers (defined as less than 5 cm), with a reduction in the larger cancers (Fig. 4.3), based on figures from Singapore National Cancer Registry. Micropapillary cancers (defined as cancers smaller than 1 cm) showed an increase of 80%; however, the percentage of micropapillary cancers diagnosed to the ratio of total cancers has remained nearly the same (about 36–38%) in Singapore. This is unlike the report from Cramer et al. [19] where they showed a consistent rate of increase for micropapillary cancers at 19% per year and larger cancers between 10 and 12% per year.

Some of the reasons attributed to the increase of smaller cancers are widespread adoption of ultrasonography and fine-needle aspiration on thyroid nodules [2, 3] and changes in pathological reporting criteria. There is evidence to suggest however that the increase of the incidence of smaller cancers may be from thyroid screening as shown in the epidemiological data from Korea and Fukushima prefecture from Japan [26, 27]. The increase in small cancers may also be due to incidental lesions picked up with medical surveillance [12].

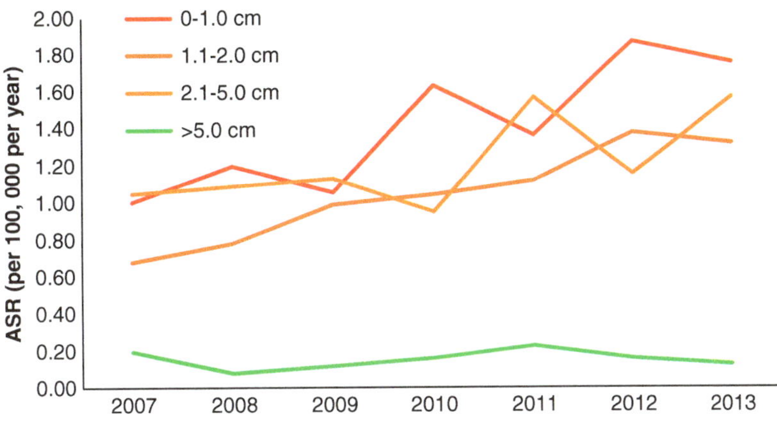

Fig. 4.3 The incidence of PTC based on the size of the tumors over the last decade (Singapore National Cancer Registry)

Is the Increased Incidence a Result of Screening with Ultrasound?

Ultrasound scan (US) is the first tool in the evaluation of thyroid nodules, especially to differentiate the benign from the malignant nodules. Small thyroid cancers that are occult, small, and indolent are seen in up to a third of adults, with no impact on survival [28]. Screening is useful in high-risk patients (positive family history, inherited mutations with high risk of thyroid cancer, distant metastasis, and history of irradiation). Routine screening of population deemed to be at low risk is not cost effective and leads to overdiagnosis with obvious clinical benefit.

Korea is an example where US is routinely used as a screening tool for thyroid cancer and has led to the epidemic of "overdiagnosis" of thyroid cancer [10]. Most of the cancers that were diagnosed were subclinical and rarely lethal and of microcarcinoma type [29]. As a result, patients undergoing surgery for micropapillary cancers increased from 14 to 56% from 1995 to 2015. The overprescribed surgery did have an impact on patient outcomes in the form of permanent hypoparathyroidism in 10% of patients and recurrent laryngeal nerve palsy in 2% [10]. Other potential harmful effects of US screening of small thyroid cancers and related surgery include lifelong thyroid hormone replacement [26], unnecessary lymph node dissection and radioiodine ablation, psychological morbidity [30], and higher health costs for little benefit [6].

What Is the Impact of Other Imaging Modalities on the Rising Incidence of Thyroid Cancer?

Besides US, the use of computerized tomography (CT) and magnetic resonance imaging (MRI) has increased by two- to threefold over the last two decades [31]. CT scans are now routinely used in the emergency department, with the usage increased over 200% [32]. About a fifth of images obtained by CT and MRI show incidental thyroid nodules, of which majority are small thyroid nodules [33]. These imaging modalities have contributed to a more than twofold increase in the incidence of thyroid nodules over the last 30 years [34], and a threefold increase in biopsies of the thyroid nodules [34, 35]. The increased incidence of thyroid cancer and imaging is associated with access to health care [12, 36]. Screening with CT and MRI, although picks up the small cancers, may not account for the large cancers [37].

Radiation and Thyroid Cancer

Ionizing radiation is a major risk factor for thyroid cancer, mainly papillary thyroid cancer. Thyroid is extremely radiosensitive and may be exposed to injuries from the radiation from nuclear accidents, interventional radiology, extensive imaging by CT, and radiation therapy for treatment of malignant conditions [38–40]. The definitive evidence of the association between radiation exposure and thyroid cancer risk comes from the Chernobyl nuclear accident population data [41]. There has also been an increase in background radiation from 3.6 mSv/year to 6.2 mSv/year in the US [42]. Exposure to medical X-rays increased fivefold from 0.4 to 2.2 mSv and from CT increased to 48% [42]. The latent period for developing cancer following radiation exposure to head and neck area was found to be around 28 years [33]. However cancer risk may be a possibility in patients with genetic predisposition to radiation-associated carcinogenesis [43]. Similarly diagnostic 131-iodine scanning [44, 45] and 131-I ablation for hyperthyroidism have not shown to be associated with increased incidence of thyroid cancer [45].

Other Factors

TSH and Iodine Intake

One of the major factors for growth of thyroid cancer cells is increased TSH and this may be seen in cases of iodine deficiency. Chronic iodine deficiency is considered as a risk factor for follicular thyroid cancer and goiter [46–48], and similarly excess iodine supplementation has been shown to increase the incidence of papillary thyroid cancer [49, 50]. Ever since the iodine supplementation programs, there has been a shift in the ratio of papillary to follicular thyroid cancer ratios, with higher incidence of PTCs since iodine supplementation [51, 52]. Rather than the factors mentioned above, increased surveillance and improved diagnosis have led to the increase in thyroid cancer [50, 53]. Iodine-sufficient areas have a higher incidence of BRAF-positive PTCs though this has not been causally proven [16, 54].

Hormonal and Reproductive Factors

The fact that thyroid cancers are seen more commonly in women, to almost threefold especially during the reproductive years, suggests that hormonal and reproductive factors may be involved but this has not been consistently proven in epidemiological studies [55]. Factors such as menarche, parity, pregnancy, and oral contraceptives lead to elevation of TSH and this could cause hyperplasia and possibly cancer [56–58]; however these results are not consistent.

Hashimoto's Thyroiditis

Hashimoto's thyroiditis was historically thought to be associated with increased risk of developing thyroid lymphoma [59, 60]. The first report of the association between thyroiditis and papillary thyroid cancer was in 1955 [61]. The two common hypothesis explanations for the relationship between PTC and thyroiditis include an immunological response with a cancer-impeding effect leading to a favorable outcome [62] and elevated TSH levels seen in hypothyroid patients which stimulate follicular epithelial cells leading to the development of PTC [63]. The association, though commonly described with PTC, has also been described in follicular thyroid cancer though less common [64]. Many studies have shown similar biomolecular pathways between thyroiditis and PTC and include those of RET/PTC rearrangements [65, 66], *BRAF* (V600E) mutation [67], phosphatidylinositol 3-kinase (PI3k) pathway components [68], CD98 expression [69], p63 expression [70], and human 8-oxoguanine glycosylase 1 gene [71].

Other Factors

Various other factors that have been implicated in thyroid cancer but have not been validated include obesity [72], diet and lifestyle [73, 74], increased pathological detection [11], and toxic multinodular goiter [75].

Summary

There is no doubt that the incidence of thyroid cancer worldwide is increasing and the increase is predominantly in the rise of small cancers. The reason for the increased incidence is unclear, but may be multifactorial partly accounted by early detection. Additional studies are necessary to determine whether the increased incidence is due to environmental, biological, or occupational exposures.

References

1. Shulin JH, Aizhen J, Kuo SM, Tan WB, Ngiam KY, Parameswaran R. Rising incidence of thyroid cancer in Singapore not solely due to micropapillary subtype. Ann R Coll Surg Engl. 2018;100(4):295–300.
2. Davies L, Welch HG. Increasing incidence of thyroid cancer in the United States, 1973–2002. JAMA. 2006;295(18):2164–7.
3. Kent WD, Hall SF, Isotalo PA, Houlden RL, George RL, Groome PA. Increased incidence of differentiated thyroid carcinoma and detection of subclinical disease. CMAJ. 2007;177(11):1357–61.
4. Colonna M, Guizard AV, Schvartz C, Velten M, Raverdy N, Molinie F, et al. A time trend analysis of papillary and follicular cancers as a function of tumour size: a study of data from six cancer registries in France (1983–2000). Eur J Cancer. 2007;43(5):891–900.
5. Burgess JR. Temporal trends for thyroid carcinoma in Australia: an increasing incidence of papillary thyroid carcinoma (1982–1997). Thyroid. 2002;12(2):141–9.
6. Pellegriti G, Frasca F, Regalbuto C, Squatrito S, Vigneri R. Worldwide increasing incidence of thyroid cancer: update on epidemiology and risk factors. J Cancer Epidemiol. 2013;2013:965212.
7. Aschebrook-Kilfoy B, Kaplan EL, Chiu BC, Angelos P, Grogan RH. The acceleration in papillary thyroid cancer incidence rates is similar among racial and ethnic groups in the United States. Ann Surg Oncol. 2013;20(8):2746–53.
8. Davies L, Welch HG. Current thyroid cancer trends in the United States. JAMA Otolaryngol Head Neck Surg. 2014;140(4):317–22.
9. Simard EP, Ward EM, Siegel R, Jemal A. Cancers with increasing incidence trends in the United States: 1999 through 2008. CA Cancer J Clin. 2012;62(2):118–28.
10. Ahn HS, Kim HJ, Welch HG. Korea's thyroid-cancer "epidemic"—screening and overdiagnosis. N Engl J Med. 2014;371(19):1765–7.
11. Grodski S, Brown T, Sidhu S, Gill A, Robinson B, Learoyd D, et al. Increasing incidence of thyroid cancer is due to increased pathologic detection. Surgery. 2008;144(6):1038–43. discussion 43
12. Vaccarella S, Dal Maso L, Laversanne M, Bray F, Plummer M, Franceschi S. The impact of diagnostic changes on the rise in thyroid cancer incidence: a population-based study in selected high-resource countries. Thyroid. 2015;25(10):1127–36.
13. Lee JH, Shin SW. Overdiagnosis and screening for thyroid cancer in Korea. Lancet. 2014;384(9957):1848.
14. Enewold L, Zhu K, Ron E, Marrogi AJ, Stojadinovic A, Peoples GE, et al. Rising thyroid cancer incidence in the United States by demographic and tumor characteristics, 1980–2005. Cancer Epidemiol Biomark Prev. 2009;18(3):784–91.
15. Rego-Iraeta A, Perez-Mendez LF, Mantinan B, Garcia-Mayor RV. Time trends for thyroid cancer in northwestern Spain: true rise in the incidence of micro and larger forms of papillary thyroid carcinoma. Thyroid. 2009;19(4):333–40.
16. Mathur A, Moses W, Rahbari R, Khanafshar E, Duh QY, Clark O, et al. Higher rate of BRAF mutation in papillary thyroid cancer over time: a single-institution study. Cancer. 2011;117(19):4390–5.
17. Pacini F, Castagna MG, Brilli L, Pentheroudakis G. Thyroid cancer: ESMO Clinical Practice Guidelines for diagnosis, treatment and follow-up. Ann Oncol. 2010;21(Suppl 5):v214–9.
18. Vecchia C, Malvezzi M, Bosetti C, Garavello W, Bertuccio P, Levi F, et al. Thyroid cancer mortality and incidence: a global overview. Int J Cancer. 2015;136(9):2187–95.
19. Cramer JD, Fu P, Harth KC, Margevicius S, Wilhelm SM. Analysis of the rising incidence of thyroid cancer using the Surveillance, Epidemiology and End Results national cancer data registry. Surgery. 2010;148(6):1147–52. discussion 52–3
20. Husson O, Haak HR, van Steenbergen LN, Nieuwlaat WA, van Dijk BA, Nieuwenhuijzen GA, et al. Rising incidence, no change in survival and decreasing mortality from thyroid cancer in The Netherlands since 1989. Endocr Relat Cancer. 2013;20(2):263–71.
21. Lim H, Devesa SS, Sosa JA, Check D, Kitahara CM. Trends in Thyroid Cancer Incidence and Mortality in the United States, 1974–2013. JAMA. 2017;317(13):1338–48.
22. Poljak NK, Kontic M, Colovic Z, Jeroncic I, Russo A, Mulic R. Does life along the sea carry greater risk of thyroid cancer? Coll Antropol. 2012;36(2):431–9.
23. Smailyte G, Miseikyte-Kaubriene E, Kurtinaitis J. Increasing thyroid cancer incidence in Lithuania in 1978-2003. BMC Cancer. 2006;6:284.
24. Colonna M, Grosclaude P, Remontet L, Schvartz C, Mace-Lesech J, Velten M, et al. Incidence of thyroid cancer in adults recorded by French cancer registries (1978–1997). Eur J Cancer. 2002;38(13):1762–8.
25. Roche LM, Niu X, Pawlish KS, Henry KA. Thyroid cancer incidence in New Jersey: time trend, birth cohort and socioeconomic status analysis (1979-2006). J Environ Public Health. 2011;2011:850105.
26. Ahn HS, Kim HJ, Kim KH, Lee YS, Han SJ, Kim Y, et al. Thyroid cancer screening in South Korea increases detection of papillary cancers with no impact on other subtypes or thyroid cancer mortality. Thyroid. 2016;26(11):1535–40.

27. Tsuda T, Tokinobu A, Yamamoto E, Suzuki E. Thyroid cancer detection by ultrasound among residents ages 18 years and younger in Fukushima, Japan: 2011 to 2014. Epidemiology. 2016;27(3):316–22.
28. Harach HR, Franssila KO, Wasenius VM. Occult papillary carcinoma of the thyroid. A "normal" finding in Finland. A systematic autopsy study. Cancer. 1985;56(3):531.
29. Leboulleux S, Tuttle RM, Pacini F, Schlumberger M. Papillary thyroid microcarcinoma: time to shift from surgery to active surveillance? Lancet Diabetes Endocrinol. 2016;4(11):933–42.
30. Nikiforov YE, Seethala RR, Tallini G, Baloch ZW, Basolo F, Thompson LD, et al. Nomenclature revision for encapsulated follicular variant of papillary thyroid carcinoma: a paradigm shift to reduce overtreatment of indolent tumors. JAMA Oncol. 2016;2(8):1023–9.
31. Baker LC, Atlas SW, Afendulis CC. Expanded use of imaging technology and the challenge of measuring value. Health Aff (Millwood). 2008;27(6):1467–78.
32. Rao VM, Levin DC, Parker L, Frangos AJ, Sunshine JH. Trends in utilization rates of the various imaging modalities in emergency departments: nationwide Medicare data from 2000 to 2008. J Am Coll Radiol. 2011;8(10):706–9.
33. Youserm DM, Huang T, Loevner LA, Langlotz CP. Clinical and economic impact of incidental thyroid lesions found with CT and MR. Am J Neuroradiol. 1997;18(8):1423–8.
34. Cronan JJ. Thyroid nodules: is it time to turn off the US machines? Radiology. 2008;247(3):602–4.
35. Ross DS. Editorial: predicting thyroid malignancy. J Clin Endocrinol Metab. 2006;91(11):4253–5.
36. Zagzag J, Kenigsberg A, Patel KN, Heller KS, Ogilvie JB. Thyroid cancer is more likely to be detected incidentally on imaging in private hospital patients. J Surg Res. 2017;215:239–44.
37. Morris LG. Improved detection does not fully explain the rising incidence of well-differentiated thyroid cancer: a population-based analysis. Am J Surg. 2010;200(4):454–61.
38. Ron E, Lubin JH, Shore RE, Mabuchi K, Modan B, Pottern LM, et al. Thyroid cancer after exposure to external radiation: a pooled analysis of seven studies. Radiat Res. 1995;141(3):259–77.
39. Lubin JH, Adams MJ, Shore R, Holmberg E, Schneider AB, Hawkins MM, et al. Thyroid cancer following childhood low-dose radiation exposure: a pooled analysis of nine cohorts. J Clin Endocrinol Metab. 2017;102(7):2575–83.
40. Jacob P, Bogdanova TI, Buglova E, Chepurniy M, Demidchik Y, Gavrilin Y, et al. Thyroid cancer risk in areas of Ukraine and Belarus affected by the Chernobyl accident. Radiat Res. 2006;165(1):1–8.
41. Yamashita S, Thomas G. Thyroid cancer and nuclear accidents: long-term aftereffects of Chernobyl and Fukushima. London: Academic Press; 2017.
42. Mettler FA Jr, Thomadsen BR, Bhargavan M, Gilley DB, Gray JE, Lipoti JA, et al. Medical radiation exposure in the U.S. in 2006: preliminary results. Health Phys. 2008;95(5):502–7.
43. Nikiforov YE. Is ionizing radiation responsible for the increasing incidence of thyroid cancer? Cancer. 2010;116(7):1626–8.
44. Hahn K, Schnell-Inderst P, Grosche B, Holm LE. Thyroid cancer after diagnostic administration of iodine-131 in childhood. Radiat Res. 2001;156(1):61–70.
45. Dickman PW, Holm LE, Lundell G, Boice JD Jr, Hall P. Thyroid cancer risk after thyroid examination with 131I: a population-based cohort study in Sweden. Int J Cancer. 2003;106(4):580–7.
46. Nagataki S, Nystrom E. Epidemiology and primary prevention of thyroid cancer. Thyroid. 2002;12(10):889–96.
47. Lind P, Langsteger W, Molnar M, Gallowitsch HJ, Mikosch P, Gomez I. Epidemiology of thyroid diseases in iodine sufficiency. Thyroid. 1998;8(12):1179–83.
48. Franceschi S. Iodine intake and thyroid carcinoma--a potential risk factor. Exp Clin Endocrinol Diabetes. 1998;106(Suppl 3):S38–44.
49. Delange F, Lecomte P. Iodine supplementation: benefits outweigh risks. Drug Saf. 2000;22(2):89–95.
50. Weissel M. Legal augmentation of iodine content in table salt from 10 to 20 mg KI/kg: documented effects a decade later. Exp Clin Endocrinol Diabetes. 2003;111(4):187–90.
51. Dijkstra B, Prichard RS, Lee A, Kelly LM, Smyth PP, Crotty T, et al. Changing patterns of thyroid carcinoma. Ir J Med Sci. 2007;176(2):87–90.
52. Harach HR, Escalante DA, Onativia A, Lederer Outes J, Saravia Day E, Williams ED. Thyroid carcinoma and thyroiditis in an endemic goitre region before and after iodine prophylaxis. Acta Endocrinol. 1985;108(1):55–60.
53. Verkooijen HM, Fioretta G, Pache JC, Franceschi S, Raymond L, Schubert H, et al. Diagnostic changes as a reason for the increase in papillary thyroid cancer incidence in Geneva, Switzerland. Cancer Causes Control. 2003;14(1):13–7.
54. Guan H, Ji M, Bao R, Yu H, Wang Y, Hou P, et al. Association of high iodine intake with the T1799A BRAF mutation in papillary thyroid cancer. J Clin Endocrinol Metab. 2009;94(5):1612–7.
55. Capen CC, International Agency for Research on Cancer, World Health Organization. Species differences in thyroid, kidney and urinary bladder carcinogenesis. International Agency for Research on Cancer: Lyon; 1999.
56. Truong T, Orsi L, Dubourdieu D, Rougier Y, Hemon D, Guenel P. Role of goiter and of menstrual and reproductive factors in thyroid cancer: a population-based case-control study in New Caledonia (South Pacific), a very high incidence area. Am J Epidemiol. 2005;161(11):1056–65.
57. Zhu J, Zhu X, Tu C, Li YY, Qian KQ, Jiang C, et al. Parity and thyroid cancer risk: a meta-analysis of epidemiological studies. Cancer Med. 2016;5(4):739–52.

58. Zhou YQ, Zhou Z, Qian MF, Gong T, Wang JD. Association of thyroid carcinoma with pregnancy: a meta-analysis. Mol Clin Oncol. 2015;3(2):341–6.
59. Derringer GA, Thompson LD, Frommelt RA, Bijwaard KE, Heffess CS, Abbondanzo SL. Malignant lymphoma of the thyroid gland: a clinicopathologic study of 108 cases. Am J Surg Pathol. 2000;24(5):623–39.
60. Farrell E, Heffron C, Murphy M, O'Leary G, Sheahan P. Impact of lymphocytic thyroiditis on incidence of pathological incidental thyroid carcinoma. Head Neck. 2017;39(1):122–7.
61. Dailey ME, Lindsay S, Skahen R. Relation of thyroid neoplasms to Hashimoto disease of the thyroid gland. AMA Arch Surg. 1955;70(2):291–7.
62. Jankovic B, Le KT, Hershman JM. Clinical review: Hashimoto's thyroiditis and papillary thyroid carcinoma: is there a correlation? J Clin Endocrinol Metab. 2013;98(2):474–82.
63. McLeod DS, Watters KF, Carpenter AD, Ladenson PW, Cooper DS, Ding EL. Thyrotropin and thyroid cancer diagnosis: a systematic review and dose-response meta-analysis. J Clin Endocrinol Metab. 2012;97(8):2682–92.
64. Tamimi DM. The association between chronic lymphocytic thyroiditis and thyroid tumors. Int J Surg Pathol. 2002;10(2):141–6.
65. Mechler C, Bounacer A, Suarez H, Saint Frison M, Magois C, Aillet G, et al. Papillary thyroid carcinoma: 6 cases from 2 families with associated lymphocytic thyroiditis harbouring RET/PTC rearrangements. Br J Cancer. 2001;85(12):1831–7.
66. Sheils OM, O'Eary JJ, Uhlmann V, Lattich K, Sweeney EC. ret/PTC-1 activation in Hashimoto thyroiditis. Int J Surg Pathol. 2000;8(3):185–9.
67. Kim KH, Suh KS, Kang DW, Kang DY. Mutations of the BRAF gene in papillary thyroid carcinoma and in Hashimoto's thyroiditis. Pathol Int. 2005;55(9):540–5.
68. Larson SD, Jackson LN, Riall TS, Uchida T, Thomas RP, Qiu S, et al. Increased incidence of well-differentiated thyroid cancer associated with Hashimoto thyroiditis and the role of the PI3k/Akt pathway. J Am Coll Surg. 2007;204(5):764–73. discussion 73–5
69. Anderson CE, Graham C, Herriot MM, Kamel HM, Salter DM. CD98 expression is decreased in papillary carcinoma of the thyroid and Hashimoto's thyroiditis. Histopathology. 2009;55(6):683–6.
70. Unger P, Ewart M, Wang BY, Gan L, Kohtz DS, Burstein DE. Expression of p63 in papillary thyroid carcinoma and in Hashimoto's thyroiditis: a pathobiologic link? Hum Pathol. 2003;34(8):764–9.
71. Royer MC, Zhang H, Fan CY, Kokoska MS. Genetic alterations in papillary thyroid carcinoma and Hashimoto thyroiditis: an analysis of hOGG1 loss of heterozygosity. Arch Otolaryngol Head Neck Surg. 2010;136(3):240–2.
72. Pazaitou-Panayiotou K, Polyzos SA, Mantzoros CS. Obesity and thyroid cancer: epidemiologic associations and underlying mechanisms. Obes Rev. 2013;14(12):1006–22.
73. Mack WJ, Preston-Martin S, Dal Maso L, Galanti R, Xiang M, Franceschi S, et al. A pooled analysis of case-control studies of thyroid cancer: cigarette smoking and consumption of alcohol, coffee, and tea. Cancer Causes Control. 2003;14(8):773–85.
74. Kilfoy BA, Zhang Y, Park Y, Holford TR, Schatzkin A, Hollenbeck A, et al. Dietary nitrate and nitrite and the risk of thyroid cancer in the NIH-AARP Diet and Health Study. Int J Cancer. 2011;129(1):160–72.
75. Cerci C, Cerci SS, Eroglu E, Dede M, Kapucuoglu N, Yildiz M, et al. Thyroid cancer in toxic and non-toxic multinodular goiter. J Postgrad Med. 2007;53(3):157–60.

5 Genetic Landscape of Thyroid Cancer

Samantha Peiling Yang

Introduction

Thyroid cancer incidence has been increasing over the past 40 years [1–4]. The histological and genetic profile distribution has been changing [3]. Majority of thyroid cancer are derived from thyroid follicular cells, consisting of papillary thyroid carcinoma (80%), follicular thyroid carcinoma (<10%), poorly differentiated thyroid carcinoma (7%), and anaplastic thyroid carcinoma (2%). The thyroid C cells form medullary thyroid carcinoma (3%) [1, 5, 6]. The utilisation of modern sequencing technique has enabled better correlation of clinico-pathological features with their genetic basis. The Cancer Genome Atlas (TCGA) genetic characterisation of papillary thyroid carcinoma had increased the proportion of known oncogenic drivers from 75 to 96.5% [7]. Even though the survival rate is usually high in most thyroid cancer patients, 60–70% fail to achieve complete remission (i.e. post-surgical incomplete or indeterminate treatment response) [8, 9]. About 25–50% of locally advanced or metastatic thyroid cancers become refractory to radioiodine therapy. This leads to a poorer outcome with 5-year survival of <50% and 10-year survival of <10% [10, 11]. The understanding of the genetic basis of these aggressive metastatic thyroid cancers is critical for personalised genotype-directed therapy.

Papillary Thyroid Carcinoma

The TCGA studied 496 papillary thyroid carcinoma (PTC) patients of which 69.4% had classical type, 21.2% were of follicular variant, 7.5% were of tall cell variant, 2.0% were of uncommon PTC variants, while 29 had no histological subtype classification [7]. Most of these patients did not have prior radiation exposure. The mutation density in PTC was shown to be one of the lowest, as compared to other solid tumour types, with 11 non-synonymous mutation per tumour and 0.41 mutation per Mb on the average. The mutation rate of individual patients can be different within a cancer type, and it correlates with age, risk of recurrence, and MACIS score. Bischoff et al. had reviewed the Surveillance, Epidemiology, and End Result (SEER) database and showed that the disease-specific mortality in PTC increased with age with no inflection point at age 45 [12]. Similarly, the TCGA data showed a continuum of mutation density with age, supporting that age could be viewed as a continuous variable in risk stratification instead of a binary variable of 45 years used in the TNM Staging system [7].

S. Peiling Yang
Division of Endocrinology, National University Hospital, Singapore, Singapore

Yong Loo Lin School of Medicine, National University of Singapore, Singapore, Singapore
e-mail: peiling_yang@nuhs.edu.sg

R. Parameswaran, A. Agarwal (eds.), *Evidence-Based Endocrine Surgery*,
https://doi.org/10.1007/978-981-10-1124-5_5

In previous studies of PTC, the main genetic drivers included mutations in *BRAF* (encodes serine/threonine kinase, B-raf), *RAS* (encodes small GTPases), and *RET/PTC* gene rearrangement (*RET* encodes proto-oncogene tyrosine kinase receptor, Ret); these genes signal through the mitogen-activated protein kinase (MAPK) pathway [13, 14]. Consistent with previously established genetic alterations, the TCGA study demonstrated that 74.6% of its PTC cohort harboured these significantly mutated (mutually exclusive) genes including *BRAF* (61.7% were point mutations with consequent Val600Glu mutations—V600E substitutions), *NRAS*, *HRAS*, and *KRAS* [7]. Interestingly, the $BRAF^{V600E}$ mutations correlated with classical type and tall cell variant, whereas *RAS* mutations correlated with follicular variant. From the TCGA cohort, 4.5% of PTC had 20 mutually exclusive mutations in *PTEN*, *AKT1/2*, and *PAX8-PPARG* from the PI3K and PPARG signalling pathways, 1.5% had mutations of WNT pathway-related genes, and 3.7% had mutations of tumour suppressor genes including *TP53*, *RB1*, *NF1/2*, *MEN1*, and *PTEN*. The *EIF1AX* gene was identified as driver mutation in 1.5% of the TCGA cohort that did not harbour other driver mutations, with the exception of one PTC case that had three driver mutations, *KRAS* (clonal, cancer cell fraction 100%), *EIF1AX* (subclonal, cancer cell fraction 76%), and *BRAF* (subclonal, cancer cell fraction 53%) [7, 15]. It encodes for a protein translational initiation factor required for 40S ribosome. It has been shown to activate cell proliferation and protein synthesis in mammary cell line studies [16], and its exact role in thyroid cancer tumorigenesis remains to be elucidated. Most of the *EIF1AX* mutant cases from TCGA were follicular variant PTC (5/6, 83%), except for the above case, with coexistent *BRAFV600E* mutation, which had predominant classical PTC features with some follicular components [7]. In another study by Karunamurthy et al. evaluating *EIF1AX* mutation prevalence in thyroid nodules, the gene has been described in 2.3% of PTC (all three cases were encapsulated follicular variant), 24% of anaplastic thyroid carcinoma, 7.4% of follicular adenoma, 1.3% of hyperplastic nodules, and none of the follicular thyroid carcinoma cases [17]. In some of the *EIF1AX* mutant thyroid cancer cases, coexistent *NRAS* mutation was observed, whereas none of the *EIF1AX* mutant thyroid hyperplastic nodules or follicular adenoma had coexistent gene mutations. In the TCGA study, two other significantly mutated DNA repair-related genes were *PPM1D* and *CHEK2*; these coexisted with the MAPK-pathway mutations [18]. *PPM1D* activating mutations had been previously described as a driver mutation in brain gliomas [19]. *TERT* promoter mutations (C228T and C250T) had been reported in thyroid cancer to be associated with more advanced and aggressive subtypes [20–22]. *TERT* encodes the reverse transcriptase component of telomerases that adds telomere repeats to chromosomal ends allowing for cell replication and maintaining chromosomal stability [23]. Shortened telomere length is associated with chromosomal instability, including chromosomal rearrangement, chromosomal arm gain or loss, and chromosomal fusion, deletions, or amplification that can lead to tumorigenesis [24]. Melo et al. found that *TERT*-mutant tumours were larger, associated with advance stage, distant metastases, and higher disease-specific mortality [21]. The TCGA data identified *TERT* promotor mutation in 9.4% of PTC, with C228T (7.0%), C228A (0.3%), and C250T (2.1%) substitutions [7]. It was associated with older age, higher MACIS score, and high risk of recurrence. Liu et al. also demonstrated that when TERT promoter mutations coexisted with BRAF mutations, thyroid cancer tended to be larger, associated with extra-thyroidal extension, with more advanced stage [22]. The BRAF-RAS-MAPK pathway is upstream to ETS family of transcription factor. In the setting of *BRAF/RAS* mutation, ETS transcription factor is activated. *TERT* mutations create novel consensus binding motifs for transcription factors. ETS, including GABP, binds to the binding motif, increasing TERT transcription, leading to tumour advancement [25–27]. This supports the observation of more aggressive tumours when *BRAF/RAS* and *TERT* mutations are coexistent.

Gene fusions had been shown to be gene drivers in PTC [13]. In the TCGA that studied mainly nonirradiated PTC patients, *RET* fusion genes were most frequent (6.8%), followed by *BRAF* fusion genes (2.7%). *PAX8-PPARG* fusion genes, typically described in follicular thyroid carcinoma, were also seen in PTC, especially follicular variant (0.8% of TCGA) [7]. Fusions involving *ETV6-NTRK3* and *RBPMS-NTRK3* were detected in 1.2% of the sporadic PTC in TCGA, and *THADA* fusions were found in 1.2% of PTC [7]. *ALK* fusions, including *EML4-ALK* were detected in 0.8% of TCGA cohort, indicating potential for targeted therapy with ALK inhibitors. In contrast, in a study of radiation-induced thyroid cancers, 69% were due to gene rearrangement [28], including *RET-PTC*, *ETV6-NTRK3*, *TPR-NTRK1*, *AGK-BRAF*, *AKAP9-BRAF*, *PAX8-PPARG*, and *CREB3L2-PPARG* fusions. These activate mainly MAPK signalling and less frequently PPARG-driven transcriptional program.

The TCGA found somatic copy-number alterations in PTC—9.9% had isolated loss of heterozygosity (LOH) in 22q region that encompass *NF2* and *CHEK2* genes. This group was enriched with follicular variant PTC, suggesting that the loss of tumour suppressor genes *NF2* and/or *CHEK2* might contribute to its tumorigenesis. Notably, LOH of 22q was commonly seen in *RAS*-mutant PTC (45%, especially *HRAS*) [7]. Gain of 1q, seen in 14.8% of PTC in TCGA, was enriched for *BRAF* mutations, tall cell variant PTC, higher staging, risk profile, MACIS score suggestive of association with more aggressive PTC [7]. There had been other studies with similar findings of LOH of 22q (12%) and gain of 1q (16%) reported in PTC. Consistent with TCGA data, the gain of 1q was associated with more aggressive disease and distant metastases [29, 30].

Most PTC are driven via MAPK-signalling pathway by two of the predominant driver mutations, *BRAFV600E* and mutated *RAS*. However, both driver mutations lead to different MAPK signalling output, being higher in *BRAFV600E* mutants than *RAS* mutants. Consequently, expression of genes involved in iodine uptake and tumoural behaviour differ, with *BRAFV600E*-driven tumours having reduced sodium-iodide symporter expression and more aggressive tumorigenesis [31–33]. The TCGA study team proposed using a BRAFV600E-RAS score (BRS) to determine the gene expression pattern of PTC based on exome and transcriptome data (71-gene signature). A score of −1 was assigned for BRAFV600E-like PTC, and a score of +1 was assigned for RAS-like PTC, on a continuous scale [7]. The PTC tumours that were BRAFV600E-like included those with *BRAFV600E* mutations, *BRAF* fusions, and *RET* fusions; the PTC tumours who were RAS-like included those with *BRAFK601E* mutations, *EIF1AX* mutations, and *PAX8-PPARG* fusion [7]. This is consistent with other studies where *BRAFK601E* mutations had been reported in follicular variant PTC [34] and *PAX8-PPARG* had been described in follicular variant PTC [35]. Rivera et al. showed that infiltrative follicular variant PTC were more likely to harbour *BRAFV600E* mutations or *RET-PTC* fusions and had extra-thyroidal extension and nodal metastases, like classical PTC, whereas encapsulated follicular variant PTC usually were RAS mutants, and rarely metastasise to cervical lymph nodes, like follicular thyroid carcinoma [35]. The TCGA study also developed a thyroid differentiation score based on expression of 16 thyroid metabolism and function genes. The RAS-like PTC tumours constituted mainly of follicular variant PTC and had higher thyroid differentiation score, whereas the BRAFV600E-like PTC tumours were mainly classical and tall cell variant PTC and had a wide range of thyroid differentiation score [7]. This might reflect the wide range of clinical outcome observed in *BRAFV600E* mutant PTC, leading to its uncertain prognostic value [36]. The thyroid differentiation score correlated with histological grading, risk, and MACIS score [7]. Sabra et al. had shown that radioactive iodine-avid thyroid cancers predominantly had *RAS* mutations, and radioactive iodine-refractory thyroid cancers predominantly had *BRAF* mutations [37], supporting that *BRAFV600E* mutants might have dedifferentiated to some extent. This is consistent with other studies that had shown that *BRAFV600E*-driven PTC is associated with increased MAPK signalling and downregulation of iodine uptake [32, 38]. The TCGA study had also demonstrated that RAS-like PTC had concurrent MAPK and PI3K/AKT signalling, the former through c-RAF phosphorylation [7].

Follicular Thyroid Carcinoma and Other Follicular-Patterned Neoplasm

The mutation density in follicular thyroid carcinoma (FTC) was shown to be low, similar to PTC, with 0.3 non-synonymous mutation per Mb [39]. Follicular thyroid carcinoma is predominantly driven by *RAS* mutation (*HRAS*, *KRAS*, *NRAS*; 40–50%) and *PAX8/PPARG* gene fusion (36%) [40, 41]. The *RAS* genes encode *RAS* proteins that transduce signals from cell membrane intracellularly. Its inactive form is bound to guanosine diphosphate (GDP). When it is activated, it binds to guanosine triphosphate (GTP), activating the MAPK and PI3K/AKT signalling pathway. The activated RAS-GTP protein gets deactivated by its intrinsic GTPase activity and cytoplasmic GTPase-activating proteins. For *KRAS*, most of the mutations are located at codons 12 (81.9%) and 13 (14.4%), less at codon 61 (1.6%), whereas for *NRAS*, most of the mutations occur at colon 61 (60.9%), less at codons 12 (23.4%) and 13 (11.4%). *HRAS* can have mutations at codon 12 (36.7), codon 61 (34.9%), and codon 13 (20.6%). In *RAS*-mutant neoplasm, point mutation may occur in domains of *RAS* gene that result in an increased affinity for GTP (mutations in codons 12 and 13) or inactivation of autocatalytic GTPase activity (mutation in codon 61). Consequently, the RAS protein is switched on and activates signalling pathways constitutively [41, 42]. In a study assessing clinical features of *RAS*-driven versus *BRAF*-driven thyroid cancer, the *RAS*-mutant thyroid tumours constituted follicular thyroid carcinoma and follicular variant papillary thyroid carcinoma, whereas the *BRAF*-mutant thyroid carcinoma were all classical papillary thyroid carcinoma. The *RAS*-mutant thyroid tumours tended to have isoechoic or heterogeneous thyroid parenchyma, regular margins on ultrasound evaluation, and indeterminate cytology, whereas the *BRAF*-mutant thyroid tumours tended to have hypoechoic thyroid parenchyma, irregular or lobulated margins, cytology suspicious or positive for PTC, extra-thyroidal extension, lymphovascular invasion, and lymph node metastases on histology [43].

The *PAX8-PPARG* gene fusion was less commonly detected in Asian studies of FTC (0–4.0%) and follicular adenoma (0–7.9%) [39, 44, 45]. It constitutes translocation t(2;3)(q13;p25), where the t(2;3) rearrangement introduces an in-frame fusion of the *PAX8* gene with the *PPARG* gene [40, 46, 47]. The *PAX8* gene encodes for transcriptional factor important for genesis of thyroid follicular cell lineage, while PPARG ligands had been shown to inhibit growth and promote differentiation of thyroid cancer cell lines and in mouse models [47–49]. PPARG inhibition had been shown to increase nuclear factor-KB signalling, leading to activation of cyclin D1, and repression of genes involved in apoptosis [49]. It is also possible that the *PAX8-PPARG* gene fusion deregulates PAX8 pathways in thyroid cells and promotes thyroid carcinogenesis [47].

Of note, both *RAS* mutation (*HRAS*, *KRAS*, *NRAS*; 19.5–48%) and *PAX8-PPARG* gene fusion (4–13%) have also been found in thyroid follicular adenomas, limiting their utility in diagnosis of FTC in molecular tests in FNA [40, 46, 50–52]. A study assessing thyroid nodules with *RAS*-positive thyroid FNA aspirates showed that the eventual histology could be follicular adenoma, FTC, follicular variant PTC, and anaplastic thyroid carcinoma [52]. This could support the hypothesis that *RAS* is an early driver mutational event in the stepwise progression to carcinogenesis, as supported by thyroid cancer cell line studies [53].

Yoo et al. evaluated the whole exome and whole transcriptome in follicular adenoma, minimally invasive follicular thyroid carcinoma, and PTC [54] in a Korean cohort. In the follicular adenoma and minimally invasive follicular thyroid carcinoma group, mutations in *H/K/NRAS*, *DICER1*, *EIF1AX*, *IDH1*, *PTEN*, *SOS1*, and *SPOP* were detected, and *PAX8-PPARG* gene fusion was detected only in a single case of minimally invasive follicular thyroid carcinoma. The gene expression analysis segregated according to driver genes and was categorised to BRAF-like and RAS-like; both categories are analogous to categories described in the TCGA. However, here, a third category, non-BRAF-non-RAS (NBNR) was described to be associated with *DICER1*, *EIF1AX*, *IDH1*, *PTEN*, *SOS1*, *SPOP*, and *PAX8-PPARG* genetic alterations. The BRAF-like expression was associated with *BRAFV600E*, *BRAF* fusion genes, *RET* fusion genes, and *ETV6-NTRK3* fusion gene. The RAS-like expression was associated with *H/K/NRAS*, *STRN-ALK* fusion gene, and *ETV6-NTRK3* fusion gene. There was less lymph node metastases and extra-thyroidal extension observed in RAS-like and NBNR groups as compared with BRAF-like group. Both BRAF-like and RAS-like groups were associated with MAPK and p53 signalling pathways. Amongst the NBNR group, *DICER*-mutated tumours were enriched for Wnt signalling, and *EIF1AX*-mutated tumours had predominant mTOR signalling. Interestingly, in oncocytic follicular thyroid neoplasm, there is upregulation of *ESRRA* and *PPARGC1A* that are genes associated with mitochondrial biogenesis. These are enriched for pathways associated with TCA cycle and oxidative phosphorylation [54]. In another whole exome sequencing study of FTC and follicular adenoma from Korea, *BRAF*, *TCF12*, *CNOT1*, *STAG2*, *MAP 4K3*, and *IGF2BP3* mutations were detected only in FTC, but not follicular adenoma [39]. Using a next-generation sequencing approach testing for 372 cancer genes in a Polish study of FTC and follicular thyroid carcinoma, new somatic mutations were detected in oncogenes (*MDM2*, *FLI1*, in addition to *KRAS* and *NRAS*), transcriptional factors and repressors (*MITF*, *ZNF331* in addition to *PPARG*), epigenetic enzymes (*KMT2A*, *NSD1*, *NCOA1*, *NCOA2*), and protein kinases (*JAK3*, *CHEK2*, *ALK*) [55]. These remain to be further validated in future studies.

Hurthle Cell Carcinoma

The Hurthle cell carcinoma consists of large cells with abundant granular cytoplasm rich with mitochondria and hyperchromatic nucleus [56]. Similar to FTC, Hurthle cell carcinoma is differentiated from Hurtle cell adenoma via the demonstration of capsular or vascular invasion. The extent of capsular and vascular invasion determines if Hurthle cell carcinoma is minimally or widely invasive. It had been suggested that the abundant mitochondria seen in Hurthle cells could be related to defects in mitochondrial DNA with consequent mitochondrial dysfunction and compensatory proliferation [57]. Maximo et al. detected mitochondrial common deletion in 100% of Hurthle cell adenoma, 100% in Hurthle cell follicular carcinoma, 100% in Hurthle cell papillary carcinoma, compared to 33.3% in adenoma, 18.8% in PTC, and none in FTC [57]. Mitochondrial common deletion (or mtDNA 4977 bp) deletes between nucleotides 8470 and 13,447 of the human mitochondrial DNA. This genetic alteration removes all or part of the genes encoding four complex I subunits, one complex IV subunit, two complex V subunits, and five tRNA genes that are vital for normal mitochondrial function [58]. In another study using targeted sequencing of common thyroid oncogenes and oncogenic fusions, only 11% (3/27) of Hurthle cell tumours (one minimally invasive carcinoma, two widely invasive carcinomas) had *NRAS* mutation [59]. None of the tumours had *BRAF*, *PI3KCA*, *PTEN*, *RET-PTC* fusion, or *PAX8-PPARG* fusion. The *EIF1AX* mutation was also reported in a patient with Hurtle cell carcinoma who also had *TP53* mutation [60].

Transcriptomes (analysed by microarray) of Hurthle cell adenoma, minimally invasive, and widely invasive Hurthle cell carcinoma showed differential expression on unsupervised hierarchical clustering into three groups. The gene expression set that was enriched involved beta-catenin (*CTNNB1*)-driven signature on concept module mapping using Oncomine analysis. On the Ingenuity Pathway Analysis, beta-catenin was closely involved in regulating vascular invasion. The temsirolimus-sensitive signature was also enriched on Oncomine analysis, implying potential therapeutic application of mTOR inhibitor [59]. The principal component analysis and hierarchical clustering of transcriptome of PTC and FTC varied from that of widely invasive

Hurthle cell carcinoma that had strong PI3K/Akt and Wnt/beta-catenin signatures [59]. However, in an immunohistochemistry study evaluating phosphorylated mTOR staining, Hurthle cell carcinoma and adenoma had less staining compared to follicular adenoma and FTC [61]. The genetic constitution and expression of Hurtle call neoplasm remains to be better elucidated.

Poorly Differentiated Thyroid Carcinoma and Anaplastic Thyroid Carcinoma

Poorly differentiated thyroid carcinoma (PDTC) and anaplastic thyroid carcinoma (ATC) are rare with frequency of up to 7% and 2%, respectively [5, 6]. However, patients with these carcinomas have poor 5-year survival rate of 50–60% and 1–17%, respectively [62–65]. There are two pathologic criteria for the diagnosis of PDTC. The Turin criteria needs the presence of insular, solid, or trabecular growth pattern, absence of nuclear features of PTC, and at least one of the following features: convoluted nuclei, mitotic index ≥3/10 high-power field (HPF), and tumour necrosis [65]. Whereas the Memorial Sloan Kettering Cancer Center (MSKCC) criteria requires only mitotic index ≥5/10 HPF, and/or tumour necrosis, regardless of tumour growth patterns and nuclear features [64]. The overall survival in PDTC correlated with high mitotic index and presence of tumour necrosis rather than tumour growth patterns and nuclear features [64]. The mutation burden in ATC and PDTC are high compared to PTC, with median number of mutation in ATC being 6, 2, and 1 per tumour, respectively [66]. In PDTC, the tumour mutation burden is correlated with older age, tumour size more than 4 cm, presence of distant metastases, and shorter survival [20]. Like in PTC, *BRAFV600E* and *RAS* mutations were mutually exclusive driver mutations, with *BRAFV600E* being detected in 5–33% of PDTC, 8–91% of ATC (highest rate in Korean study), and *RAS* mutation being found in 18–44% of PDTC and 9–31% of ATC [27, 66–72]. Amongst PDTC, 92% of *RAS* mutation was detected in PDTC fulfilling the Turin criteria, and 81% of *BRAFV600E* mutation was found in PDTC fulfilling the MSKCC criteria [66, 73]. *RAS*-mutant PDTC was noted to be larger and had a higher tendency for distant metastases; *BRAFV600E*-mutant PDTC was noted to be smaller and associated with nodal metastases and extra-thyroidal extension instead [66, 72]. *RET-PTC* rearrangement was found in 17% of PDTC but none in ATC. The *RET*-positive PDTC were associated with extra-thyroidal extension [72].

The *TERT* promoter mutation is more frequently detected in PDTC (38–52%) and ATC (43–73%), as compared to PTC (9–23%) and FTC (11%) [7, 20, 66, 74]. PDTC with *TERT* mutation was associated with distant metastases, and ATC with *TERT* mutation had shorter survival especially in the presence of coexistent *BRAF* or *RAS* mutation [66]. *EIF1AX* mutation had been reported to be more frequent in PDTC (11%) and ATC (9–14%) as compared to PTC (1.5% in TCGA study) [7, 66]. Most (93.3%) of the *EIF1AX* mutant PDTC and ATC coexist with *RAS* mutations [66, 67]. PDTC with *EIF1AX* mutation were noted to be larger and have poorer survival [66]. Tumour suppressor genes played a significant role in tumorigenesis of PDTC and ATC. Inactivating mutation of *TP53* tumour suppressor gene is more frequently found in ATC (27–80%) than in PDTC (8–67%) [66–71, 75, 76]. *ATM* is a cell cycle checkpoint and DNA damage response gene [77], and its mutation had been noted in 7% of PDTC and 9–40% of ATC [66, 68]. *ATM*-mutant tumours were noted to have higher mutation burden; this is likely related to the loss of DNA repair function in the setting of *ATM* mutation [66]. Loss of function *NF2* mutation had been reported in up to 27% of ATC and 22% of PDTC [66, 67, 70, 78]. *NF2* encodes for merlin protein that links transmembrane receptors and intracellular effectors to regulate signalling pathways that control cell proliferation and survival, such as receptor tyrosine kinase, mTOR, PI3K/Akt, Hippo pathways, small GTPase, and cell adhesion [79]. Loss of heterozygosity (LOH) in the chromosome 22q region encompassing *NF2* is often observed in *NF2* mutant neoplasm. Chromosomal 22q LOH was associated with 50% of *RAS*-mutant PDTC (similar to PTC), but none in *BRAFV600E*-mutant PDTC. Hippo is a kinase cascade that inhibits tissue overgrowth via phosphorylation of YAP, reducing its ability to promote transcriptional enhancer activation domain (TEAD)-dependent gene transcription for proliferation and survival. In mouse models, *NF2* deletion or *HRAS* mutation in isolation did not lead to tumorigenesis; however, when present in combination, increased MAPK signalling is induced with formation of PDTC. *NF2* deletion with consequent merlin loss led to increased *RAS* signalling through Hippo inhibition that activates YAP-TEAD transcriptional program. The presence of *NF2* loss in *RAS*-mutant tumours increases dependency on MAPK pathway. In treatment with MEK inhibitors in murine models with *RAS*-mutant, *NF2* loss tumours led to reduction in tumour volume. In *NF2*-null cell lines, inhibition of YAP-TEAD with verteporfin reduces *RAS* transcription and signalling and inhibited cell growth. These represent potential therapeutic options in *RAS*-mutant tumours with *NF2* loss [78]. Tumour suppressor gene *NF1* (neurofibromin 1) is detected in 9–40% of ATC, as opposed to none in PDTC and 0.5% in PTC from the TCGA data [7, 68, 71, 78]. Majority of *NF1* mutant ATC tended to coexist with other mutations [68, 71]. *NF1* has been shown to cause neurofibromatosis type 1. However, ATC is not a typical malignancy observed in this condition. This suggests that *NF1* is unlikely to be the main driver mutation in ATC. It is likely that additional loss of *NF1* tumour suppressor gene can lead to progression of thyroid cancer to ATC [71]. In both PDTC and ATC, inactivating mutations were also infrequently observed in other tumour suppressor genes, including *RB1* and *MEN1* [27, 66, 68]. Mutation in anaplastic lymphoma kinase (*ALK*) gene was observed in 20% of ATC mostly in association with *TP53* and *NF1* [71]. The striatin (*STRN*) gene and *ALK* gene fusion (*STRN-ALK*) had been described in 1.3% of PTC, 9% of PDTC, and 4% of ATC. *STRN-ALK* gene had been shown to stimulate MAPK activation and induce tumour formation in mouse models [80]. In ATC thyroid cancer cell lines, *ALK* mutation increased signalling of the PI3K/AKT and MAPK pathways [81]. ALK inhibitor, crizotinib, had led to inhibition of *STRN-ALK* expressing thyroid cancer cell line growth [80] and clinical response in ATC patient with *STRN-ALK* gene fusion [82].

Mutations of *PIK3CA*, *PTEN*, *PIK3C2G*, *PIK3CG*, *PIK3C3*, *PIK3R1*, *PIK3R2*, *AKT3*, *TSC1*, *TSC2*, and *mTOR* of the PIK3CA-AKT-mTOR pathway is present at higher frequency in PDTC (11–20%) and ATC (4–39%), compared to PTC (1.4%) [7, 66, 67, 69, 70]. Similarly, mutations in the SWI/SNF nucleosome remodelling complex (such as *ARID1A*, *ARID1B*, *ARID2*, *ARID5B*, *SMARCB1*, *PBRM1*, and *ATRX*) were more frequent in ATC (5–36%) compared to PDTC (6%) [66, 67]. This is consistent with reports of mutations of subunits of the SWI/SNF chromatin remodelling complex being associated with carcinogenesis [83]. Mutations of the histone methyltransferases (such as *KMT2A*, *KMT2C*, *KMT2D*, and *SETD2*) were seen in 5–24% of ATC and 7% of PDTC [66, 67, 70]. The presence of *KMT2D* mutation was associated with poorer survival in ATC [70]. These mutations in epigenetic factors were less frequently reported in PTC from TCGA (1–2%, *ARID1B*, *KMT2A*, *KMT2C*) [7]. DNA mismatch repair gene (such as *MSH2*, *MSH6*, and *MLH1*) mutations were observed in 12–20% of ATC and 2% of PDTC. ATC and PDTC associated with these mutations were associated with higher mutational burden, likely related to the dysfunction of DNA repair [66–68]. Wnt signalling pathway (including *CTNNB1* [beta-catenin], *APC*, and *AXIN1*) had been reported to be more frequent in aggressive thyroid cancer (ATC more than PDTC). Beta-catenin is important for E-cadherin-mediated cell adhesion and signal transduction in the Wnt pathway. It is usually on the cell membrane, and the free cytoplasmic beta-catenin level is low due to its rapid ubiquitin-proteasome degradation. When Wnt binds to cell surface receptors, it antagonises beta-catenin degradation, so that beta-catenin localises to the nucleus to stimulate target gene expression of *cyclin D1* and *c-myc*. The process of degradation of beta-catenin is facilitated by a multi-protein destruction complex including adenomatous polyposis coli (APC) protein and axin [84]. In earlier studies using single-strand conformational polymorphism (PCR-SSCP) technique, the presence of activating beta-catenin gene (*CTNNB1*) mutation, which stabilises beta-catenin, was found in 25% of PDTC and 61–66% of ATC, and aberrant nuclear beta-catenin immunochemical staining was observed in 21% of PDTC and 43% of ATC, but not in follicular adenoma, PTC, or FTC [85, 86]. These indicated Wnt activation in these PDTC and ATC, and that *CTNNB1* was a late event in cancer progression since it was not observed in well-differentiated thyroid cancer. The presence of aberrant nuclear beta-catenin localisation correlated with lymph node metastases and poor survival. *CTNNB1* mutation also correlated with poor survival [85]. In a subsequent Japanese ATC study, beta-catenin immunochemical staining was positive in the nucleus in 41% of ATC and positive in the cytoplasm in 67% (five cases had both cytoplasmic and nuclear staining). The mutational analysis by direct PCR sequencing of *CTNNB1* gene showed mutation in only 4.5% of ATC, *APC* gene mutation in 9%, and *AXIN* gene mutation in 82% of ATC [87]. The difference in rates of *CTNNB1* mutation might be due to different sequencing techniques. In recent whole exome sequencing or targeted sequencing studies, *CTNNB1* (5% in PDTC and 0–4.5% in ATC), *APC*, and *AXIN1* (8% in PDTC and 6% in ATC) mutations had been rare [66, 67, 69]. Mutations in cyclin-dependent kinase (*CDK1*) family (including *CDKN2A*, *CDKN2B*, *CDKN2C*, *CDKN1A*, *CDKN1B*) were detected in 20% in PDTC and 9–14% of ATC [67, 69]. In ATC and PDTC, downregulation of *CDH1* gene (E-cadherin) and gain of mesenchymal markers (such as fibronectin and WNT5A) were shown, indicating activation of epithelial-to-mesenchymal transition (EMT), where epithelial cells lost contact and developed cytoskeleton remodelling [68, 69]. Gene expression of TGF-β signalling components (*TGFB1*, *LTBP1*, *TGFBR1*) had been shown to be upregulated, likely related to its promotion of EMT [69]. The overexpression of *SNA12* gene had also been described in ATC [69]. *SNA12* gene encoded for zinc-finger transcription factor that repressed expression of E-cadherin, and it is activated by TGF-β [88].

Medullary Thyroid Carcinoma (Sporadic)

Medullary thyroid carcinoma (MTC) arises from the calcitonin-producing parafollicular C cell of thyroid gland and is sporadic in up to 75% of cases. The main gene driver in sporadic and hereditary MTC had been the *RET* proto-oncogene, occurring in 12–100% of sporadic MTC depending on series [89, 90]. The *RET* gene encoded for a receptor tyrosine kinase and its activating mutation increased *RET* kinase activity, leading to activation of intracellular signalling and tumour growth. Hereditary form of MTC displayed close genotype-phenotype correlation—MEN2A was mainly related to mutations in exons 10 or 11, while MEN2B (more aggressive) was mainly related to p.Met918Thr mutation in exon 16 [91]. The p.Met918Thr *RET* mutation had been the commonest form of mutation in sporadic MTC; however, its detection rate was highly variable 5–66% [92]. In a study of sporadic MTC, where patients were categorised by risk levels [group 1 with mutations in *RET* exons 15 and 16 (that includes somatic p.Met918Thr and p.Ala883Phe RET mutation cases—these represent level D mutations in American Thyroid Association guidelines, with highest risk of early development and growth of MTC [91]), group 2 with other *RET* mutations, and group 3 having no *RET* mutations], group 1 had higher prevalence, more lymph node metastases, more multi-focal tumours, stage IV disease, and more persistent disease [92]. Patients with other *RET* mutations had the most indolent course, whereas those with no *RET* mutation (regardless of *RAS* mutational status) were at intermediate risk [89]. *NF-kB* that is transcription factor involved in cell growth, differentiation, and apoptosis was detected on immunohistochemical staining more frequently in sporadic or germline MTC with *RET* mutation [93], indicating that *RET* mutation had likely led to *NF-kB* overexpression.

Increasingly, in *RET* wild-type MTC, *RAS* mutation had been reported to be the gene driver, with prevalence of *HRAS* ranging from 0 to 41.2%, that of *KRAS* ranging from 0 to 40.9% and that of *NRAS* from 0 to 1.8% as summarised by a review by Moura et al. [89, 94]. According to the COSMIC (catalogue of somatic mutations in cancer) database, in *RAS*-mutant MTC, *HRAS* occurred at the highest frequency (9.3%), followed by *KRAS* (3.0%), and rarely *NRAS* (0.6%). This was contrary to the distribution observed in carcinoma, arising from thyroid follicular cells, where *NRAS* occurred more frequently (4.2% in PTC, 15.7% in FTC, 15.4% in ATC), followed by *KRAS* (1.2% in PTC, 3.9% in FTC, 8.1% in ATC), and *HRAS* (1.8% in PTC, 6.3% in FTC, 4.6% in ATC). In a MTC study including 56 sporadic cases and 8 familial cases, there was significant nuclear *PDCD4* downregulation. Programmed cell death 4 (*PDCD4*) was a tumour suppressor gene involved in apoptosis, consistently downregulated in cancers. Of this cohort, 36% (20/56) had somatic *RET* mutations. Six *RAS*-mutant (11% of sporadic MTC) MTC cases had higher nuclear *PDCD4* expression than *RET*-positive or *RET/RAS* wild-type cases, as well as increased phospho-AKT on western blot analysis, indicating activation of PI3K-AKT-mTOR pathway [95]. It had been hypothesised that in *RAS*-mutant sporadic MTC, *AKT* caused phosphorylation of *PDCD4*, inhibiting its tumour suppressor effect [96]. Agrawal et al. performed whole exome sequencing of 17 sporadic MTC and then validated the frequency of recurrently mutated genes and genes of interest in a separate cohort of 19 sporadic MTC and 21 hereditary MTC [90]. In the discovery set, 71% of sporadic MTC had *RET* mutation. In the combined *RET*- and *RAS*-negative sporadic MTC, 8% had *MDC1* mutation (two cases in the discovery set and one case in the validation set) [90]. *MDC1* (mediator of DNA damage checkpoint protein 1) is part of the DNA damage response [97]. Inactivating mutation of *MDC1* could lead to dysfunction of homologous recombination and non-homologous end point repair pathways [97].

Summary

The genetic landscape of thyroid cancer has been better understood with the availability of newer genetic testing techniques (Fig. 5.1). This unravelled data could be utilised in the molecular

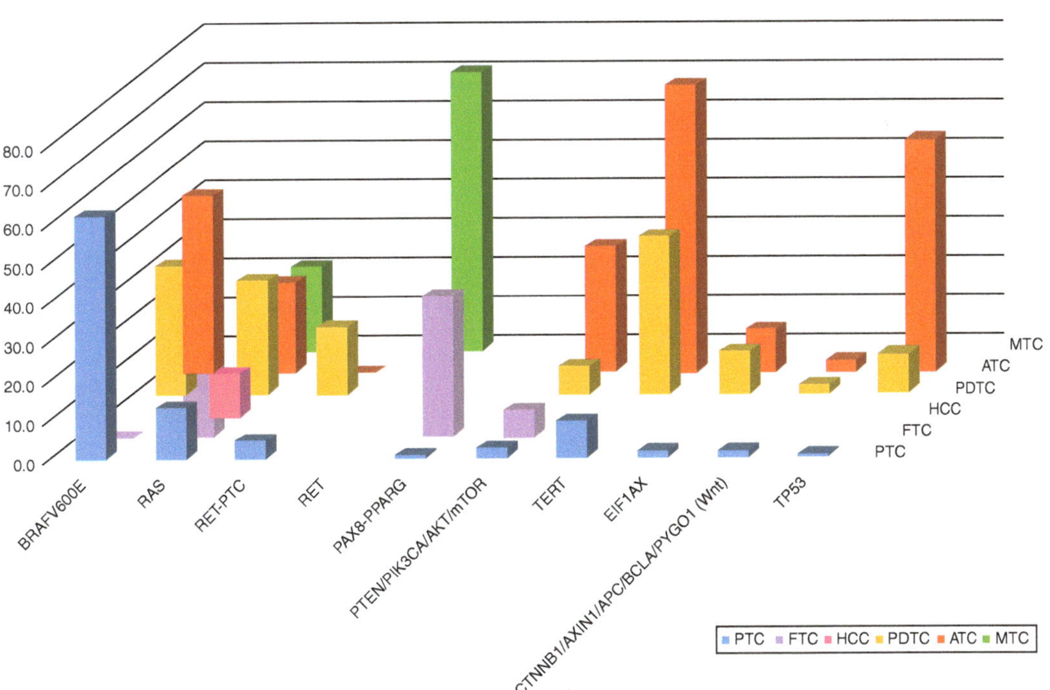

Fig. 5.1 Genetic landscape of thyroid cancer. *PTC* papillary thyroid carcinoma, *FTC* follicular thyroid carcinoma, *HCC* Hurthle cell carcinoma, *PDTC* poorly differentiated thyroid carcinoma, *ATC* anaplastic thyroid carcinoma, *MTC* medullary thyroid carcinoma. Prevalence data from references 7, 27, 40, 54, 59, 72, 89, 90

characterisation of thyroid nodules with indeterminate cytology for better prediction of thyroid malignancy. It could be also utilised to guided personalised genotype-directed systemic therapy in radioiodine-refractory advanced thyroid cancer.

References

1. Davies L, Welch H. Increasing incidence of thyroid cancer in the United States, 1973–2002. JAMA. 2006;295(18):2164–7.
2. Davies L, Welch H. Current thyroid cancer trends in the United States. JAMA Otolaryngol Head Neck Surg. 2014;140(4):317–22.
3. Jung CK, et al. The increase in thyroid cancer incidence during the last four decades is accompanied by a high frequency of BRAF mutations and a sharp increase in RAS mutations. J Clin Endocrinol Metab. 2014;99(2):E276–85.
4. National Registry of Diseases Office (NRDO). Singapore Cancer Registry Interim Annual Report. Trends in Cancer Incidence in Singapore 2010–2014. 2015
5. World Health Organization (WHO) Classification. PathologyOutlines.com website. http://www.pathologyoutlines.com/topic/thyroidwho.html. Accessed 10 Sept 2017.
6. Kondo T, Ezzat S, Asa SL. Pathogenetic mechanisms in thyroid follicular-cell neoplasia. Nat Rev Cancer. 2006;6(4):292–306.
7. Network CGAR. Integrated genomic characterization of papillary thyroid carcinoma. Cell. 2014;159(3):676–90.
8. Vaisman F, et al. Spontaneous remission in thyroid cancer patients after biochemical incomplete response to initial therapy. Clin Endocrinol. 2012;77(1):132–8.
9. Tuttle RM, et al. Estimating risk of recurrence in differentiated thyroid cancer after total thyroidectomy and radioactive iodine remnant ablation: using response to therapy variables to modify the initial risk estimates predicted by the new American Thyroid Association staging system. Thyroid. 2010;20(12):1341–9.
10. Martin S, et al. Long-term results of treatment of 283 patients with lung and bone metastases from differentiated thyroid carcinoma. J Clin Endocrinol Metabol. 1986;63(4):960–7.
11. Durante C, et al. Long-term outcome of 444 patients with distant metastases from papillary and follicular thyroid carcinoma: benefits and limits of radioiodine therapy. J Clin Endocrinol Metabol. 2006;91(8):2892–9.
12. Bischoff L, et al. Is above age 45 appropriate for upstaging well-differentiated papillary thyroid cancer? Endocr Pract. 2013;19(6):995–7.
13. Kimura ET, et al. High prevalence of BRAF mutations in thyroid cancer: genetic evidence for constitutive activation of the RET/PTC-RAS-BRAF signaling pathway in papillary thyroid carcinoma. Cancer Res. 2003;63(7):1454–7.
14. Cohen Y, et al. BRAF mutation in papillary thyroid carcinoma. J Natl Cancer Inst. 2003;95(8):625–7.
15. Chai L, Li J, Lv Z. An integrated analysis of cancer genes in thyroid cancer. Oncol Rep. 2016;35(2):962–70.
16. Yu C, et al. Molecular network including eIF1AX, RPS7, and 14-3-3γ regulates protein translation and cell proliferation in bovine mammary epithelial cells. Arch Biochem Biophys. 2014;564:142–55.
17. Karunamurthy A, et al. Prevalence and phenotypic correlations of EIF1AX mutations in thyroid nodules. Endocr Relat Cancer. 2016;23(4):295–301.
18. Oliva-Trastoy M, et al. The Wip1 phosphatase (PPM1D) antagonizes activation of the Chk2 tumour suppressor kinase. Oncogene. 2007;26(10):1449–58.
19. Zhang L, et al. Exome sequencing identifies somatic gain-of-function PPM1D mutations in brainstem gliomas. Nat Genet. 2014;46(7):726–30.
20. Landa I, et al. Frequent somatic TERT promoter mutations in thyroid cancer: higher prevalence in advanced forms of the disease. J Clin Endocrinol Metabol. 2013;98(9):E1562–6.
21. Melo M, et al. TERT promoter mutations are a major indicator of poor outcome in differentiated thyroid carcinomas. J Clin Endocrinol Metabol. 2014;99(5):E754–65.
22. Liu X, et al. TERT promoter mutations and their association with BRAF V600E mutation and aggressive clinicopathological characteristics of thyroid cancer. J Clin Endocrinol Metabol. 2014;99(6):E1130–6.
23. Fu D, Collins K. Purification of human telomerase complexes identifies factors involved in telomerase biogenesis and telomere length regulation. Mol Cell. 2007;28(5):773–85.
24. De Lange T. Telomere-related genome instability in cancer. Cold Spring Harb Symp Quant Biol. 2005;70:197–204.
25. Akincilar SC, Unal B, Tergaonkar V. Reactivation of telomerase in cancer. Cell Mol Life Sci. 2016;73(8):1659–70.
26. Bell RJ, et al. The transcription factor GABP selectively binds and activates the mutant TERT promoter in cancer. Science. 2015;348(6238):1036–9.
27. Xu B, Ghossein R. Genomic landscape of poorly differentiated and anaplastic thyroid carcinoma. Endocr Pathol. 2016;27(3):205–12.
28. Ricarte-Filho JC, et al. Identification of kinase fusion oncogenes in post-Chernobyl radiation-induced thyroid cancers. J Clin Invest. 2013;123(11):4935.
29. Kjellman P, et al. Gain of 1q and loss of 9q21. 3-q32 are associated with a less favorable prognosis in papillary thyroid carcinoma. Genes Chromosomes Cancer. 2001;32(1):43–9.
30. Wreesmann VB, et al. Genome-wide profiling of papillary thyroid cancer identifies MUC1 as an independent prognostic marker. Cancer Res. 2004;64(11):3780–9.

31. Durante C, et al. BRAF mutations in papillary thyroid carcinomas inhibit genes involved in iodine metabolism. J Clin Endocrinol Metabol. 2007;92(7):2840–3.
32. Franco AT, et al. Thyrotrophin receptor signaling dependence of Braf-induced thyroid tumor initiation in mice. Proc Natl Acad Sci. 2011;108(4):1615–20.
33. Charles R-P, et al. Mutationally activated BRAF^{V600E} elicits papillary thyroid cancer in the adult mouse. Cancer Res. 2011;71(11):3863–71.
34. Park JY, et al. BRAF and RAS mutations in follicular variants of papillary thyroid carcinoma. Endocr Pathol. 2013;24(2):69–76.
35. Rivera M, et al. Molecular genotyping of papillary thyroid carcinoma follicular variant according to its histological subtypes (encapsulated vs infiltrative) reveals distinct BRAF and RAS mutation patterns. Mod Pathol. 2010;23(9):1191–200.
36. Xing M, et al. Association between BRAF v600e mutation and mortality in patients with papillary thyroid cancer. JAMA. 2013;309(14):1493–501.
37. Sabra M, et al. Clinical outcomes and molecular profile of differentiated thyroid cancers with radioiodine-avid distant metastases. J Clin Endocrinol Metabol. 2013;98(5):E829–36.
38. Chakravarty D, et al. Small-molecule MAPK inhibitors restore radioiodine incorporation in mouse thyroid cancers with conditional BRAF activation. J Clin Invest. 2011;121(12):4700.
39. Jung S-H, et al. Mutational burdens and evolutionary ages of thyroid follicular adenoma are comparable to those of follicular carcinoma. Oncotarget. 2016;7(43):69638.
40. Nikiforova MN, et al. RAS point mutations and PAX8-PPARγ rearrangement in thyroid tumors: evidence for distinct molecular pathways in thyroid follicular carcinoma. J Clin Endocrinol Metabol. 2003;88(5):2318–26.
41. Nikiforov YE. Thyroid carcinoma: molecular pathways and therapeutic targets. Mod Pathol. 2008;21(Suppl 2):S37–43.
42. Campbell SL, et al. Increasing complexity of Ras signaling. Oncogene. 1998;17(11):1395–413.
43. Kakarmath S, et al. Clinical, sonographic, and pathological characteristics of RAS-positive versus BRAF-positive thyroid carcinoma. J Clin Endocrinol Metabol. 2016;101(12):4938–44.
44. Jeong SH, et al. Analysis of RAS mutation and PAX8/PPARγ rearrangements in follicular-derived thyroid neoplasms in a Korean population: frequency and ultrasound findings. J Endocrinol Investig. 2015;38(8):849–57.
45. Mochizuki K, et al. Low frequency of PAX8-PPARγ rearrangement in follicular thyroid carcinomas in Japanese patients. Pathol Int. 2015;65(5):250–3.
46. Nikiforova MN, et al. PAX8-PPARγ rearrangement in thyroid tumors: RT-PCR and immunohistochemical analyses. Am J Surg Pathol. 2002;26(8):1016–23.
47. Kroll TG, et al. PAX8-PPARgamma 1 fusion oncogene in human thyroid carcinoma. Science. 2000;289(5483):1357–60.
48. Park J-W, et al. Troglitazone, the peroxisome proliferator-activated receptor-γ agonist, induces antiproliferation and redifferentiation in human thyroid cancer cell lines. Thyroid. 2005;15(3):222–31.
49. Kato Y, et al. PPAR[gamma] insufficiency promotes follicular thyroid carcinogenesis via activation of the nuclear factor-[kappa]B signaling pathway. Oncogene. 2005;25(19):2736–47.
50. Marques AR, et al. Expression of PAX8-PPARγ1 rearrangements in both follicular thyroid carcinomas and adenomas. J Clin Endocrinol Metabol. 2002;87(8):3947–52.
51. Vasko V, et al. Specific pattern of RAS oncogene mutations in follicular thyroid tumors. J Clin Endocrinol Metab. 2003;88(6):2745–52.
52. Gupta N, et al. RAS mutations in thyroid FNA specimens are highly predictive of predominantly low-risk follicular-pattern cancers. J Clin Endocrinol Metabol. 2013;98(5):E914–22.
53. Burns JS, et al. Stepwise transformation of primary thyroid epithelial cells by a mutant Ha-ras oncogene: an in vitro model of tumor progression. Mol Carcinog. 1992;6(2):129–39.
54. Yoo S-K, et al. Comprehensive analysis of the transcriptional and mutational landscape of follicular and papillary thyroid cancers. PLoS Genet. 2016;12(8):e1006239.
55. Swierniak M, et al. Somatic mutation profiling of follicular thyroid cancer by next generation sequencing. Mol Cell Endocrinol. 2016;433:130–7.
56. Montone KT, Baloch ZW, LiVolsi VA. The thyroid Hürthle (oncocytic) cell and its associated pathologic conditions: a surgical pathology and cytopathology review. Arch Pathol Lab Med. 2008;132(8):1241–50.
57. Máximo V, et al. Mitochondrial DNA somatic mutations (point mutations and large deletions) and mitochondrial DNA variants in human thyroid pathology: a study with emphasis on Hürthle cell tumors. Am J Pathol. 2002;160(5):1857–65.
58. Peng T-I, et al. Visualizing common deletion of mitochondrial DNA-augmented mitochondrial reactive oxygen species generation and apoptosis upon oxidative stress. Biochim Biophys Acta. 2006;1762(2):241–55.
59. Ganly I, et al. Genomic dissection of Hurthle cell carcinoma reveals a unique class of thyroid malignancy. J Clin Endocrinol Metabol. 2013;98(5):E962–72.
60. Topf MC, et al. EIF1AX mutation in a patient with Hürthle cell carcinoma. Endocr Pathol. 2018;29:27–9.
61. Covach A, et al. Phosphorylated mechanistic target of rapamycin (p-mTOR) and noncoding RNA expression in follicular and Hurthle cell thyroid neoplasm. Endocr Pathol. 2017;28:207–12.
62. Kebebew E, et al. Anaplastic thyroid carcinoma. Cancer. 2005;103(7):1330–5.
63. Carcangiu ML, Zamp G, Rosai J. Poorly differentiated ("insular") thyroid carcinoma: a reinterpretation of Langhans' "wuchernde Struma". Am J Surg Pathol. 1984;8(9):655–68.

64. Hiltzik D, et al. Poorly differentiated thyroid carcinomas defined on the basis of mitosis and necrosis. Cancer. 2006;106(6):1286–95.
65. Volante M, et al. Poorly differentiated thyroid carcinoma: the Turin proposal for the use of uniform diagnostic criteria and an algorithmic diagnostic approach. Am J Surg Pathol. 2007;31(8):1256–64.
66. Landa I, et al. Genomic and transcriptomic hallmarks of poorly differentiated and anaplastic thyroid cancers. J Clin Invest. 2016;126(3):1052–66.
67. Kunstman JW, et al. Characterization of the mutational landscape of anaplastic thyroid cancer via whole-exome sequencing. Hum Mol Genet. 2015;24(8):2318–29.
68. Sykorova V, et al. Search for new genetic biomarkers in poorly differentiated and anaplastic thyroid carcinomas using next generation sequencing. Anticancer Res. 2015;35(4):2029–36.
69. Pita JM, et al. Cell cycle deregulation and TP53 and RAS mutations are major events in poorly differentiated and undifferentiated thyroid carcinomas. J Clin Endocrinol Metabol. 2014;99(3):E497–507.
70. Jeon MJ, et al. Genomic alterations of anaplastic thyroid carcinoma detected by targeted massive parallel sequencing in a BRAFV600E mutation-prevalent area. Thyroid. 2016;26(5):683–90.
71. Latteyer S, et al. Targeted next-generation sequencing for TP53, RAS, BRAF, ALK and NF1 mutations in anaplastic thyroid cancer. Endocrine. 2016;54(3):733–41.
72. Ricarte-Filho JC, et al. Mutational profile of advanced primary and metastatic radioactive iodine-refractory thyroid cancers reveals distinct pathogenetic roles for BRAF, PIK3CA, and AKT1. Cancer Res. 2009;69(11):4885–93.
73. Volante M, et al. RAS mutations are the predominant molecular alteration in poorly differentiated thyroid carcinomas and bear prognostic impact. J Clin Endocrinol Metabol. 2009;94(12):4735–41.
74. Liu X, et al. Highly prevalent TERT promoter mutations in aggressive thyroid cancers. Endocr Relat Cancer. 2013;20(4):603–10.
75. Fagin JA, et al. High prevalence of mutations of the p53 gene in poorly differentiated human thyroid carcinomas. J Clin Investig. 1993;91(1):179–84.
76. Ito T, et al. Unique association of p53 mutations with undifferentiated but not with differentiated carcinomas of the thyroid gland. Cancer Res. 1992;52(5):1369–71.
77. Cremona CA, Behrens A. ATM signalling and cancer. Oncogene. 2014;33(26):3351–60.
78. Garcia-Rendueles ME, et al. NF2 loss promotes oncogenic RAS-induced thyroid cancers via YAP-dependent transactivation of RAS proteins and sensitizes them to MEK inhibition. Cancer Discov. 2015;5(11):1178–93.
79. Petrilli AM, Fernández-Valle C. Role of Merlin/NF2 inactivation in tumor biology. Oncogene. 2016;35(5):537–48.
80. Kelly LM, et al. Identification of the transforming STRN-ALK fusion as a potential therapeutic target in the aggressive forms of thyroid cancer. Proc Natl Acad Sci U S A. 2014;111(11):4233–8.
81. Murugan AK, Xing M. Anaplastic thyroid cancers harbor novel oncogenic mutations of the ALK gene. Cancer Res. 2011;71(13):4403–11.
82. Godbert Y, et al. Remarkable response to crizotinib in woman with anaplastic lymphoma kinase–rearranged anaplastic thyroid carcinoma. J Clin Oncol. 2014;33(20):e84–7.
83. Helming KC, Wang X, Roberts CW. Vulnerabilities of mutant SWI/SNF complexes in cancer. Cancer Cell. 2014;26(3):309–17.
84. Miller JR, et al. Mechanism and function of signal transduction by the Wnt/beta-catenin and Wnt/Ca2+ pathways. Oncogene. 1999;18(55):7860–72.
85. Garcia-Rostan G, et al. β-catenin dysregulation in thyroid neoplasms: down-regulation, aberrant nuclear expression, and CTNNB1 exon 3 mutations are markers for aggressive tumor phenotypes and poor prognosis. Am J Pathol. 2001;158(3):987–96.
86. Garcia-Rostan G, et al. Frequent mutation and nuclear localization of β-catenin in anaplastic thyroid carcinoma. Cancer Res. 1999;59(8):1811–5.
87. Kurihara T, et al. Immunohistochemical and sequencing analyses of the Wnt signaling components in Japanese anaplastic thyroid cancers. Thyroid. 2004;14(12):1020–9.
88. Peinado H, Olmeda D, Cano A. Snail, Zeb and bHLH factors in tumour progression: an alliance against the epithelial phenotype? Nat Rev Cancer. 2007;7(6):415.
89. Moura MM, Cavaco BM, Leite V. RAS proto-oncogene in medullary thyroid carcinoma. Endocr Relat Cancer. 2015;22(5):R235–52.
90. Agrawal N, et al. Exomic sequencing of medullary thyroid cancer reveals dominant and mutually exclusive oncogenic mutations in RET and RAS. J Clin Endocrinol Metabol. 2012;98(2):E364–9.
91. Kloos RT, et al. Medullary thyroid cancer: management guidelines of the American Thyroid Association. Thyroid. 2009;19(6):565–612.
92. Moura M, et al. Correlation of RET somatic mutations with clinicopathological features in sporadic medullary thyroid carcinomas. Br J Cancer. 2009;100(11):1777.
93. Gallel P, et al. Nuclear factor–κB activation is associated with somatic and germ line RET mutations in medullary thyroid carcinoma. Hum Pathol. 2008;39(7):994–1001.
94. Moura MM, et al. High prevalence of RAS mutations in RET-negative sporadic medullary thyroid carcinomas. J Clin Endocrinol Metabol. 2011;96(5):E863–8.
95. Pennelli G, et al. The PDCD4/miR-21 pathway in medullary thyroid carcinoma. Hum Pathol. 2015;46(1):50–7.
96. Palamarchuk A, et al. Akt phosphorylates and regulates Pdcd4 tumor suppressor protein. Cancer Res. 2005;65(24):11282–6.
97. Coster G, Goldberg M. The cellular response to DNA damage: a focus on MDC1 and its interacting proteins. Nucleus. 2010;1(2):166–78.

6 Updates in Thyroid Cytology

Min En Nga

Introduction

Fine needle aspiration cytology (FNAC) is undisputedly one of the most clinically useful methods of preoperative diagnosis of thyroid nodules. A combined approach of clinical examination, ultrasonography and FNAC forms the main elements of the diagnostic workup of thyroid nodules.

The last decade has seen worldwide efforts at standardisation of diagnostic terminology amongst pathologists, in order for a more evidence-based approach to the management of thyroid nodules. We will discuss various classification systems, with particular attention to the Bethesda System for Reporting Thyroid Cytology (TBSRTC) and its updates [1–3].

Recent years have also seen a much greater understanding of the molecular profiles of thyroid neoplasms, with an appreciation of the differences between classical papillary thyroid carcinoma (PTC) and follicular-patterned neoplasms. Practical aspects of molecular testing on cytologic specimens will be discussed, although a more detailed expansion on the various molecular alterations and available platforms will be covered in the chapter on Genetic Landscape of Thyroid Cancer.

M. E. Nga
Department of Pathology, National University of Singapore and National Univeristy Hospital, Singapore, Singapore
e-mail: min_en_nga@nuhs.edu.sg

Lastly, in 2016, significant ripples were caused by the coining of a new term, "Non-invasive follicular thyroid neoplasm with papillary-like nuclear features (NIFTP)" [4]. NIFTPs fall within what was previously considered a subset of follicular variant papillary thyroid carcinoma (FVPTC), namely fully encapsulated, non-invasive tumours with an exclusively follicular architecture. The impact of this new diagnostic term on TBSRTC will be discussed, with particular attention to the implications for preoperative diagnosis and surgical management and the impact on rates of malignancy in TBSRTC.

Summary of points for discussion:

1. Standardising thyroid cytology reporting: The Bethesda Catalyst and Beyond
2. Molecular testing in thyroid cytology: Feasibility and Clinical Utility
3. NIFTP: Implications for Preoperative Diagnosis and Surgical Management

1. Standardising Thyroid Cytology Reporting: The Bethesda Catalyst and Beyond

Although FNAC is well established as a robust diagnostic test for thyroid nodules, a reliable, logical and reproducible reporting language is also of utmost importance. This language must be shared by both diagnosticians (pathologists and

R. Parameswaran, A. Agarwal (eds.), *Evidence-Based Endocrine Surgery*,
https://doi.org/10.1007/978-981-10-1124-5_6

radiologists) and clinicians, such that clear management plans can be followed. Therein lies the worldwide move for a standardised and universal thyroid cytology reporting classification system.

The Bethesda System for Reporting Thyroid Cytology (TBSRTC) was the catalyst that provided the impetus for a collective move towards a more unified classification system across the globe [1]. This was borne out of the 2-day multidisciplinary discussion on thyroid cytology reporting at the National Cancer Institute Thyroid Fine Needle Aspiration State of the Science Conference in Bethesda, Maryland, in October 2007, organised by Dr. Andrea Abati and moderated by Drs Edmund Cibas and Susan J. Mandel.

TBSRTC has enjoyed wide uptake since its formal publication in 2009 and the publication of the monograph in 2010 [1, 5]. It has also been endorsed in the 2015 American Thyroid Association Guidelines, which recommend that thyroid FNACs be reported according to the categories defined by TBSRTC [6].

Other classification systems in use include the Papanicolaou Society classification system [7], the British Thyroid Association/Royal College of Pathologists' Thy 1–5 reporting system which was first published in 2002 and underwent revision in 2009 and 2016 [8, 9] and the Australasian classification system which was jointly endorsed by the Royal College of Pathologists of Australasia (RCPA) and the Australian Society of Cytology (ASC) [10, 11].

The main classification systems in use are summarised in Table 6.1. Clear management guidelines are suggested but not compulsory in TBSRTC and the Australasian classification system, while the British system provides some explanatory suggestions within each category. Both the 2009 and 2017 versions of TBSRTC are presented.

Since the publication of TBSRTC, there has been a proliferation of literature on the follow-up of thyroid nodules within each Bethesda category, particularly in the indeterminate categories of atypia of undetermined significance/follicular lesion of undetermined significance (AUS/FLUS), as well as follicular neoplasm/suspicious for follicular neoplasm (FN/SFN) [10–17]. These indeterminate nodules pose difficulties for two main reasons: limited diagnostic reproducibility and a broad spectrum of cytologic scenarios with a corresponding range of histologic outcomes spanning benign to malignant entities.

Firstly, reproducibility is limited—there is a degree of subjectivity in interpreting architectural and nuclear atypia. Indeed, Padmanabhan et al. found an agreement of only 36.4% (78/196 cases) in the AUS/FLUS category amongst 7 qualified cytopathologists with 5–30 years of diagnostic experience [12].

Secondly, TBSRTC itself provides several example scenarios within AUS/FLUS, amongst which are the presence of architectural or nuclear atypia, suboptimally preserved smears with questionable atypia and lymphoid-rich smears [5]. It is thus not surprising that the rate of malignancy varies widely in follow-up studies within this category [13–17]. We will be focusing primarily on the indeterminate category of AUS/FLUS in the following discussion. Recommendations and risks of malignancy in other Bethesda categories are reflected in Table 6.1.

Incidence Rate of AUS/FLUS

TBSRTC has recommended the frequency of AUS/FLUS to be in the range of approximately 7% of all thyroid FNACs [5]. Since the initial publication of the monograph, the literature has abounded with articles documenting the incidence of the various diagnostic categories. Bongiovanni et al., in their meta-analysis of a total number of 22.445 thyroid FNACs, found that the incidence of AUS/FLUS ranged from 0.8% to 27.2% with a mean incidence of 9.6% [13]. Ohori et al.'s meta-analysis also found the incidence to range between 0.7% and 18% amongst 7 studies from 6 laboratories [18]. In the present author's diagnostic service, the incidence of AUS/FLUS was found to be 6.4% within a 7-year period.

The Bethesda panel have been working on proposed modifications and updates based on cumulative literature. In 2016, specific discussions on each diagnostic category were presented at a symposium entitled "TBSRTC: Past, Present and Future" at the International Cytology Congress (ICC) in Yokohama, Japan, in May 2016, moderated by Drs. Syed Ali and Philippe Vielh, at which the current author was present. Thereafter, the Proposed Modifications and Updates for TBSRTC were published in *Acta Cytologica* in October 2016 [2]. The 2017 TBSRTC have now been published and the second edition of TBSRTC book was published in 2018 [3].

In the 2017 TBSRTC, the expected frequency of AUS/FLUS has been revised to up to 10%, a little above the original recommended range [3].

Interestingly, the Proposed Modifications and Updates briefly mentioned a potential quality control measure that was initially suggested by Krane et al. to evaluate individual laboratories' usage of the AUS/FLUS category [19]. This was the AUS/M ratio, where "M" includes both the suspicious for malignancy and malignant

Table 6.1 Major thyroid cytology reporting classification systems

Reporting system	BTA/RCPath classification (2016 revision) [8]	RCPA/ASC Australasian classification 2014 [8]	TBSRTC (2009) [1]	TBSRTC (2017) [3]
Categories	Non-diagnostic for cytological diagnosis—Thy 1/Thy 1c ("c" refers to cystic lesions)	Non-diagnostic (includes cyst contents only without sufficient colloid or well preserved follicular cells) *Recommendation: Repeat FNAC with ultrasound guidance*	Non-diagnostic or unsatisfactory (includes lesions showing cyst fluid only without ample colloid or sufficient well preserved follicular cells) *Recommendation: Repeat FNAC with ultrasound guidance*	Non-diagnostic or unsatisfactory *Recommendation: Repeat FNAC with ultrasound guidance*
	Non-neoplastic—Thy 2/ Thy 2c	Benign	Benign *Recommendation: Clinical follow-up*	Benign *Recommendation: Clinical follow-up and correlate with sonographic findings*
	Neoplasm possible—Thy3 Two subcategories: 1. Thy3a: samples that exhibit cytological/ nuclear or architectural atypia and raise the possibility of neoplasia; or suboptimal samples with mild cytologic atypia *Note: "In many cases, a repeat thyroid cytology sample is able to be placed into a more definitive category"* and 2. Thy 3f: samples suggesting follicular neoplasms *Note: "… a repeat may help clarify the exact diagnostic category. Review of the cytology and/or MDT discussion locally or centrally may be of use to help in patient Management"*	Indeterminate/follicular lesion of undetermined significance *Estimated risk of malignancy: Very low* *Recommendation: Repeat FNA after 3 months or shorter, depending on clinical circumstances* *In cases with a concerning lymphoid population, repeat the FNA with material for flow cytometry*	Atypia of undetermined significance/ follicular lesion of undetermined significance *Estimated risk of malignancy 5–15%* *Recommendation: Repeat FNA after an appropriate interval*	Atypia of undetermined significance/follicular lesion of undetermined significance *Risk of malignancy:* *— 10–30% pre-NIFTP* *— 6–18% post-NIFTP* *Recommendation: Repeat FNA, molecular testing or lobectomy*

(continued)

Table 6.1 (continued)

Reporting system	BTA/RCPath classification (2016 revision) [8]	RCPA/ASC Australasian classification 2014 [8]	TBSRTC (2009) [1]	TBSRTC (2017) [3]
	–	Suggestive of a follicular neoplasm *Recommendation: Refer to specialist surgeon*	Follicular neoplasm/ suspicious for follicular neoplasm *Estimated risk of malignancy 15–30%* *Recommendation: Lobectomy*	Follicular neoplasm/ suspicious for follicular neoplasm *Risk of malignancy* *– 25–40% pre-NIFTP* *– 10–40% post-NIFTP* *Recommendation: Lobectomy or molecular testing*
	Suspicious of malignancy—Thy4	Suspicious of malignancy *Recommendation: Specialist referral*	Suspicious for malignancy *Recommendation: Near total thyroidectomy or lobectomy*	Suspicious for malignancy *Risk of malignancy* *– 50–75% pre-NIFTP* *– 45–60% post-NIFTP* *Recommendation: Near total thyroidectomy or lobectomy*
	Malignant—Thy5	Malignant *Recommendation: Specialist referral as appropriate*	Malignant *Recommendation: Near total thyroidectomy*	Malignant *Recommendation: Near total thyroidectomy or lobectomy*

BTA British Thyroid Association
RCPath Royal College of Pathologists, United Kingdom
RCPA Royal College of Pathologists of Australasia
ASC Australian Society of Cytology
HN hyperplastic nodule, *FA* follicular adenoma, *FC* Follicular carcinoma (well differentiated), *FVPTC* follicular variant papillary thyroid carcinoma, *HCA* Hurthle cell adenoma, *HCC* Hurthle cell carcinoma

categories. Krane et al. found that this ratio posed the least amount of variability in their analysis of results from 8 series and recommended a ratio within the range of 1.0–3.0. Further meta-analytic studies are required to evaluate the usefulness of this ratio as a performance measure.

Follow-Up of AUS/FLUS

Repeat FNAC

TBSRTC recommends repeat FNAC in the majority of AUS/FLUS cases [1, 5]. This is also in line with the Australasian system, in the parallel category of the "indeterminate nodule" [11]. There is substantial literature that supports this recommendation, showing that repeat FNAC yields a more definitive result in AUS/FLUS or equivalent categories in 56–80% of the time [13, 17–22]. In the present author's institution, a more definitive FNAC result (defined as one that directs management more definitively, i.e. any category other than non-diagnostic or AUS/FLUS) was seen in 67.1% of repeat FNACs (n = 73), with majority falling into the benign category (60.3%) [21].

Molecular Testing

The 2017 TBSRTC has also included the recommendation of molecular testing, particularly using the Afirma rule-out gene expression classifier test, where a negative result would justify observation

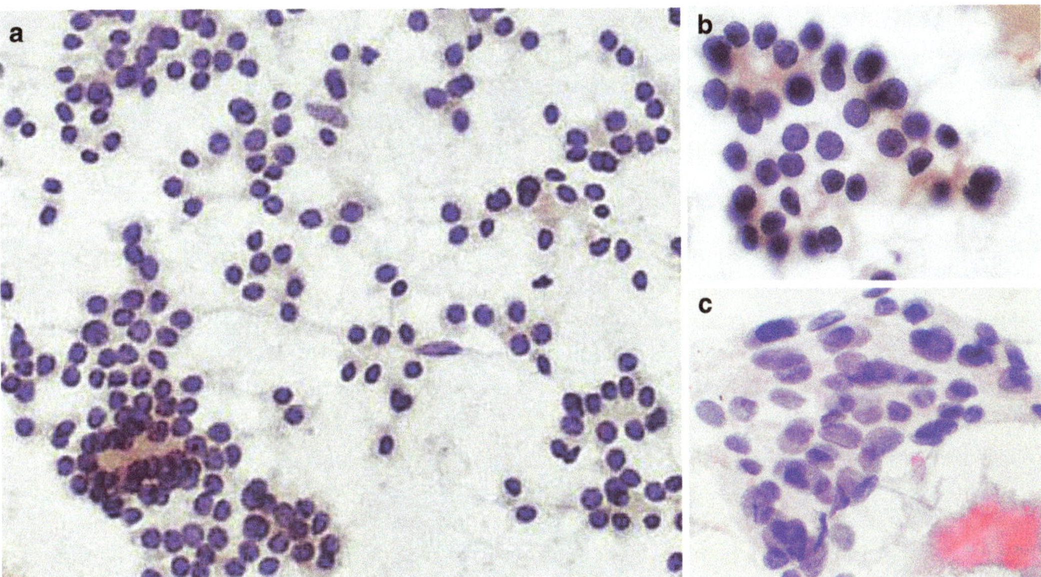

Fig. 6.1 FLUS/AUS with and without nuclear atypia. (**a**) FLUS/AUS with architectural atypia—both microfollicles and flat sheets are seen (Pap, 400×); (**b**) Same case, showing no significant nuclear atypia (Pap, 600×); (**c**) FLUS/AUS case showing nuclear atypia with enlargement and occasional nuclear grooves; histology showed a follicular adenoma with atypical nuclear features. (Pap, 600×)

rather than a repeat FNA or surgery [3]. An overview of the commercially available molecular tests is provided in the following section.

Surgical Outcomes

Amongst surgically resected nodules, several meta-analyses focusing on malignant outcomes have been performed in the recent literature [13, 17]. Straccia et al. documented malignancy rates in AUS/FLUS of 12.5–69.1%, with an overall malignancy rate of 27% (n = 4474) [17]. In contrast, Bongiovanni et al. found an overall malignancy rate of 15.9% (n = 2441) [13]. More recently, Gan et al. from our institution presented a meta-analysis of 12 studies, of malignancy rates of AUS/FLUS nodules that were triaged directly to surgery, finding an overall malignancy rate of 34% (n = 1946), with individual studies' rates ranging from 15.7% to 81.0% [14]. Within our institution, the malignancy rate amongst all AUS/FLUS nodules that were surgically excised was 27% from 2008 to 2014 [14]. In the 2017 TBSRTC, the overall risk of malignancy is stated as approximately 10–30%, before the consideration of NIFTP [3].

Regardless of published rates of malignancy, it cannot be overemphasised that in order for a clinically meaningful thyroid cytology reporting system to be in place, individual laboratories should perform regular and robust follow-up studies of malignancy rates within all diagnostic categories, with particular attention to the indeterminate categories. Findings should be communicated regularly to the multidisciplinary team of radiologists, surgeons, endocrine physicians, pathologists and radiation oncologists.

Substratification of Risk Within AUS/FLUS

Some evidence in the recent literature has emerged in support of further substratification of the AUS/FLUS category into different risk categories [14, 16, 23–25]. While some authors propose multiple subcategories within AUS/FLUS [16, 24, 25], we realise that it is difficult to further substratify a category in which there already exists significant inter-observer variability and propose a more simple means of subclassification of non-lymphoid lesions into cases in which nuclear atypia predominates versus those which only harbour architectural atypia [14]. This is illustrated in Fig. 6.1, which shows an example of AUS/FLUS with and without nuclear atypia.

Our findings showed that out of 137 AUS/FLUS nodules that were surgically excised, 132 could be readily stratified into those with predominantly nuclear atypia (n = 57) versus those with architectural atypia (n = 75), while the rest showed atypical lymphoid cells (n = 5). Nodules with both nuclear and architectural atypia were stratified into the "nuclear atypia" group. We found that the rate of malignancy was significantly higher in the nuclear atypia group (36.8%) than that with architectural atypia (14.7%), $p < 0.01$ [14]. Other studies have consistently documented similar findings, with malignancy rates in nodules with only architectural atypia ranging from 6.9% to 25% while rates in nodules with nuclear atypia ranged from 28% to 65.8% [16, 23–25].

While evidence mounts in support of substratifying the AUS/FLUS category by cytomorphological criteria, there is still no unified agreement on the **management** guidelines for these subcategories. In view of the high rates of malignancy amongst surgically excised AUS/FLUS nodules with nuclear atypia, a case could potentially be made for direct triage to surgery or for molecular testing within this subcategory.

It may logically follow that the architectural atypia subcategory (presence of a mixed microfollicular/trabecular and macrofollicular pattern, where a follicular neoplasm is not excluded) may benefit from repeat FNAC more than the nuclear atypia subgroup. To this end, our analysis showed that repeat FNAC yielded a higher rate of benign diagnoses within the architectural atypia group (24 of 34 [70.6%]) vs. the nuclear atypia group (19 of 39 [48.7%]); however, the results were not statistically significant ($p > 0.05$). It is tempting to recommend repeat FNAC in nodules with architectural atypia alone and surgical excision in those with nuclear atypia; however, prospective large cohort studies are required to validate this proposed route of management.

In the 2017 TBSRTC, it is mentioned that the mean risk of malignancy is 47% in cases with cytologic atypia and that cytologic atypia does convey a higher risk than architectural atypia alone. Several subclasses are provided featuring cytological atypia, architectural atypia, Hurthle cell aspirates, and atypical lymphoid cells. However, there is no specific recommendation to substratify this category based on the presence of nuclear/cytologic atypia [3]. While some authors have been using the terms "FLUS" to denote architectural atypia and "AUS" to indicate nuclear atypia, this splitting of terminology ithin Bethesda category III is not encouraged by TBSRTC [2, 3, 26].

Summary Points

- *A standardised reporting system for thyroid cytology is highly recommended.*
- *Robust institutional audits should be conducted regularly and results communicated within the multidisciplinary team.*
- *Within TBSRTC AUS/FLUS category, there is mounting evidence that nodules with nuclear atypia have higher rates of malignancy than those with architectural atypia.*
- *No clear guidelines on management have yet been established within the AUSFLUS subgroups.*
- *Repeat FNA or molecular testing may be recommended for AUS/FLUS.*

2. Molecular Testing in Thyroid Cytology: Feasibility and Clinical Utility

The ultimate aim of preoperative assessment of thyroid nodules is to triage nodules for surgical management, i.e. identify nodules which require surgery while minimising unnecessary surgery in nodules with indolent behaviour. While significant strides have been made towards a standardised reporting system for thyroid cytology, the indeterminate categories still leave much to be desired in terms of achieving high sensitivity and specificity in triaging malignant nodules for surgery.

While some degree of cytomorphological triage is possible within the AUS/FLUS category as discussed above, much work is still required to achieve a more robust system of surgical triage, when considering the attendant risks of surgery. In recent years, this has fallen into the realm of molecular testing [27–40]. A detailed description of the specific molecular aberrations in various types of thyroid neoplasms will be covered in the chapter on Genetic Landscape of Thyroid Cancer.

Our discussion will focus more on the practical feasibility and clinical utility of performing molecular tests on cytologic material. An important question to ask is—how reliable is a positive or negative molecular result in terms of safely dictating surgical vs. conservative management? Positive and negative predictive values vary between diagnostic categories, and it is important that clinicians have a full understanding of which categories would benefit most from molecular testing, when used as a means to decide on which nodules should come under the knife.

Briefly, the main molecular abnormalities in PTC include *BRAF* mutation and *RET/PTC* gene rearrangements, while in FPNs, they include *RAS* mutations (*N-RAS, H-RAS, K-RAS*) and *PAX8/PPAR*γ chromosomal rearrangements. An important point for clinicians to note is that *not all molecular aberrations correlate with malignant neoplasms*. Indeed, *RAS* mutations can be found even in lesions with histologic features of hyperplastic nodules [32]. This is where the divide between papillary thyroid carcinoma (PTC) and follicular-patterned neoplasms (FPNs) occurs. *In general, molecular aberrations found in PTC are far more specific for malignancy than those found in follicular-patterned lesions.* The latter may be seen in both benign and malignant entities (hyperplastic nodule, follicular adenoma, follicular carcinoma and follicular variant papillary thyroid carcinoma [FVPTC]).

Methodology for detecting molecular aberrations varies amongst centres; however, it would be useful to note that single gene mutations (e.g. *BRAF*, *RAS*) are easier to test and hence more readily accessible in laboratories with molecular testing facilities, while gene rearrangements pose more of a challenge in terms of specimen collection and test methodology.

BRAF

In PTC, one of the commonest and most highly specific molecular abnormalities is the *BRAF* V600E mutation, which is seen in approximately 40–45% of PTC in the Western population [31]. Interestingly, the incidence is higher in Asian cohorts, with a mean incidence of 68.7% in a meta-analysis by Song et al. [41]. Nikiforov et al. initially demonstrated that the *BRAF* mutation was only found in PTC, and not encountered in benign thyroid nodules (n = 111) or in non-PTC malignancies (n = 45) [42]. This specificity is further borne out in a review article by the same authors, who documented a specificity for PTC of 99.8% (580/581 cases), both from existing literature and their own work [43].

Specific methods of sequencing are beyond the scope of this chapter. It is, however, important to note that *BRAF* mutation testing has been shown to be feasible on a variety of types of cytologic material, including snap-frozen needle washings, residual liquid-based cytology material, needle rinse material in saline and even scrapings performed from previously stained smears [29, 35, 44–46]. Immunohistochemistry is also available specifically for the *BRAF* V600E mutation using the BRAF VE1 antibody clone, which has been shown to correlate well with molecular testing and thus could potentially be applied to cell block material from thyroid FNAC samples [47].

Therefore, the rationale of performing *BRAF* mutation testing on cytologic material, particularly in diagnostically indeterminate cases, appears sound. However, in practice, does this actually provide a clear management pathway, e.g. total thyroidectomy for *BRAF* mutation-positive cases? Also, are there sufficient cases that will test positive in the indeterminate categories to warrant reflex testing? Several meta-analyses have concluded that in the majority of indeterminate nodules, *BRAF* mutation testing alone does not significantly contribute to more definitive management, largely due to the low pickup rate, particularly in AUS/FLUS nodules [28, 46, 48, 49]. There may be limited usefulness in the suspicious for malignancy (SM) category, with a somewhat higher *BRAF* mutation-positive rate of 42–58% [48, 50, 51]. Hence, *BRAF* mutation testing alone may have limited practical utility in indeterminate nodules, while more potential lies in combining this with a panel of other molecular tests [28].

Commercially Available Testing Platforms

There are currently three commercially available testing panels: Afirma (by Veracyte), ThyGenX (Interpace Diagnostics) and ThyroSeq (University of Pittsburgh Medical Center, via CBLPath). These are summarised in Table 6.2. We will briefly discuss them in turn.

Table 6.2 Main commercially available molecular testing platforms

	Afirma by Veracyte	ThyGenX (previously miRInform)	ThyroSeq and ThyroSeq v2
Sample collection	2 dedicated passes (collected in RNA preservative; −20 °C stable up to 1 year)	1 dedicated FNA (collected in nucleic acid preservative solution; stable in room temperature for up to 6 weeks)	1–2 drops from first pass if sufficiently cellular (sample stability is 24 h at 4 °C and 6 h at room temperature)
Reporting FNAC	Separate diagnostic passes, reported by a central laboratory	Local laboratory	Local laboratory (with option to be reported in centralised laboratory)
Cost[a]	$4875	$1675	$3200
Utility	"Rule out" malignancy Initial validation study: NPV in AUS/FLUS 95% and FN/SFN 94% Combined sensitivity 90%, specificity 52% [52]	"Rule in" malignancy. Largest validation study: PPV in AUS/FLUS 88% and FN/SFN 87% [60]	ThyroSeq v2 Initial validation study NPV in FN/SFN 96%; PPV 83%, Sensitivity 90% and specificity 93% [67]
Remarks	Limited PPV	Limited NPV in categories with higher malignancy outcome rates (based on individual institutional results)	Limited utility in AUS/FLUS [40]

[a]Cost is in USD, as of June 2015

Afirma

The Afirma Gene Expression Classifier (GEC) test is based on a 167-gene mRNA detection panel, which also includes testing for metastatic malignancies and medullary thyroid carcinoma (MTC)-related genetic aberrations. This is marketed as a "rule out" test with a high negative predictive value (NPV) following a benign result. In the initial validation study, a "benign GEC result" (benign gene expression profile) had a NPV of 95% and 94% in AUS/FLUS and FN/SFN nodules, respectively, corresponding to a 5–6% risk of malignancy ($n = 265$ nodules). In contrast, for a "suspicious GEC" result, the positive predictive value (PPV) was only 38% for AUS/FLUS and 37% for FN/SFN, which is comparable to cytology alone in some institutions [52].

To translate this into practice, which Bethesda categories would benefit most from the Afirma test? Its usefulness is clear in FN/SFN nodules in which a benign GEC result has a high predictive value for benign histology, where the clinician may then reasonably choose to adopt a more conservative approach of close follow-up rather than immediate surgery. This is also reflected in the 2017 TBSRTC recommendations [3].

The 2017 TBSRTC has included this test as a possible management recommendation for AUS/FLUS [3]. However, in actual practice, the utility in this category is perhaps more controversial, due to a significant proportion of cases benefiting from a repeat FNAC, as discussed above, which is a much cheaper alternative.

The disadvantages of the Afirma test lie in the cost (refer to Table 6.2) as well as the specimen collection protocol. The test protocol requires *two* dedicated FNAC passes, with the samples washed in RNA preservative material and frozen for storage. In addition, the test also requires more diagnostic passes to be made and smears sent to a central laboratory for cytologic reporting, upon which reflex Afirma testing is performed in cases with indeterminate cytology results.

Post-validation studies performed by independent laboratories showed that amongst AUS/FLUS or FN/SFN nodules, the NPV ranged from 75% to 100%, while the sensitivity ranged from 83% to 100% [53–59]. Amongst all these studies, a total of only 363 nodules with a "benign" GEC result were excised, of which there were 3 false negatives (2 PTCs and 1 follicular carcinoma).

ThyGenX

In contrast to Afirma, ThyGenX is a "rule in" test that has a high positive predictive value for malignancy. The test is currently provided by Interpace Diagnostics (Parsippany, New Jersey,

United States) and was previously known as the miRInform test (Asuragen, Austin, Texas). It is a 7-gene panel that detects mutations in *BRAF, KRAS, HRAS, NRAS*, and chromosomal translocations resulting in *RET/PTC1, RET/PTC3* and *PAX8/PPARγ* fusions.

A dedicated FNAC pass is required, with material washed into nucleic acid preservative solution while other passes are made for diagnostic cytologic evaluation. The latter are performed in the local laboratory, with cytologically indeterminate nodules proceeding to the ThyGenX test.

In the largest validation study featuring 513 excised cytologically indeterminate nodules (AUS/FLUS and FN/SFN), Nikiforov et al. documented that the PPV for malignancy was 88% in AUS/FLUS nodules ($n = 247$), 87% in FN/SFN nodules ($n = 214$) and 95% in suspicious for malignancy (SM) nodules ($n = 52$) [60]. The NPVs were 84%, 86% and 72%, respectively. For AUS/FLUS, the sensitivity and specificity were 63% and 99%, respectively, while for FN/SNF they were 57% and 7%, respectively. Other smaller validation studies have yielded similar results [30, 53, 61–65].

The clinician should note, however, that non-PTC-related genetic aberrations should be interpreted with caution, due to their relative lack of specificity for malignancy. Eszlinger M et al. showed that while a positive result for *BRAF* mutation or *RET/PTC* rearrangement correlated with a 100% malignancy rate on histology, *RAS* mutation or *PAX8/PPARγ* rearrangement only showed malignant histology in 12% and 50% of surgical samples, respectively, with most of the benign outcomes being follicular adenomas [63]. Whether or not these follicular adenomas represent "preinvasive" forms of follicular thyroid carcinoma remains to be proven. This further highlights the lack of specificity for known genetic aberrations in follicular neoplasms.

A disadvantage of the ThyGenX test is its relatively limited ability to rule out malignancy. In the series of 513 indeterminate nodules, the NPV was lower in Bethesda diagnostic categories with higher malignant outcome rates on resection (94% in AUS/FLUS, 86% in FN/SFN and only 72% in SM) [60]. Therefore, in categories with significant rates of malignancy (e.g. greater than 20–25%) on cyto-histologic follow-up, a negative result should be interpreted with caution, in view of a significant percentage of false negatives.

An advantage of ThyGenX, though, is its practical feasibility. It is one of the more robust testing platforms because it is a DNA-based test. Thus it is feasible on residual liquid-based cytology preparations (e.g. ThinPrep) as well as even scrapings from air-dried smears [63, 64, 66].

ThyroSeq and ThyroSeq2

ThyroSeq, developed at the University of Pittsburgh Medical Center and commercially offered by CBL Path (Rye Brook, New York, United States), is a test that aims to maximise both PPV and NPV, using next-generation sequencing (NGS), a high-throughput molecular analytic platform [38]. In addition to the 7 genetic loci tested in ThyGenX, this test also incorporates hotspot mutations in *PIK3CA, PTEN, TP53, TSHR, CTNNB1, RET, AKT1* and *TERT*, as well as a gene fusions involving *RET, BRAF, NTRK1, NTRK3, AKT, PPARγ* and *THADA* to various partner genes, as well as a *GNAS* mutation test that is associated with benignity.

Laboratories have the option of submitting material for both cytologic interpretation and ThyroSeq molecular testing or just molecular testing alone. One advantage of employing NGS technology is that only 10 ng of DNA is required for this expanded test panel.

Initial validation for Thyroseq v2 was performed on 143 FN/SFN nodules [65]. The combined sensitivity and specificity for malignancy was 90% and 93%, respectively. PPV was 83% and NPV was 96%. Of note was that some specific mutations (*KRAS, HRAS, NRAS, TSHR and* BRAF K601E) were seen in benign entities, namely follicular adenoma (including Hurthle cell adenoma) and hyperplastic nodules.

In 2017, Valderrabano et al. performed an independent validation study of ThyroSeq v2 [40]. 102 cytologically indeterminate AUS/FLUS and FN/SFN nodules were analysed, all of which underwent surgical excision. In AUS/FLUS ($n = 52$), the sensitivity and specificity were 43% and 71% while the PPV was only 19% and the NPV was 89%. The results suggested that this test may have limited clinical utility in this diagnostic category. A possible reason is the inclusion in the panel of genetic alterations that were less specific for malignancy.

The FN/SFN category (n = 50) yielded more promising results. The sensitivity and specificity were 95% and 84%, respectively, while the PPV and NPV were 65% and 94%. Based on the high NPV, the authors concluded that the test was likely to be helpful in ruling out malignancy, but less predictive of ruling *in* malignancy. Nevertheless, more large-scale prospective studies are required to better understand the clinical utility of this new NGS-based platform.

American Thyroid Association Recommendations on Molecular Testing

The 2015 American Thyroid Association (ATA) Guidelines provide some recommendations regarding molecular testing within specific TBSRTC diagnostic categories [6].

- AUS/FLUS: "… after consideration of worrisome clinical and sonographic features, investigations such as repeat FNA or molecular testing may be used to supplement malignancy risk assessment in lieu of proceeding directly with a strategy of either surveillance or diagnostic surgery…" (Recommendation 15. Weak recommendation, Moderate-quality evidence).
- FN/SFN: "… after consideration of clinical and sonographic features, molecular testing may be used to supplement malignancy risk assessment data in lieu of proceeding directly with surgery. Informed patient preference and feasibility should be considered in clinical decision-making." (Recommendation 16. Weak recommendation, Moderate-quality evidence).
- SM: "… After consideration of clinical and sonographic features, mutational testing for BRAF or the seven-gene mutation marker panel (BRAF, RAS, RET/PTC, PAX8/PPARγ) may be considered … if such data would be expected to alter surgical decision making." (Recommendation 17. Weak recommendation, Moderate-quality evidence).

The Guidelines also recommend that should molecular testing be considered, patients should be clearly counselled regarding the "potential benefits and limitations of testing".

Ultimately, long-term outcome data is required to evaluate if molecular testing is sufficiently beneficial to be incorporated into routine preoperative investigations of thyroid nodules. Cost-efficiency is also a consideration that needs to be included in the equation. Currently, there is no single reliable molecular test that can effectively rule in or rule out malignancy in indeterminate nodules.

Summary Points

- *Molecular testing for classical PTC is more specific for malignancy than for follicular-patterned neoplasms.*
- *Sensitivity, specificity and negative and positive predictive values of test results vary between diagnostic categories due to varying rates of malignant outcomes.*
- *Three main commercially available tests include Afirma gene expression classifier ("rule out malignancy"), ThyGenX ("rule in malignancy") and ThyroSeq next-generation sequencing test.*
- *The Afirma gene expression classifier has been included in the 2017 TBSRTC for AUS/FLUS and FN/SFN categories.*
- *Technical feasibility on collected material, accessibility and cost are important considerations.*
- *Long-term outcome studies are still required to ultimately evaluate clinical utility.*

3. NIFTP: Implications for Preoperative Diagnosis and Surgical Management

In the April issue of the Journal of the American Medical Association (JAMA), Nikiforov et al. formally described the "non-invasive follicular thyroid neoplasm with papillary-like nuclear features (NIFTP)" [4]. This caused a stir in the community of thyroid surgeons, pathologists and even patients. The reclassification of this entity as a non-malignant neoplasm garnered sufficient publicity to be featured in the New York Times in a passage entitled "It's Not Cancer: Doctors Reclassify a Thyroid Tumor" [68].

The rationale behind this reclassification is the indolent behaviour of NIFTP. Long-term follow-up of 109 cases (median 13 years, range 10–25 years) showed no evidence of disease [4]. None of the 109 cases received radioiodine (RAI) therapy, while 67 cases were treated conservatively with lobectomy. In contrast, amongst the 101 cases of encapsulated FVPTC with either capsular or vascular invasion, 12% developed an adverse event (metastatic disease, persistent disease, nodal recurrence or biochemical evidence of disease) after a minimum follow-up of at least 1 year. Other corroborating follow-up studies also suggest indolent clinical behaviour in NIFTP, including large tumours measuring at least 4 cm in maximal dimension [69, 70].

Prior to this revised nomenclature, NIFTP was considered a subset of FVPTV—encapsulated FVPTC without capsular or vascular invasion. In the Western population, they comprise approximately 20–25% of thyroid neoplasms previously designated as malignant [69, 71, 72]. The diagnostic criteria for NIFTP are strict and are based on histologic examination of *surgically excised nodules* with adequate sampling of the lesional capsule. These criteria are summarised in Table 6.3.

NIFTP is a diagnosis that should not be made on frozen section evaluation. This is for two reasons—adequate capsular sampling is required to confirm the absence of capsular or vascular invasion, and nuclear artefacts can occur in frozen sections that can mimic the nuclear features of PTC. Hence, histologic examination of thoroughly sampled, well-fixed lesional tissue is necessary for the diagnosis of NIFTP.

Due to its indolent behaviour, it is recommended that NIFTP be treated with simple lobectomy without RAI. Hence treatment is similar to that of a follicular neoplasm rather than FVPTC.

Can NIFTP be diagnosed on cytology? The short answer is no. The diagnosis of NIFTP by definition requires histologic evaluation of the capsule–thyroid interface, which cannot be reliably achieved on cytology. *Hence it is not possible to make a definitive preoperative diagnosis of NIFTP, although the possible differential of NIFTP may be suggested.* This then raises the question of which Bethesda categories NIFTP will fall into, and how this will impact management of these nodules. In addition, in the post-NIFTP era, malignancy rates can also be expected to fall in most TBSRTC categories, based on the removal of NIFTPs from the malignant outcome cohort.

Table 6.3 Diagnostic criteria for NIFTP

Criteria
1. Encapsulation or clear demarcation • Thick, thin, or partial capsule or • Well circumscribed nodule with a clear demarcation from adjacent thyroid tissue
2. Follicular growth pattern • Microfollicular, normofollicular, or macrofollicular architecture with abundant colloid • <1% papillae • No psammoma bodies • Less than 30% solid/trabecular/insular growth pattern
3. Nuclear score of 2 or 3 (of the following 3 points) • Size/shape (enlargement, elongation, overlapping) • Membrane (irregularity, presence of grooves and pseudoinclusions) • Chromatin (clear, glassy, marginated)
4. No vascular or capsular invasion • Requires adequate sampling and microscopic examination of the tumour capsule interface
5. No tumour necrosis
6. No high mitotic activity • High mitotic activity defined as at least 3 mitoses per 10 high-powered fields (400×)

Several recent publications have documented the cytologic characterisation of NIFTP based on retrospective analysis of histologically confirmed cases [71, 73, 74]. NIFTPs were found in most Bethesda diagnostic categories, from benign to malignant. The findings are summarised in Table 6.4. The most frequent categories harbouring NIFTP are AUS/FLUS, FN/SFN and SM.

It is concerning to note that there are significant numbers of NIFTPs within the outright malignant category (ranging from 2% to 20% of NIFTPs)—this could potentially result in unnecessary total thyroidectomies for patients who eventually turn out to have NIFTP, accompanied by a drop in specificity for malignancy in this category. Indeed, both Strickland and Faquin et al. found a decrease in rate of malignancy (ROM) in all TBSRTC categories when NIFTPs were removed from malignant outcome cohorts. In the malignant category, the rates dropped from close to 100% to 93.6%–95.7% [71, 72]. In the 2017 TBSRTC, the risks of malignancy pre- and post-NIFTP have been estimated, and these are shown in Table 6.1.

Pathologists and surgeons alike would rightfully be concerned about the possibility of false positive

Table 6.4 Cytologic categories of preoperative diagnosis of NIFTP and Decrease in ROM

	NIFTP cytologic categories			Decrease in ROM	
	Strickland et al. [71]	Maletta et al. [73]	Hahn et al. [74]	Strickland et al. (%) [71]	Faquin et al. (%) [72]
Non-diagnostic (%)	1 (1.2)	0	2 (6)	18.9 to 17	25.3 to 23.9
Benign (%)	13 (15)	0	5 (14)	13.2 to 5.4	9.3 to 5.8
AUS/FLUS (%)	17 (20)	14 (15)	9 (26)	39.2 to 21.6	31.2 to 17.6
FN/SFN (%)	7 (8)	54 (56)	2 (6)	45.5 to 37.5	33.2 to 18
SM (%)	39 (46)	26 (27)	10 (29)	87.2 to 45.7	82.6 to 59.2
Malignant (%)	8 (9)	2 (2)	7 (20)	98.7 to 93.6	99.1 to 95.7
Total no. of cases	85	96	34	655	1826

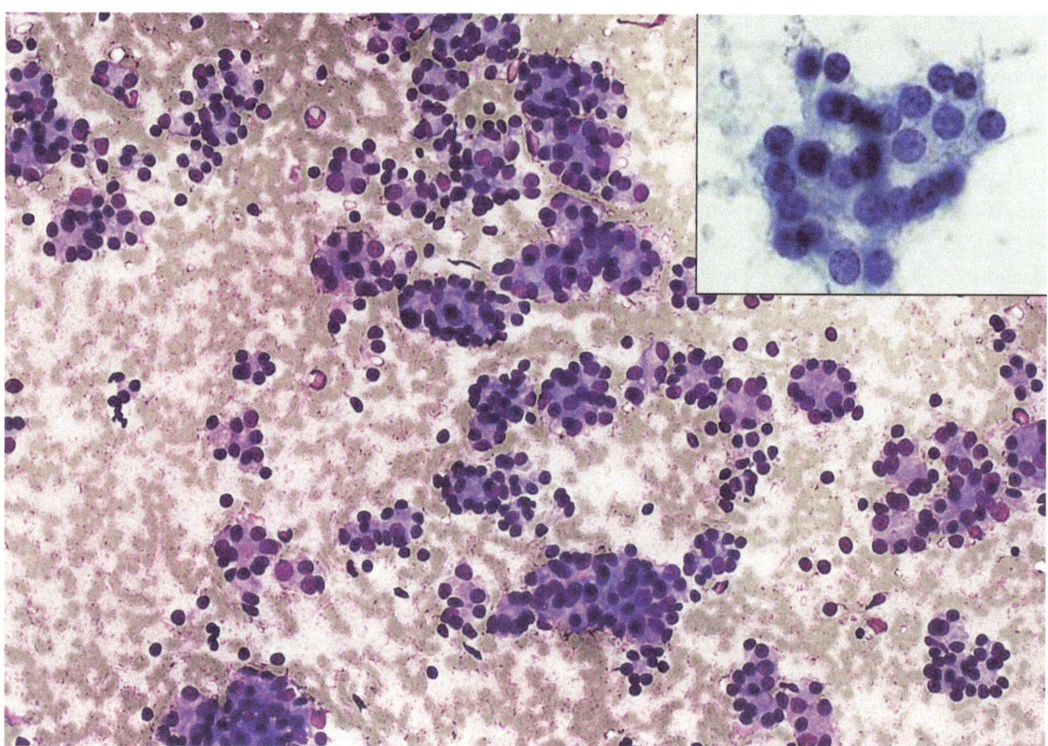

Fig. 6.2 FN/SFN. Follicular neoplasm showing repetitive microfollicular structures (Hemacolor, 200×). Inset shows round, normochromatic nuclei without significant nuclear atypia. (Pap, 600×)

cytologic malignant diagnosis in cases of NIFTP. There are several points of practice that can reduce false positives to some extent—the diagnostic cytopathologist should pay strict attention to specific cytologic features when rendering a malignant cytologic diagnosis. In order to maximise the diagnostic specificity of PTC on cytology, definite cytologic features of classical PTC should be sought, such as syncytial sheets and fibrovascular cores, and well-defined intranuclear pseudoinclusions.

Cytologic features raising the possibility of NIFTP are described in Krane's commentary on NIFTP and the Bethesda Proposed Modifications and Updates, and include microfollicular architecture and subtle nuclear features of PTC without overtly obvious nuclear pseudoinclusions, and the absence of true papillary structures, fibrovascular cores and psammomatous calcifications [2, 75]. *In short, NIFTP would be a viable differential diagnostic consideration whenever the possibility of FVPTC is raised on cytology.*

Figure 6.2 illustrates a case classified as FN/SFN, which does not show significant nuclear atypia. In contrast, Fig. 6.3 shows a case falling

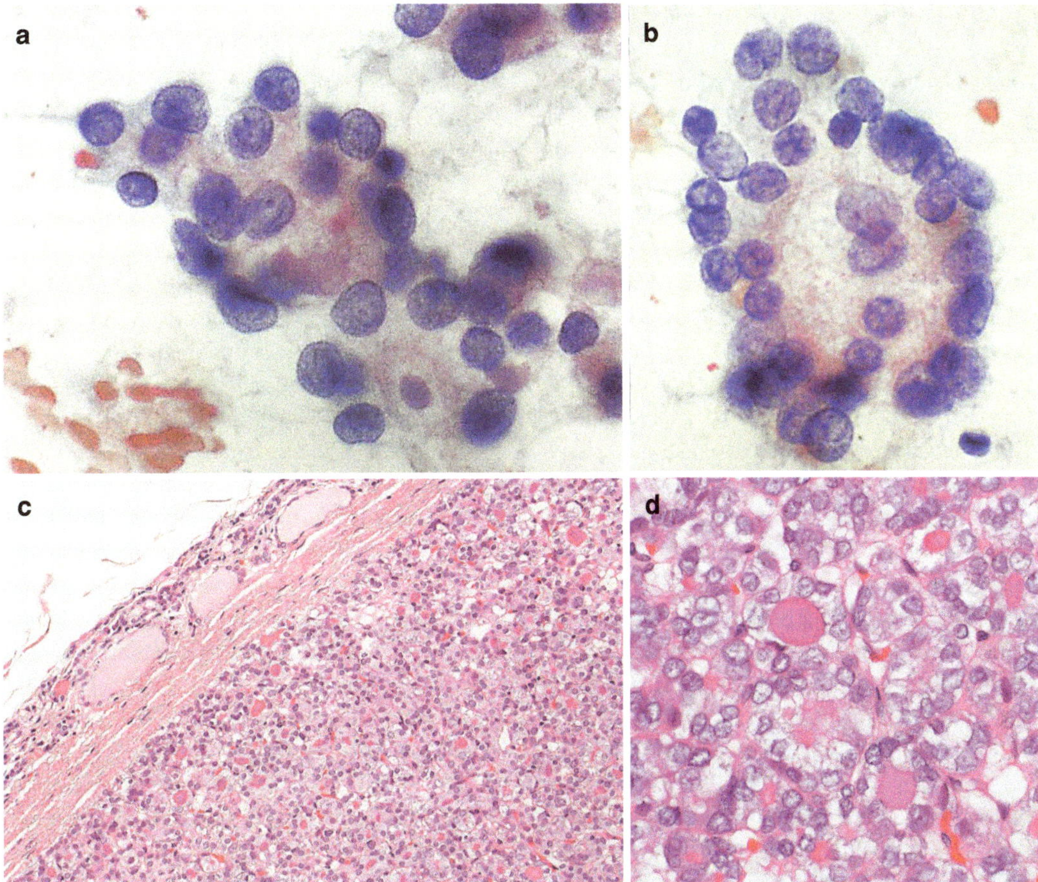

Fig. 6.3 FN/SFN with nuclear atypia. (**a**, **b**) Follicular patterned lesion showing nuclear enlargement, pale chromatin and occasional grooves without pseudoinclusions. Lesion classified as FN/SFN, possibilities include FVPTC or NIFTP (Pap, 600×). (**c**) Low-power histology showing encapsulated nodule (HE, 100×); (**d**) High-power microscopy showing microfollicles lined by cells with nuclear atypia, consistent with NIFTP (HE, 300×)

into the same category, but with nuclear atypia. In the comments section, it should be noted that FVPTC and NIFTP would be differentials for this case. Histology showed a NIFTP.

In terms of a practical approach to cytology of NIFTP, several suggestions have been made, which generally include exercising caution when making a malignant diagnosis (as highlighted above) and erring on the side of FN/SFN rather than SM in nodules in which NIFTP is being considered. Another viable suggestion, as stated in the 2017 TBSRTC, is to include NIFTP as a possible differential diagnosis in the notes or comments of the cytology report where appropriate [2, 3, 75, 76]. The latter should be applied judiciously to cases in which there is genuine concern about NIFTP, i.e. nodules with a predominant microfollicular architecture and with some nuclear atypia. Although some have suggested including an optional explanatory comment in the malignant category (regarding the possibility of NIFTP and stating the reduced in ROM as a result of NIFTP), the current author feels that this may not be necessary if strict diagnostic criteria for classical PTC are applied when making such a cytologic diagnosis.

Based on the histologic features of NIFTP, we expect that in many instances, the cytologic features will fall into the FN/SFN, and, less commonly, the AUS/FLUS categories. This is reassuring as in most cases the management will be fairly conservative.

It would be logical to argue that close attention should be paid to sonographic findings of nodules in which cytology raises the possibility of NIFTP, because one of the main diagnostic criteria is encapsulation and/or circumscription. As yet, though, the current literature holds a paucity of work documenting specific sonographic features of NIFTP [74, 77, 78]. Hahn et al. documented the finding of circumscription in 85.3% of NIFTP ($n = 34$), with most cases falling into the low to intermediate suspicion group [74]. Similarly, Rosario et al. documented that amongst 120 NIFTPs, the sonographic features mostly fell within the ATA low to intermediate suspicion categories (91%) while only 5% of cases were in the high suspicion category [78]. However, in contrast, Jeon et al. analysed sonographic features of 39 NIFTPs and found suspicious features in 51% of cases; however, they did not further substratify these into specific features such as lesional margins [77]. Further studies are required to ascertain if the radiologic features of NIFTP can help further strengthen the cytologic impression on FNAC, thereby providing more specific guidance for subsequent management.

The role of molecular testing in the preoperative diagnosis of NIFTP is not yet established. The molecular profile of NIFTP is distinct from classical PTC, but, rather, exhibit changes seen more often in follicular neoplasms, such as *RAS* mutations, *PAX8/PPARγ* fusion and other abnormalities [4, 79].

Summary Points

- *NIFTP was previously considered a subset of encapsulated FVPTC. It is now no longer classified as a malignant tumour.*
- *The behaviour is indolent and recommended treatment is lobectomy.*
- *The diagnosis of NIFTP requires surgical excision; it cannot be diagnosed on frozen section or cytology.*
- *On cytology, NIFTP would be most represented in the FN/SFN. SM and AUS/FLUS categories and may be considered whenever FVPTC is a possibility.*
- *Where significant preoperative concern for NIFTP exists, conservative surgery should be considered* (i.e. *lobectomy).*
- *The rates of malignancy in TBSRTC categories have fallen when NIFTPs are reclassified as non-malignant* (Table 6.1).

Conclusion

With the widespread adoption of globally recognised reporting systems for thyroid cytology, institutional multidisciplinary teams are in a better place to perform robust audits within their respective diagnostic services. This is a positive step towards evidence-based management of the thyroid nodule.

Although there is much literature on the outcomes of indeterminate nodules, in particular showing a higher malignancy rate in nodules with nuclear atypia, it must be emphasised that *individual institutions must actively establish rational management protocols based on local follow-up studies.*

Molecular testing can provide additional information that contributes to management of thyroid nodules; however, currently there is no single "magic bullet" that is able to accurately rule in and rule out malignancy in indeterminate nodules. Also, it should be noted that the practical utility of molecular testing varies with each diagnostic category, with the AUS/FLUS and FN/SFN categories perhaps benefitting the most. However, cost and accessibility remain important issues, although this may change over time, as lower cost platforms are developed.

Finally, in the reclassification of NIFTP to a non-malignant entity, malignancy rates have been reduced in all Bethesda cytologic diagnostic categories, in particular, the indeterminate and suspicious categories. Clinicians and pathologists should be aware of this possibility when planning surgical management of thyroid nodules. Studies on specific radiologic features of NIFTP would be helpful in ascertaining the role of imaging in the distinction between invasive FVPTC, encapsulated FVPTC and NIFTP.

References

1. Cibas ES, Ali SZ, NCI Thyroid FNA. State of the science conference. The Bethesda system for reporting thyroid cytopathology. Am J Clin Pathol. 2009;132(5):658–65.
2. Pusztaszeri M, Rossi ED, Auger M, Baloch Z, Bishop J, Bongiovanni M, et al. The Bethesda

system for reporting thyroid cytopathology: proposed modifications and updates for the second edition from an international panel. Acta Cytol. 2016;60(5):399–405.
3. Ali SZ, Cibas E, editors. The Bethesda system for reporting thyroid cytopathology: definitions, criteria, and explanatory notes [Internet]. 2nd ed. New York: Springer; 2018. http://www.springer.com/gp/book/9783319605692. Accessed 18 Jun 2018.
4. Nikiforov YE, Seethala RR, Tallini G, Baloch ZW, Basolo F, Thompson LDR, et al. Nomenclature revision for encapsulated follicular variant of papillary thyroid carcinoma: a paradigm shift to reduce overtreatment of indolent tumors. JAMA Oncol. 2016;2(8):1023–9.
5. Ali SZ, Cibas E, editors. The Bethesda system for reporting thyroid cytopathology: definitions, criteria and explanatory notes. 2010th ed. New York: Springer; 2010. p. 174.
6. Haugen BR, Alexander EK, Bible KC, Doherty GM, Mandel SJ, Nikiforov YE, et al. American Thyroid Association Management Guidelines for Adult Patients with Thyroid Nodules and Differentiated Thyroid Cancer: The American Thyroid Association Guidelines Task Force on Thyroid Nodules and Differentiated Thyroid Cancer. Thyroid. 2015;26(1):1–133.
7. Guidelines of the Papanicolaou Society of Cytopathology for the Examination of Fine-Needle Aspiration Specimens from Thyroid Nodules. The Papanicolaou Society of Cytopathology Task Force on Standards of Practice. Mod Pathol. 1996;9(6):710–5.
8. Guidance on the reporting of thyroid cytology specimens [Internet]. 2017. http://www.rcpath.org/resourceLibrary/g089-guidancereportingthyroidcytology-jan16.html. Accessed 8 Mar 2017.
9. Lobo C, McQueen A, Beale T, Kocjan G. The UK Royal College of Pathologists thyroid fine-needle aspiration diagnostic classification is a robust tool for the clinical management of abnormal thyroid nodules. Acta Cytol. 2011;55(6):499–506.
10. Kumarasinghe MP, Cummings MC, Raymond W, Shield P, Judge M, Beaty A, et al. Approach to thyroid cytology: rationale for standardisation. Pathology (Phila). 2015;47(4):285–8.
11. RCPA - Cancer Protocols [Internet]. 2017. http://www.rcpa.edu.au/Library/Practising-Pathology/Structured-Pathology-Reporting-of-Cancer/Cancer-Protocols. Accessed 8 Mar 2017.
12. Padmanabhan V, Marshall CB, Akdas Barkan G, Ghofrani M, Laser A, Tolgay Ocal I, et al. Reproducibility of atypia of undetermined significance/follicular lesion of undetermined significance category using the Bethesda system for reporting thyroid cytology when reviewing slides from different institutions: a study of interobserver variability among cytopathologists. Diagn Cytopathol. 2017;45(5):399–405.
13. Bongiovanni M, Spitale A, Faquin WC, Mazzucchelli L, Baloch ZW. The Bethesda system for reporting thyroid cytopathology: a meta-analysis. Acta Cytol. 2012;56(4):333–9.
14. Gan TRX, Nga ME, Lum JHY, Wong WM, Tan WB, Parameswaran R, et al. Thyroid cytology-nuclear versus architectural atypia within the "Atypia of undetermined significance/follicular lesion of undetermined significance" Bethesda category have significantly different rates of malignancy. Cancer. 2017;125(4):245–56.
15. Ho AS, Sarti EE, Jain KS, Wang H, Nixon IJ, Shaha AR, et al. Malignancy rate in thyroid nodules classified as Bethesda category III (AUS/FLUS). Thyroid. 2014;24(5):832–9.
16. Önder S, Firat P, Ates D. The Bethesda system for reporting thyroid cytopathology: an institutional experience of the outcome of indeterminate categories. Cytopathology. 2014;25(3):177–84.
17. Straccia P, Rossi ED, Bizzarro T, Brunelli C, Cianfrini F, Damiani D, et al. A meta-analytic review of the Bethesda system for reporting thyroid cytopathology: has the rate of malignancy in indeterminate lesions been underestimated? Cancer Cytopathol. 2015;123(12):713–22.
18. Ohori NP, Schoedel KE. Variability in the atypia of undetermined significance/follicular lesion of undetermined significance diagnosis in the Bethesda system for reporting thyroid cytopathology: sources and recommendations. Acta Cytol. 2011;55(6):492–8.
19. Krane JF, Vanderlaan PA, Faquin WC, Renshaw AA. The atypia of undetermined significance/follicular lesion of undetermined significance: malignant ratio: a proposed performance measure for reporting in the Bethesda system for thyroid cytopathology. Cancer Cytopathol. 2012;120(2):111–6.
20. Gocun PU, Karakus E, Bulutay P, Akturk M, Akin M, Poyraz A. What is the malignancy risk for atypia of undetermined significance? Three years' experience at a university hospital in Turkey. Cancer Cytopathol. 2014;122(8):604–10.
21. Dincer N, Balci S, Yazgan A, Guney G, Ersoy R, Cakir B, et al. Follow-up of atypia and follicular lesions of undetermined significance in thyroid fine needle aspiration cytology. Cytopathology. 2013;24(6):385–90.
22. Yassa L, Cibas ES, Benson CB, Frates MC, Doubilet PM, Gawande AA, et al. Long-term assessment of a multidisciplinary approach to thyroid nodule diagnostic evaluation. Cancer. 2007;111(6):508–16.
23. Rossi M, Lupo S, Rossi R, Franceschetti P, Trasforini G, Bruni S, et al. Proposal for a novel management of indeterminate thyroid nodules on the basis of cytopathological subclasses. Endocrine. 2017;57(1):98–107.
24. Wu HH, Inman A, Cramer HM. Subclassification of "atypia of undetermined significance" in thyroid fine-needle aspirates. Diagn Cytopathol. 2014;42(1):23–9.
25. VanderLaan PA, Marqusee E, Krane JF. Usefulness of diagnostic qualifiers for thyroid fine-needle aspirations with atypia of undetermined significance. Am J Clin Pathol. 2011;136(4):572–7.
26. Kim SJ, Roh J, Baek JH, Hong SJ, Shong YK, Kim WB, et al. Risk of malignancy according to sub-clas-

sification of the atypia of undetermined significance or follicular lesion of undetermined significance (AUS/FLUS) category in the Bethesda system for reporting thyroid cytopathology. Cytopathology. 2017;28(1):65–73.
27. Salvatore G, Giannini R, Faviana P, Caleo A, Migliaccio I, Fagin JA, et al. Analysis of BRAF point mutation and RET/PTC rearrangement refines the fine-needle aspiration diagnosis of papillary thyroid carcinoma. J Clin Endocrinol Metab. 2004;89(10):5175–80.
28. Pusztaszeri MP, Krane JF, Faquin WC. BRAF testing and thyroid FNA. Cancer Cytopathol. 2015;123(12):689–95.
29. Poller DN, Glaysher S. BRAF V600 co-testing is technically feasible in conventional thyroid fine needle aspiration (FNA) cytology smears and can reduce the need for completion thyroidectomy. Cytopathology. 2014;25(3):155–9.
30. Nikiforov YE, Steward DL, Robinson-Smith TM, Haugen BR, Klopper JP, Zhu Z, et al. Molecular testing for mutations in improving the fine-needle aspiration diagnosis of thyroid nodules. J Clin Endocrinol Metab. 2009;94(6):2092–8.
31. Nikiforov YE, Nikiforova MN. Molecular genetics and diagnosis of thyroid cancer. Nat Rev Endocrinol. 2011;7(10):569–80.
32. Nikiforov YE. Molecular diagnostics of thyroid tumors. Arch Pathol Lab Med. 2011;135(5):569–77.
33. Nikiforov YE. Thyroid cancer in 2015: molecular landscape of thyroid cancer continues to be deciphered. Nat Rev Endocrinol. 2016;12(2):67–8.
34. Mehta V, Nikiforov YE, Ferris RL. Use of molecular biomarkers in FNA specimens to personalize treatment for thyroid surgery. Head Neck. 2013;35(10):1499–506.
35. Kwon H, Kim WG, Eszlinger M, Paschke R, Song DE, Kim M, et al. Molecular diagnosis using residual liquid-based cytology materials for patients with nondiagnostic or indeterminate thyroid nodules. Endocrinol Metab (Seoul Korea). 2016;31(4):586–91.
36. Kloos RT. Molecular profiling of thyroid nodules: current role for the Afirma gene expression classifier on clinical decision making. Mol Imaging Radionucl Ther. 2016;26(Suppl 1):36–49.
37. Hsiao SJ, Nikiforov YE. Molecular approaches to thyroid cancer diagnosis. Endocr Relat Cancer. 2014;21(5):T301–13.
38. Nikiforova MN, Wald AI, Roy S, Durso MB, Nikiforov YE. Targeted next-generation sequencing panel (ThyroSeq) for detection of mutations in thyroid cancer. J Clin Endocrinol Metab. 2013;98(11):E1852–60.
39. Nikiforov YE, Carty SE, Chiosea SI, Coyne C, Duvvuri U, Ferris RL, et al. Impact of the multi-gene ThyroSeq next-generation sequencing assay on cancer diagnosis in thyroid nodules with atypia of undetermined significance/follicular lesion of undetermined significance cytology. Thyroid. 2015;25(11):1217–23.
40. Valderrabano P, Khazai L, Leon ME, Thompson ZJ, Ma Z, Chung CH, et al. Evaluation of ThyroSeq v2 performance in thyroid nodules with indeterminate cytology. Endocr Relat Cancer. 2017;24(3):127–36.
41. Song YS, Lim JA, Park YJ. Mutation profile of well-differentiated thyroid Cancer in Asians. Endocrinol Metab (Seoul Korea). 2015;30(3):252–62.
42. Nikiforova MN, Kimura ET, Gandhi M, Biddinger PW, Knauf JA, Basolo F, et al. BRAF mutations in thyroid tumors are restricted to papillary carcinomas and anaplastic or poorly differentiated carcinomas arising from papillary carcinomas. J Clin Endocrinol Metab. 2003;88(11):5399–404.
43. Nikiforova MN, Nikiforov YE. Molecular diagnostics and predictors in thyroid cancer. Thyroid. 2009;19(12):1351–61.
44. Ohori NP, Nikiforova MN, Schoedel KE, LeBeau SO, Hodak SP, Seethala RR, et al. Contribution of molecular testing to thyroid fine-needle aspiration cytology of "follicular lesion of undetermined significance/atypia of undetermined significance". Cancer Cytopathol. 2010;118(1):17–23.
45. Chung SY, Lee JS, Lee H, Park SH, Kim SJ, Ryu HS. Cytomorphological factors and BRAF mutation predicting risk of lymph node metastasis in preoperative liquid-based fine needle aspirations of papillary thyroid carcinoma. Acta Cytol. 2013;57(3):252–8.
46. Koh J, Choi JR, Han KH, Kim E-K, Yoon JH, Moon HJ, et al. Proper indication of BRAF(V600E) mutation testing in fine-needle aspirates of thyroid nodules. PLoS One. 2013;8(5):e64505.
47. Ilie MI, Lassalle S, Long-Mira E, Bonnetaud C, Bordone O, Lespinet V, et al. Diagnostic value of immunohistochemistry for the detection of the BRAF(V600E) mutation in papillary thyroid carcinoma: comparative analysis with three DNA-based assays. Thyroid. 2014;24(5):858–66.
48. Jinih M, Foley N, Osho O, Houlihan L, Toor AA, Khan JZ, et al. BRAF(V600E) mutation as a predictor of thyroid malignancy in indeterminate nodules: a systematic review and meta-analysis. Eur J Surg Oncol. 2017;43(7):1219–27.
49. Trimboli P, Treglia G, Condorelli E, Romanelli F, Crescenzi A, Bongiovanni M, et al. BRAF-mutated carcinomas among thyroid nodules with prior indeterminate FNA report: a systematic review and meta-analysis. Clin Endocrinol (Oxf). 2016;84(3):315–20.
50. Su X, Jiang X, Xu X, Wang W, Teng X, Shao A, et al. Diagnostic value of BRAF (V600E)-mutation analysis in fine-needle aspiration of thyroid nodules: a meta-analysis. Onco Targets Ther. 2016;9:2495–509.
51. Kleiman DA, Sporn MJ, Beninato T, Crowley MJ, Nguyen A, Uccelli A, et al. Preoperative BRAF(V600E) mutation screening is unlikely to alter initial surgical treatment of patients with indeterminate thyroid nodules: a prospective case series of 960 patients. Cancer. 2013;119(8):1495–502.
52. Alexander EK, Kennedy GC, Baloch ZW, Cibas ES, Chudova D, Diggans J, et al. Preoperative diagnosis of benign thyroid nodules with indeterminate cytology. N Engl J Med. 2012;367(8):705–15.
53. Nishino M. Molecular cytopathology for thyroid nodules: a review of methodology and test performance. Cancer Cytopathol. 2016;124(1):14–27.
54. Alexander EK, Schorr M, Klopper J, Kim C, Sipos J, Nabhan F, et al. Multicenter clinical experience

with the Afirma gene expression classifier. J Clin Endocrinol Metab. 2014;99(1):119–25.
55. Harrell RM, Bimston DN. Surgical utility of Afirma: effects of high cancer prevalence and oncocytic cell types in patients with indeterminate thyroid cytology. Endocr Pract. 2014;20(4):364–9.
56. Lastra RR, Pramick MR, Crammer CJ, LiVolsi VA, Baloch ZW. Implications of a suspicious Afirma test result in thyroid fine-needle aspiration cytology: an institutional experience. Cancer Cytopathol. 2014;122(10):737–44.
57. McIver B, Castro MR, Morris JC, Bernet V, Smallridge R, Henry M, et al. An independent study of a gene expression classifier (Afirma) in the evaluation of cytologically indeterminate thyroid nodules. J Clin Endocrinol Metab. 2014;99(11):4069–77.
58. Brauner E, Holmes BJ, Krane JF, Nishino M, Zurakowski D, Hennessey JV, et al. Performance of the Afirma gene expression classifier in Hürthle cell thyroid nodules differs from other indeterminate thyroid nodules. Thyroid. 2015;25(7):789–96.
59. Marti JL, Avadhani V, Donatelli LA, Niyogi S, Wang B, Wong RJ, et al. Wide inter-institutional variation in performance of a molecular classifier for indeterminate thyroid nodules. Ann Surg Oncol. 2015;22(12):3996–4001.
60. Nikiforov YE, Ohori NP, Hodak SP, Carty SE, LeBeau SO, Ferris RL, et al. Impact of mutational testing on the diagnosis and management of patients with cytologically indeterminate thyroid nodules: a prospective analysis of 1056 FNA samples. J Clin Endocrinol Metab. 2011;96(11):3390–7.
61. Beaudenon-Huibregtse S, Alexander EK, Guttler RB, Hershman JM, Babu V, Blevins TC, et al. Centralized molecular testing for oncogenic gene mutations complements the local cytopathologic diagnosis of thyroid nodules. Thyroid. 2014;24(10):1479–87.
62. Cantara S, Capezzone M, Marchisotta S, Capuano S, Busonero G, Toti P, et al. Impact of proto-oncogene mutation detection in cytological specimens from thyroid nodules improves the diagnostic accuracy of cytology. J Clin Endocrinol Metab. 2010;95(3):1365–9.
63. Eszlinger M, Krogdahl A, Münz S, Rehfeld C, Precht Jensen EM, Ferraz C, et al. Impact of molecular screening for point mutations and rearrangements in routine air-dried fine-needle aspiration samples of thyroid nodules. Thyroid. 2014;24(2):305–13.
64. Eszlinger M, Piana S, Moll A, Bösenberg E, Bisagni A, Ciarrocchi A, et al. Molecular testing of thyroid fine-needle aspirations improves presurgical diagnosis and supports the histologic identification of minimally invasive follicular thyroid carcinomas. Thyroid. 2015;25(4):401–9.
65. Labourier E, Shifrin A, Busseniers AE, Lupo MA, Manganelli ML, Andruss B, et al. Molecular testing for miRNA, mRNA, and DNA on fine-needle aspiration improves the preoperative diagnosis of thyroid nodules with indeterminate cytology. J Clin Endocrinol Metab. 2015;100(7):2743–50.
66. Krane JF, Cibas ES, Alexander EK, Paschke R, Eszlinger M. Molecular analysis of residual ThinPrep material from thyroid FNAs increases diagnostic sensitivity. Cancer Cytopathol. 2015;123(6):356–61.
67. Nikiforov YE, Carty SE, Chiosea SI, Coyne C, Duvvuri U, Ferris RL, et al. Highly accurate diagnosis of cancer in thyroid nodules with follicular neoplasm/suspicious for a follicular neoplasm cytology by ThyroSeq v2 next-generation sequencing assay. Cancer. 2014;120(23):3627–34.
68. Kolata G. It's Not Cancer: Doctors Reclassify a Thyroid Tumor. The New York Times [Internet]. 2016. https://www.nytimes.com/2016/04/15/health/thyroid-tumor-cancer-reclassification.html. Accessed 3 Mar 2017.
69. Thompson LD. Ninety-four cases of encapsulated follicular variant of papillary thyroid carcinoma: a name change to noninvasive follicular thyroid neoplasm with papillary-like nuclear features would help prevent overtreatment. Mod Pathol. 2016;29(7):698–707.
70. Xu B, Tallini G, Scognamiglio T, Roman BR, Tuttle RM, Ghossein R. Outcome of large noninvasive follicular thyroid neoplasm with papillary-like nuclear features (NIFTP). Thyroid. 2017;27(4):512–7.
71. Strickland KC, Howitt BE, Marqusee E, Alexander EK, Cibas ES, Krane JF, et al. The impact of noninvasive follicular variant of papillary thyroid carcinoma on rates of malignancy for fine-needle aspiration diagnostic categories. Thyroid. 2015;25(9):987–92.
72. Faquin WC, Wong LQ, Afrogheh AH, Ali SZ, Bishop JA, Bongiovanni M, et al. Impact of reclassifying noninvasive follicular variant of papillary thyroid carcinoma on the risk of malignancy in The Bethesda System for Reporting Thyroid Cytopathology. Cancer Cytopathol. 2016;124(3):181–7.
73. Maletta F, Massa F, Torregrossa L, Duregon E, Casadei GP, Basolo F, et al. Cytological features of "noninvasive follicular thyroid neoplasm with papillary-like nuclear features" and their correlation with tumor histology. Hum Pathol. 2016;54:134–42.
74. Hahn SY, Shin JH, Lim HK, Jung SL, Oh YL, Choi IH, et al. Preoperative differentiation between noninvasive follicular thyroid neoplasm with papillary-like nuclear features (NIFTP) and non-NIFTP. Clin Endocrinol (Oxf). 2017;86(3):444–50.
75. Krane JF, Alexander EK, Cibas ES, Barletta JA. Coming to terms with NIFTP: a provisional approach for cytologists. Cancer. 2016;124(11):767–72.
76. Baloch ZW, Seethala RR, Faquin WC, Papotti MG, Basolo F, Fadda G, et al. Noninvasive follicular thyroid neoplasm with papillary-like nuclear features (NIFTP): a changing paradigm in thyroid surgical pathology and implications for thyroid cytopathology. Cancer Cytopathol. 2016;124(9):616–20.
77. Jeon MJ, Song DE, Jung CK, Kim WG, Kwon H, Lee Y-M, et al. Impact of reclassification on thyroid nodules with architectural atypia: from non-invasive encapsulated follicular variant papillary thyroid carcinomas to non-invasive follicular thyroid neoplasm with papillary-like nuclear features. PLoS One. 2016;11(12):e0167756.
78. Rosario PW, Mourão GF, Nunes MB, Nunes MS, Calsolari MR. Noninvasive follicular thyroid neo-

plasm with papillary-like nuclear features. Endocr Relat Cancer. 2016;23(12):893–7.
79. Zhao L, Dias-Santagata D, Sadow PM, Faquin WC. Cytological, molecular, and clinical features of noninvasive follicular thyroid neoplasm with papillary-like nuclear features versus invasive forms of follicular variant of papillary thyroid carcinoma. Cancer. 2017;125(5):323–31.

Imaging in Differentiated Thyroid Cancer

7

Sabaretnam Mayilvaganan, Aromal Chekavar, Roma Pradhan, and Amit Agarwal

It cannot be overemphasized that manual palpation of thyroid nodules is extremely variable between even experienced clinicians and as such imaging with ultrasound, especially surgeon-performed ultrasound, has become essential to the evaluation of the thyroid gland. Surgeon-performed ultrasound is rapidly becoming an extension of the physical examination, adding images containing objective information to the subjective palpation by the surgeon's hands. Various imaging tools play key roles in various phases in treatment of thyroid cancer. Various imaging modalities comprise of:

- High-resolution ultrasonography
- Contrast-enhanced computerized tomography
- Magnetic resonance tomography
- Radioiodine scans
- Positron emission tomography

Selection of appropriate modality in appropriate time is of paramount importance in thyroid carcinoma management.

The initial application of sonography for the evaluation of the neck, more than 30 years ago, was to differentiate cystic and solid thyroid nodules. With improvements in technology, ultrasound has been applied to characterize distinct features in the appearance of thyroid nodules. More recently, its function has been expanded to assess cervical lymph nodes for metastatic thyroid cancer. Most recent guidelines by the ATA, US is the imaging study of choice for characterization of thyroid nodules, surveillance of multinodular goiter, and preoperative evaluation in known DTC [1]. Even though USG can be used to do cervical lymph node staging in patient with palpable cervical lymph node, USG will miss mediastinal and retropharyngeal regions, so cross-sectional imaging will be more appropriate in these cases.

Ultrasound Imaging of Thyroid Nodules

When examined by ultrasound, rather than by palpation, thyroid nodules are commonly detected with a prevalence of 40–50% in the general population [2]. However, only 5–10% of thyroid nodules are malignant, even if found incidentally; while fine-needle aspiration is the cornerstone of the evaluation of thyroid nodules, ultrasound contributes significantly both to identify and to evaluate thyroid nodules. Multiple reports have examined the sonographic features of thyroid nodules as predictors of malignancy

S. Mayilvaganan · A. Chekavar · A. Agarwal (✉)
Department of Endocrine Surgery, Sanjay Gandhi Post Graduate Institute of Medical Sciences, Lucknow, India

R. Pradhan
Department of Endocrine Surgery, Dr Ram Manohar Lohia Institute of Medical Sciences, Lucknow, India

R. Parameswaran, A. Agarwal (eds.), *Evidence-Based Endocrine Surgery*,
https://doi.org/10.1007/978-981-10-1124-5_7

list the reported sensitivities and specificities of these features from 11 studies that analyzed over 100 nodules. Unfortunately, there is significant variability among these studies because of differing methodologies and because report of ultrasound features is highly operator dependent [3].

The echogenicity of a thyroid nodule is its brightness relative to the normal thyroid parenchyma or which is homogeneously hyperechoic compared with the surrounding strap muscles of the neck. Hypoechoic nodules are darker than the surrounding normal thyroid tissue. Hypoechogenecity results from the increased cellularity and cellular compaction seen in papillary thyroid cancer [4]. But in follicular neoplasm, either a benign follicular adenoma or follicular carcinoma is composed of small microfollicles with variable amounts of colloid. Therefore, the echogenicity of follicular carcinomas may depend on the colloid content and images as more hyperechoic [5]. Fifty-five percent of nodules have some cystic composition which requires identification of the solid component to determine echogenicity.

The vascularity of a thyroid nodule is demonstrated with color flow Doppler (CFD) or power Doppler (PD) imaging. CFD is a measure of the directional component of the velocity of blood moving through the sample volume [6]. The technical issue of CFD includes interference by noise and dependence on the angle of the probe. PD imaging is relatively independent of the angle of the probe, and the sound beam and noise can be assigned to a homogeneous background rather than appearing as random color, and since PD does not reflect directional flow, it is more sensitive for the detection of flow in small vessels. Nodule vascularity is categorized as absent, perinodular, or intranodular. Using PD, some authors have further subdivided intranodular flow into regular versus chaotic patterns. Increased intranodular flow is associated with malignancy and has good interobserver variability (Figs. 7.1, 7.2, 7.3, and 7.4).

Calcifications are noted up to 30% of thyroid nodules. Microcalcifications image as echogenic foci smaller than 2 mm and are associated with malignancy. The interobserver variability for the identification of microcalcifications is very good. Microcalcifications are thought to represent aggregates of psammoma bodies, the laminated spherical concretions characteristic of many papillary cancers, and are rarely found in benign nodules or follicular neoplastic lesions. Coarse or dense calcifications are larger than 2 mm and cause posterior acoustic shadowing. These

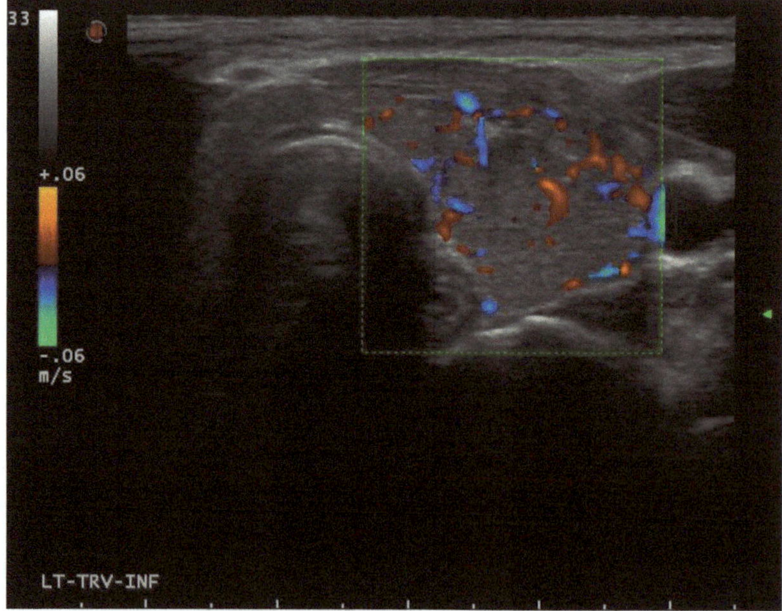

Fig. 7.1 High Resolution Ultrasound thyroid showing thyroid nodule with increased vascularity

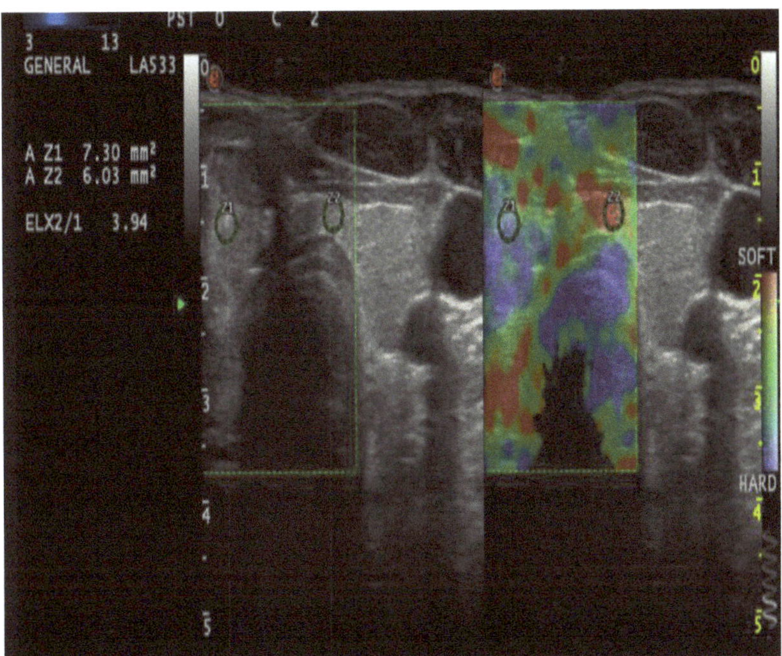

Fig. 7.2 Strain-Elastography of the thyroid nodule showing comparison between Normal lobe and the nodule

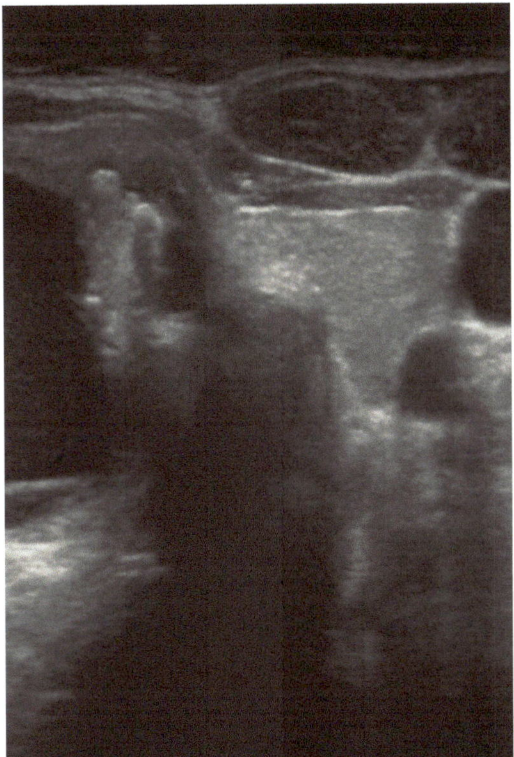

Fig. 7.3 High Resolution Ultrasound of thyroid showing isthumic hypoechoic lesion with illdefined border and microcalcification

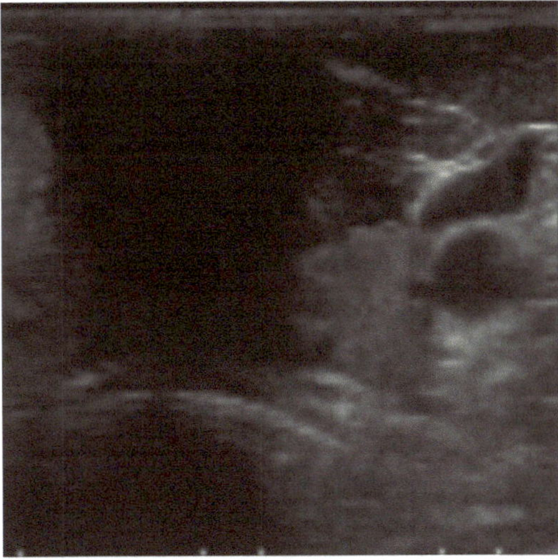

Fig. 7.4 High Resolution Ultrasound of thyroid showing hypoechoic lesion with illdefined borders

dystrophic calcifications occur in both benign and malignant lesions in areas of fibrosis, tissue degeneration, and necrosis. Coarse calcifications may be associated with malignancy nodules. Peripheral calcifications surround a thyroid nodule and were once thought to indicate a benign process. However, this finding can be seen in malignant nodules, sometimes with interruption of the circumferential calcific rim that suggests malignant invasion of thyroid parenchyma. Coarse calcifications are associated with malignancy when they appear with microcalcifications or in the center of a hypoechoic nodule [7].

The margins of a thyroid nodule can be regular and well defined or irregular and microlobulated, and interobserver variability for classification of nodule borders is the greatest of all sonographic features. Irregular margins are seen with invasion of a malignant nodule into the surrounding thyroid parenchyma. The irregular margin is less commonly observed with encapsulated as a thin hypoechoic rim that surround a nodule and is thought to represent compression of the extranodular blood vessels as a benign nodule slowly grows. An invasive malignancy, such as unencapsulated papillary cancer of medullary cancer, lacks a halo. However, follicular and Hurthle cell adenomas and cancers are surrounded by a fibrous avascular capsule. This capsule images sonographically as a thick, irregular hypoechoic rim, which is now recognized as a more worrisome, second type of halo. Hypoechoic rims are more frequent for follicular cancers (87%) rather than for papillary cancers (26% $P < 0.05$) [8].

Other additional sonographic features of thyroid nodules that have been shown to be associated with are shape of the nodule by looking at the ratio of the anteroposterior to transverse diameter (A/T). When the A/T ratio is greater than 1.0, indicating a spherical nodule, Cappelli and colleagues found that this kind of detected thyroid cancer has a sensitivity of 84% and a specificity of 82%, but these require further validation studies [9]. Tissue stiffness is a risk factor for malignancy in a subset of nodules with indeterminate cytology using a technique called elastography. High elasticity scores, indicating stiffness, point toward malignant histology and low scores to benign lesions. Finally, extrathyroidal invasion may be occasionally seen when the tumor growth extends through either the anterior or posterior thyroid capsule, which normally appears as a bright white outline surrounding the thyroid. In such instances, the margin of the tumor has an ill-defined edge that interrupts this capsule. Because individual sonographic feature has limited utility in predicting malignancy, some series have explored the association of combinations of features with cancer risk. In most series, as the specificity of a combination increases, the sensitivity decreases. But sonographic features with high-risk characteristics of malignancy can be selected for FNAC. The combination of sonographic features that maximizes sensitivity and specificity is a solid, hypoechoic nodule, which identifies approximately 70% of all cancers but still describes the appearance of 30% of benign nodules. Additionally, as many as 66% of papillary thyroid cancers have at least one sonographic feature not typically associated with malignancy, and 69% of benign nodules have one sonographic predictor of malignancy. Decision-making for FNA based on suspicious sonographic features of hypoechogenicity, microcalcifications, irregular margins, or increased vascularity is superior to using an arbitrary size cutoff of larger than 1 cm. In hypoechoic, solid small nodules, with or without microcalcifications, it is critical to examine the ipsilateral cervical lymph nodes for metastases. If an abnormal lymph node is present, it is this lymph node that should be targeted for FNA.

Lymph Nodes

In addition to providing excellent imaging for thyroid nodules, high-frequency (10–14 MHz) ultrasound transducers allow for high-resolution imaging of small anatomic structures such as cervical lymph nodes. Of the approximately 800 lymph nodes in the human body, about 300 are located in the neck, varying in size from 3 to 30 mm. Most neck lymph nodes are located superficially and are accessible to ultrasound imaging. Because of the frequent metastatic involvement of these lymph nodes by differentiated thyroid cancer (DTC), specifically papillary or Hurthle cell carcinoma, for these DTC patients, ultrasound provides an inexpensive and available means both to evaluate the lateral cervical lymph nodes before thyroidectomy and to monitor for recurrence in the central and lateral compartment lymph nodes and in the thyroid bed. In addition, ultrasound can also be a complementary modality in the surveillance of medullary thyroid cancer. For imaging the cervical neck lymph nodes, a hyperextended neck position facilitates visualization of the low level IV and VI lymph nodes, and a pillow may be placed under the patient's neck for support. The procedure for examining the lateral compartment regions of the neck is to orient the transducer in the transverse plane. The transducer is placed over the submandibular gland and then moved inferiorly along the external carotid artery to the bifurcation of the common carotid artery. It is then centered over the jugulocarotid sheath and moved inferiorly until the carotid is visualized joining the subclavian artery on the right or disappears under the clavicle to enter the aortic arch on the left. The supraclavicular fossa and posterior triangle of the neck (level V) are then examined by moving the probe laterally along the supraclavicular region and then posteriorly and superiorly to the mastoid region along the course of the imputed track of the spinal accessory nerve, which approximates the posterior edge of the sternocleidomastoid muscle. For imaging the central neck, the transducer is placed in transverse orientation above the tracheal cartilage at the approximate level of the hyoid bone and moved inferiorly along the anterior border of the trachea to the sternal notch. The more focused examination of the left and right paratracheal regions requires centering the probe between the trachea and respective carotid artery just inferior to the tracheal cartilage and scanning inferiorly to the sternal notch. Longitudinal imaging should be performed for any identified abnormal lymph node.

Ultrasound Imaging of Normal and Metastatic Lymph Nodes

Normal lymph node morphology is characterized by a connective tissue capsule surrounding an outer cortex with the densely packed lymphocytes forming lymphoid follicles and an inner medulla containing the blood vessel, lymphatic sinuses, and connective tissue that provide guidance for the blood vessels to the more peripheral regions of the lymph node. The main artery to the lymph node enters at this central hilus and subsequently branches into smaller arterioles as it flows to the cortex. The frequency of lymph node detection did not vary based on age, gender, or even recent infection. Therefore, since detection of normal cervical lymph nodes is common and thyroid cancer often metastasizes to these same lymph nodes, it is essential to appreciate the different imaging characteristics of benign and malignant lymph nodes.

The evaluated parameters should include:

1. Size
2. Shape
3. Presence of an echogenic hilus
4. Hypoechoic cortex
5. Vascularity
6. Echogenicity
7. Cystic change and calcifications

Therefore, since detection of normal cervical lymph nodes is common and thyroid cancer often metastasizes to these same lymph nodes, it is essential to appreciate the different imaging characteristics of benign and malignant lymph nodes. The size of normal lymph nodes may vary depending on neck region, with submandibular or level II lymph nodes tending to be larger, perhaps due to reactive hyperplasia from repeated oral cavity inflammation. Furthermore, thyroid cancer patients with radioiodine-induced sialadenitis may also develop large hyperplastic level II lymph nodes found in the submandibular and parotid regions. Large reactive lymph nodes in this area may exhibit a long axis measurement of up to 18 mm. The short axis diameter varies less, and the maximal short axis for a normal lymph node is reported to be 8 mm in level II and less than 5 mm in the other cervical regions.

The shape of a lymph node is assessed in numerical terms by the short-to-long axis ratio (S:L). A normal lymph node is oval, which translates into an S:L less than 0.5. Since neoplastic infiltration of lymph node begins in the cortex, malignant lymph nodes generally have a larger transverse diameter and a rounder shape, with an S:L of 0.5 or higher. A round shape is suggestive of malignancy, but its specificity may depend on the region of the neck. Submandibular and parotid lymph nodes may be round, as defined by the S:L. Furthermore, round reactive central neck lymph nodes just inferior to the thyroid are often imaged in patients with chronic autoimmune thyroiditis. Sonographic imaging of a normal lymph node demonstrates an echogenic central hilus surrounded by a hypoechoic cortex. The echogenic hilus is more commonly present in larger (>5 mm transverse diameter) rather than smaller lymph nodes. The echogenicity reflects two features: intranodal fatty tissue, which becomes more prominent with age, and the presence of intranodal arteries, veins, and lymphatic sinuses presenting acoustic interfaces that reflect sound waves. The likelihood of visualizing the fatty hilus increases with age reflecting the increased fatty deposition. Thyroid cancer metastases to lymph nodes begin with peripheral neoplastic infiltration and subsequent loss of the hypoechoic cortex that may be replaced by a hyperechoic appearance. Early in the nodal invasion by thyroid cancer, the echogenic hilus may be preserved, and the malignant cells are apparent as a small peripheral hyperechoic area in the otherwise normal hypoechoic cortex. As the lymph node is progressively replaced by thyroid cancer, it assumes a more heterogeneous appearance and may demonstrate intranodal calcifications (both in papillary and medullary cancer) and cystic necrosis. Because metastatic lymph nodes in levels II to IV are situated adjacent to the carotid and jugular vessels, jugular compression or displacement of the jugular vein from the carotid artery suggests malignancy.

Color or power Doppler examination of cervical lymph nodes allows for determination of vascularity patterns. To maximize sensitivity, Doppler settings should use both a low wall filter and a pulse repetition frequency of 850 Hz or lower to allow detection of low-flow vessels. Since hilar vascularity is detected in about 90% of normal lymph nodes with a transverse diameter larger than 5 mm and smaller normal lymph nodes which usually appear avascular. Capillaries arising from these hilar vessels feed the nodal cortex. Interestingly, the detection rate of hilar vascularity is higher in the elderly, which is thought to be caused by decreased vessel compressibility because of higher vessel stiffness in this group. Furthermore, reactive lymph nodes may have prominent hilar vascularity because of both increased blood flow and vessel diameter. In malignant lymph nodes, the vascular pattern is either peripheral or diffuse (hilar and peripheral), often with irregular distribution. The increase in peripheral nodal vascularity occurs because of initial deposition of the malignant cells in the marginal sinuses and the tumor-induced angiogenesis causes subsequent neovascularization. As tumor infiltration proceeds, increased vascularity is apparent throughout the lymph node. Currently, the role of vascular resistance indices for determination of metastatic lymph node involvement is not well defined. Newer modalities like sonoelastography help differentiate malignant from benign lymph nodes based on their relatively higher tissue stiffness. This technique is relatively time intensive involving over 30 min of post-data acquisition analysis and requires further validation; therefore, its current applicability is limited of cystic areas (100%), presence of hyperechoic punctations representing either colloid or microcalcifications (100%), and peripheral vascularity (82%). Of these, the only one with sufficient sensitivity was peripheral vascularity (86%). All of the others had sensitivities less than 60% and would not be adequate to use as a single criterion for identification of malignant involvement. As shown by earlier studies, the feature with the highest sensitivity was absence of a hilus (100%), but this had a low specificity of only 29%.Therefore, a reasonable approach to identify suspicious lymph nodes for further investigation would be to submit those without a fatty hilus to a careful Doppler examination for evaluation of vascularity. Peripheral or diffuse vascularization is worrisome. However, a rounded shape, an absent hilus, and heterogeneous echogenicity raise the suspicion of malignancy, especially when they coexist in the same lymph node. Last lymph nodes with cystic change or microcalcifications should be considered as metastatic thyroid cancer [10].

Ultrasonography Adjuncts

Thyroid Imaging Reporting and Data System

"Thyroid imaging reporting and data system" is proposed for the first time by Horvath et al. (2009).

TI-RADS assessment is based on five high-risk characteristics:

1. Hypoechoic
2. Taller than wider
3. Irregular margins
4. Microcalcification
5. Predominantly solid

   Based on the abovementioned findings, suspicious US features were classified as:

TI-RADS category 3 (no suspicious features)
TI-RADS category 4a (with one suspicious US feature)
TI-RADS category 4b (with two suspicious US features)
TI-RADS category 4c (with three or four suspicious US features)
TI-RADS category 5 (with five suspicious US features), respectively

The malignancy risks of categories 3, 4a, 4b, 4c, and 5 nodules were 0% (0/9), 4.0% 131 (1/25), 12.5% (4/32), 62.2% (28/45), and 100% (10/10), respectively ($P < 0.001$) [11, 12].

Elastography

Elastography is a newer technique to evaluate stiffness of lesion and compare it from normal tissue. It is also considered as "electronic palpation" of thyroid nodule. Clinical application of thyroid elastography was first reported in 2007 by Rago et al. [13]. There are two types of elastography strain and shear wave elastography.

- Strain *use*
  - Tissues are deformed mechanically by the operator.
  - Relative displacement (strain) is greater in soft compared to stiff tissues.
- Shear wave elastography
  - Focused acoustic impulses from the transducer induce laterally propagating shear waves
  - Whose velocities are higher in stiffer tissues

Elastography reported as different patterns

- Pattern 1: the entire nodule section is diffusely elastic
- Pattern 2: the formation appears to be largely elastic with the inconstant appearance of anelastic areas during the real-time examination
- Pattern 3: constant presence of large anelastic areas is seen at the periphery (Pattern 3A) or center (Pattern 3B) of the formation
- Pattern 4: uniformly displayed anelasticity throughout the whole nodule

- Lesions that present Pattern 1 or 2 are classified as probably benign, while Patterns 3 and 4 are indicative of probable malignancy

Assessment of strain ratio will also help in risk assessment in thyroid nodule.

- Strain ratio is calculated as the ratio of stiffness between nodular tissue and surrounding normal thyroid.
  - ELX Ratio or SR = Z2/Z1
  - Z2 = strain value of nodular tissue
  - Z1 = strain value of normal thyroid
  - ELXR/SR >3 high probability of malignancy

Clinical Scenarios for Ultrasound Lymph Node Evaluation Pre-thyroidectomy

At initial diagnosis of DTC, up to 30% of patients have clinically detected lymph node metastases. However, centers performing routine ipsilateral and central neck dissections have documented lymph node metastases in up to 60% of patients. Before thyroidectomy, the thyroid itself limits sonographic visualization of central neck lymph nodes, but level VI lymph nodes inferior to the lower lobes of the thyroid can be assessed. Ultrasound can evaluate the lateral neck compartments. Although the reported sensitivity for sonographic identification of metastatic lymph nodes in this setting may only be about 40%, ultrasound-detectable lymphadenopathy is clinically relevant. Sonographically identified lateral metastatic lymph nodes, but not those recognized microscopically only after pathologic examination of the resected specimen, are associated with worse relapse-free and overall survival.

Surveillance for Recurrent Differentiated Thyroid Cancer

The primary goal of follow-up in DTC patients is the early discovery of persistent or recurrent disease. The overall risk of local recurrence of papillary thyroid cancer, either in cervical lymph nodes or in the thyroid bed, is up to 30% but is as high as 25% even in low-risk (stage I and II) patients. In the past, a radioiodine whole-body scan was considered the main tool for disease detection during surveillance, but this has recently been discredited. Three studies have confirmed that whole-body scans fail to identify the presence of metastatic cervical lymph nodes in almost 80% of cases when neck sonography accurately detects these abnormal lymph nodes. The American Thyroid Association DTC Guidelines suggest that "cervical ultrasound to evaluate the thyroid bed and central and lateral cervical nodal compartments should be performed at 6 and 12 months and then annually for at least 3–5 years, depending on the patients' risk for recurrent disease and thyroglobulin status" and the distribution of persistent or recurrent lymph node metastases is most commonly the central compartment (35–50%), followed by the ipsilateral lateral neck (20–30%). Only rarely (8–15%) is the contralateral lateral neck compartment involved. Within the levels of the lateral neck, a recent study reported that the pattern of metastatic lymph node involvement was approximately 50% for levels II and III, 40% for level IV, and only 20% for level V.

Computed Tomography and Magnetic Resonance Imaging Role in Thyroid Cancer

Whereas ultrasound is the imaging study of choice in evaluation of the thyroid gland, CT also has an important role. Even though high-resolution ultrasound can be accurate in preoperative evaluation for extrathyroidal tumor extension and lateral lymph node metastasis, contrast-enhanced CT scan had greater sensitivity than ultrasound alone in the detection of central lymph node metastasis for all lesions [14]. CT is best used as an adjunct modality in imaging advanced thyroid pathology when there is substernal, intrathoracic, or retrotracheal pathology/ extension of the gland suspected. As noted earlier areas in which ultrasound imaging is limited as a result of acoustic distortion because of bone or air. In these situations, a CT scan can be very helpful in the preoperative assessment, discerning the development of lymphadenopathy as well as determining invasion/compression of the aerodigestive tracts. Magnetic resonance imaging can perform the same imaging as CT although at a much higher cost. CT scan is a common mechanism for the discovery of incidental thyroid nodules. According to prior studies, 16% of cervical or thoracic CT scans will yield a diagnosis of an incidental thyroid nodule [15]. However, although CT scans are good at detecting thyroid nodules, they have several pitfalls. First, CT can often underestimate the size of nodules. According to ATA Guidelines, preoperative use of cross-sectional imaging studies (CT, MRI) with intravenous (IV) contrast is recommended as an adjunct to US for patients with clinical suspicion for advanced disease, including invasive primary tumor, or clinically apparent multiple or bulky lymph node involvement [16] (Fig. 7.5).

Risk factors for thyroid cancer based on history and physical examination which necessitates CECT/MRI are:

- Prior personal history of thyroid cancer
- Family history of thyroid cancer, including papillary and medullary thyroid cancer (multiple endocrine neoplasia syndrome, type IIA and IIB)
- History of head and neck or upper chest radiation exposure
- Fixed palpable mass in the thyroid gland
- Palpable cervical lymphadenopathy in a patient with a thyroid nodule
- Hoarseness of the voice (representing invasion of the recurrent laryngeal nerve)

Important radiological signs to look for in CECT and MRI [17–20] are best seen by the three-step check list:

- ***Central structures around which the thyroid normally drapes***
  - Trachea, esophagus, larynx, pharynx, and RLN
- Esophagus: deformity of lumen, focal mucosal irregularity, mucosal thickening, surrounds the circumference > 180°
- RLN: invasion of RLN can be predicted by effaced fatty tissue inT-0 groove for >3 axial images and signs of VC dysfunction
- ***Structures immediately surrounding thyroid gland***
- Vascular structures, strap muscles, prevertebral space.
- IJV (can be occluded or effaced by tumor without invasion).
- Arteries are more resistant to compression.

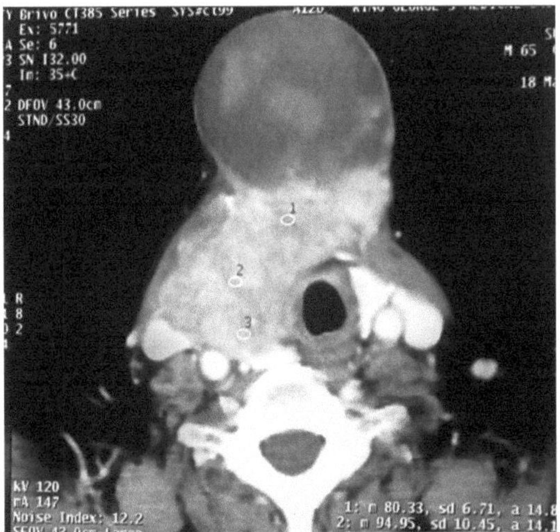

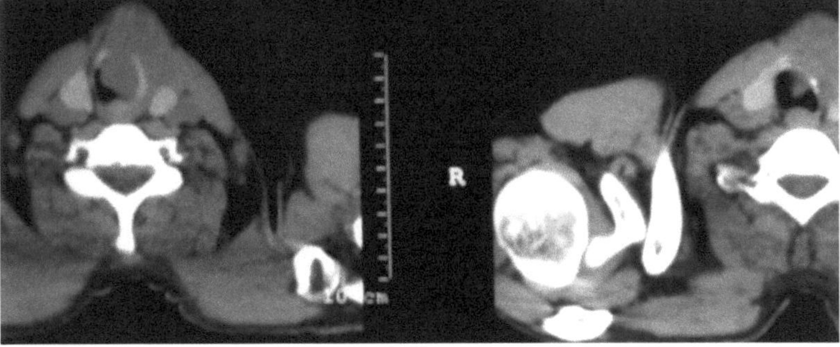

Fig. 7.5 CECT Scan findings. A: Exophytic Thyroid lobe arising from Left lobe of thyroid, B: Locally advanced thyroid cancer with intraluminal extension, C:Intraluminal Extension of thyroid cancer (polypoidal growth)

- Another sign of invasion is tumor contacting the circumference of the artery by >180°.
- Carotid artery, mediastinal vessels should also be assessed.
- If invaded it becomes T4b disease.
- Best sign of strap muscle invasion is asymmetry and tumor on external surface of the muscle.
- Prevertebral musculature invasion is more difficult to evaluate because large tumors can compress the muscle and even result in signal changes on MR imaging without invasion.
- ***Assessment of metastatic disease***
- LN
- Lungs
- Bone

CECT
Tracheal infiltration signs are:

- ≥180° circumferential contact
- Lumen deformity
- Mucosal abnormality

Esophagus

- ≥180° circumferential contact
- Abnormal wall or lumen

Recurrent laryngeal nerve

- Effaced fatty tissue in tracheoesophageal groove
- >25% of tumor abutting posterior portion of the thyroid
- Signs of ipsilateral vocal cord palsy

Carotid and IJV

- ≥180° circumferential contact

MRI
Tracheal infiltration signs are:

- ≥180° circumferential contact
- Soft tissue signal in cartilage
- Intraluminal mass

Esophagus infiltration sign is:

- Outer layer invasion

RLN infiltration sign is:

- Effaced fatty tissue in tracheoesophageal groove on at least one axial image

Carotid and IJV infiltration sign is:

- Circumferential encasement

Key Points for CT Scan Detected Incidental Thyroid Nodules

- 16% of all cervical and thoracic CT scans will identify an incidental thyroid nodule.
- CT scans do not reliably predict the correct size or number of thyroid nodules.
- The risk of malignancy in an incidentally discovered thyroid nodule (found by CT) is 3.9–11.3%.
- Incidental thyroid nodules found on CT scan should undergo a dedicated thyroid US and referral to an endocrine specialist.

CECT	Sensitivity	Specificity
CECT trachea	59	91
Esophagus	29	96
RLN	78	90
Carotid vessels	75	99
IJV	33	99
MRI trachea	100	84
Esophagus	82	94
RLN	94	82
Carotid vessels	100	88
IJV	–	–

Limitations of CECT are:

CECT may overestimate or underestimate the number of thyroid nodules. In a 3-year study (1998–2001), Shetty and colleagues examined all cervical and thoracic CT scans performed at the Massachusetts General Hospital in Boston. They identified 230 patients with a CT-based thyroid abnormality that subsequently underwent thyroid

US. They found that CECT scan findings agreed with US for lesion size only 53% of the time; CECT identified the dominant nodule but missed multinodularity 30% of the time and had a false positive identification of a thyroid nodule 4.3% of the time. Other limitations of CECT include "CECT scans of the chest often do not image the entire thyroid gland" (thus a false negative for nodules may occur); routine CT cuts of 3–5 mm may miss lesions; and during chest CECT, patients arms are positioned over the head, which often results in beam hardening artifacts in the thyroid." Nonetheless, CECT is the most likely radiographic test to detect incidental thyroid nodules. In regard to CECT's ability to detect malignancy in a thyroid nodule, Shetty and colleagues found that the overall risk of malignancy based on CECT identification of an incidental nodule was 3.9–11.3% [21].

Therefore, although CT is a common mechanism for detecting incidental thyroid nodules, it is quite limited, by itself, in measuring nodule size accurately, predicting the correct number of thyroid nodules, or assessing for the risk of malignancy. Therefore it is currently recommended that incidental thyroid nodules discovered on CT scan should undergo a dedicated thyroid US and referral to an endocrine specialist (endocrine surgeon, endocrinologist, ENT, or general surgeons with high-volume practices of thyroid disease) to determine the next step in nodule evaluation. Finally CT scan plays a role in the evaluation of thyroid disease, but should not be used as a "screening tool" for thyroid nodules for many of the reasons listed above. The role of CT scan in thyroid disease is generally confined to (1) evaluation of the extent of substernal goiters for surgical planning (need for sternotomy, intubation risks); (2) assessment of large thyroid cancers suspicious for local invasion into the trachea, great vessels, and others that again may alter surgical planning or extent of resection; (3) stating of thyroid cancer and looking for metastatic disease; and (4) follow-up evaluation of the thyroid bed or lymph nodes after thyroidectomy for cancer (may be used as an adjunct to neck US).

Evidence-Based Discussion on Intravenous Iodinated Contrast on RAI

Iodinated Contrast

The quantity of iodine from iodinated contrast is huge when compared to iodine in normal duet. 100 mL of intravenous contrast contains at best 150 mg of iodine per ml of contrast. When exposed to such magnitude of load, body stores of iodine in interstitial fluids, in colloid and other organs are expanded. This is a major hued when a patient is prepared for I-131 therapy or a radioiodine scan. Theoretically iodine-rich diet and iodine contrast medium in imaging procedures skew radioactive iodine scan testing significantly [22–26].

S. No.	Authors	Title	Patients	Recommendations
1.	Nimmons Grace L[22]	Urinary iodine excretion after contrastcomputed tomography scan	21 patients Level 4	Normalized 43 days
2.	Seo Young Sohn[23]	The impact of iodinated contrast agent administeredduring preoperative computed tomography scan on bodyIodine pool in patients with differentiated thyroid cancerpreparing for radioactive iodine treatment	1023 patients Level 6	1–3 months
3.	Rosa' lia P. Padovani[24]	One month is sufficientfor urinary iodine to return to its baseline valueafter the use of water-soluble iodinated contrast agentsin post-thyroidectomy patients requiring radioiodine therapy	25 patients Level 4	1 month
4.	Anjali Mishra[25]	Preoperative contrast-enhanced computerizedtomography should not delay radioiodine ablationin differentiated thyroid carcinoma patients	32 patients Level 4	4 to 6 weeks
5.	Sun Y. Lee[26]	Urinary iodine excretion and serum thyroid functionin adults after iodinated contrast administration	54 patients Level 4	Normalized 5.2 weeks

PET CT Scan in Thyroid Carcinoma

PET scan is commonly performed as cancer surveillance and staging tools. Thus the finding of an incidental thyroid nodule can be a source of stress for patients already diagnosed with another primary malignancy. Fluorodeoxyglucose or FDG-PET relies on the principle that tissue with a high metabolic demand (cancer, inflammation, infection) will uptake more of the tracer. PET scan uptake patterns for thyroid disease generally come in two forms. The first form is diffuse uptake throughout the thyroid gland. This uptake is generally representative of thyroiditis or Graves' disease. As such, this pattern generally indicates benign disease of the thyroid. The second pattern of uptake is that of a solitary focus that corresponds to a nodule in the thyroid and raises suspicion for malignancy.

Although the prevalence of incidental thyroid nodules found on CT scan is 16% as outlined above, the prevalence of thyroid nodules discovered on PET scan is much lower. A large meta-analysis recently reviewed 22 articles pertaining to PET and thyroid nodules. Of more than 125,000 patients who underwent FDG-PET for varying indications, only 1.6% had a thyroid incidentaloma discovered. Despite the lower overall incidence of thyroid nodules found during PET scan (compared with CT scan), there is much greater concern of malignancy, based on the pattern of tracer uptake. As mentioned above, diffuse uptake on PET scan is much more consistent with benign disease and has been demonstrated in multiple studies, including a large US-based study and a large Korean study that included more than 5000 patients each. A diffuse uptake pattern only yielded a rate of malignancy of 4.4%, which is again almost identical to palpable nodules at 5%. However, focal uptake has been found to correlate with a cancer rate of 30–50% in most studies and was 34.8% in the meta-analysis.

Our current recommendation for the evaluation of the thyroid incidentaloma detected by PET scan are a detailed history and a physical examination (looking for risk factors for cancer, such as radiation exposure, family history of thyroid cancer), thyroid function testing (including anti-TPO antibody to look for thyroiditis manifesting as diffuse uptake on PET), and a dedicated thyroid US with FNABx. The American Thyroid Association Guidelines, as mentioned above, dictate that nodules greater than 1 cm in size be biopsied. However, they also include a suggestion that lesions less than 1 cm in size with atypical or worrisome characteristics should be considered for biopsy. As such, in the setting of an isolated nodules detected by positive PET scan, biopsy can be considered even at a size less than 1 cm due to the high risk of malignancy.

Key Points for PET Scan Detected Incidental Thyroid Nodules

- The prevalence of thyroid incidentalomas found during PET scan is 1.6%.
- Risk of malignancy in a PET thyroid incidentaloma varies with PET uptake pattern but is highest with a solitary uptake pattern (30%–50%).
- Decreasing the biopsy size threshold for focal PET and thyroid incidentalomas should be considered.

Summary

- Excessive work-up of ITN is a costly healthcare problem. Three-tiered system can be used to guide the evaluation of ITN.
- USG is ideal for characterizing thyroid nodules.
- Innovative advances in high-resolution US now enable detailed anatomical characterization and accurate differentiation of benign from malignant disease.
- Adoption of TI-RADS system of reporting would avoid unnecessary FNAC/surgery in Bethesda 3 and 4.
- The large evidence base for *use* indicates that the assessment of nodule stiffness can improve the imaging evaluation of thyroid lesions and potentially avoids unnecessary FNAC/surgery

for benign nodules, particularly if integrated with TI-RADS.

- The potential for 3D and CEUS has not yet been realized.
- CT and MR imaging is required preoperatively in invasive thyroid cancers to guide operative approach or decide whether surgery is possible.
- Imaging recurrent thyroid cancer involves nuclear medicine modalities.

References

1. Cooper DS, Doherty GM, Haugen BR, et al. Revised American Thyroid Association management guidelines for patients with thyroid nodules and differentiated thyroid cancer. Thyroid. 2009;19:1167–214.
2. Ezzat S, Sarti DA, Cain DR, Braunstein GD. Thyroid incidentalomas. Prevalence by palpation and ultrasonography. Arch Intern Med. 1994;154(16):1838–40.
3. Anil G, Hegde A, Chong FH. Thyroid nodules: risk stratification for malignancy with ultrasound and guided biopsy. Cancer Imaging. 2011;11:209–23. https://doi.org/10.1102/1470-7330.2011.0030. Review
4. Papini E, Guglielmi R, Bianchini A, et al. Risk of malignancy in nonpalpable thyroid nodules: predictive value of ultrasound and color-Doppler features. J Clin Endocrinol Metab. 2002;87(5):1941–6.
5. Wienke JR, Chong WK, Fielding JR, et al. Sonographic features of benign thyroid nodules: interobserver reliability and overlap with malignancy. J Ultrasound Med. 2003;22(10):1027–31.
6. Cerbone G, Spiezia S, Colao A, et al. Power Doppler improves the diagnostic accuracy of color Doppler ultrasonography in cold thyroid nodules: follow-up results. Horm Res. 1999;52(1):19–24.
7. Fish SA, Langer JE, Mandel SJ. Sonographic imaging of thyroid nodules and cervical lymph nodes. Endocrinol Metab Clin North Am 2008;37(2):401–417., ix. doi: https://doi.org/10.1016/j.ecl.2007.12.003. Review.
8. Jeh SK, Jung SL, Kim BS, et al. Evaluating the degree of conformity of papillary carcinoma and follicular carcinoma to the reported ultrasonographic findings of malignant thyroid tumor. Korean J Radiol. 2007;8(3):192–7.
9. Cappelli C, Pirola I, Cumetti D, et al. Is the anteroposterior and transverse diameter ratio of nonpalpable thyroid nodules a sonographic criteria for recommending fine-needle aspiration cytology? Clin Endocrinol (Oxf). 2005;63(6):689–93.
10. Kuna SK, Bracic I, Tesic V, et al. Ultrasonographic differentiation of benign from malignant neck lymphadenopathy in thyroid cancer. J Ultrasound Med. 2006;25(12):1531–7. quiz 1538–40
11. Horvath E, Majlis S, Rossi R, Franco C, Niedmann JP, Castro A, et al. An ultrasonogram reporting system for thyroid nodules stratifying cancer risk for clinical management. J Clin Endocrinol Metab. 2009;94(5):1748–51.
12. Kwak JY, Han KH, Yoon JH, Moon HJ, Son EJ, Park SH, et al. Thyroid imaging reporting and data system for 257 US features of nodules: a step in establishing better stratification of cancer risk. Radiology. 2011;260(3):892–9.
13. Rago T, Santini F, Scutari M, Pinchera A, Vitti P. Elastography: new developments in ultrasound for predicting malignancy in thyroid nodules. J Clin Endocrinol Metab. 2007;92(8):2917–22. Epub 2007 May 29
14. Choi JS, Kim J, Kwak JY, Kim MJ, Chang HS, Kim EK. Preoperative staging of papillary thyroid carcinoma: comparison of ultrasound imaging and CT. Am J Roentgenol. 2009;193(3):871–8. https://doi.org/10.2214/AJR.09.2386.
15. Yoon DY, Chang SK, Choi CS, Yun EJ, Seo YL, Nam ES, Cho SJ, Rho YS, Ahn HY. The prevalence and significance of incidental thyroid nodules identified on computed tomography. J Comput Assist Tomogr. 2008;32(5):810–5. https://doi.org/10.1097/RCT.0b013e318157fd38.
16. Haugen BR, Alexander EK, Bible KC, Doherty GM, Mandel SJ, Nikiforov YE, Pacini F, Randolph GW, Sawka AM, Schlumberger M, Schuff KG, Sherman SI, Sosa JA, Steward DL, Tuttle RM, Wartofsky L. 2015 American Thyroid Association Management Guidelines for adult patients with thyroid nodules and differentiated thyroid cancer: the American Thyroid Association Guidelines Task Force on thyroid nodules and differentiated thyroid cancer. Thyroid. 2016;26(1):1–133. https://doi.org/10.1089/thy.2015.0020. Review
17. Takashima S, Takayama F, Wang J, Kobayashi S, Kadoya M. Using MR imaging to predict invasion of the recurrent laryngeal nerve by thyroid carcinoma. Am J Roentgenol. 2003;180:837–42. https://doi.org/10.2214/ajr.180.3.1800837.
18. Wang JC, Takashima S, Takayama F, et al. Tracheal invasion by thyroid carcinoma: prediction using MR imaging. Am J Roentgenol. 2001;177:929–36. https://doi.org/10.2214/ajr.177.4.1770929.
19. Roychowdhury S, Loevner LA, Yousem DM, Chalian A, Montone KT. MR imaging for predicting neoplastic invasion of the cervical esophagus. Am J Neuroradiol. 2000;21:1681–7.
20. Yousem DM, Hatabu H, Hurst RW, et al. Carotid artery invasion by head and neck masses: prediction with MR imaging. Radiology. 1995;195:715–20.
21. Shetty SK, Maher MM, Hahn PF, Halpern EF, Aquino SL. Significance of incidental thyroid lesions detected on CT: correlation among CT, sonography, and pathology. Am J Roentgenol. 2006;187(5):1349–56. Erratum in: Am J Roentgenol. 2007;188(1):8.

22. Nimmons GL, Funk GF, Graham MM, Pagedar NA. Urinary iodine excretion after contrast computed tomography scan: implications for radioactive iodine use. JAMA Otolaryngol Head Neck Surg. 2013;139(5):479–82. https://doi.org/10.1001/jamaoto.2013.2552.
23. Sohn SY, Choi JH, Kim NK, Joung JY, Cho YY, Park SM, Kim TH, Jin SM, Bae JC, Lee SY, Chung JH, Kim SW. The impact of iodinated contrast agent administered during preoperative computed tomography scan on body iodine pool in patients with differentiated thyroid cancer preparing for radioactive iodine treatment. Thyroid. 2014;24(5):872–7. https://doi.org/10.1089/thy.2013.0238. Epub 2014 Mar 6
24. Padovani RP, Kasamatsu TS, Nakabashi CC, Camacho CP, Andreoni DM, Malouf EZ, Marone MM, Maciel RM, Biscolla RP. One month is sufficient for urinary iodine to return to its baseline value after the use of water-soluble iodinated contrast agents in post-thyroidectomy patients requiring radioiodine therapy. Thyroid. 2012;22(9):926–30. https://doi.org/10.1089/thy.2012.0099. Epub 2012 Jul 24
25. Mishra A, Pradhan PK, Gambhir S, Sabaretnam M, Gupta A, Babu S. Preoperative contrast-enhanced computerized tomography should not delay radioiodine ablation in differentiated thyroid carcinoma patients. J Surg Res. 2015;193(2):731–7. https://doi.org/10.1016/j.jss.2014.07.065. Epub 2014 Aug 12
26. Lee SY, Chang DL, He X, Pearce EN, Braverman LE, Leung AM. Urinary iodine excretion and serum thyroid function in adults after iodinated contrast administration. Thyroid. 2015;25(5):471–7. https://doi.org/10.1089/thy.2015.0024. Epub 2015 Mar 23

Management of Locally Advanced Thyroid Cancer

8

Andrea R. Marcadis, Jennifer Cracchiolo, and Ashok K. Shaha

Introduction

Cancer staging allows patients to be stratified based on aggressiveness of their disease and provides important prognostic information to both the patient and clinician. The tumor-nodal-metastasis (TNM) system from the American Joint Committee on Cancer (AJCC) is the most commonly used staging system for many cancers, including thyroid cancer, and has been shown to predict differentiated thyroid cancer-related death [1]. While most patients with thyroid carcinoma have well-differentiated tumors that have an excellent prognosis, there are certain characteristics that carry a worse prognosis, including older age, larger primary tumor size, aggressive tumor histology, extrathyroidal tumor extension (ETE), and distant metastasis [2].

In 1993, the Mayo Clinic published on the prognostic factors for papillary thyroid carcinoma (PTC), using the acronym MACIS (distant metastasis, age, completeness of resection, local/vascular invasion, tumor size), adding completeness of resection to the known prognostic factors for thyroid cancer [3]. In 2012, Memorial Sloan Kettering Cancer Center created a similar acronym, GAMES (tumor grade, age, distant metastasis, extrathyroidal extension, size of tumor) [4]. Of these prognostic factors, ETE has a significant negative impact, conferring a greater risk of local recurrence, regional spread, and distant metastasis [5], and with 10-year survival rates of 45%, as compared to 91% in patients with no ETE [6]. Patients with ETE often have several of these adverse prognostic factors, with many being older in age and having tumors with aggressive histological features [5].

Locally advanced thyroid cancer (LATC) occurs when there is either ETE from the primary tumor or from extracapsular extension from involved lymph nodes into the surrounding structures [5]. The structures that are in closest proximity to the thyroid and cervical lymph nodes are the most susceptible to local invasion, with a study of 262 patients with invasive thyroid cancer over 50 years showing involvement of the strap muscles in 53%, recurrent laryngeal nerve (RLN) in 47%, trachea in 37%, great vessels/vagus nerve in 30%, esophagus in 21%, and larynx in 12% [7].

Tumor histology affects the surgical decision-making in patients with LATC. Patients with well-differentiated thyroid carcinoma (WDTC) of follicular origin, including papillary and follicular thyroid cancer, are generally candidates for surgical intervention, even if they have known metastatic disease, as it is the local/regional disease rather than distant metastasis that causes morbidity and mortality in these patients.

A. R. Marcadis · J. Cracchiolo · A. K. Shaha (✉)
Memorial Sloane Kettering Centre,
New York, NY, USA
e-mail: marcadia@mskcc.org; shahaa@mskcc.org; cracchij@mskcc.org

R. Parameswaran, A. Agarwal (eds.), *Evidence-Based Endocrine Surgery*,
https://doi.org/10.1007/978-981-10-1124-5_8

Additionally, patients with metastatic WDTC generally respond better to adjuvant therapy after local disease has been fully excised. However, patients with locally advanced poorly differentiated thyroid carcinoma (PDTC) and anaplastic thyroid carcinoma (ATC), generally have more aggressive tumors in which primary surgical resection may be more difficult and cause higher morbidity and mortality [8]. In these patients, management plans differ and should depend on the patient's overall health and disease burden.

Importantly, the 8th edition of the AJCC staging system was published in October 2016, and among other changes, made significant modifications with regard to the staging of ETE in differentiated LATC. ETE that is only detected microscopically no longer has an impact on the staging of thyroid cancer, and a new "T" sub-category, T3b, has been created for tumors of any size demonstrating gross ETE into strap muscles alone, with tumors that show gross ETE into major neck structures remaining in the T4 category. Additionally, N1 nodal disease is no longer stage III and is now considered stage I in patients <55 years of age, and stage II in patients ≥55 years [9]. The overall effect of these changes is a downstaging of patients with only *microscopic* ETE and regional lymph node involvement, reemphasizing the importance of *gross* (radiologic and/or clinical) ETE as a poor prognostic factor in thyroid cancer [9].

In patients with locally aggressive WDTC, the principles of surgical management are removal of all gross tumor, preservation of functioning and vital structures, and appropriate use of adjuvant therapies [5]. While all agree that gross disease should be fully resected, there are two general approaches to the management of microscopic disease left behind on vital structures: one being to resect the invaded structures to obtain clean margins, and the other to perform shave or tangential excision procedures followed by adjuvant therapy for residual disease [8]. The approach depends on the extent of disease and the functional status of vital structures, for which a thorough preoperative evaluation is paramount.

Preoperative Evaluation/Anesthesia Considerations

Preoperative evaluation of a patient with a newly diagnosed thyroid nodule or thyroid carcinoma involves a thorough history and physical to evaluate for signs or symptoms of LATC. Symptoms of invasive thyroid cancer include voice changes or hoarseness from invasion of the RLN, cough, stridor, or hemoptysis from intraluminal invasion of the larynx or trachea, or dysphagia from tumor compression or invasion of the pharynx or esophagus [8]. Patients may experience neck pain or stiffness and on physical exam can exhibit tenderness or a firm mass which may be fixed to the surrounding structures [5]. Many of these findings are seen late in the disease process [5].

Most patients with LATC are asymptomatic at presentation. Patients with an affected RLN may have had gradual compensation from the contralateral functioning vocal cord such that there is no noticeable voice change. This underscores the importance of routine preoperative fiber-optic or indirect office laryngoscopy on all patients undergoing workup for thyroid surgery [2]. Patients with signs or symptoms of LATC should also have, in addition to their routine fine needle aspiration (FNA) and thyroid ultrasound (US), preoperative cross-sectional imaging such as CT or MRI for optimal identification and localization of aerodigestive tract invasion [8]. The added information gained from the use of iodinated contrast with a neck CT scan far outweighs once accepted concerns about IV contrast causing a delay in subsequent radioactive iodine (RAI) administration. Contrast neck CT scans provide high-quality preoperative imaging, which may enhance the likelihood of achieving a complete surgical resection of disease. An upper GI contrast study may be useful in evaluating suspected esophageal invasion [2]. Vocal cord abnormalities, as well as fullness, ulceration, or a mass seen in the lumen of the larynx or trachea on imaging or indirect laryngoscopy, should prompt further workup, including direct laryngoscopy, bronchoscopy, or rigid esophagoscopy as necessary in order to best guide surgical management [8]. When performing rigid esophagoscopy, the surgeon can move the mucosa over the mass to confirm that esophageal mucosa is not involved.

Patients with LATC have a higher risk of distant metastasis, and a full metastatic workup is essential, as this can significantly change management [5]. RAI scanning is generally the best test in assessing for distant metastasis in those with WDTC cancers of follicular origin. If medullary thyroid cancer (MTC) or PDTC is suspected, metastatic workup is best undertaken with a PET scan, as thyroid cancers of non-follicular origin and PDTC are usually non-RAI avid [5].

Because of the risk of a distorted airway, paralyzed vocal cords, or tracheal intraluminal tumor in patients with LATC, extra precautions need to be taken when planning and administering anesthesia [2]. While for most patients, general endotracheal anesthesia is safe and effective, in patients with significant airway involvement, awake/fiberoptic nasotracheal intubation can be used [2]. Tracheotomy should be avoided unless absolutely necessary, as this can introduce secretions into the surgical bed and delay wound healing. If tracheotomy is performed, it should be carefully placed, taking into account the altered anatomy from the resection and planned reconstruction [2].

Discussion of Structures Involved in LATC

The presentation, workup, management, and prognosis of patients with LATC differ depending on the particular structure invaded. Therefore, the discussion of the structures will be undertaken individually.

Strap Muscle Invasion

The strap muscles (sternohyoid, sternothyroid, and omohyoid) are the most common structures involved in LATC due to their close anatomical relationship to the thyroid. Management of strap muscle invasion entails resection of the involved portion of strap muscle to obtain negative margins, generally with no significant morbidity. After resection, patients with strap muscle invasion alone have an excellent prognosis, similar to those with no invasion [5].

Recurrent Laryngeal Nerve Invasion

The RLN is one of the most common structures affected by LATC, usually from invasion by the primary tumor or extracapsular spread from involved lymph nodes, and occasionally by external compression [5] (Fig. 8.1). While voice changes and vocal cord impairment can point to RLN pathology, there are many patients with an invaded RLN who have normally functioning vocal cords [8]. This was clearly demonstrated in a study by Nishida and colleagues which found that 51% of patients with known LATC and no vocal cord impairment during preoperative workup in fact had RLN involvement [10].

When evaluating a patient with LATC and an affected RLN, the management algorithm depends, in part, on the preoperative vocal cord function. In the simplest case of a patient whose RLN is preoperatively known to be paralyzed and confirmed intraoperatively to be invaded, the nerve should be resected [5]. In a patient with a preoperatively paralyzed nerve that intraoperatively is found to be compressed but *not* invaded, it is acceptable to remove the gross disease and preserve the nerve, as there is some potential for vocal cord recovery postoperatively [11, 12].

In a patient with WDTC and RLN invasion who had intact vocal cord function preoperatively, the decision to resect versus spare the nerve becomes more difficult. Most agree that if nerve preservation requires gross disease to be left behind, the nerve should be resected. However, if the tumor can be peeled off of the functioning nerve in order to achieve a gross total (R1) resection, this may be attempted [5]. Several groups

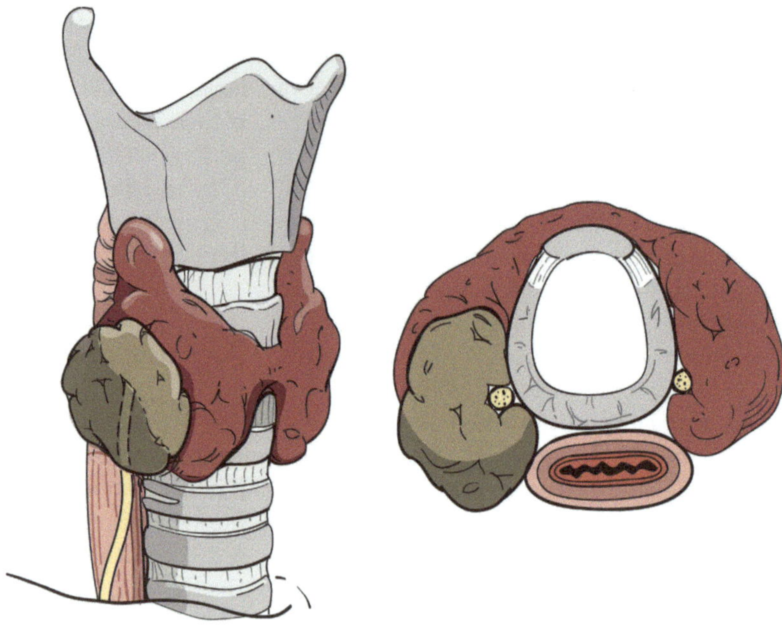

Fig. 8.1 Schematic of recurrent laryngeal nerve invasion (courtesy of Memorial Sloan Kettering Cancer Center)

have shown no difference in survival and local recurrence in patients with microscopic disease left behind on the RLN compared to those who undergo nerve resection for microscopic disease, as long as those with the preserved nerve receive postoperative RAI [2, 10, 12], or external beam radiation therapy (EBRT) in the case of poorly differentiated, non-RAI-avid tumors [13]. It is important to note that before any RLN resection, the opposite nerve should be carefully checked to assure function, as bilateral vocal cord paralysis generally leads to tracheostomy dependence with a high aspiration risk and should be avoided at all costs. Nerve monitoring is a very useful tool for assuring RLN function intraoperatively and can be helpful in planning the extent of the operation as well as anticipating postoperative function [2].

After unilateral RLN sacrifice, immediate nerve repair can be performed by either primary anastomosis of resected RLN or nerve graft with the great auricular nerve, ansa cervicalis, or sural nerve [14, 15]. Yumoto and colleagues studied 22 patients with LATC involving the RLN and found that patients who had immediate nerve repair with either interposition nerve graft or primary anastomosis had better postoperative phonation than those who did not have nerve reconstruction [14]. If the patient is not a candidate for nerve repair, postoperative vocal cord medicalization with implants and/or arytenoid adduction can assist with voice power and projection, as well as decrease risk of aspiration. Vocal fold augmentation can also be performed with fillers such as Cymetra, Gelfoam, or fat [5].

Laryngotracheal Invasion

As opposed to strap muscle and RLN invasion, laryngotracheal invasion by WDTC has been shown to be independently and significantly associated with decreased survival [16, 17]. Because of the difference in incidence and approach to treatment, laryngeal and tracheal invasion will be discussed separately.

Laryngeal Invasion

Unlike tracheal invasion which is common in patients with LATC, laryngeal invasion is relatively rare, occurring in about 12% [7]. Because of its rarity, there are no clearly established guidelines with regard to management, with surgical options ranging from peeling or shave procedures to partial or total laryngectomy, depending on the extent of invasion [2].

With a completely extraluminal tumor, the general recommendation is to perform a shave procedure, defined by McCaffrey and colleagues as removal of all gross tumor by resection of a partial thickness of the aerodigestive tract wall [18], with the assumption that microscopic foci of tumor remain [19]. Several retrospective studies show no difference in survival between those who undergo radical resection and those who undergo shave procedures when all gross disease is completely resected [7, 16, 20].

In contrast to those with only extraluminal involvement, in patients with intraluminal invasion, an open procedure is necessary [5]. Attempts should be made to preserve laryngeal function; however, this is not always possible. Often, the laryngeal framework needs to be resected [5]. If only unilateral laryngeal invasion is present, a partial laryngectomy may be sufficient [5]. A total laryngectomy is rarely needed for patients with LATC; however, it may be necessary in patients with recurrent disease involving the laryngeal lumen or cricothyroid cartilage, or may be performed in patients with lack of laryngeal function preoperatively [21]. If the tumor has invaded through the thyroid cartilage into the paraglottic space, it is usually unilateral and amenable to a vertical laryngectomy because of the lateral location of most thyroid tumors [17].

With regard to cartilaginous invasion, management depends on the extent of cartilage involved and differs between the cricoid and thyroid cartilage. With cricoid cartilage invasion, up to one-third can generally be resected without the need for a complex reconstruction or tracheotomy [2, 22]. In these cases, reconstruction with a cartilage graft can be useful if necessary [8]. With greater than one-third of the cricoid cartilage involved or destructed by tumor, a more extensive intervention is necessary, with some authors advocating total laryngectomy to avoid airway stenosis, and others suggesting that partial laryngeal resection with formal laryngotracheal reconstruction can be performed without significant airway stenosis [16, 21]. Those with subglottic involvement, either from invasion directly through the cricoid cartilage or through the cricothyroid membrane, generally need a total laryngectomy [5]. Invasion of the thyroid cartilage is slightly more forgiving, with up to one-half of cases able to be resected without the need for complex reconstruction or tracheotomy [2, 22].

Tracheal Invasion

More common than laryngeal invasion is tracheal invasion, which is seen in one-third of patients with LATC and is the third most commonly invaded structure in LATC after the strap muscles and the RLN [7]. It is generally involved by direct tumor extension either anteriorly or posteriorly, and tumor can invade through the tracheal ring cartilage and the intercartilaginous spaces into the tracheal lumen [5]. Because it is more common than laryngeal invasion, there is more discussion in the literature regarding optimal management, though with conflicting recommendations. Shin and colleagues have created a staging system (stages I–IV) for tracheal invasion (Fig. 8.2), where stage I disease invades through the capsule of the thyroid gland and abuts but does not invade the external perichondrium of the trachea, stage II disease invades into the cartilage or causes cartilage destruction, stage III disease extends into the lamina propria of the tracheal mucosa with no elevation or penetration of the mucosa, and stage IV disease is full-thickness invasion with expansion of the tracheal mucosa that is visible bronchoscopically as a bulge or an ulcerated mass [23].

For stage I disease with no intraluminal invasion of the trachea, some report that shave excision is sufficient; however, others recommend a more extensive resection. The advocates of shave excision point to the morbidity associated with tracheal resection as well as the risk of complications such as tracheal stenosis [19]. Nishida and colleagues evaluated patients with stage I tracheal invasion who underwent shave procedures compared to those who had LATC with no airway involvement and found no difference in local or regional recurrence, distant metastasis, or overall survival [24]. Several others have had similar findings [16, 20, 25], including Segal and colleagues, who noted an equivalent 5-year survival between patients who underwent radical resection to excise all microscopic disease and

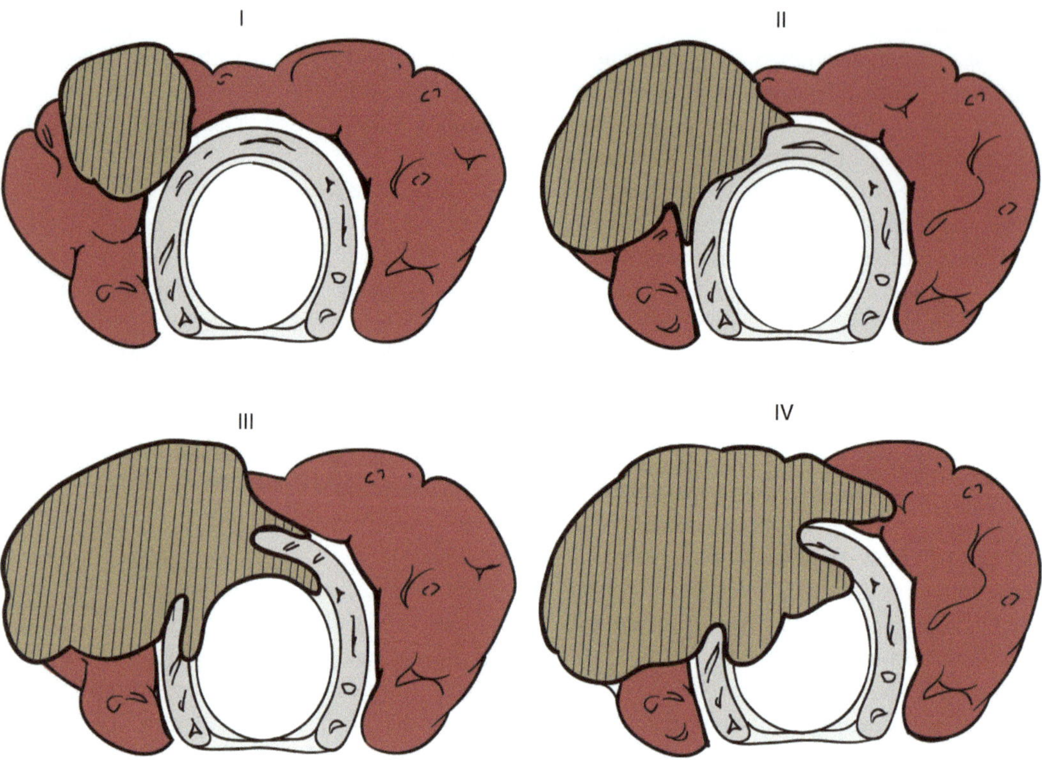

Fig. 8.2 Classification of tracheal invasion as proposed by Shin et al. [23] (courtesy of Memorial Sloan Kettering Cancer Center)

those who underwent shave resection of macroscopic disease and RAI for microscopic residual disease [25].

In contrast to these proponents of shave resection, advocates of complete resection for extraluminal tracheal disease cite higher recurrence rates and worse survival associated with shave procedures [22, 26–28]. A commonly cited paper by Gaissert and colleagues reports that patients who initially undergo shave procedures and later develop laryngotracheal recurrence have worse disease-free and overall survival than those who undergo complete resection at initial presentation [28]. Additionally, the authors note that segmental airway resection for LATC is generally well tolerated and can relieve airway obstruction, with good overall voice preservation [28].

It is also important, even in these patients with only extraluminal tracheal disease, to consider the histology of the particular thyroid cancer. Those with aggressive PTC variants which may not be RAI-avid or those with Hurthle cell cancer, MTC, or PDTC may be better candidates for a formal resection instead of a shave procedure [2]. Additionally, the patients' comorbidities and disease burden should be considered when deciding extent of resection [2].

When the LATC does more than simply abut the trachea (stage II and above), a shave procedure is not sufficient to control disease. In fact, Nishida and colleagues, who recommend shave procedure for stage I disease, found that patients with stage II and higher tracheal invasion (at least into cartilage or cartilaginous destruction) who underwent tracheal resection had lower local recurrence rates (8% vs. 79%) and longer overall survival (8.7 vs. 1.5 years) compared to patients who had a subtotal operation with no airway resection [24].

Patients with intraluminal tracheal extension of their thyroid cancer require a formal resection, but the extent of operation depends on the circumference and extent of the trachea that is involved. In those with more limited involvement of an anteriorly or laterally located tumor, or those with involvement of less than one-third the circumference of the trachea, a wedge resection with primary closure may be possible [5], or a window resection with muscle patch closure such as a strap muscle or sternocleidomastoid patch may be appropriate [19]. Anterior tumor extension can occasionally be managed by converting the surgical defect into a tracheostomy which can be postoperatively downsized and eventually capped and decannulated, with the tracheal window healing spontaneously [19]. Even in these patients with less aggressive resections and reconstructions, however, there are reports of tracheal stenosis, and therefore many continue to recommend circumferential resection [19].

In cases of involvement of greater than one-third of the circumference of the trachea [5] or those requiring resection of at least one tracheal ring [2], a circumferential segmental resection of the trachea is necessary. A primary anastomosis can be performed with a circumferential or sleeve resection of as many as seven to eight tracheal rings [5] or 5–6 cm; however this varies from patient to patient and requires some degree of neck flexion [2]. To ensure a tension-free anastomosis, a supralaryngeal release with division of the thyrohyoid membrane and musculature can be performed if necessary to gain an additional approximately 2 cm, and if extra length is necessary, division of the suprahyoid muscles can be performed [2]. In the rare case that there is still not enough length for tracheal reanastomosis, a sternotomy with hilar mobilization can provide the last several centimeters [2, 19]. Additionally, as the extent of intraluminal mucosal disease sometimes exceeds the extent of extraluminal disease, intraoperative frozen sections are advised by some, in order to ensure negative intraluminal margins before reconstruction [8].

When performing tracheal resection, it is important to keep the plane of dissection along the anterior tracheal wall [5] and to avoid circumferential mobilization of the trachea [2] in order to prevent devascularization of the trachea from the laterally entering blood supply, and also to avoid injuring the RLN [2]. It is important to constantly be aware of glottis function throughout the procedure, especially in patients who have involvement of one of their RLNs, so as to avoid disrupting the contralateral nerve [2].

Pharyngeal/Esophageal Invasion

Pharyngeal or esophageal invasion is found in about one-fifth of patients with LATC [2, 7]. It most commonly occurs by direct extension in patients with tracheal invasion, however can also occur by extension from paratracheal or paraesophageal lymph nodes [2]. As with laryngotracheal invasion, pharyngoesophageal invasion is a poor prognostic factor and is associated with a significantly decreased overall survival [2, 7, 24]. Most commonly, pharyngoesophageal invasion is confined to the muscularis layer without extension into the submucosa or mucosa (Fig. 8.3), as

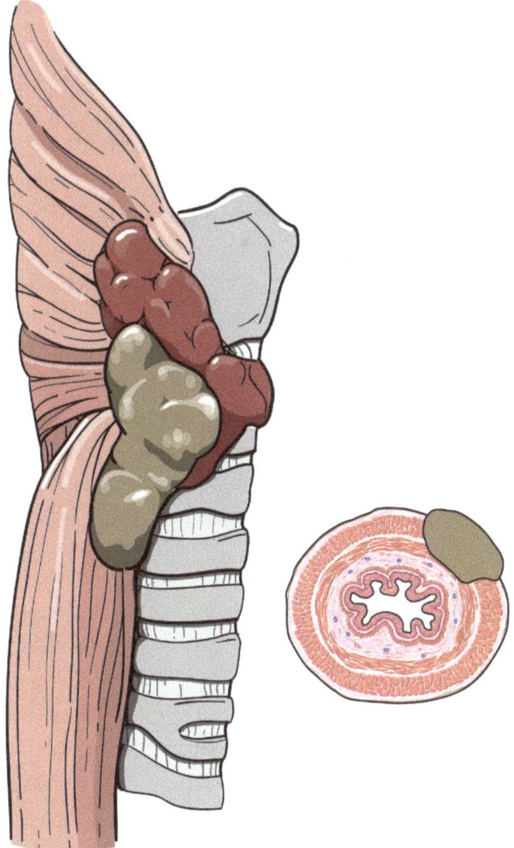

Fig. 8.3 Schematic of esophageal invasion (courtesy of Memorial Sloan Kettering Cancer Center)

the mucosa of the pharynx and esophagus is somewhat resistant to direct invasion [5, 19]. In cases of suspected pharyngoesophageal invasion, it is important to have good preoperative imaging to determine thickness of invasion and allow appropriate surgical planning [8]. Endoscopic ultrasound may also be useful for this purpose.

Treatment of pharyngeal or esophageal invasion depends on the thickness of invasion. When the invasion is confined to the muscularis with no submucosal or mucosal invasion, a simple resection of involved muscularis can be undertaken in order to obtain negative margins, taking caution not to tear the mucosa [5]. When there is full-thickness or circumferential involvement, a segmental resection should be performed [5]. If a full-thickness defect is created to excise the tumor, a primary closure can be performed, as long as the tissue is healthy and non-radiated and the closure is not under tension. This primary closure must be water-tight and multilayer [2].

When there is pharyngeal involvement, a resection of the pyriform sinus by a lateral pharyngotomy that includes a portion of the thyroid lamina can sometimes be performed, allowing for a complete resection without sacrificing voice or swallowing [8]. Extensive pharyngeal tumors with luminal invasion, however, may require total laryngopharyngectomy [8]. Reconstruction options for the more extensive esophageal resections not amenable to primary closure include free tissue transfer, myo- or fascio-cutaneous pedicled flaps, gastric pull-up, or gastric, colonic, or jejunal tissue transfer [5, 19]. Esophageal stents may be used for palliation in patients who are not candidates for surgical resection [19].

Carotid Artery Invasion

Management of carotid artery involvement depends on the circumferential degree of involvement. In patients with less than 270° of tumor involvement of the carotid artery, it is acceptable to carefully peel the tumor off of the artery. In those with greater than 270° of involvement, however, surgical management of the carotid is often not indicated. Though it is technically feasible to ligate or bypass the common carotid artery, these patients often have such advanced disease that this is rarely curative. Additionally, any involvement of the aerodigestive tract requiring repair or anastomosis is a strict contraindication for carotid resection [8].

Adjuvant Therapy

Patients with LATC are at an increased risk for local recurrence and distant metastasis, and therefore most will require adjuvant therapy [5]. The general recommendation is for adjuvant RAI and thyroid-stimulating hormone (TSH) suppression to treat residual and/or metastatic disease after total thyroidectomy and other necessary resections have been performed [5].

These recommendations are backed by several studies. Cooper and colleagues found that in patients with stage III or IV PTC, a higher degree of TSH suppression was associated with decreased disease progression [29], and a meta-analysis by McGriff and colleagues found a decrease in postoperative adverse clinical events including disease progression, recurrence, and mortality in patients who had TSH suppression [30]. Mazzaferri and colleagues found that in patients with locally invasive thyroid cancers of follicular origin, postoperative RAI therapy combined with TSH suppression reduced tumor recurrence and disease-related mortality enough to compensate for the increased risk in those patients due to their locally invasive disease [31, 32]. Samaan and colleagues showed postoperative RAI therapy is the most important indicator for increased disease-free and overall survival [33].

While RAI treatment is effective in patients with WDTC, many patients with LATC have poorly differentiated tumors which may not be RAI-avid. Many studies have been reported about the use of EBRT in these patients [34–36]. In patients with WDTC and gross residual disease, retrospective studies have shown EBRT to be effective for locoregional control [13, 37, 38]. Romesser and colleagues demonstrated a 90% locoregional progression-free survival in patients with advanced or recurrent non-anaplastic, non-medullary thyroid cancer with combination chemotherapy and EBRT, which was a nonsignificant improvement over the 73% locoregional progression-free survival with EBRT alone. A significant improvement with chemoradiotherapy was observed in those with poorly differentiated histology; however this was associated with a significantly worse distant metastasis-free survival. Though this study showed benefits with chemoradiotherapy in advanced thyroid cancer, it did have limitations including its retrospective nature and small/heterogeneous group of patients with LATC [39]. While these benefits of EBRT have been shown with WDTC and gross residual disease, the use of EBRT after adequately resected WDTC and in patients with RAI-avid, microscopic residual disease remains unclear. Oftentimes the combination of RAI scan and PET scan results may help select patients most likely to benefit from EBRT.

The effect of EBRT seems to be dose-dependent, with better local control seen with doses greater than 50 Gy [40]. These higher doses, however, also come with increased side effects and late complications, and therefore some are choosing to use intensity-modulated radiotherapy (IMRT), which allows radiation to be delivered to the thyroid bed while decreasing the risk for complications such as spinal cord injury [5, 41].

With regard to adjuvant chemotherapy, there have been several studies about its use in patients with LATC; however none have shown a significant benefit. The most commonly used agent is doxorubicin, either alone or in combination with other agents, with partial response rates in 30–40% but poor long-term results [2, 42].

Targeted Therapy in Locally Advanced and Metastatic Thyroid Cancer

Over the past decade, we have observed significant advancement in the medical treatment of advanced thyroid cancer. Two multikinase inhibitors, lenvatinib [43] and sorafenib [44], have been approved by the FDA for the treatment of patients with progressive, recurrent, or metastatic thyroid cancer that does not respond to treatment with RAI. Quality of life and the long-term cumulative toxicities of therapy remain areas in need of further research. A comprehensive picture of how these systemic therapies benefit patients in the long term is still open to question. Other drugs such as tyrosine kinase inhibitors and BRAF mutation targeting agents have been used to redifferentiate and restore tumor RAI-avidity [45].

On a final note, patients who have undergone treatment for LATC need to continue to have close follow-up after their primary treatment has ended. This generally involves monitoring thyroglobulin levels, RAI scans in patients with RAI-avid tumors, and PET scans as needed for those with non-RAI active tumors. It is very important for these patients to maintain close follow-up with their surgeon and/or endocrinologist to monitor for recurrence [5].

Conclusion

Management of LATC must include an understanding of tumor biology, as well as a detailed knowledge of anatomy. Rapidity of growth and location of disease will affect management. Anatomic imaging is critical for treatment and surgical planning. While surgery represents the mainstay in treatment of resectable LATC, use of other therapies including EBRT and targeted therapy also plays a role in the adjuvant setting as well as in patients with unresectable disease.

References

1. Tanase K, Thies E-D, Mäder U, Reiners C, Verburg FA. The TNM system (version 7) is the most accurate staging system for the prediction of loss of life expectancy in differentiated thyroid cancer. Clin Endocrinol (Oxf). 2015;[Epub ahead of print].
2. Price DL, Wong RJ, Randolph GW. Invasive thyroid cancer: management of the trachea and esophagus. Otolaryngol Clin N Am. 2008;41(6):1155–68. ix–x
3. Hay ID, Bergstralh EJ, Goellner JR, Ebersold JR, Grant CS. Predicting outcome in papillary thyroid carcinoma: development of a reliable prognostic scoring system in a cohort of 1779 patients surgically

treated at one institution during 1940 through 1989. Surgery. 1993;114(6):1050–7. discussion 1057–8

4. Ibrahimpasic T, Nixon IJ, Palmer FL, Whitcher MM, Tuttle RM, Shaha A, et al. Undetectable thyroglobulin after total thyroidectomy in patients with low- and intermediate-risk papillary thyroid cancer—is there a need for radioactive iodine therapy? Surgery. 2012;152(6):1096–105.
5. Patel KN, Shaha AR. Locally advanced thyroid cancer. Curr Opin Otolaryngol Head Neck Surg. 2005;13(2):112–6.
6. Andersen PE, Kinsella J, Loree TR, Shaha AR, Shah JP. Differentiated carcinoma of the thyroid with extrathyroidal extension. Am J Surg. 1995;170(5):467–70.
7. McCaffrey TV, Bergstralh EJ, Hay ID. Locally invasive papillary thyroid carcinoma: 1940–1990. Head Neck. 1994;16(2):165–72.
8. Ark N, Zemo S, Nolen D, Holsinger FC, Weber RS. Management of locally invasive well-differentiated thyroid cancer. Surg Oncol Clin N Am. 2008;17(1):145–55. ix
9. Tuttle RM, Haugen B, Perrier ND. Updated American Joint Committee on Cancer/Tumor-Node-Metastasis Staging System for Differentiated and Anaplastic Thyroid Cancer (Eighth Edition): What Changed and Why? Thyroid. 2017;27(6):751–6.
10. Nishida T, Nakao K, Hamaji M, Kamiike W, Kurozumi K, Matsuda H. Preservation of recurrent laryngeal nerve invaded by differentiated thyroid cancer. Ann Surg. 1997;226(1):85–91.
11. Chiang F-Y, Wang L-F, Huang Y-F, Lee K-W, Kuo W-R. Recurrent laryngeal nerve palsy after thyroidectomy with routine identification of the recurrent laryngeal nerve. Surgery. 2005;137(3):342–7.
12. Falk SA, McCaffrey TV. Management of the recurrent laryngeal nerve in suspected and proven thyroid cancer. Otolaryngol Head Neck Surg. 1995;113(1):42–8.
13. Tsang RW, Brierley JD, Simpson WJ, Panzarella T, Gospodarowicz MK, Sutcliffe SB. The effects of surgery, radioiodine, and external radiation therapy on the clinical outcome of patients with differentiated thyroid carcinoma. Cancer. 1998;82(2):375–88.
14. Yumoto E, Sanuki T, Kumai Y. Immediate recurrent laryngeal nerve reconstruction and vocal outcome. Laryngoscope. 2006;116(9):1657–61.
15. Miyauchi A, Inoue H, Tomoda C, Fukushima M, Kihara M, Higashiyama T, et al. Improvement in phonation after reconstruction of the recurrent laryngeal nerve in patients with thyroid cancer invading the nerve. Surgery. 2009;146(6):1056–62.
16. Czaja JM, McCaffrey TV. The surgical management of laryngotracheal invasion by well-differentiated papillary thyroid carcinoma. Arch Otolaryngol Head Neck Surg. 1997;123(5):484–90.
17. McCaffrey JC. Aerodigestive tract invasion by well-differentiated thyroid carcinoma: diagnosis, management, prognosis, and biology. Laryngoscope. 2006;116(1):1–11.
18. McCaffrey JC. Evaluation and treatment of aerodigestive tract invasion by well-differentiated thyroid carcinoma. Cancer Control. 2000;7(3):246–52.
19. An S-Y, Kim KH. Surgical management of locally advanced thyroid cancer. Curr Opin Otolaryngol Head Neck Surg. 2010;18(2):119–23.
20. McCaffrey TV, Lipton RJ. Thyroid carcinoma invading the upper aerodigestive system. Laryngoscope. 1990;100(8):824–30.
21. Donnelly MJ, Timon CI, McShane DP. The role of total laryngectomy in the management of intraluminal upper airway invasion by well-differentiated thyroid carcinoma. Ear Nose Throat J. 1994;73(9):659–62.
22. Friedman M, Danielzadeh JA, Caldarelli DD. Treatment of patients with carcinoma of the thyroid invading the airway. Arch Otolaryngol Head Neck Surg. 1994;120(12):1377–81.
23. Shin DH, Mark EJ, Suen HC, Grillo HC. Pathologic staging of papillary carcinoma of the thyroid with airway invasion based on the anatomic manner of extension to the trachea: a clinicopathologic study based on 22 patients who underwent thyroidectomy and airway resection. Hum Pathol. 1993;24(8):866–70.
24. Nishida T, Nakao K, Hamaji M. Differentiated thyroid carcinoma with airway invasion: indication for tracheal resection based on the extent of cancer invasion. J Thorac Cardiovasc Surg. 1997;114(1):84–92.
25. Segal K, Shpitzer T, Hazan A, Bachar G, Marshak G, Popovtzer A. Invasive well-differentiated thyroid carcinoma: effect of treatment modalities on outcome. Otolaryngol Head Neck Surg. 2006;134(5):819–22.
26. Park CS, Suh KW, Min JS. Cartilage-shaving procedure for the control of tracheal cartilage invasion by thyroid carcinoma. Head Neck. 1993;15(4):289–91.
27. Kasperbauer JL. Locally advanced thyroid carcinoma. Ann Otol Rhinol Laryngol. 2004;113(9):749–53.
28. Gaissert HA, Honings J, Grillo HC, Donahue DM, Wain JC, Wright CD, et al. Segmental laryngotracheal and tracheal resection for invasive thyroid carcinoma. Ann Thorac Surg. 2007;83(6):1952–9.
29. Cooper DS, Specker B, Ho M, Sperling M, Ladenson PW, Ross DS, et al. Thyrotropin suppression and disease progression in patients with differentiated thyroid cancer: results from the National Thyroid Cancer Treatment Cooperative Registry. Thyroid. 1998;8(9):737–44.
30. McGriff NJ, Csako G, Gourgiotis L, Lori CG, Pucino F, Sarlis NJ. Effects of thyroid hormone suppression therapy on adverse clinical outcomes in thyroid cancer. Ann Med. 2002;34(7–8):554–64.
31. Mazzaferri EL, Jhiang SM. Long-term impact of initial surgical and medical therapy on papillary and follicular thyroid cancer. Am J Med. 1994;97(5):418–28.
32. Mazzaferri EL. Treating high thyroglobulin with radioiodine: a magic bullet or a shot in the dark? J Clin Endocrinol Metab. 1995;80(5):1485–7.
33. Samaan NA, Schultz PN, Hickey RC, Goepfert H, Haynie TP, Johnston DA, et al. The results of various

modalities of treatment of well differentiated thyroid carcinomas: a retrospective review of 1599 patients. J Clin Endocrinol Metab. 1992;75(3):714–20.

34. Tubiana M, Haddad E, Schlumberger M, Hill C, Rougier P, Sarrazin D. External radiotherapy in thyroid cancers. Cancer. 1985;55(9 Suppl):2062–71.
35. Lee N, Tuttle M. The role of external beam radiotherapy in the treatment of papillary thyroid cancer. Endocr Relat Cancer. 2006;13(4):971–7.
36. Kiess AP, Agrawal N, Brierley JD, Duvvuri U, Ferris RL, Genden E, et al. External-beam radiotherapy for differentiated thyroid cancer locoregional control: a statement of the American Head and Neck Society: external-beam RT for differentiated thyroid cancer. Head Neck. 2016;38(4):493–8.
37. O'Connell ME, A'Hern RP, Harmer CL. Results of external beam radiotherapy in differentiated thyroid carcinoma: a retrospective study from the Royal Marsden Hospital. Eur J Cancer. 1994;30A(6):733–9.
38. Farahati J, Reiners C, Stuschke M, Müller SP, Stüben G, Sauerwein W, et al. Differentiated thyroid cancer. Impact of adjuvant external radiotherapy in patients with perithyroidal tumor infiltration (stage pT4). Cancer. 1996;77(1):172–80.
39. Romesser PB, Sherman EJ, Shaha AR, Lian M, Wong RJ, Sabra M, et al. External beam radiotherapy with or without concurrent chemotherapy in advanced or recurrent non-anaplastic non-medullary thyroid cancer. J Surg Oncol. 2014;110(4):375–82.
40. Ford D, Giridharan S, McConkey C, Hartley A, Brammer C, Watkinson JC, Glaholm J. External beam radiotherapy in the management of differentiated thyroid cancer. Clin Oncol. 2003;15(6):337–41.
41. Urbano TG, Clark CH, Hansen VN, Adams EJ, Miles EA, Mc Nair H, et al. Intensity modulated radiotherapy (IMRT) in locally advanced thyroid cancer: acute toxicity results of a phase I study. Radiother Oncol. 2007;85(1):58–63.
42. Sarlis NJ. Metastatic thyroid cancer unresponsive to conventional therapies: novel management approaches through translational clinical research. Curr Drug Targets Immune Endocr Metab Disord. 2001;1(2):103–15.
43. Schlumberger M, Tahara M, Wirth LJ, Robinson B, Brose MS, Elisei R, et al. Lenvatinib versus placebo in radioiodine-refractory thyroid cancer. N Engl J Med. 2015;372(7):621–30.
44. Brose MS, Nutting CM, Jarzab B, Elisei R, Siena S, Bastholt L, et al. Sorafenib in radioactive iodine-refractory, locally advanced or metastatic differentiated thyroid cancer: a randomised, double-blind, phase 3 trial. Lancet. 2014;384(9940):319–28.
45. Ho AL, Grewal RK, Leboeuf R, Sherman EJ, Pfister DG, Deandreis D, et al. Selumetinib-enhanced radioiodine uptake in advanced thyroid cancer. N Engl J Med. 2013;368(7):623–32.

Neck Dissection in Well-Differentiated Thyroid Cancer

9

Kwok Seng Loh and Donovon Kum Chuen Eu

Introduction

Surgery is considered to be the primary modality of treatment in well-differentiated thyroid cancers. The principles of surgery are to remove the tumor in the thyroid gland and the involved lymph nodes as well as to preserve functions of breathing, speech, and swallowing. Thyroid cancers, particularly papillary thyroid cancers, have a propensity to metastasize to cervical lymph nodes. The first echelon of lymph nodes that are affected are the level VI and VII nodes, known commonly as the central neck nodes. Subsequent echelon of lymph nodes may include the other levels of the neck, collectively known as the lateral neck nodes.

The surgical procedure to remove the cervical lymph nodes in thyroid cancer is neck dissection. In thyroid cancers, neck dissection can either be central neck dissection alone or together with lateral neck dissection. Central neck dissection refers to removing lymph nodes in levels VI and VII. In thyroid cancers, lateral neck dissection very often refers to removing lymph nodes in levels II–V.

K. S. Loh (✉)
Department of Otolaryngology,
National University of Singapore,
Singapore, Singapore
e-mail: entv5@nus.edu.sg

D. K. C. Eu
Department of Otolaryngology Head and Neck Surgery,
National University Hospital,
Singapore, Singapore

Surgical Anatomy

Central Neck Nodes

Central neck nodes refer to the pre-laryngeal, pre-tracheal, paratracheal, and superior mediastinal nodes. These are considered to be the first echelon of nodes. The lymph nodes correspond to level VI and VII nodes in the classification of level of lymph nodes [1]. Level VI nodes are defined as pre-laryngeal, pre-tracheal, and paratracheal nodes from the level of the hyoid bone superiorly to the level of the sternal notch inferiorly with the carotid arteries forming the lateral boundaries. It may be divided arbitrarily by the midline into left and right level VI nodes. Level VII nodes are the lymph nodes in the region of the superior mediastinum. It is bounded inferiorly by the innominate artery and extends superiorly to the level of the sternal notch. On the right, the lateral border of level VII is the right carotid artery as it arises from the innominate artery, while the left common carotid artery arising from the aorta forms the left lateral border. Together, level VI and VII nodes form the central neck nodes that are removed in central neck dissection. The boundaries of the central neck dissection as well as the important structures within the compartment are listed in Table 9.1.

R. Parameswaran, A. Agarwal (eds.), *Evidence-Based Endocrine Surgery*,
https://doi.org/10.1007/978-981-10-1124-5_9

Table 9.1 Central neck dissection: surgical boundaries and contents

	Central neck dissection boundaries	Contents
Level VI	Superior: hyoid Inferior: sternal notch Lateral: carotid artery	Pre-laryngeal, pre-tracheal, paratracheal nodes, external branch of superior laryngeal nerve, recurrent laryngeal nerve, parathyroids, trachea, esophagus
Level VII	Superior: sternal notch Inferior: innominate artery Lateral: carotid artery	Superior mediastinum nodes, thymus fat, thyroidea ima vessels

Table 9.2 Surgical boundaries of levels I–VII

Levels of neck	Surgical boundaries
Level IA	Between anterior bellies of digastric and hyoid inferiorly
Level IB	Body of mandible superiorly, anterior belly digastric anteriorly, stylohyoid muscle posteriorly
Level II	Skull base superiorly, inferior border hyoid inferiorly, posterior border of sternocleidomastoid muscle (SCM) posteriorly, stylohyoid muscle anteriorly
Level IIA	Anterior inferior to accessory nerve
Level IIB	Posterior superior to accessory nerve
Level III	Inferior border of hyoid superiorly, inferior border cricoid cartilage inferiorly, posterior border of SCM posteriorly, sternohyoid muscle anteriorly
Level IV	Inferior border of cricoid cartilage superiorly, clavicle inferiorly, posterior border of SCM posteriorly, sternohyoid muscle anteriorly
Level V	Posterior border of SCM anteriorly, anterior border of trapezius posteriorly, clavicle inferiorly
Level Va	Superior to an imaginary transverse line at level of inferior border of cricoid cartilage
Level Vb	Inferior to an imaginary transverse line at level of inferior border of cricoid cartilage
Level VI	Hyoid superiorly, sternal notch inferiorly, medial border carotid arteries bilaterally
Level VII	Sternal notch superiorly to innominate artery inferiorly

Lateral Neck Nodes

The definitions for the group of lymph nodes in the neck termed levels I–V have been widely used and are well accepted [2]. The boundaries of the levels of the neck are outlined in Table 9.2. The most common levels of lymph nodes that well-differentiated thyroid cancers metastasize to are level VI/VII nodes followed by levels III, IV, and II. Metastasis to level I nodes is very uncommon [3, 4]. It is considered in general to be unnecessary to remove level I nodes in well-differentiated thyroid cancer. In thyroid cancers, neck dissection of these groups of lymph nodes can take the form of radical neck dissection, modified radical neck dissection, or selective neck dissection. In most instances, it is possible to perform selective neck dissection. This selective neck dissection is synonymous with the term lateral neck dissection. Hence lateral neck dissection in thyroid cancer usually refers to removal of lymph nodes in levels II–V.

Indications

Central Neck Dissection

Central neck dissection is indicated when there is presence of enlarged or suspicious level VI/VII nodes at the time of thyroidectomy. While intra-operative assessment may not be very accurate [5], it is generally accepted that any nodes in level VI or VII that is 0.5 cm or more should be considered suspicious. In particular, multiple obvious level VI nodes seen in the paratracheal groove during thyroidectomy for thyroid cancer are often suggestive of metastasis. These metastatic nodes may also be pigmented. In these situations, the central neck dissection is termed therapeutic. Central neck dissection is also indicated if lateral neck dissection is planned.

Prophylactic or elective central neck dissection remains controversial. No prospective data exists to support or refute its role in thyroid cancer patients with no clinical evidence of lymph

Table 9.3 Indications for neck dissection

Neck dissection	Indications
Central neck (therapeutic)	(a) Presence of malignant nodes or suspicious nodes in level VI/VII (b) Presence of malignant lateral neck nodes
Lateral neck (therapeutic)	Presence of metastatic lateral nodes on clinical examination or on imaging
Central neck (elective)	(a) Primary thyroid tumor >4 cm (b) Extra-capsular invasion Other parameters that may be used: (c) Aggressive variants (d) BRAF V600E positive thyroid cancer (e) Age < 45 years (f) Male gender (g) Multifocal tumors

node metastasis [6, 7]. Proponents of elective central neck dissection argue that it reduces the risk of local regional recurrence as well as the risks of morbidity in reoperation. It can also assist in the decision-making process for post-thyroidectomy radioiodine. Multiple systematic reviews and meta-analysis of retrospective cohort studies [8–13] indicate fairly consistent parameters that are associated with central nodal metastasis (Table 9.3). Primary tumors larger than 1 cm, male gender, age less than 45 years, extrathyroidal extension, aggressive variants, multifocality, inferior pole tumors, and BRAF V600E mutation have been reported to be associated with a higher risk of central nodal metastasis. While the data suggests that these factors are associated with central nodal metastasis, what has not been shown conclusively is whether the addition of the central neck dissection provides benefits in terms of overall survival and reduced recurrence rates. If we were to base the decision on performing central neck dissection on these parameters, we will likely be advocating it in the majority of thyroid cancer patients. As an example of how wide the net is cast if we were to use tumor size as an indicator for central neck dissection, even micro-papillary carcinomas of 0.5 cm have been associated with higher risks of central node metastasis. Aggressive pathological variants such as diffuse sclerosing and tall cell variants as well as insular carcinoma may be associated with higher risks of central node metastasis [14, 15]. However, these aggressive variants together with other pathological parameters such as lymphovascular invasion and multifocality can only be determined conclusively after the thyroidectomy. Hence these parameters are not always useful for decision-making to perform the central neck dissection. BRAF V600E has been reported to be a useful test in the fine needle aspirate (FNA) [16] to assist decision-making process. However, this arguably is costly and is a test that is not readily available in most centers. It is therefore understandable that the American Thyroid Association confined its recommendations that elective central neck dissection may be performed if the thyroid cancer is more than 4 cm (T3/T4 tumors) and/or has extrathyroidal extension [11]. Extrathyroidal extension includes invasion of the strap muscles, recurrent laryngeal nerve, tracheal invasion, and esophageal invasion.

Lateral Neck Dissection

Lateral neck dissection is indicated if there is clinical evidence of a metastasis in any lateral node [17]. The evidence of a metastatic node may be because of a clinically palpable neck node or a suspicious node on radiological imaging. The suspicious features of malignancy in the lymph node are best determined by ultrasound [18]. A needle biopsy is often advocated to determine the presence of metastasis preoperatively. Where it is not feasible by the needle biopsy to determine metastasis, another approach may be to perform frozen section of the lymph node at the time of planned thyroidectomy and neck dissection.

Lateral neck dissection is not indicated when there is no evidence of metastasis. Prophylactic lateral neck dissection is not indicated because the yield of occult metastatic lymph nodes when there are no clinical or imaging evidence of metastasis in the lateral nodes has been shown to be low [19]. Systematic reviews of data in the literature suggest that there is no benefit in reducing nodal recurrences by performing prophylactic lateral neck dissection [20]. Lateral neck dissection has possible side effects, and this has to be considered if one advocates performing it prophylactically.

Preoperative Investigations

Thyroid Function

The majority of patients with well-differentiated thyroid cancers are euthyroid. It is however not uncommon to detect subclinical hypothyroidism in these patients [21]. Hyperthyroidism is uncommon. It will be wise to ensure that these patients undergoing treatment should be assessed with regard to thyroid function and if necessary to be controlled before the operation.

Ultrasound of the Neck

This has become a standard investigation of the patient with thyroid cancer. Besides assessing the thyroid gland, ultrasound affords excellent analysis of the size and shape of the lymph nodes in the neck. The patient is not exposed to radiation. It is also relatively less costly than a MRI. It is however difficult to assess the central neck in the presence of the thyroid gland. Suspicious lateral nodes include size of 1.5 cm or greater as well as rounded, hypoechoic signals, microcalcifications, and loss of fatty hilum [22].

CT Scan/MRI

The major role of CT scan and/or MRI is to define the primary tumor in the thyroid gland with respect to local invasion. It may also be useful for assessing the relationship of the metastatic lymph nodes with the carotid artery and internal jugular vein. Its role in defining nodal metastasis is not superior to that of ultrasound [23]. In fact, it is believed that the use of ultrasound to detect metastatic lymph nodes results in reduced regional recurrences and return to the operating room [24].

Surgical Technique

Central Neck Dissection

This is performed after the thyroidectomy is completed. The key to the procedure is identification of the recurrent laryngeal nerves. Central neck dissection technically is defined as complete removal of all level VI and VII nodes (Fig. 9.1). At the end of a central neck dissection, there should be no tissue between the carotid artery and esophagus. The recurrent laryngeal nerve is preserved, and possibly the parathyroids are preserved or reimplanted (Fig. 9.2). By dissecting the tissue in both paratracheal areas, the parathyroids and recurrent laryngeal nerves will be exposed to a higher risk of damage. In clinical situations where bilateral paratracheal lymph nodes are seen, this will have to be done. However it may be reasonable to perform ipsilateral paratracheal lymph node (level VI) dissection if the thyroid cancer is confined to one lobe and there are no enlarged level VI nodes on the contralateral side. This will reduce the risks of serious morbidity such as chronic hypocalcemia and bilateral vocal cord paralysis.

(a) Start out by identifying the common carotid artery. Fascia is dissected off the carotid artery from level of the hyoid bone to behind the sternoclavicular joint. The tissue with its lymph nodes is dissected medially.
(b) The recurrent laryngeal nerve is identified and is gently freed away from the soft tissue along its length, thus skeletonizing the nerve.
(c) The parathyroid glands in particular the superior parathyroid may be identified and

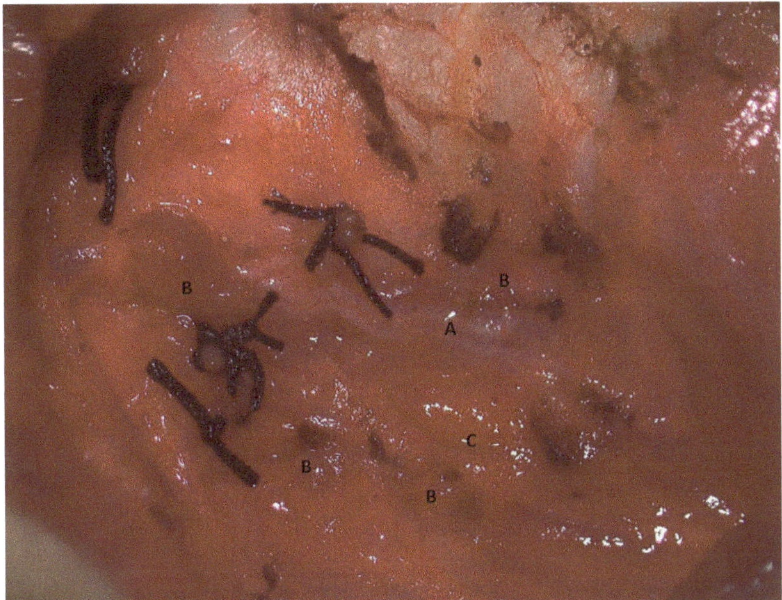

Fig. 9.1 Left level VI with metastatic nodes. *A* left recurrent laryngeal nerve, *B* metastatic lymph nodes, *C* left superior parathyroid gland

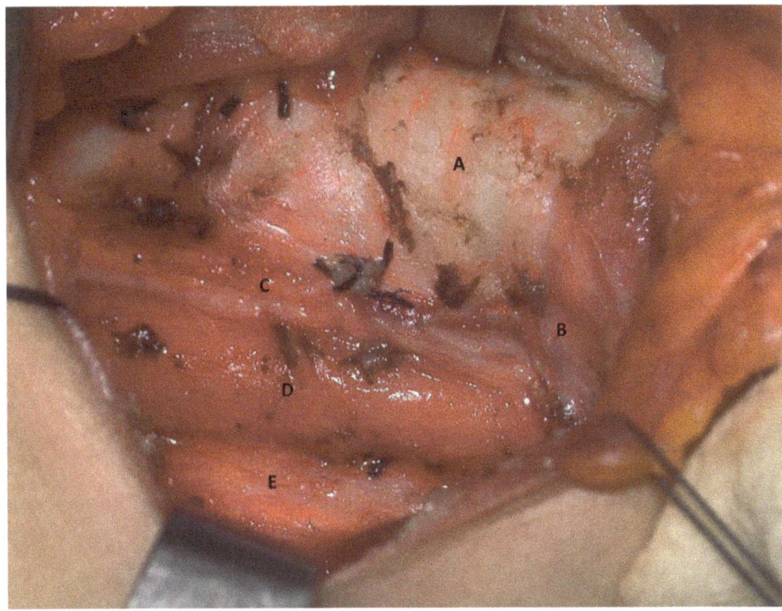

Fig. 9.2 Left levels VI and VII dissected. *A* trachea, *B* cricothyroid joint, *C* left recurrent laryngeal nerve, *D* esophagus, *E* carotid artery

part of it removed for confirmation by frozen section (Fig. 9.3). Occasionally, with multiple nodes in level VI, it may be difficult to be certain of the superior parathyroid. If it is actually dissected off the paratracheal bed, a small part of it is removed, and confirmation is obtained on frozen section. This is to ensure it is parathyroid tissue and not harboring metastatic cells. The tissue is kept in saline. Parathyroid will sink to the bottom of the container, as opposed to fatty tissue which will float. At the end of the operation, the parathyroid tissue is divided with a scalpel. A pocket is created on the ipsilateral sternocleidomastoid muscle and the finely

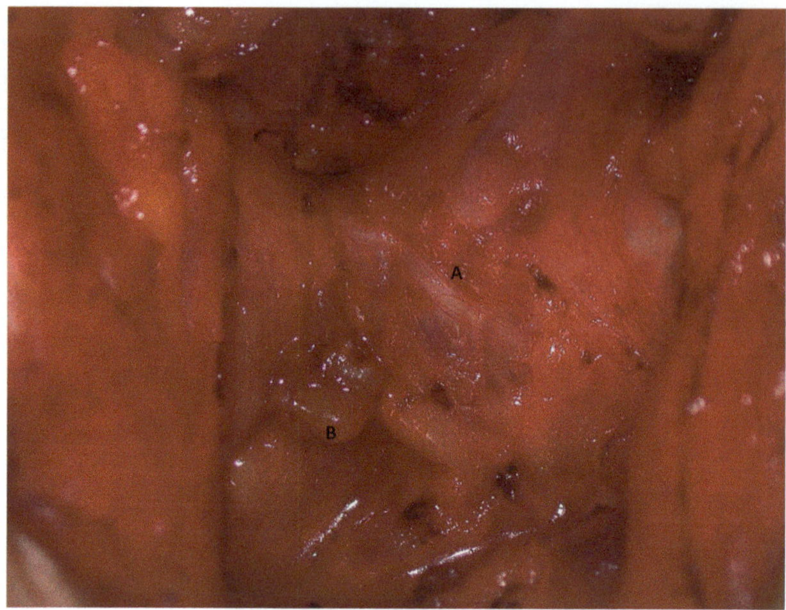

Fig. 9.3 Right level VI before dissection. *A* right recurrent laryngeal nerve, *B* right superior parathyroid

divided pieces are placed into it. The pocket of the muscle is closed with a 2.0 silk suture.

(d) Dissection is continued in a superior to inferior direction, ensuring the recurrent laryngeal nerve is dissected free of the lymph nodes along its length, including anterior and posterior to the plane of the nerve.
(e) The posterior limit of the dissection medially is the esophagus. The esophageal wall is identified, and the fascia with the lymph nodes is separated from it.
(f) Eventually the entire packet of tissue is brought medial to the plane of the recurrent laryngeal nerve and onto the anterior-lateral tracheal wall. It may then be connected with the tissue from the superior mediastinum.
(g) The key to dissecting the superior mediastinum tissue is to have superior traction and good exposure provided by counter traction of the strap muscles inferiorly. By blunt and sharp dissection, the innominate artery is palpated and exposed. Thymus tissue may be encountered. The tissue with its lymph nodes is brought superiorly and connected with the level VI tissue, thus completing the central neck dissection.

Lateral Neck Dissection

Lateral neck dissection for thyroid surgery largely involves levels II–V (Fig. 9.4). An extended Kocher's incision is made, with a short vertical limb extending toward the mastoid tip. Sub-platysma skin flaps are raised. There are others who will extend the transverse thyroidectomy incision laterally without extending it vertically.

(a) Fascia overlying the sternocleidomastoid muscle is dissected to expose the anterior border of the muscle. Dissection of the fascia sheath continues along the length of the muscle from the lateral to the medial aspect.
(b) The spinal accessory nerve is identified and skeletonized. To remove level IIb, the fibrofatty tissue superior to the accessory nerve is dissected off the floor of the neck.
(c) The floor of the neck is delineated and the overlying fascia dissected off the muscle bed. This is carried from levels II to IV. The omo-

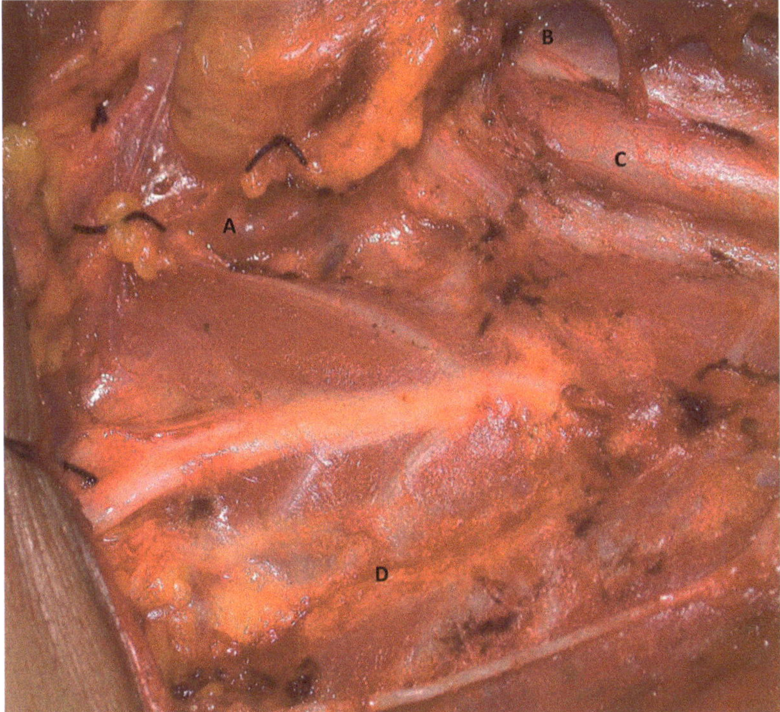

Fig. 9.4 Left level IV (Chassaignac's triangle). Area predisposed to chyle leak. *A* thoracic duct, *B* left internal jugular vein, *C* left common carotid artery, *D* level Vb

hyoid muscle is divided at the tendon thereby allowing exposure of the internal jugular vein. The phrenic nerve is identified approximately 1 cm lateral to the inferior aspect of the internal jugular vein (Fig. 9.4).

(d) The spinal accessory nerve is skeletonized in the posterior triangle, and fibrofatty tissue is dissected off the floor of the neck.

(e) Supraclavicular and posterior triangle soft tissue (level V) are then dissected off the floor of the neck superficial to the prevertebral fascia. Together with the levels II–IV tissue, the entire tissue is then dissected off the carotid sheath. Tributaries to the internal jugular vein are ligated, with the vagus nerve and the carotid artery visualized and preserved.

(f) The submandibular gland forms the superior extent of the neck dissection. The hypoglossal nerve is identified and preserved.

(g) When completed, level II–V lymph nodes are removed but preserving the sternocleidomastoid muscle, internal jugular vein, and the accessory nerve. (Fig. 9.5).

Complications

Central Neck Dissection

The main complications of central neck dissection are related to the recurrent laryngeal nerve, parathyroid glands, carotid artery, innominate artery, and esophagus.

Hemorrhage

Vascular injury though infrequent may lead to catastrophic results. The lateral boundary of the central neck dissection is the carotid artery that may be injured during dissection. It may be avoided by good exposure of the carotid along the length of dissection as well as careful dissection of the fascia away from the wall of the artery. Inferiorly, a high-riding innominate artery may

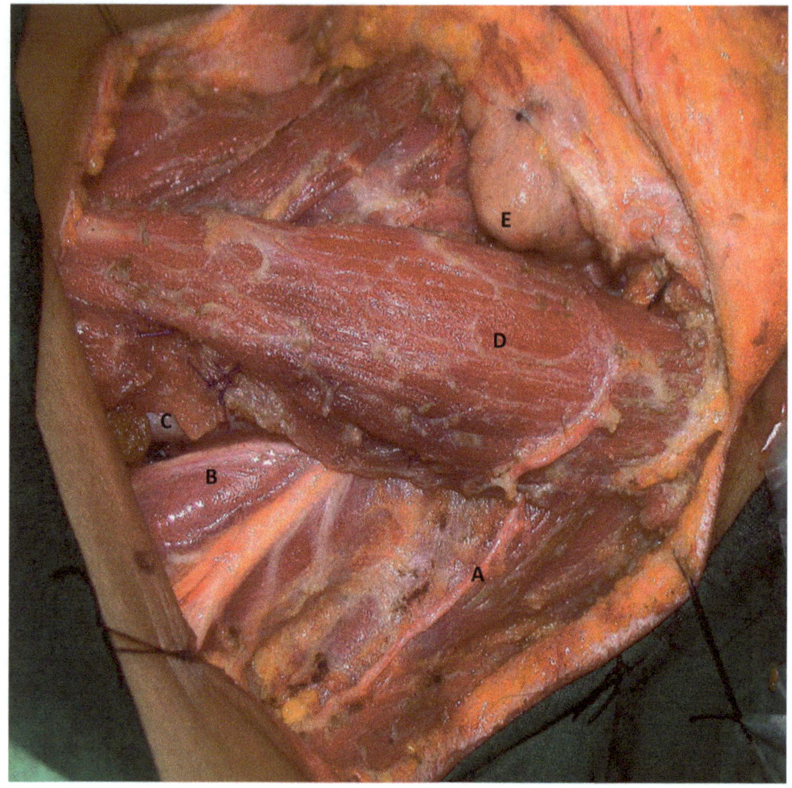

Fig. 9.5 Neck dissection (levels II–V). *A* accessory nerve dissected free of lymph nodes and preserved, *B* phrenic nerve preserved, *C* internal jugular vein (level IV), *D* sternocleidomastoid muscle preserved, *E* submandibular gland (level I) preserved

also be encountered. Careful palpation within the superior mediastinum for transmitted pulsations of a high-riding innominate artery will possibly reduce the risk of injury to the artery. More commonly encountered though are the thyroidea ima artery and its branches as well as the veins draining into the brachiocephalic vein. Small branches of the inferior thyroid artery may also be a cause of bleeding. As dissection progresses in level VII, it may be prudent to ligate where appropriate to reduce the risk of primary hemorrhage in this area.

Recurrent Laryngeal Nerve Injury

Central neck dissection puts the recurrent laryngeal nerve at risk due to the intimate relationship between the lymph nodes and the nerve. In order to minimize the chance of local and regional recurrences within the central neck compartment, meticulous dissection should be performed to remove all fibrofatty tissue surrounding the recurrent laryngeal nerve. This will inevitably involve skeletonizing the recurrent laryngeal nerve. The potential for either neuropraxia or transection of the nerve is significant. Thermal or traction injury may be the cause of recurrent laryngeal nerve palsy. Recurrent laryngeal nerve monitoring has been advocated in thyroidectomy. However, multiple reviews conclude that vocal fold palsy rates may not be significantly different from visual localization [25]. In central neck dissection, the recurrent laryngeal nerve will have been exposed following the thyroidectomy. Hence the utility of laryngeal nerve monitoring in reducing recurrent laryngeal nerve injury in central neck dissection is uncertain and may be of limited benefit. The risk of temporary or permanent (unilateral or bilateral) vocal fold paralysis in central neck dissection has been reported to be similar to total thyroidectomy alone [26, 27]. Even if the injury was a neuropraxia, patients who develop bilateral vocal fold palsy may take some time before sufficient movements return. Either keeping the patient intubated or a tracheostomy may be required to reestablish the airway. In addition, these patients may also have significant risks for aspiration and may require enteral feeding until recovery occurs.

Hypocalcemia/Hypoparathyroidism

Accidental removal or devascularization of the parathyroid glands may result in significant postoperative hypocalcemia. This can either be transient or permanent. Severe hypocalcemia may lead to tetany and prolonged hospitalization. Central neck dissection has been associated with transient hypocalcemia and permanent hypocalcemia [7, 28, 29]. The best way to reduce the risk of hypocalcemia is to identify the parathyroids, followed by frozen section confirmation. Alternatively the parathyroids may be reimplanted into the ipsilateral sternocleidomastoid muscle. Preservation of the branches of the inferior thyroid artery is helpful.

Lateral Neck Dissection

The various complications of neck dissection have been well described [30, 31]. In lateral neck dissection for thyroid cancers, the specific complications relate mainly to the spinal accessory nerve, vagus nerve, phrenic nerve, sympathetic trunk, and the thoracic duct.

Spinal Accessory Nerve

Transection of the nerve invariably leads to weakness in abduction of the arm. Chronic shoulder pain is experienced in some patients following devascularization of the nerve, leading to significant stiffness, discomfort, and sometimes intense pain for these patients. This forms the basis for advocating that levels Va and IIb may be spared to reduce devascularization risk to the accessory nerve.

Vagus Nerve Injury

The vagus nerve lies within the carotid sheath. Vagal nerve injury will result in vocal fold paralysis. It can be difficult to locate the vagus nerve in patients with bulky matted level III and IV nodes. The safest way is to begin identifying the vagus nerve more proximally in the region of level II and meticulously dissecting the bulky nodes away from the carotid sheath. Visualization of the vagus nerve is crucial to avoiding injury, in particular in the region of left level IV. In this area of neck dissection, it is always prudent to ligate tissues systematically to avoid thoracic duct chyle leak. Hence, knowing the path of the vagus nerve will help avoid accidentally ligating it when level IV nodes are dissected. If vagus nerve injury does occur, these patients will not only present with hoarseness but will also have significant aspiration due to reduced sensation, affecting the afferent feedback that is necessary to close off the larynx during swallowing.

Chyle Leak

Chyle leak has been estimated to occur in 1.4–8.3% of neck dissections in thyroid cancers [30, 32, 33]. It can occur with left or right lateral neck dissection [32, 33]. The right lymphatic duct drains into the right internal jugular vein or right subclavian vein. The thoracic duct ascends to the root of the neck and subsequently drains into the subclavian vein on the left side of the neck (Fig. 9.4). In particular, the thoracic duct lies in a precarious position during dissection of left level IV nodes. Thoracic duct injuries may be prevented by meticulous ligation during dissection of the fibrofatty tissue in level IV. In patients with large nodes or multiple nodes in level IV, the risk of thoracic duct injury is higher [32]. In the event of inadvertent tears of the thoracic duct or its tributaries, compressive figure of eight sutures can be applied. It is best to deal with a chyle leak once it is discovered. If the chyle leak is discovered post operation, the major decision on how it should be managed depends on the daily volume of chyle in the drain bottle. If this is more than 300 mL or more every 24 h and not reducing in the next few days despite conservative measures, the patient will benefit from re-exploration to stop the chyle leak. Conservative measures include a complete fat-free diet such as glucose drinks, medium chain triglyceride diet, and parenteral octreotide. More invasive measures include intravenous total parenteral nutrition and surgical exploration.

Phrenic Nerve and Cervical Sympathetic Trunk Injury

The phrenic nerve lies anteriorly on the belly of the scalenus anterior muscle. It is covered by a layer of prevertebral fascia. Metastatic nodes do not usually breach this fascia. Nevertheless dissection of level IV and III nodes may accidentally breach this fascia and injure the nerve. This may occur in patients with large bulky nodes, or it may be simply an iatrogenic injury. The consequence is often clinically silent. The injury results in a raised hemidiaphragm, and it may affect the respiratory effort in obese patients or those with pre-existing lung problems.

The cervical sympathetic trunk lies posterior to the carotid sheath. It is in an anatomical position that is not within the boundaries of neck dissections. However, in patients with large metastatic nodes, which may extend lateral and posterior to the carotid artery, the cervical sympathetic trunk may be injured. This results in Horner's syndrome which does not recover.

> Prophylactic central neck dissection (PCND) remains controversial. The current literature is divided between authors who perform PCND routinely and those who selectively perform PCND.

> The view of proponents of PCND include improvements in thyroglobulin levels post central neck dissection, a more accurate staging of patients, and the belief that performing PCND at the initial surgery improves loco-regional control. Furthermore, PCND decreases the potential morbidity of re-operation. There has however been no high level evidence to directly correlate PCND with improvements in loco-regional control or overall survival. This is due to inherent difficulties in performing quality clinical trials for a condition that in general has low mortality and morbidity risks.

> Authors who propose a selective approach for PCND reasoned that the role of central neck dissections do not clearly improve patient survival. In addition, with adjuvant radioactive iodine, loco-regional control as well as thyroglobulin levels reach similar levels to that of patients undergoing routine PCND. Furthermore, routine PCND are not without significant morbidity even if the risks are low. Several reports have attributed central neck dissections with a significantly greater risk of transient hypocalcemia compared to a total thyroidectomy.

> The recent guidelines by the American Thyroid Association published in 2015 states that prophylactic neck dissections may be considered in patients with advanced T3/T4 primary tumours, clinically involved lateral neck nodes or if the information gathered will aid in further management. This was however backed by low-quality evidence and was graded as a weak recommendation. Conversely, in patients with small T1/T2 papillary thyroid cancers with no evidence of nodal disease and patients with follicular carcinoma, the guideline gives strong recommendations total thyroidectomy without PCND is appropriate.

References

1. Carty SE, Cooper DS, Doherty GM, Duh QY, Kloos RT, Mandel SJ, Randolph GW, Stack BC Jr, Steward DL, Terris DJ, Thompson GB, Tufano RP, Tutle RM, Udelsman R. Consensus statement on the terminology and classification of central neck dissection for thyroid cancer. Thyroid. 2009;19:1153–8.

2. Robbins KT, Medina JE, Wolfe GT, Levine PA, Sessions RB, Pruet CW. Standardizing neck dissection terminology. Arch Otolaryngol Head Neck Surg. 1991;117:601–5.
3. Kupferman ME, Patterson M, Mandel SJ, LiVolsi V, Weber RS. Patterns of lateral neck metastasis in papillary thyroid carcinoma. Arch Otolaryngol Head Neck Surg. 2004;130:857–60.
4. Sivanandan R, Soo KC. Pattern of cervical lymph node metastases from papillary carcinoma of the thyroid. Br J Surg. 2001;88(9):1241–4.
5. Ji YB, Lee DW, Song CM, Kim KR, Prk CW, Tae K. Accuracy of intraoperative determination of central node metastasis by the surgeon in papillary thyroid carcinoma. Otolaryngol Head Neck Surg. 2014;150(4):542–7.
6. Nixon IJ, Wang LY, Ganly I, Patel SG, Morris LG, Migliacci JC, Tuttle RM, Shah JP, Shaha AR. Outcomes for patients with papillary thyroid cancer who do not undergo prophylactic central neck dissection. Br J Surg. 2016;103:218–25.
7. Lang BH, Ng SH, Lau LL, Cowling BJ, Wong KP, Wan KY. A systematic review and meta-analysis of prophylactic central neck dissection on short-term locoregional recurrence in papillary thyroid carcinomaafter total thyroidectomy. Thyroid. 2013;23(9):1087–98.
8. Qu H, Sun GR, Liu Y, He QS. Clinical risk factors for central lymph node metastasis in papillary carcinoma: a systematic review and meta-analysis. Clin Endocrinol. 2015;83(1):124–32.
9. Suman P, Wang CH, Abadin SS, Moo-Young TA, Prinz RA, Winchester DJ. Risk factors for central lymph node metastasis in papillary thyroid carcinoma: a National Cancer Data Base (NCDB) study. Surgery. 2016;159:31–9.
10. Mitchell AL, Gandhi A, Scott-Coombes D, Prros P. Management of thyroid cancer: United Kingdom National Multidisciplinary Guidelines. J Laryngol Otol. 2016;130:S150–60.
11. Haugen BR, Alexander EK, Bible KC, Doherty GM, Mandel SJ, Nikiforov YE, Pacini F, Randolph GW, Sawka AM, Schlumberger M, Schuff KG, Sherman SI, Sosa JA, Steward DL, Tuttle RM, Wartofsky L. 2015 American Thyroid Association Management Guidelines for adult patients with thyroid nodules and differentiated thyroid cancer: the American Thyroid Association Guidelines Task Force on thyroid nodules and differentiated thyroid cancer. Thyroid. 2016;26(1):1–133.
12. Su W, Lan X, Zhang H, Dong W, Wang Z, He L, Zhang T, Liu S. Risk factors for central lymph node metastasis in cN0 papillary thyroid carcinoma. A systematic review and meta-analysis. PLoS One. 2015;10(10):e0139021.
13. Ma B, Wang Y, Yang S, Ji Q. Predictive factors for central lymph node metastasis in patients with cN0 paillary thyrod carcinoma: a systematic review and meta-analysis. Int J Surg. 2016;28:153–61.
14. Kazure HS, Roman SA, Sosa JA. Aggressive variants of papillary thyroid cancer: incidence, characteristics and predictors of survival among 43,738 patients. Ann Surg Oncol. 2012;19(6):1874–80.
15. Pezzi TA, Sandulache VC, Pezzi CM, Turkeltaub AE, Feng L, Cabillanas ME, Williams MD, Lai SY. Treatment and survival of patients with insular thyroid carcinoma: 508 cases from the National Cancer Data Base. Head Neck. 2016;38(6):906–12.
16. Joo JY, Park JY, Yoon YH, Choi B, Kim JM, Jo YS, Shong M, Koo BS. Prediction of occult centra lymph node metastasis in papillary thyroid carcinoma by preoperative BRAF analysis using fine-needle aspiration biopsy: prospective study. J Clin Endocrinol Metab. 2012;97(11):3996–4003.
17. Stack BC, Ferris RL, Goldenburg D, Hayman M, Shaha A, Sheth S, Sosa JA, Tufano RP. American Thyroid Association consensus review and statement regarding anatomy, terminology and rationale for lateral neck dissection in differentiated thyroid cancer. Thyroid. 2012;22(5):501–8.
18. Hwang HS, Orloff LA. Efficacy of preoperative neck ultrasound in the detection of cervical lymph node metastasis from thyroid cancer. Laryngoscope. 2011;121(30):487–91.
19. Randolph GW, Duh QY, Heller KS, LiVolsi VA, Mandel SJ, Steward DL, Tufaano RP, Tuttle RM. The prognostic significance of nodal metastases from papillary thyroid carcinoma can be stratified based on the size and number of metastatic lymph nodes, as well as the presence of extranodal extension. Thyroid. 2012;22(11):1144–52.
20. Madenei AL, Caragaciance D, Boeckmann JO, Stack BC Jr, Shin JJ. Lateral neck dissection for well differentiated thyroid carcinoma: a systematic review. Laryngoscope. 2014;124(7):1724–34.
21. Ahn D, Sohn JH, Kim JH, Shin CM, Jeon JH, Park JY. Preoperative subclinical hypothyroidism in patients with papillary thyroid carcinoma. Am J Otolaryngol. 2013;34(4):312–9.
22. Ahuja AT, Ying M. Sonographic evaluation of cervical lymph nodes. Am J Roentgenol. 2005;184(5):1691–9.
23. Morita S, Mizoguchi K, Suzuki M, Lizuka K. The accuracy of (18)[F]-fluoro-2-deoxy-D-glucose-positron emission tomography/computed tomography, ultrasonography, and enhanced computed tomography alone in the preoperative diagnosis of cervical lymph node metastasis in patients with papillary thyroid carcinoma. World J Surg. 2010;34(11):2564–9.
24. Wang LY, Palmer FL, Thomas D, Shaha AR, Shah JP, Patel SG, Tuttle RM, Ganly I. Pre-operative neck ultrasound in clinical node-negative differentiated thyroid cancer. J Clin Endocrinol Metab. 2014;99(10):3686–93.
25. Dralle H, Sekulla C, Lorenz K, Brauckhoff M, Machens A. German IONM study group. Intraoperative monitoring of the recurrent laryngeal nerve in thyroid surgery. World J Surg. 2008;32(7):1358–66.
26. Chisholm EJ, Kulinskava E, Tolley NS. Systematic review and meta-analysis of the adverse effects of thyroidectomy combined with central neck dissection as

compared with thyroidectomy alone. Laryngoscope. 2009;119(6):1135–9.

27. Shan CX, Zhang W, Jiang DZ, Zheng XM, Liu S, Qiu M. Routine central neck dissection in differentiated thyroid carcinoma: a systematic review and meta-analysis. Laryngoscope. 2012;122(4):797–804.
28. Kim SK, Woo JW, Lee JH, Park I, Choe JH, Kim JH, Kim JS. Prophylactic central neck dissection might not be necessary in papillary thyroid carcinoma: analysis of 11,569 cases from a single institution. J Am Coll Surg. 2016;222(5):853–64.
29. Zhao W, You L, Hou X, Chen S, Ren X, Chen G, Zhao Y. The effect of prophylactic central neck dissection (pCND) on locoregional recurrence in papillary thyroid cancer after total thyroidectomy: systematic review and meta-analysis: pCND for the locoregional recurrence of papillary thyroid cancer. Ann Surg Oncol. 2017;24:2189–98.
30. Polistena A, Monacelli M, Lucchini R, Tviola R, Conti C, Avenia S, Barillaro I, Sanguinetti A, Avenia N. Surgical morbidity of cervical lymphadenopathy for thyroid cancer: a retrospective cohort study over 25 years. Int J Surg. 2015;21:128–34.
31. McMullen C, Rocke D, Freeman J. Complications of bilateral neck dissection in thyroid cancers from a single high-volume center. JAMA Otolaryngol Head Neck Surg. 2017;143:376–81.
32. Ahn D, Sohn JH, Jeong JY. Chyle fistula after neck dissection: an 8-year, single-center, prospective study of incidence, clinical features, and treatment. Ann Surg Oncol. 2015;22(Suppl):S1000–6.
33. Roh JL, Kim DH, Park CI. Prospective identification of chyle leakage in patients undergoing lateral neck dissection for metastatic thyroid cancer. Ann Surg Oncol. 2008;15(2):424–9.

Radioiodine Therapy for Well-Differentiated Thyroid Cancer

10

Sue Ping Thang and David Chee-Eng Ng

Different Functions of Radioiodine for Thyroid Cancer

It has become clearer over the last decade that radioiodine can be deemed to have several fairly distinct clinical functions. The understanding of these functions has helped to define how radioiodine is used clinically.

1. Ablative—to ablate small normal thyroid remnants or residues in the thyroid bed after near-total or total thyroidectomy. This allows the thyroglobulin levels to reflect more accurately the absence/presence of disease as well as the disease burden. After ablation, detection of recurrent disease is rendered more accurate in the absence of significant focal uptake in the neck on the whole-body scan.
2. Adjuvant—to reduce the risk of recurrence post-operatively and disease-specific mortality by presumably destroying low-volume disease. This function is of more relevance in the group of intermediate-risk thyroid cancers than in the low-risk group.
3. Therapy—this role of radioiodine is to treat known local disease or distant metastases.
4. Diagnostic—the role of radioiodine serves to perform a diagnostic scan for detection of iodine-avid disease in a surveillance setting.

From a practical point of view, it is sometimes difficult to distinguish these separate roles of ablation and adjuvant therapy in the use of the first dose of radioiodine, and in fact the roles of ablative and adjuvant were often considered together, even within a single term of "radioiodine ablation" (RAI). Nonetheless, recognising these distinct functions of radioiodine allows a more rational and scientific use of radioiodine for thyroid cancer management.

Evidence for Use of Radioiodine in Thyroid Cancer and Indications

There is a reasonably large body of data supporting the use of radioiodine in thyroid cancer. The interpretation of the evidence for radioiodine is compounded by various factors: the risk stratification of the thyroid cancer in the study population, dose activity of the iodine-131 given, definition of ablation success, length of follow-up and definition of recurrence or ablation success. Despite these differences, there is considerable consensus that patients who are in

S. P. Thang · D. C.-E. Ng (✉)
Department of Nuclear Medicine and Molecular Imaging, Singapore General Hospital, Singapore, Singapore
e-mail: thang.sue.ping@singhealth.com.sg; david.ng.c.e@singhealth.com.sg

R. Parameswaran, A. Agarwal (eds.), *Evidence-Based Endocrine Surgery*,
https://doi.org/10.1007/978-981-10-1124-5_10

the intermediate- or high-risk group would benefit from radioiodine. What is less certain is the role of radioiodine in the low-risk group. Another related question is the dose activity of the radioiodine used.

Sawka et al. [1] provided an early review of the effectiveness of radioactive iodine remnant ablation for well-differentiated thyroid cancer. Out of 1543 English references, pooled analysis were suggestive of a statistically significant treatment effect of ablation for 10-year outcome in loco-regional recurrence (relative risk of 0.31). It was noted that there are conflicting results for some outcomes, and the incremental benefit of remnant ablation in low-risk patients is not clear. In a large cohort study, for patients with primary tumour >1.5 cm or cervical nodal metastases, Mazzaferri and Jhiang [2] showed that there was significant benefit in overall survival in 1004 patients whose recurrence rates were one-third when radioiodine ablation was performed compared to no ablation, and the rates for distant metastases were also reduced. DeGroot also demonstrated that the use of radioiodine ablation reduced the recurrence rate in what is deemed to be stage II/III disease [3].

Jonklaas et al. [4] classified patients as low risk (stages I and II) or high risk (stages III and IV). Treatments employed included near-total thyroidectomy, administration of radioactive iodine and thyroid hormone suppression therapy. Outcome measures were overall survival, disease-specific survival and disease-free survival. Near-total thyroidectomy, radioactive iodine and aggressive thyroid hormone suppression therapy were each independently associated with longer overall survival in high-risk patients. The relative risk of death in the absence of post-operative radioiodine therapy was 43% higher in high-risk patients (stages III and IV in the National Thyroid Cancer Treatment Cooperative Study Group staging system) but not low-risk patients. Near-total thyroidectomy followed by radioactive iodine therapy and moderate thyroid hormone suppression therapy both predicted improved overall survival in stage II patients. They concluded that radioactive iodine therapy is beneficial for stage II, III and IV patients.

The indications for radioiodine treatment are largely based on risk stratification. There are several of such stratification schemes, ranging from the AMES and MACIS scores to various guidelines from different countries and professional societies, such as the British Thyroid Association, the European Society of Medical Oncology and the European Association of Nuclear Medicine to the American Thyroid Association (ATA) Guidelines. As regards the AJCC TNM staging system, it is well known that it stratifies patients into stages based on mortality data. The other risk stratification schemes mentioned are more inclusive of recurrences and hence provide a more overall risk of both recurrence and death. For example, the ATA Guidelines (2015) take into account resection status, histological subtypes and vascular invasion as part of the risk assessment. The use of AJCC TNM classification along with other more inclusive stratification systems such as the American Thyroid Association (ATA) risk stratification classification would more likely provide a more complete characterisation of the risk profile of the patient to guide management and prognostication.

More recently, more emphasis is given to a dynamic risk stratification system as post-ablation management of patients requires an approach to estimate risk change over time based on response to therapy and course of the disease. Tuttle showed that when the ATA guidelines (2009) were used to risk stratify patients, the change in risk estimates as a function of response to therapy is most notable in the ATA intermediate-risk group where an estimated risk of recurrent or persistent structural disease of 18% dropped to as little as 2% in patients having an excellent response to therapy [5]. This is useful for making decisions about radioiodine therapy on follow-up management. It also indirectly suggests that radioiodine has clinical impact on intermediate-risk thyroid cancer and that dynamic risk stratification is helpful in revising the risk status of patients and guiding future management.

In view of these published data and others, ATA guidelines (2015) [6] recommend the following regarding the use of radioiodine in different groups of patients, who are stratified by two systems—the ATA risk stratification system and the TNM stage—to provide guidance as to whether radioiodine ablation is indicated:

ATA risk category and TNM stage	Description of TNM stage	Radioiodine ablation indicated?
ATA low risk T1a	T ≤1 cm	No
ATA low risk T1b, T2	T 1–4 cm	Not routine+
ATA low and intermediate risk T3	T >4 cm or minimal ETE	Consider—generally favoured for minimal ETE
ATA low and intermediate risk T1–3 N1a or N1b	Central compartment or lateral compartment nodes	Consider—generally favoured
ATA high risk T4	Gross ETE	Yes
ATA high risk M1	Distant metastases	Yes

Based on the ATA guidelines, for patients that fulfil the criteria for low-risk thyroid cancer predominantly those with unifocal intra-thyroidal papillary microcarcinoma without any other adverse features, the evidence appears to support the concept that there is no need for radioiodine ablation (RAI). In other low-risk tumours with adverse features, radioiodine ablation may be considered on a case-by-case basis, perhaps with a low radioiodine dosing (eg: 30 mCi). In general, however, it appears reasonable at the current time to consider radioiodine ablation and treatment for intermediate-risk and high-risk thyroid cancer.

Radioactive Dosing

There are typically two major methodologies for deciding radioiodine dosing. Most centres use the empirical method which has standardised ranges of prescribed activity for different categories of patients, as described earlier. A few centers use lesional and body dosimetry to estimate the maximum tolerated absorbed dose to the bone marrow or whole body and calculate the radioiodine dose activity to be given in individual patients.

Current empirical dosing depends to a large extent on the risk stratification of patients.

Specifically for relatively low-risk thyroid cancer, two major clinical trials [7, 8] attempted to test the hypothesis that 30 mCi is non-inferior to 100 mCi and in a thyroxine withdrawal versus a recombinant thyroid-stimulating hormone (TSH) group. The follow-up is less than 9 months, and in both the end points were ablation success. The data cannot nor should it be extrapolated to the risk of recurrence. The results showed that as far as ablation success is concerned, 30 mCi is not statistically inferior to 100 mCi. Although the evidence is not strongly conclusive for the use of a “low dose” of 30 mCi, in general it would appear fairly reasonable to consider such a lower dose activity of radioiodine in the treatment of low-risk thyroid cancer. The NCCN guidelines have a similar recommendation for the use of 30 mCi in low-risk thyroid cancer.

For intermediate-risk thyroid cancer, the evidence for the effective dose activity is more varied and less uniform, due to various factors: the number of patients studied and patient selection, type of risk stratification classification of the thyroid cancer in the study population, different ranges of dose activity of the iodine-131 given, definition of ablation success, duration of follow-up and definition of recurrence. A summary of the findings is given in the table.

Study	Definition of risk and subjects studied	Results after radioiodine ablation
DeGroot et al. (1990) [3]	All risk groups (n = 269 (total))	30 mCi vs. 50–60 mCi Better ablation with higher dose Average follow-up 12 years from diagnosis
Mazzaferri and Jhiang (1994) [2]	All risk groups (n = 1355)	29–50 mCi vs. 51–200 mCi No difference recurrence rate Follow-up was 15.7 years (median)
Bal et al. (1996) [9]	All risk groups (n = 149)	30 mCi vs. 50 mCi vs. 90 mCi vs. 155 mCi Dose-response plateaus after 50 mCi ablation Evaluation was performed 6–12 months after radioiodine ablation
Verburg et al. (2014) [10]	Low risk: T1/2 High risk: T3/4 and/or N1 M1 disease included (n = 1298)	Mortality higher in <54 mCi, than in 54–81 mCi or >81 mCi in those >45 years old especially in high risk group. Follow-up at least 5 years
Kruijff et al. (2013) [11]	T1–T3 No mention of N stage (n = 970)	No difference in recurrence rate between <75 mCi vs. >75 mCi. Follow-up was 60 months (mean)
Castagna et al. (2013) [12]	T3 and/or N1 (n = 225)	No difference in ablation success between 30 and 50 mCi vs. >100 mCi. Follow-up was 6–18 months (median 9 months)
Sabra et al. (2014) [13]	N1b disease (n = 181)	Not significant for young, but plausible significant better response for older patients with higher dosing. 100 mCi vs. 150 mCi vs. >200 mCi. Follow-up was 3.6 years (median)
Han et al. (2014) [14]	T3 ETE (n = 176)	No difference in recurrence or ablation success by 30 mCi vs. 150 mCi. Follow-up was 7.2 years (median)

For intermediate-risk thyroid cancer, ATA guidelines (2015) considers it reasonable to consider dosing activity of between 30 and 150 mCi, although the evidence is clearly heterogeneous due to the many variables present in the clinical literature. Based on the currently available evidence and various practice guidelines, it may generally be recommended that a generally higher dose activity such as 100 mCi be considered for intermediate-risk thyroid cancer, particularly when an adjuvant function of radioiodine is deemed important for the particular patient.

For high-risk thyroid cancer patients, there is more consensus opinion for the range of dose activity to be administered, particularly for those with iodine-avid distant metastases. For pulmonary metastases, it is recommended that patients should be treated with radioiodine in the primary consideration, unless there are clinical concerns, as long as the disease continues to concentrate radioiodine and respond clinically. For iodine-avid bone metastases, typical dose activities range from 100 to 200 mCi or more, or as determined by dosimetry. For lung metastases, it is recommended that the dose activity should be limited to a whole-body retention of below 80 mCi at 48 h or 2 Gy to the bone marrow. Lung function tests may be useful as an adjunct to follow-up on patients with extensive iodine-avid pulmonary metastases given radioiodine in large dosing and where the uptake of the radioiodine is clearly significant. It is also well known that in renal failure, the retention time of radioiodine in the body can be significantly increased and the dosing should be correspondingly adjusted lower.

For paediatric individuals, the dosing of radioiodine should be adjusted accordingly. For radioiodine ablation in children, some centres adjust activity by body weight (e.g. to 1.85–7.4 MBq/kg) or surface area or by age (e.g. to 1/3 the adult activity in a 5-year-old, 1/2 the adult activity in a 10-year-old or 5/6 the adult activity in a 15-year-old). Another approach, recommended in the German procedure guidelines for radioiodine therapy in paediatric DTC patients, is to adjust the ablation activity according to the 24-h thyroid bed uptake of a test activity of radioiodine as well as according to body weight: <5% uptake would warrant an activity of 50 MBq/kg, 5–10% uptake would warrant an activity of 25 MBq/kg and 10–20% uptake would warrant an activity of 15 MBq/kg. Because it maximises the degree of individualisation, flexible ablation dosing according to one or more individual patient body characteristics, i.e. weight, surface area and thyroid bed radioiodine uptake, appears to be a preferable strategy to fixed dosing or to flexible dosing based on age [15].

Practical aspects include the avoidance of iodine-rich foodstuff and confounding substances such as IV contrast and amiodarone that may inhibit the uptake of radioiodine. There is controversy regarding the necessity of a low-iodine diet, with some centres and guidelines recommending different durations of avoidance and types of foodstuff. A few centres measure urinary iodine to determine if the radioiodine administration should be postponed. The TSH should be elevated to >30 U/L through either thyroxine withdrawal or rhTSH administration.

Procedure

Patient Preparation

Thyroid-Stimulating Hormone Stimulation

The effectiveness of radioiodine therapy depends on the patient's serum TSH level being adequately elevated. A TSH level of at least 30 mU/L is believed to increase sodium-iodide symporter (NIS) expression and thereby optimise radioiodine uptake [16]. In cases where TSH stimulation is difficult, such as when completion thyroidectomy is technically impossible or undesired in patients with large thyroid remnants, or in patients with functional metastatic thyroid disease, endogenous TSH level of less than 30 mU/L is acceptable [15].

The TSH elevation can be achieved via two main ways:

1. Thyroid hormone withdrawal (THW)
2. Recombinant human thyrotropin (rhTSH, trade name Thyrogen) administration

Comparison between the two techniques has been performed in multiple studies [7, 8, 17–23] in the setting of thyroid remnant ablation (Table 10.1). These studies showed that rhTSH for preparation for remnant ablation is associated with similar rates of successful remnant ablation but superior short-term quality of life compared to THW.

The 2015 ATA guidelines [6] suggest that the use of rhTSH is an acceptable alternative to THW in patients with low to intermediate risk without extensive lymph node involvement (i.e. T1–T3, N0/Nx/N1a, M0). The use of rhTSH may also be considered in patients with intermediate-risk differentiated thyroid cancer (DTC) who have extensive lymph node disease in the absence of distant metastasis. However, in patients with high-risk DTC with higher risks of disease-related mortality and morbidity, more RCT data from long-term outcome studies are needed before rhTSH preparation can be recommended. rhTSH preparation can nevertheless be considered in patients with DTC of any risk level with significant comorbidity that may preclude thyroid hormone withdrawal prior to RAI administration. This includes patients who are unable to produce an adequate endogenous TSH rise (e.g. hypopituitarism) and those with significant medical (e.g. cardiac failure) or psychiatric comorbidity which could be exacerbated by hypothyroidism induced with THW.

Clinical caution is advised during TSH stimulation (especially with rhTSH) in patients with known sites of metastatic disease involving the central nervous system, lungs or bones. Extreme or prolonged elevations of TSH from either thyroid hormone withdrawal or rhTSH may acutely stimulate tumour growth and compromise function of structures adjacent to these sites [24–27]. High-dose steroid co-administration to prevent tumour swelling is therefore recommended. Dexamethasone has been used in doses of 2–4 mg every 8 h starting 6–12 h prior to rhTSH and RAI dosing or after 10–12 days of thyroid hormone withdrawal, with the steroids continued in a tapering dosage schedule for 1 week post-therapy, for 48–72 h after rhTSH administration, or for 72 h after reinstitution of thyroxine therapy in the setting of thyroid hormone withdrawal [28]. A reduced dose of rhTSH or an attenuated degree and duration of endogenous TSH elevation after thyroid hormone withdrawal (achieved by the temporary addition of triiodothyronine (LT_3) therapy to thyroxine replacement prior to RAI and to recommence thyroxine (LT_4) therapy once the dose of RAI is administered) should be considered (Table 10.1).

Table 10.1 Thyroid hormone withdrawal (THW) vs rhTSH administration

	Thyroid hormone withdrawal (THW)	rhTSH administration
Regimen	(a) LT_4 withdrawal (b) LT_4 withdrawal with substitution of LT_3 in initial weeks • For those on hormone replacement therapy, withdrawal of LT_4 should be at least 3–4 weeks and LT_3 at least 2 weeks prior to radioiodine administration • For those post-thyroidectomy and not on hormone replacement therapy, waiting for at least 3 weeks after surgery is recommended prior to radioiodine administration • Thyroid hormone should be initiated or resumed 2–3 days after radioiodine administration • Serum thyroglobulin should be obtained under TSH stimulation, e.g. on the day of and prior to radioiodine administration	• Two consecutive daily intramuscular injections of 0.9 mg. Subcutaneous injection may be used in patients on oral anticoagulants to reduce the risk of injection site haematoma • Radioiodine is given 1 day after the second rhTSH injection • Patient can continue with hormone replacement therapy • Serum thyroglobulin should be checked at the time of maximal TSH stimulation, i.e. 3 days after the last rhTSH injection
Clinical use	• High-risk DTC	• Low- to intermediate-risk DTC with or without extensive neck lymphadenopathy • Presence of hypothyroidism-related comorbidities, or unable to raise endogenous TSH, irrespective of risk level
Advantages	• Low cost • No Intramuscular/Subcutaneous injections • May improve lesion detection for metastatic disease	• No hypothyroid symptoms • Produce more rapid and predictable TSH elevation • Improved or preserved renal function under euthyroid status may decrease radiation exposure of extra-thyroidal tissues and blood • Treatment can be given at any time, although a 2-week recovery period is advisable in post-operative setting
Disadvantages	• Hypothyroid symptoms potentially resulting in deterioration of existing medical condition and quality of life • Potential delay of treatment for at least 3–4 weeks to allow for adequate TSH stimulation	• Relatively higher cost • Requires Intramuscular/Subcutaneous injections • May be associated with mild nausea, headache and general lethargy with rhTSH injections

Table 10.2 Recommended time of withdrawal for pharmaceuticals blocking radioiodine uptake [29]

Type of medication	Recommended time of withdrawal
Thionamide medications (e.g. propylthiouracil, methimazole carbimazole)	3 days
Multivitamins containing iodide	7–10 days
Natural or synthetic thyroid hormones	10–14 days for triiodothyronine, 3–4 weeks for thyroxine
Kelp, agar, carrageenan, Lugol solution	2–3 weeks, depending on iodide content
Saturated solution of potassium iodide	2–3 weeks
Topical iodine (e.g. surgical skin preparation)	2–3 weeks
Intravenous radiographic contrast agents:	
Water soluble	6–8 weeks, assuming normal renal function
Lipophilic	1–6 months
Amiodarone	3–6 months or longer

Avoidance of Iodine Excess

Iodine excess may result in competitive handling by NIS of non-radioactive iodine rather than radioiodine, and potentially resulting in reduced efficacy of RAI therapy.

Patients should be advised to avoid iodine-containing medications prior to RAI therapy (Table 10.2). As thyroid hormone also contains iodine, some clinicians stop thyroid hormones for about 4 days before RAI therapy if rhTSH is used [29]. The half-life of thyroxine of 7 days however makes this recommendation of uncertain value.

The use of low-iodine diet (LID) is also recommended. The optimal stringency and duration of LID prior to RAI therapy are not known. Systematic review of observational studies showed that LIDs (≤50 μg/day of iodine) for 1–2 weeks appeared to be associated with reduction in urinary iodine excretion as well as increase in radioiodine uptake [30]. The recommendation for a low-iodine diet can be found on www.thyroid.org/faq-low-iodine-diet/.

Urinary iodine excretion can be measured in doubtful cases. Levels above an arbitrary institutional cut-off in the range of 150–200 μg/L are believed to reflect clinically relevant iodine excess and should lead to postponement of RAI therapy [15].

Others

Food intake may alter the absorption of orally administered radioiodine. The patient should not take any food or water by mouth for approximately 2 h before and 1–2 h after the oral administration of RAI [15, 29].

Radiation Safety Advice

Depending on the dose of radioiodine administered, the patient may require hospitalisation during RAI therapy to avoid unnecessary radiation exposure to family members and members of the public. Inpatient stay may be required when the administered activity is more than a certain threshold eg: 1.22 GBq (33 mCi) [29] in some countries. The patient will be discharged when the radiation exposure is less than a prescribed threshold which may vary from country to country.

Written instructions on how to reduce radiation exposure should be given to patients. These typically include the following after therapy [29] although some centres may have slightly differing practices:

- Prolonged use of public transportation is generally discouraged for the first 24 h after RAI therapy.
- Patient is to sleep alone and should abstain close contact for approximately 1 week after therapy.
- Alternative care arrangements for up to a week may be necessary for patients with infants and small children. Close contact of approximately 10 min daily is allowed but patients should otherwise maintain a distance of about 0.9–1.8 m (3–6 ft) from pregnant women and children.
- Exposure of family members from items contaminated by patient's saliva or urine must be prevented, e.g. dishes and utensils should not

be shared before washing, toilet should be flushed twice after use followed by adequate hand washing and men may urinate sitting down to avoid contamination in the toilet area.

Pregnancy, Breastfeeding and Conception

Pregnancy must be excluded within a few days before each RAI therapy, by a beta-hCG-based test preferably. Adjunctive use of ultrasound to rule out pregnancy may also be considered. A falsely negative urinary pregnancy test during a late (midterm) pregnancy is potentially possible due to both a decreased production of beta-hCG and a decreased degree of salinisation, which results in a shorter half-life of beta-hCG due to its breakdown in the liver [31, 32].

As radioiodine can accumulate in the breasts, RAI therapy should be deferred until lactating women have stopped breastfeeding or expressing for at least 3 months.

Most experts recommend that both men and women use effective contraception for 6–12 months after RAI therapy before trying to conceive. A 12-month interval also allows for follow-up imaging to evaluate the effectiveness of the treatment and for retreatment if deemed appropriate.

Post-therapy Scintigraphy

Patients who received RAI therapy should undergo whole-body scintigraphy (WBS) approximately 3–10 days after treatment. This is to document the iodine uptake of any structural disease as well as to stage the disease. Studies have shown that post-therapy scan has been reported to discover new lesions as well as alter disease stage [33–36]. In some cases, single-photon emission computed tomography (SPECT) or hybrid SPECT/CT scan (if available) may be performed. The three-dimensional images provided by SPECT, and the additional morphological information provided by SPECT/CT, often have incremental value especially for situations in which there is a diagnostic uncertainty, or when disease was advanced and two-dimensional WBS was inconclusive [37, 38].

Avoidance of "Stunning"

Stunning is defined as diminution of RAI uptake and efficacy following recent diagnostic radioiodine administration. In cases where RAI therapy is clearly necessary, pre-therapeutic ^{131}I diagnostic scan may be avoided because their results will not modify the indication for RAI therapy and this procedure may potentially induce stunning. To reduce the possibility of stunning when it is not yet known whether RAI therapy is indicated, ^{131}I diagnostic WBS or thyroid uptake quantification of low activities should be performed. Recommended quantities are approximately 10–185 MBq for WBS and 3–10 MBq for uptake quantification. Alternatively, use of 40–200 MBq of 123-iodine (^{123}I) for diagnostic imaging can minimise the risk of stunning. 124-Iodine (^{124}I) PET/CT is emerging as an attractive modality for pre-RAI therapy imaging and dosimetry [39–41]. The extent of stunning effects with ^{124}I is still unknown, but as a precaution activities of this radioisotope should be kept to a minimum.

Side Effects

In general, RAI is a reasonably safe therapy, associated with low-risk cumulative dose-related early- and late-onset complications as shown in Table 10.3.

Most long-term follow-up studies report very low risks of secondary malignancies (bone and soft-tissue malignancies, including breast, colorectal, kidney and salivary cancers, and leukaemia) in long-term survivors [42, 43]. The 2015 ATA guidelines [6] have stated that the absolute increase in risk of developing a second primary malignancy attributable to RAI treatment is considered small and does not warrant specific screening to any extent greater than age-appropriate general population health screening.

Table 10.3 Early- and late-onset complications of RAI therapy

	Side effects	Management
Early onset	Sialadenitis may result in alteration of taste and dental caries in long term [54]	Prevention: good hydration; sour candies and lemon juice increase salivary flow and reduce radiation exposure of the salivary glands. The recommended use of sour candy/lemon juice is at 24 h post-therapy, as when given within 1 h of therapy it may increase salivary gland damage [55] Treatment: Acute pain: local application of ice, anti-inflammatory non-steroidal medication, or steroids Chronic dry mouth/dental caries: cholinergic agents may have a role [56]. Interventional sialendoscopy may be helpful if refractory to medical therapy [57–59] Discussion on preventive strategies with dental/oral health professional is advised to prevent dental caries
	Nasolacrimal duct obstruction [60]	Surgical correction may be considered with excessive tearing which may predispose to infection
	Nausea, occasional vomiting	Prophylactic anti-emetics before starting therapy
	Transient decrease in white blood cell and platelet counts May occur up to 6–10 weeks following ^{131}I activity more than 5.55–7.4 GBq (150–200 mCi) [29] or with multiple therapies	Full blood count and renal function should be routinely performed prior to treatment Reduced renal function can result in reduced iodine excretion from the body and hence increase radiation to bone marrow Normal pre-therapy profile makes these side effects unlikely. If these blood test results are abnormal, dosimetry is advised to determine the highest safe ^{131}I activity while delivering less than 2 Gy to the blood and bone marrow [29]
Late onset	Secondary malignancies	Use of laxatives may decrease radiation exposure of the bowel, particularly in patients treated after prolonged withdrawal of thyroid hormone with increased risk of constipation. Vigorous oral hydration will reduce exposure of the bladder and gonads
	Male infertility	Good hydration to reduce gonadal radiation exposure, frequent micturition to empty the bladder and avoidance of constipation Sperm banking may be considered in men who receive cumulative RAI activities ≥400 mCi [47]

No threshold for radiation-induced carcinogenesis has been firmly established [44]. The excess risk of secondary malignancy is greater in young individuals compared to older individuals [45] and is dose related [43]. Cumulative ^{131}I activities above 500–600 mCi may be associated with a significant increase in risk of secondary malignancies [43] although the current evidence is not conclusive. However, the low risk of secondary malignancies should not deter the patient from receiving RAI therapy when the benefits of therapy clearly outweigh the risks.

In men, RAI therapy may be associated with a transient diminished spermatogenesis and elevated serum follicle-stimulating hormone levels [46, 47]. Higher cumulative activities (500–800 mCi) in men are associated with an increased risk of persistent elevation of serum follicle-stimulating hormone levels, but fertility and risks of miscarriage or congenital abnormalities in subsequent pregnancies are not changed with moderate RAI activities (~200 mCi) [48, 49]. Permanent male infertility is unlikely with a single ablative activity of RAI, but theoretically there could be cumulative damage with multiple treatments. In women, a modestly earlier onset of menopause has been described after repeated courses of RAI [50].

More importantly, the long-term rates of infertility, miscarriage and foetal malformation do not appear to be elevated in women after RAI therapy [51–53].

References

1. Sawka AM, et al. A systematic review and mataanalysis of the effectiveness of radioactive iodine renmant ablation for well-differentiated thyroid cancer. J Clin Endocrinol Metab. 2004;89:3668–76.
2. Mazzaferri EL, Jhiang SM. Long-term impact of initial surgical and medical therapy on papillary and follicular thyroid cancer. Am J Med. 1994;97:418–28.
3. DeGroot LJ, et al. Natural history, treatment and course of papillary thyroid cancer. J Clin Endocrinol Metab. 1990;71:414–24.
4. Jonklaas J, et al. Outcomes of patients with differentiated thyroid carcinoma after initial therapy. Thyroid. 2006;16:1229–42.
5. Tuttle RM, et al. Estimating risk of recurrence in differentiated thyroid cancer after total thyroidectomy and radioactive iodine remnant ablation: using response to therapy variable to modify the initial risk estimates predicted by the new American Thyroid Association staging system. Thyroid. 2010;20:1341–9.
6. Haugen BR, Alexander EK, Bible KC, Doherty GM, Mandel SJ, Nikiforov YE, Pacini F, Randolph GW, Sawka AM, Schlumberger M, Schuff KG, Sherman SI, Sosa JA, Steward DL, Tuttle RM, Wartofsky L. 2015 American Thyroid Association management guidelines for adult patients with thyroid nodules and differentiated thyroid cancer: the American Thyroid Association guidelines task force on thyroid nodules and differentiated thyroid cancer. Thyroid. 2016;26:1–133.
7. Mallick U, et al. Ablation with low-dose radioiodine and thyrotropin alfa in thyroid cancer. N Engl J Med. 2012;366:1674–85.
8. Schlumberger M, et al. Strategies in radioiodine ablation in patients with low-risk thyroid cancer. N Engl J Med. 2012;366:1663–73.
9. Bal C, et al. Prospective Randomized Clinical Trial to evaluate the optimal dose of 131I for remnant ablation in patients with differentiated thyroid carcinoma. Cancer. 1996;77:2574–80.
10. Verburg FA, et al. Long-term survival in differentiated thyroid cancer is worse after low-activity initial post-surgical 131I therapy in both high- and low-risk patients. J Clin Endocrinol Metab. 2014;99:4487–96.
11. Kruijff S, et al. Decreasing the dose of radioiodine for remant ablation does not increase structural recurrence rates in papillary thyroid carcinoma. Surgery. 2013;154:1337–44.
12. Castagna MG, et al. Post-surgical thyroid ablation with low or high radioiodine activities results in similar outcomes in intermediate risk differentiated thyroid cancer patients. Eur J Endocrinol. 2013;169:23–9.
13. Sabra MM, et al. Higher administered activities of radioactive iodine are associated with less structural persistent response in older but not younger papillary thyroid cancer patients with lateral neck lymph node metastases. Thyroid. 2014;24:1088–95.
14. Han JM, et al. Effects of low-dose and high-dose postoperative radioiodine therapy on the clinical outcome in patients with small differentiated thyroid cancer having microscopic extrathyroidal extension. Thyroid. 2014;24(5):820.
15. Luster M, et al. Guidelines for radioiodine therapy of differentiated thyroid cancer. Eur J Nucl Med Mol Imag. 2008;3:1941–59.
16. Edmonds CJ, Hayes S, Kermode JC, Thompson BD. Measurement of serum TSH and thyroid hormones in the management of treatment of thyroid carcinoma with radioiodine. Br J Radiol. 1977;50:799–807.
17. Lee J, Yun MJ, Nam KH, Chung WY, Soh EY, Park CS. Quality of life and effectiveness comparisons of thyroxine withdrawal, triiodothyronine withdrawal, and recombinant thyroid-stimulating hormone administration for low-dose radioiodine remnant ablation of differentiated thyroid carcinoma. Thyroid. 2010;20:173–9.
18. Chianelli M, Todino V, Graziano FM, Panunzi C, Pace D, Guglielmi R, Signore A, Papini E. Low-activity (2.0 GBq; 54 mCi) radioiodine post-surgical remnant ablation in thyroid cancer: comparison between hormone withdrawal and use of rhTSH in low-risk patients. Eur J Endocrinol. 2009;160:431–6.
19. Pacini F, Ladenson PW, Schlumberger M, Driedger A, Luster M, Kloos RT, Sherman S, Haugen B, Corone C, Molinaro E, Elisei R, Ceccarelli C, Pinchera A, Wahl RL, Leboulleux S, Ricard M, Yoo J, Busaidy NL, Delpassand E, Hanscheid H, Felbinger R, Lassmann M, Reiners C. Radioiodine ablation of thyroid remnants after preparation with recombinant human thyrotropin in differentiated thyroid carcinoma: results of an international, randomized, controlled study. J Clin Endocrinol Metab. 2006;91:926–32.
20. Taieb D, Sebag F, Cherenko M, Baumstarck-Barrau K, Fortanier C, Farman-Ara B, de Micco C, Vaillant J, Thomas S, Conte-Devolx B, Loundou A, Auquier P, Henry JF, Mundler O. Quality of life changes and clinical outcomes in thyroid cancer patients undergoing radioiodine remnant ablation (RRA) with recombinant human TSH (rhTSH): a randomized controlled study. Clin Endocrinol (Oxf). 2009;71:115–23.
21. Emmanouilidis N, Muller JA, Jager MD, Kaaden S, Helfritz FA, Guner Z, Kespohl H, Knitsch W, Knapp WH, Klempnauer J, Scheumann GF. Surgery and radioablation therapy combined: introducing a 1-weekcondensed procedure bonding total thyroidectomy and radioablation therapy with recombinant human TSH. Eur J Endocrinol. 2009;161:763–9.
22. Tu J, Wang S, Huo Z, Lin Y, Li X, Wang S. Recombinant human thyrotropin-aided versus thyroid hormone withdrawal-aided radioiodine treatment for differentiated thyroid cancer after total thyroidectomy: a meta-analysis. Radiother Oncol. 2014;110:25–30.

23. Pak K, Cheon GJ, Kang KW, Kim SJ, Kim IJ, Kim EE, Lee DS, Chung JK. The effectiveness of recombinant human thyroid-stimulating hormone versus thyroid hormone withdrawal prior to radioiodine remnant ablation in thyroid cancer: a meta-analysis of randomized controlled trials. J Korean Med Sci. 2014;29:811–7.
24. Lippi F, Capezzone M, Angelini F, Taddei D, Molinaro E, Pinchera A, Pacini F. Radioiodine treatment of metastatic differentiated thyroid cancer in patients on Lthyroxine, using recombinant human TSH. Eur J Endocrinol. 2001;144:5–11.
25. Vargas GE, Uy H, Bazan C, Guise TA, Bruder JM. Hemiplegia after thyrotropin alfa in a hypothyroid patient with thyroid carcinoma metastatic to the brain. J Clin Endocrinol Metab. 1999;84:3867–71.
26. Robbins RJ, Voelker E, Wang W, Macapinlac HA, Larson SM. Compassionate use of recombinant human thyrotropin to facilitate radioiodine therapy: case report and review of literature. Endocr Pract. 2000;6:460–4.
27. Braga M, Ringel MD, Cooper DS. Sudden enlargement of local recurrent thyroid tumor after recombinant human TSH administration. J Clin Endocrinol Metab. 2001;86:5148–51.
28. Luster M, Lassmann M, Haenscheid H, Michalowski U, Incerti C, Reiners C. Use of recombinant human thyrotropin before radioiodine therapy in patients with advanced differentiated thyroid carcinoma. J Clin Endocrinol Metab. 2000;85:3640–5.
29. Silberstein EB, Alavi A, Balon HR, Clarke SE, Divgi C, Gelfand MJ, Goldsmith SJ, Jadvar H, Marcus CS, Martin WH, Parker JA, Royal HD, Sarkar SD, Stabin M, Waxman AD. The SNMMI practice guideline for therapy of thyroid disease with 131I 3.0. J Nucl Med. 2012;53:1633–51.
30. Sawka AM, Ibrahim-Zada I, Galacgac P, Tsang RW, Brierley JD, Ezzat S, Goldstein DP. Dietary iodine restriction in preparation for radioactive iodine treatment or scanning in well-differentiated thyroid cancer: a systematic review. Thyroid. 2010;20:1129–38.
31. Berg G, et al. Consequences of inadvertent radioiodine treatment of Graves' disease and thyroid cancer in undiagnosed pregnancy. Can we rely on routine pregnancy testing? Acta Oncol. 2008;47:145–9.
32. Schlumberger M, et al. Exposure to radioactive iodine-131 for scintigraphy or therapy does not preclude pregnancy in thyroid cancer patients. J Nucl Med. 1996;37:606–12.
33. Avram AM, Fig LM, Frey KA, Gross MD, Wong KK. Preablation 131-I scans with SPECT/CT in postoperative thyroid cancer patients: what is the impact on staging? J Clin Endocrinol Metab. 2013;98:1163–71.
34. Sherman SI, Tielens ET, Sostre S, Wharam MD Jr, Ladenson PW. Clinical utility of posttreatment radioiodine scans in the management of patients with thyroid carcinoma. J Clin Endocrinol Metab. 1994;78:629–34.
35. Fatourechi V, Hay ID, Mullan BP, Wiseman GA, Eghbali-Fatourechi GZ, Thorson LM, Gorman CA. Are posttherapy radioiodine scans informative and do they influence subsequent therapy of patients with differentiated thyroid cancer? Thyroid. 2000;10:573–7.
36. Souza Rosario PW, Barroso AL, Rezende LL, Padrao EL, Fagundes TA, Penna GC, Purisch S. Post I-131 therapy scanning in patients with thyroid carcinoma metastases: an unnecessary cost or a relevant contribution? Clin Nucl Med. 2004;29:795–8.
37. Kohlfuerst S, Igerc I, Lobnig M, Gallowitsch HJ, Gomez-Segovia I, Matschnig S, Mayr J, Mikosch P, Beheshti M, Lind P. Posttherapeutic (131)I SPECTCT offers high diagnostic accuracy when the findings on conventional planar imaging are inconclusive and allows a tailored patient treatment regimen. Eur J Nucl Med Mol Imaging. 2009;36:886–93.
38. Chen L, Luo Q, Shen Y, Yu Y, Yuan Z, Lu H, Zhu R. Incremental value of 131I SPECT/CT in the management of patients with differentiated thyroid carcinoma. J Nucl Med. 2008;49:1952–7.
39. Freudenberg L, Jentzen W, Goerges R, Petrich T, Marlowe RJ, Knust J, Bockisch A. 124 I-PET dosimetry in advanced differentiated thyroid cancer. Therapeutic impact. Nuklearmedizin. 2007;46:121–8.
40. Pentlow KS, et al. Quantitative imaging of iodine-124 with PET. J Nucl Med. 1996;37:1557–62.
41. Sgouros G, et al. Patient-specific dosimetry for 131I thyroid cancer therapy using 124I PET and 3-dimensional-internal dosimetry (3D-ID) software. J Nucl Med. 2004;45:1366–72.
42. Brown AP, Chen J, Hitchcock YJ, Szabo A, Shrieve DC, Tward JD. The risk of second primary malignancies up to three decades after the treatment of differentiated thyroid cancer. J Clin Endocrinol Metab. 2008;93:504–15.
43. Rubino C, de Vathaire F, Dottorini ME, Hall P, Schvartz C, Couette JE, Dondon MG, Abbas MT, Langlois C, Schlumberger M. Second primary malignancies in thyroid cancer patients. Br J Cancer. 2003;89:1638–44.
44. National Research Council. Health risks from exposure to low levels of ionizing radiation: BEIR VII, Phase 2. Chapter 12. Washington, DC: The National Academies Press; 2006.
45. Iyer NG, Morris LG, Tuttle RM, Shaha AR, Ganly I. Rising incidence of second cancers in patients with low-risk (T1N0) thyroid cancer who receive radioactive iodine therapy. Cancer. 2011;117:4439–46.
46. Wichers M, Benz E, Palmedo H, Biersack HJ, Grunwald F, Klingmuller D. Testicular function after radioiodine therapy for thyroid carcinoma. Eur J Nucl Med. 2000;27:503–7.
47. Hyer S, Vini L, O'Connell M, Pratt B, Harmer C. Testicular dose and fertility in men following I(131) therapy for thyroid cancer. Clin Endocrinol (Oxf). 2002;56:755–8.
48. Lushbaugh CC, Casarett GW. The effects of gonadal irradiation in clinical radiation therapy: a review. Cancer. 1976;37:1111–25.
49. Sarkar SD, Beierwaltes WH, Gill SP, Cowley BJ. Subsequent fertility and birth histories of children

and adolescents treated with 131I for thyroid cancer. J Nucl Med. 1976;17:460–4.
50. Ceccarelli C, et al. 131I therapy for differentiated thyroid cancer leads to an earlier onset of menopause: results of a retrospective study. J Clin Endocrinol Metab. 2001;86:3512–5.
51. Vini L, Hyer S, Al-Saadi A, Pratt B, Harmer C. Prognosis for fertility and ovarian function after treatment with radioiodine for thyroid cancer. Postgrad Med J. 2002;78:92–3.
52. Dottorini ME, Lomuscio G, Mazzucchelli L, Vignati A, Colombo L. Assessment of female fertility and carcinogenesis after iodine-131 therapy for differentiated thyroid carcinoma. J Nucl Med. 1995;36:21–7.
53. Sawka AM, Lakra DC, Lea J, Alshehri B, Tsang RW, Brierley JD, Straus S, Thabane L, Gafni A, Ezzat S, George SR, Goldstein DP. A systematic review examining the effects of therapeutic radioactive iodine on ovarian function and future pregnancy in female thyroid cancer survivors. Clin Endocrinol (Oxf). 2008;69:479–90.
54. Walter MA, Turtschi CP, Schindler C, Minnig P, MullerBrand J, Muller B. The dental safety profile of highdose radioiodine therapy for thyroid cancer: long-term results of a longitudinal cohort study. J Nucl Med. 2007;48:1620–5.
55. Nakada K, Ishibashi T, Takei T, Hirata K, Shinohara K, Katoh S, Zhao S, Tamaki N, Noguchi Y, Noguchi S. Does lemon candy decrease salivary gland damage after radioiodine therapy for thyroid cancer? J Nucl Med. 2005;46:261–6.
56. Mandel SJ, Mandel L. Radioactive iodine and the salivary glands. Thyroid. 2003;13:265–71.
57. Bomeli SR, Schaitkin B, Carrau RL, Walvekar RR. Interventional sialendoscopy for treatment of radioiodine induced sialadenitis. Laryngoscope. 2009;119:864–7.
58. Prendes BL, Orloff LA, Eisele DW. Therapeutic sialendoscopy for the management of radioiodine sialadenitis. Arch Otolaryngol Head Neck Surg. 2012;138:15–9.
59. Bhayani MK, Acharya V, Kongkiatkamon S, Farah S, Roberts DB, Sterba J, Chambers MS, Lai SY. Sialendoscopy for patients with radioiodine-induced sialadenitis and xerostomia. Thyroid. 2015;25:834–8.
60. Kloos RT, Duvuuri V, Jhiang SM, Cahill KV, Foster JA, Burns JA. Nasolacrimal drainage system obstruction from radioactive iodine therapy for thyroid carcinoma. J Clin Endocrinol Metab. 2002;87:5817–20.

Management of Distant Metastasis in Differentiated Thyroid Cancer

11

David A. Pattison, Julie A. Miller, Bhadrakant Khavar, and Jeanne Tie

Introduction

There has been a well-documented increase in the incidence of DTC diagnosis—particularly relating to incidental asymptomatic small tumours—despite stable or declining overall mortality over recent decades [1]. As a result there are important diverging trends in management at opposite ends of the thyroid cancer spectrum with adoption of a risk-adapted, individualised approach to treatment [2]. This involves a 'de-escalation' of treatment for those with low-risk disease including observation [3], fewer indications for use of RAI remnant ablation in the recent American Thyroid Association (ATA) consensus guidelines for DTC [4] and reclassification of encapsulated follicular variant of papillary thyroid carcinoma (fv-PTC) as a benign tumour [5]. Conversely there is ongoing development of improved diagnostics (including genetic profiling and molecular imaging) and targeted therapies to provide better disease characterisation and effective treatment for patients at highest risk of death with metastatic disease which will be the focus of this chapter.

It is important to consider the significant variability in prognosis amongst patients with distant metastatic disease, largely determined by individual tumour biology. A proportion of patients with indolent metastatic disease enjoy long-term survival without ongoing treatment after initial surgery and radioiodine therapy [6], whilst others require aggressive multimodality therapy. Three distinct groups with markedly different overall survivals have been defined from a series of 444 patients with RAI-avid metastatic disease [7]. Young patients (<40 years of age) with biochemical disease not visible on structural imaging demonstrated a 10-year survival rate of 95%, whilst older patients with macroscopic pulmonary metastases (>1 cm) or multiple osseous metastases had a 10-year survival of only 14%. An intermediate 10-year survival of 64% was identified in young patients with macroscopic disease and

D. A. Pattison (✉)
Department of Nuclear Medicine & Specialised PET Service, Royal Brisbane & Women's Hospital, Brisbane, Australia
e-mail: David.Pattison@health.qld.gov.au

B. Khavar · J. A. Miller
Department of Surgery, University of Melbourne, Melbourne, Australia

Endocrine Surgery Unit, The Royal Melbourne Hospital, Melbourne, Australia

Department of Neurosurgery, The Royal Melbourne Hospital, Melbourne, Australia

J. Tie (✉)
Department of Medical Oncology, Peter MacCallum Cancer Centre, Melbourne, Australia

Department of Medicine, University of Melbourne, Melbourne, Australia
e-mail: Jeanne.Tie@mh.org.au

R. Parameswaran, A. Agarwal (eds.), *Evidence-Based Endocrine Surgery*,
https://doi.org/10.1007/978-981-10-1124-5_11

older patients with subcentimetre pulmonary nodules. Thus risk stratification of patients with metastatic DTC is required to determine the optimum management approach, given the risks of both under- and overtreatment associated with an increasing array of potential therapies.

Background: Increasing Role of Genomics and Personalised Therapy

Significant progress has been made in our understanding of the molecular pathogenesis of thyroid cancer, uncovering new therapeutic targets for a disease with a disappointing response to conventional cytotoxic chemotherapy. Central to the development of thyroid cancer is the accumulation of mutations leading to the activation of the mitogen-activated protein kinase (MAPK) and phosphoinositide 3-kinase (PI3K) signalling pathways. Studies in PTC have reported a high rate (~70%) of mutually exclusive activating mutations in genes encoding the effectors of the MAPK pathway, such as point mutations in BRAF (most commonly the $BRAF^{V600E}$ mutation) and RAS [8–14], and rearrangements of the RET-PTC and NTRK1 tyrosine kinase [15–17]. Although H-, N- and K-RAS mutations are found in only a small proportion of classic PTC, they are the most commonly found mutations in follicular thyroid cancer (FTC) and fv-PTC. Other genetic changes in FTCs are PTEN deletion/mutation, paired box 8-peroxisome proliferator-activated receptor-gamma (PAX8/PPARg) rearrangement, PIK3CA and IDH1 mutations.

Over the past decade, the development of massively parallel sequencing technologies has enabled large-scale systematic effort (e.g. The Cancer Genome Atlas, International Cancer Genome Consortium and Slim Initiative for Genomic Medicine) to further characterise the genomic landscapes of human malignancies, including thyroid cancer [18]. The Cancer Genome Atlas (TCGA) project performed a comprehensive multiplatform analysis of 496 PTC and confirmed that 80% of driver genetic events, mostly somatic point mutations and fusions, were concentrated in four genes (BRAF, NRAS, KRAS and RET), whilst the remaining 20% were low-frequency mutations spread across at least 30 genes (known as 'long-tail' mutations) [19]. Importantly, this effort discovered new driver mutations in PTC, either entirely novel driver in PTC (EIF1AX) or novel changes of known drivers (BRAF, RET and ALK fusions), exposing potential new molecular therapeutic targets. This multidimensional genomic approach also illustrated that $BRAF^{V600E}$ PTC is a heterogeneous group of tumours, consisting of at least four molecular subtypes with variable differentiation and potentially clinical outcome. Collectively, this study highlights the genetic diversity of PTC and the importance of precision medicine in the optimal management of individual patients.

Presentations

The vast majority of DTC is confined to the thyroid with or without regional lymphadenopathy at presentation. Distant metastases occur during follow-up in approximately 6–20% of patients [20–22] whilst a smaller number of patients (approximately 3%) have metastatic disease identified at presentation. Of the 3.4% of patients that presented with metastatic disease in a recent large Korean study, 59.6% of cases were identified radiologically and 40.4% presented clinically [23]. Presenting symptoms relate to the predominant sites of distant metastases, including pain due to osseous metastasis (17.3%), pathologic fracture (5.8%), paralysis of lower extremities (5.8%), cough and/or dyspnoea (5.8%), and haemoptysis, pleural effusion and palpable mass (1.9% for each). Typical sites of metastases in this cohort included lungs only (including pleura) in 61.5%, and bone only in 21.2%. Multiple sites were involved in 17.3% of cases. Brain metastases occur in approximately 1%, and are associated with a worse prognosis [24]. Brain metastases are most commonly detected on screening imaging, but patients may present with headache, nausea, vomiting, visual changes, focal or generalised seizures or a neurological deficit.

The pathology of the primary tumour also has implications on the likelihood and distribution of metastatic disease. In this cohort of patients, PTC comprised 69.2%, FTC 17.5% and poorly differentiated components of the primary thyroid tumour 3.8% each for diffuse sclerosing variant, Hurthle cell carcinoma and insular carcinoma, and tall cell variant in 1.9%. PTC is typically associated with regional nodal and pulmonary metastases, whilst FTC is associated with osseous metastatic disease [25].

Investigations

There are numerous potential investigations for evaluation of distant metastatic disease. Paired thyroglobulin (Tg) and thyroglobulin antibodies (TgAb) remain the mainstay of biochemical disease surveillance and treatment response in metastatic disease. Although useful for investigation of disease in the neck, ultrasound has limited role in the evaluation of distant metastatic disease and won't be discussed in this section. There is greater role of cross-sectional (CT and magnetic resonance imaging [MRI]) and molecular imaging using iodine isotopes and FDG PET/CT.

Thyroglobulin

Serum thyroglobulin is the biochemical tumour marker utilised in the monitoring of differentiated thyroid carcinoma. The development of more sensitive (second generation) thyroglobulin immunometric assay measurements has resulted in a much higher functional sensitivity (<0.1 μg/L) than older first-generation tests (~1.0 μg/L) [26] and has essentially removed the need for TSH-stimulated thyroglobulin testing [27]. Consequently, measurement of the basal Tg—using the same assay—trend and doubling time provide important prognostic information for both disease recurrence and response to therapy. However, interference from both TgAb and heterophile antibodies is the major limitation of immunometric assays. In the presence of TgAb, the trend in TgAb levels can be used as a surrogate tumour marker [28].

In the setting of known metastatic disease, the basal Tg has been shown to directly correlate with the number of lesions, and is highest in patients with bone metastases and FTC, and lowest in cervical metastases and PTC, respectively [29]. In contrast, the response to recombinant human (rh)-TSH stimulation varies by histological type of cancer, being highest in PTC and lowest in Hurthle cell carcinoma, likely reflecting the relative differentiation of malignancy. However a small proportion of cases with clinically significant metastatic disease do not have measurable thyroglobulin levels [30]. Thyroglobulin has recently been shown to be a useful biomarker when compared to Response Evaluation Criteria in Solid Tumours (RECIST) response assessment during treatment with sorafenib, and is particularly useful in patients with non-measurable disease [31].

CT and MRI

In patients with elevated or rising Tg or TgAb and no evidence of structural disease on cervical US, CT imaging of the neck and chest should be considered. In advanced regional disease, intravenous contrast is important for assessment of the neck and mediastinum to facilitate surgical planning if required. The majority of iodinated contrast will have been excreted within 4–8 weeks in most patients, such that radioiodine can still be administered. A random urine iodine-to-creatinine ratio can be used to exclude high iodine retention if there is clinical concern. MRI is particularly useful for exclusion of brain metastases or spinal cord compression when clinically suspected. Imaging of symptomatic sites with either CT or MRI is also recommended, particularly if Tg is elevated >10 ng/mL [4].

Diagnostic RAI Imaging

There are three radioactive isotopes of iodine utilised in nuclear medicine imaging (Table 11.1). I-131 emits high-energy beta-particles for effective radionuclide therapy of thyroid cancer, but it's high-energy gamma emissions have relatively

Table 11.1 Table outlining the physical characteristics of three iodine isotopes used in nuclear medicine imaging and therapy for thyroid cancer

Characteristics	I-123	I-124	I-131
Role	*Imaging*	*Imaging*	*Therapy* (and imaging)
Emission	Gamma (159 keV)	Positron	Gamma (364 keV) and beta-particle
Modality	Gamma/SPECT	PET	Gamma/SPECT
Path length (tissue)	N/A	N/A	1–2 mm
Stunning	No	Uncertain	Likely
Half-life	13.2 h	4.2 days	8 days
Imaging time post-injection	24 h (DxWBS)	24–120 h (PET)	<72 h (DxWBS) 5–7 days (RxWBS)

SPECT single-photon emission computed tomography, *PET* positron emission tomography, *DxWBS* diagnostic whole-body scan, *RxWBS* post-treatment whole-body scan

poor imaging characteristics for diagnostic imaging. In contrast, I-123 has much better imaging characteristics and the lack of significant beta-particle emission eliminates the risk of stunning, but I-123 has limited availability due to cost. I-124 is a positron emitter with excellent image resolution, and imaging on a PET camera enables assessment of prospective dosimetry to facilitate RAI therapy. There is an emerging body of literature supporting the use of I-124 but availability is currently limited to large academic referral centres.

The recent ATA guidelines [4] outline three primarily accepted clinical roles for a *diagnostic* whole-body scan (WBS): (1) patients with abnormal uptake outside the thyroid bed on *post-therapy* WBS, (2) patients with poorly informative post-ablation WBS because of large thyroid remnants with high uptake of I-131 (>2% administered activity) potentially limiting the visualisation of faint uptake in cervical lymph nodes and (3) patients with thyroglobulin antibodies (or discordant uptake on post-ablation WBS despite negative Tg) at risk of false-negative Tg measurement. Other groups utilise routine pre-therapy diagnostic WBS imaging to risk-stratify and direct the decision to proceed with therapy.

I-131 and I-123 imaging may be performed with either traditional 2-dimensional planar imaging or use of 3-dimensional SPECT/CT which enables direct superimposition of functional and anatomic imaging, providing much greater specificity and anatomic localisation of focal iodine uptake. Numerous studies confirm the superior management impact of SPECT/CT imaging (either diagnostic or post-therapy) compared with traditional planar imaging, including increased diagnosis of metastatic lymph nodes, a decrease in equivocal findings, change in management in approximately 1/3 of patients and a potential reduction in the need for further cross-sectional imaging studies [32, 33].

I-124 PET/CT is particularly useful for dosimetry to quantify the uptake and retention of I-124 within each lesion and estimate the expected dose of radiation per unit of administered I-131 therapy. As expected, I-124 is reported to have a significantly higher sensitivity than diagnostic I-131 planar WBS [34] and a recent retrospective study confirmed a high level of agreement (95%) between pre-therapeutic I-124 PET and post-therapy I-131 imaging in detection of iodine-avid thyroid cancer metastases in 137 patients [35].

FDG PET/CT

The enhanced uptake of glucose (or it's analogue FDG) by cancer cells due to inefficient aerobic glycolysis—termed the Warburg effect [36]—is the hallmark of *in vivo* cancer imaging with FDG PET/CT. Suggested indications for FDG PET/CT in differentiated thyroid carcinoma are listed in Table 11.2 [37]. Numerous studies have demonstrated a correlation between increasing FDG avidity and poor prognosis in thyroid cancer. In a retrospective series of 400 patients with metastatic thyroid cancer followed for a median of 7.9 years, only age and FDG PET results

Table 11.2 Suggested indications for FDG PET/CT in differentiated thyroid carcinoma [37]

Staging of patients with higher risk of metastatic disease
– Hurthle cell and aggressive subtypes of thyroid cancer (tall cell, poorly differentiated subtypes)
Assessment of patients with metastatic disease
– Theranostic tool to determine suitability for radionuclide therapy by excluding spatially discordant iodine-negative/FDG-positive disease
– Prognostic tool to identify sites of disease at the highest risk for rapid disease progression and also risk of patient mortality
Assessment of increasing thyroglobulin level with negative radioiodine imaging
Evaluation of post-treatment response of FDG PET-positive lesions

(SUVmax of the most active lesion and number of FDG-avid lesions) were strong predictors of survival [38]. Notably the AJCC cancer stage was not significant under multivariate analysis. Consequently it was proposed that the real-time prognostic value of FDG PET/CT be utilised at diagnosis of metastatic differentiated thyroid cancer to guide the aggressiveness of therapy.

It is also important to recognise that not all intensely FDG-avid lesions represent poorly differentiated disease. Oncocytic tumours—defined histologically by the presence of a granular cytoplasm due to mitochondrial hyperproliferation and described in the thyroid (Hurthle cell), salivary gland (Warthin's), kidney and other organs—are a group of tumours for which intense FDG avidity represents inherent constitutive activation of glycolytic pathways rather than a poorly differentiated phenotype. Loss of the mitochondrial respiratory chain complex I has been shown to be a molecular marker of the oncocytic phenotype [39], leading to mitochondrial dysfunction, inhibition of oxidative phosphorylation and upregulation of glycolytic metabolism. The specific mechanism of observed intense FDG uptake is not elucidated in these tumours; however numerous large series [40] and case reports [41] of FDG-avid incidentalomas have clearly defined very intense FDG uptake in both benign and malignant Hurthle cell tumours of the thyroid.

A flip-flop phenomenon is also described whereby well-differentiated thyroid carcinoma retains activity of the sodium iodide symporter and iodine avidity (with low-glucose requirements similar to normal cells) with subsequent loss of iodine avidity and increased FDG avidity in sites of poorly differentiated disease [42]. The dedifferentiation process represents a spectrum rather than a binary switch, with a substantial proportion of patients (33%) [43] with FDG-avid disease still retaining Na/I symporter activity. Whilst not recommended for all patients, pre-therapeutic imaging with combined iodine (preferably I-123 or I-124) and FDG PET/CT can be utilised in high-risk patients with metastatic disease to determine the most appropriate therapeutic strategy directed to the highest grade (i.e. FDG avid) disease elements. If all disease sites are FDG/iodine avid, then I-131 therapy is recommended; however local therapy or systemic tyrosine kinase inhibitors should be considered for patients with discordant FDG-avid disease [44].

In the context of a negative iodine scan and increasing Tg level, FDG PET/CT has high accuracy for detection of residual or recurrent disease. A meta-analysis of 165 patients from 6 studies identified a pooled sensitivity of 93.5% and specificity of 83.9% of PET/CT for detecting disease recurrence which was superior to conventional techniques [45]. The ATA guidelines recommend a threshold stimulated Tg level of 10 ng/mL for performing FDG PET/CT as a good compromise between sensitivity and specificity [4]. The potential impact of TgAb should also be considered with lower levels of Tg.

Treatment Options

There are an increasing variety of available treatment options for metastatic differentiated thyroid carcinoma which can be tailored to need of the individual. Personalised medicine involves the stratification of patients into different groups on the basis of the risk of underlying disease or predicted response to therapies, with the choice depending upon clinical, biochemical, radiologic, molecular imaging and genetic factors of the patient and their disease. The ATA guidelines recommended that the hierarchy of treatment for metastatic disease is surgical excision of locoregional disease in potentially curable patients, I-131 therapy for RAI-responsive disease, external beam radiation or other directed treatment (such as surgery) for symptomatic, solitary or otherwise sites at high risk of local complications, TSH-suppressive thyroid hormone therapy alone for patients with stable or slowly progressive asymptomatic disease, and addition of systemic therapy with multikinase inhibitor therapy for patients with significantly progressive or symptomatic macroscopic refractory disease. The rationale, indications and potential side effects of these treatments are outlined below.

TSH Suppression

TSH suppression is an effective well-tolerated treatment for metastatic thyroid carcinoma. It is defined as the administration of thyroid hormone, usually in the form of oral levothyroxine (LT4), at doses sufficient to decrease serum thyroid-stimulating hormone (TSH) below the limit of the normal range without symptomatic thyrotoxicosis. The rationale behind this approach is based upon the assumption that the growth of residual malignant thyroid carcinoma foci is TSH dependent and thus lower levels of TSH will improve the outcome of disease. No large prospective randomised controlled trial has been performed, but a large meta-analysis demonstrated a reduced risk of major adverse clinical events (disease recurrence or death) in TSH-suppressed patients with thyroid cancer after initial therapy [46]. Similarly, analysis of the US National Thyroid Cancer Treatment Cooperative Study Group by Jonklaas et al. [47] clearly demonstrated a significant association between TSH suppression and overall survival and disease-specific survival in stage III/IV high-risk patients. Whilst the risk/benefit of TSH suppression must be carefully considered in low-risk patients, the current ATA guidelines recommend complete TSH suppression (target <0.1 mU/L) in all patients with metastatic disease except in the presence of atrial fibrillation, when milder suppression to 0.1–0.5 mU/L may be acceptable.

Radioactive Iodine

RAI is selectively taken up via the sodium-iodide symporter within thyroid (or well-differentiated thyroid carcinoma) cells and undergoes organification. During the radioactive decay process with a half-life of 8 days, emitted beta-particles deposit energy into adjacent tissue with a mean path length of 1–2 mm causing radiation-induced cell death. This combination of exquisite biochemical targeting and physical radioactive properties has ensured the ongoing role of RAI in the treatment of thyroid cancer since its first reported use by Seidlin et al. in 1948 [48] for a patient with metastatic functional thyroid carcinoma. There are three indications for I-131 therapy in thyroid carcinoma: (1) thyroid remnant ablation to destroy residual thyroid tissue and facilitate follow-up, (2) adjuvant therapy to treat suspected residual thyroid carcinoma and (3) therapy of known residual or metastatic disease, the focus of this chapter.

Optimising I-131 Uptake

Iodine uptake by the tumour may be optimised by minimising levels of competing elemental iodine, via avoidance of large iodine loads (e.g. iodinated contrast) for 4–8 weeks, and adherence to a low-iodine diet for 2 weeks prior to therapy. TSH stimulation (TSH > 30 mU/L) is utilised to increase expression of Na/I symporter expression. Whilst there is high-quality evidence confirming non-inferiority for remnant ablation of normal thyroid tissue (and significantly improved quality of life) using rh-TSH and T4WD stimulation [49], similar data is not available for TSH stimulation to facilitate I-131 therapy of metastatic disease. In fact, case reports [50] demonstrate much greater iodine uptake assessed by I-124 PET using T4WD than rh-TSH stimulation in the setting of metastatic disease. Furthermore, the recent THYROPET study demonstrated reduced iodine uptake on I-124 PET studies performed under rh-TSH stimulation compared to T4WD stimulation of post-I-131 therapy scans [51]. This is considered more likely to reflect differences in biologic tumour response to TSH stimulation, rather than technical differences in scan resolution [52]. In the setting of metastatic disease the ATA guidelines recommend the use of rh-TSH stimulation in patients with pituitary dysfunction who are unable to raise their serum TSH, those unable to safely tolerate thyroxine withdrawal (including psychiatric disturbance or active cardiovascular disease) or those in whom a delay in therapy may be deleterious. Patients administered rh-TSH should receive the same or higher activity than they would receive if prepared with hypothyroidism.

Empiric Versus Dosimetric Therapy

Although there is extensive data supporting the effectiveness of I-131 therapy for metastatic thyroid cancer, there is no consensus regarding the optimal administered activity of I-131. The case for a dose-response relationship in thyroid cancer was established two decades ago by Maxon et al. [53] demonstrating that an absorbed dose of 85 Gy in nodal metastatic disease and 300 Gy in thyroid remnants was associated with complete response rates of 80–90%. More recent data using I-124 PET/CT has confirmed similar findings for both nodal and pulmonary metastatic diseases at a dose threshold of 85 Gy [54]; however lower response rates were observed for bone metastases. In fact, doses of 350–650 Gy are required to achieve complete response rates of 70–80% in bone metastases (at 6 months) attributable to spatial non-uniformity of these lesions and higher tissue density [55]. Complete responses in bone metastases are still achievable in practice as demonstrated in Fig. 11.1. However

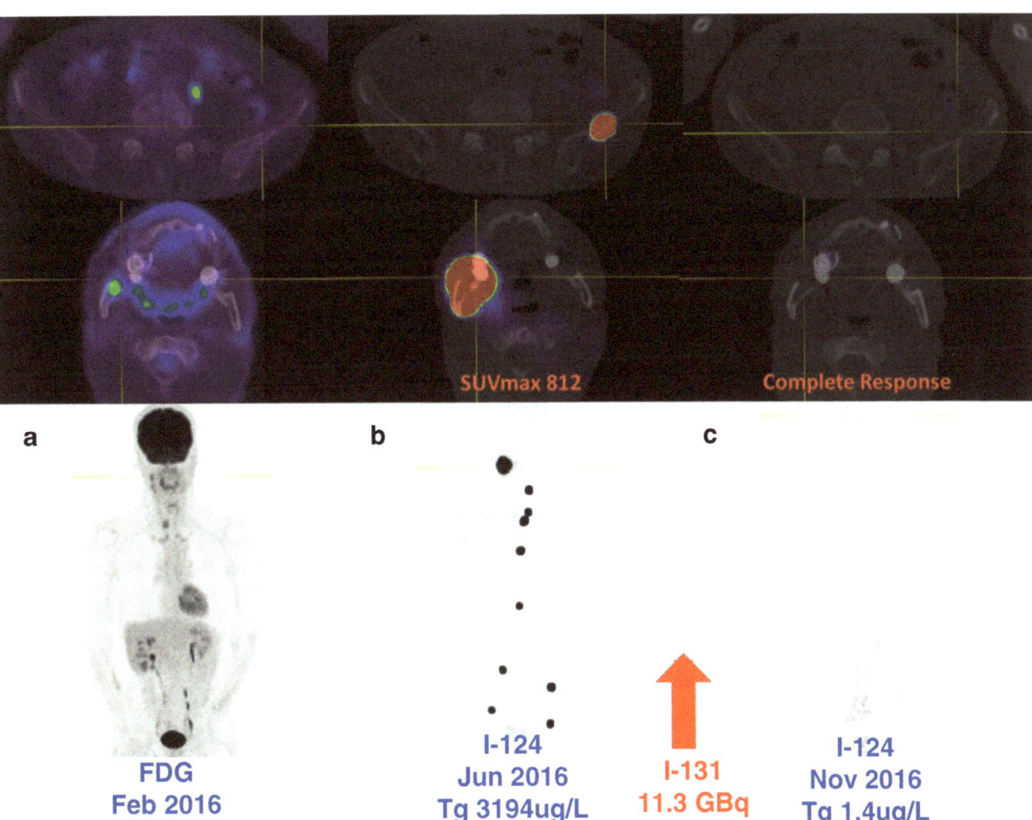

Fig. 11.1 Multiple osseous metastases demonstrate complete response to I-131 therapy. Fifty-seven-year-old man presented with painful right mandible lesion confirmed as follicular thyroid carcinoma metastasis. Upper row and middle row demonstrate fused axial PET/CT images through the pelvis and mandible, respectively, whilst lowest row demonstrates PET maximum intensity projections. Staging FDG PET/CT (**a**) only demonstrates mild FDG uptake in right thyroid nodule in addition to right mandible. Many more intensely iodine-avid lesions identified on I-124 PET/CT (**b**) which were all successfully treated with a complete response to I-131 therapy as evident on follow-up I-124 PET/CT (**c**) and thyroglobulin response

a focus upon complete response does not recognise that partial response or stabilisation of previously progressive disease represents a favourable outcome, or that response to radionuclide therapy may be incomplete at 6 months.

Despite these theoretical advantages, empiric amounts of I-131 are used in most centres for pragmatic reasons in the absence of prospective randomised controlled trials comparing different dosimetric approaches for treatment of metastatic disease. Furthermore, a recent large retrospective study comparing a dosimetric approach (maximal tolerable activity) to an empiric activity approach in patients with metastatic thyroid cancer showed no significant difference in overall survival [56]. However, whilst laudable in its scope, interpretation of these findings is limited by differences in rh-TSH stimulation (83% of cases treated with dosimetric approach received rh-TSH stimulation) and significantly different baseline criteria in a selected population (67% of patients receiving empiric therapy were excluded from analysis) of this retrospective study.

There are three approaches to I-131 therapy of metastatic disease:

1. Empiric fixed amounts of I-131
2. Maximal tolerable dose (activity determined by the upper limit of blood and body dosimetry)
3. Lesional dosimetry (activity determined by threshold dose to sites of disease)

Recommended empiric I-131 therapy activity is 100–200 mCi, or 100–150 mCi in patients >70 years or with renal impairment. A limitation of administering a fixed activity is the variability in tumour uptake and physiologic clearance, such that patients are at risk of either inadequate lesional dosimetry or exceeding the maximal tolerated dose of 200 cGy to bone marrow. In particular, empiric activity of 7.4 GBq (200 mCi) has been estimated to exceed the MTA in 22–38% of patients aged >70 years [57]. Therapy may be repeated (typically at intervals of 3–9 months) when there is objective evidence of response including decrease in size of lesions or falling Tg.

In centres with specialised nuclear medicine expertise, use of dosimetry to identify a maximal tolerable activity aims to limit the dose to the bone marrow to 200 cGy, and typically involves blood samples and whole-body imaging performed at multiple time points to calculate the clearance of the radionuclide from the blood pool. Lesional dosimetry is best performed using I-124 PET/CT to quantitatively identify the absorbed dose of radiation per unit of administered I131 activity, again requiring multiple time-point imaging. A combination of these two approaches can prospectively identify the expected dose to key lesions and ensure that required administered activities of I-131 do not exceed the limit to bone marrow. If adequate tumoricidal dosimetry is not anticipated at critical sites (e.g. spinal canal), this can be prospectively identified and treated with adjuvant external beam radiotherapy. In such cases it is preferable to administer EBRT after I-131, because EBRT can damage tumour microvasculature and thus limit the delivery of I-131 to tumour. Use of dosimetry is favoured when treating patients with diffuse pulmonary metastatic disease to limit the whole-body retention to 80 mCi at 48 h to reduce the potential risk of pulmonary fibrosis [58].

The ATA guidelines provide a weak recommendation to consider empiric therapy with 100–200 mCi I-131 in patients with significantly elevated serum Tg levels (>10 ng/mL), rapidly rising Tg levels or rising Tg antibody levels in whom conventional imaging has failed to reveal a tumour source [4]. Inherent to this approach is a recognition of the poor quality of I-131 diagnostic WBS, such that this approach is less desirable in centres where I-124 PET/CT imaging is available. If the post-therapy scan is negative, the patient should be considered to have RAI-refractory disease and no RAI should be administered. This requires a balance of risk of high cumulative administered activities and uncertain long-term benefits. Although there is no maximum allowable cumulative activity, the risk of the incidence of secondary malignancy (increasing after 600 mCi) [59] should be balanced against the clinical benefit.

Surgery

Primary Thyroid Surgery in the Setting of Metastatic Differentiated Thyroid Cancer

DTC is one of the few cancers for which there is strong evidence supporting resection of the primary cancer in the setting of metastatic disease. Total thyroidectomy in the setting of metastatic DTC not only achieves local control, but also maximises delivery of radioactive iodine (RAI) to iodine-avid metastases.

Cornerstones of optimal local treatment include:

1. Adequate preoperative nodal staging with high-resolution ultrasound in all cases, and contrast CT of the neck in cases with evidence of locally advanced disease
2. Meticulous surgical technique to resect all normal thyroid tissue, close inspection of or resection of the central lymph nodes and dissection of lateral nodes when lateral metastases are present

Areas deserving special attention during total thyroidectomy include the following key anatomic sites most commonly responsible for radioiodine uptake in the thyroid bed: the upper poles, pyramidal lobe, Berry's ligament and thyrothymic tract. The occasional patient will have lingual thyroid tissue of which the thyroid surgeon is not aware until the post-treatment radioiodine scan.

Upper poles: The terminal branches of the superior thyroid arteries should be divided on the thyroid capsule, taking care not to amputate any of the superior pole, including thyroid tissue commonly present postero-supero-medial to the anterior fascial layer containing the superior vessels.

The pyramidal lobe can easily be left behind if not stringently searched for. All connective tissue should be removed from the anterior surface of the thyroid cartilage to the level of the hyoid bone during every thyroid operation, including isthmusectomy, hemithyroidectomy or total thyroidectomy.

Berry's ligament often contains a tongue of thyroid tissue extending laterally, deep to the insertion of the recurrent laryngeal nerve under the cricopharyngeus muscle. With careful dissection, the recurrent laryngeal nerve can be released and gently displaced laterally with a peanut swab, allowing all thyroid tissue to be resected.

The thyrothymic ligaments and tracheo-oesophageal grooves may contain, in addition to the central nodes, separate rests of thyroid tissue in up to 50% of patients. Surgeons who perform selective, rather than routine, central neck dissection must take care to open the pretracheal fascia enveloping the recurrent laryngeal nerves, as well as the thyrothymic tracts, and carefully inspect the central compartment for pathological lymph nodes and thyroid rests, while preserving the inferior parathyroid glands when possible.

Careful and meticulous surgical technique during total thyroidectomy for DTC, especially in the setting of distant metastases, will optimise diagnosis and treatment of distant metastatic disease.

Surgery for Metastatic Disease

Complete surgical excision of cerebral and spinal metastases is associated with a better prognosis and best option for solitary lesions in non-eloquent areas [60]. If surgery is deemed to be very high risk—stereotactic radiosurgery is an effective option [61]. For multiple brain lesions, RAI (if there is I-131 uptake) or whole-brain irradiation should be considered [62].

Spinal metastases may be asymptomatic and found incidentally on imaging [63, 64], such as in the patient described in the introduction. With progression of the disease there is likely to be pain and eventually neurological sequelae like dysaesthesia, radiculopathy, myelopathy, numbness and/or weakness and potentially sphincter dysfunction.

Depending on the anatomy of the lesion and extent of other disease, treatment can be curative if possible or palliative at best. Options include selective embolisation, surgery, radioactive ablation, bisphosphonates and small molecular therapy [65]. Depending on the structural integrity of the spine, surgical decompression may be adequate, but if the vertebral body is affected spinal stabilisation is likely to be required. Ramadan et al. have noted that there is increased survival with RAI avidity and complete bone metastasis resection, and support aggressive treatment especially for patients younger than 45 years [66].

Lung metastases are typically multiple and bilateral, and hence there is no role for surgical resection.

External Radiotherapy for Distant Metastases

Local treatment modalities such as external radiotherapy (stereotactic radiotherapy or external beam radiotherapy) have important selected roles in the treatment of metastatic disease prior to initiation of systemic treatment in the setting of individual symptomatic metastases or those at high risk of local complications. External radiotherapy may also potentially be utilised in the setting of progression of a single lesion with otherwise controlled disease on systemic therapy. The principle of external radiotherapy is selective treatment of a lesion for local disease control with relatively few side effects. This may be selectively utilised in treatment of metastases to the brain, lung, liver and bone. If safe and practical, it is recommended that RAI therapy is administered prior to external radiotherapy to augment the local radiation dose.

Management of Radioactive-Iodine Refractory Disease

Systemic Therapy

Cytotoxic chemotherapies based on doxorubicin and cisplatin have yielded little clinical benefit and significant toxicities in patients with metastatic DTC [67, 68]. Recent advances in our understanding of the major signalling pathways and various tyrosine kinases implicated in DTC tumorigenesis have led to the development of multiple tyrosine kinase inhibitors (TKI) in RAI-refractory (RIA-R) DTC. Thyroid cancers are highly vascularised and the angiogenesis pathway is a major player in the pathogenesis of thyroid cancer. Elevated levels of vascular endothelial growth factor (VEGF) are associated with larger tumour size, lymphatic metastasis and poorer prognosis in DTC [69, 70]. In addition to targeting the MAPK and the PI3K-AKT pathways, VEGF inhibition is also a common target for most of the TKIs that have been evaluated in DTC.

Approved Tyrosine Kinase Inhibitors for RAI-Refractory DTC

To date, the US Food and Drug Administration (FDA) has approved two multi-targeted TKI, sorafenib and lenvatinib, for the treatment of RAI-R advanced DTC based on improvement in progression-free survival in two pivotal randomised placebo-controlled phase III trials (Table 11.3) [71, 72]. Notably, neither of these studies has demonstrated a significant overall survival benefit of TKI treatment, likely due to a large proportion of the patients in the placebo arm who crossed over to receive active treatment after disease progression.

Sorafenib

Sorafenib is the first TKI to be evaluated in a randomised phase III trial (DECISION trial) for RAI-R locally advanced or metastatic DTC. Sorafenib is an oral multi-targeted TKI of VEGFR-1, VEGFR-2 and VEGFR-3; RET (including RET/PTC); RAF (including $BRAF^{V600E}$); and platelet-derived growth factor receptor β [73, 74]. The efficacy of this agent for the treatment of advanced or metastatic thyroid cancer was evaluated in two open-label phase II studies, showing promising response rates of 15–23% and median progression-free survival (PFS) of over 12 months [75, 76]. This led to the landmark international randomised placebo-controlled phase III DECISION trial, where 417 TKI-naïve patients with RAI-R locally advanced or metastatic differentiated thyroid cancer that had progressed within the past 14 months were randomised on a 1:1 ratio to sorafenib (400 mg twice daily) or placebo. Upon protocol-defined progression, patients from both groups were allowed to be treated with open-label sorafenib at investigator's discretion.

Table 11.3 Summary of completed phase III clinical trials with tyrosine kinase inhibitors in RAI-refractory DTC

Characteristics	DECISION trial (sorafenib)	SELECT trial (lenvatinib)
Sample size	417	392
Randomisation	1:1	2:1
Primary outcome	Progression-free survival	Progression-free survival
Key inclusion criteria	RECIST progression within 14 months confirmed by local radiologists	RECIST progression within 12 months confirmed by independent central review
Prior anti-VEGFR treatment	Not allowed	One prior TKI allowed
Crossover post-progression	Open-label sorafenib allowed for both active and placebo arms	Open-label lenvatinib allowed for placebo arm only
Median progression-free survival (TKI vs. placebo)	10.8 vs. 5.8 months (HR 0.59; 95% CI 0.45–0.76)	18.3 vs. 3.6 months (HR 0.21; 95% CI 0.14–0.31)
Overall survival (TKI vs. placebo)	No difference	No difference
Objective response rate (TKI vs. placebo)	12.2% vs. 0.5%	64.8% vs. 1.5%
Median treatment duration active arm	10.6 months (5.3–15.7)	13.8 months
Drug dose	Start dose 800 mg/day Mean dose 651 mg/day	Start dose 24 mg/day Mean dose 17.2 mg/day
Drug interruption, active arm	66.2%	82.4%
Dose reduction, active arm	64.3%	67.8%
Serious AE, treatment related	37.2%	30.3%
Fatal AE, treatment related	0.5%	2.3%
Most common AE occurring in ≥30% of patients in active arm (all grade/≥G3)	Hand-foot skin reaction (76.3/20.3%) Diarrhoea (68.6/5.8%) Alopecia (67.1%/-) Rash or desquamation (50.2/4.8%) Fatigue (49.8/5.3%) Weight loss (46.9/5.8%) Hypertension (40.6/9.7%) Anorexia (31.9/2.4%)	Hypertension (67.8/41.8%) Diarrhoea (59.4/8.0%) Fatigue (59.0/9.2%) Decreased appetite (50.2/5.4%) Decreased weight (46.4/9.6%) Nausea (41.0/2.3%) Stomatitis (35.6/4.2%) Hand-foot skin reaction (31.8/3.4%) Proteinuria (31.0/10.0%)
Most common reason for drug interruptions or reductions	Hand-foot skin reaction	Diarrhoea

The DECISION study demonstrated a significant improvement in median PFS of 5 months for patients treated with sorafenib compared with placebo (10.8 vs. 5.8 months; HR 0.59, 95% CI 0.45–0.76). Objective response rates of 12.2% and 0.5% were observed in the sorafenib and placebo groups, respectively. The median duration of response for patients who achieved a partial response to sorafenib was 10.2 months. A large proportion of patients (71.4%) receiving placebo subsequently crossed over to receive sorafenib at disease progression. A subsequent exploratory analysis of the outcomes of patients treated with open-label sorafenib after protocol-defined progression provided some insights into delayed treatment and treatment beyond radiographic progression [77]. For patients initially treated with placebo and then crossed over to receive open-label sorafenib, the observed response rate of 9.5% and median PFS of 9.6 months were comparable to patients who received sorafenib at the beginning of the trial (response rate of 12.2% and PFS of 10.8 months). Though not definitive, this finding suggests that delaying treatment initiation may not significantly impact the clinical benefit derived from sorafenib treatment. Interestingly, patients who continued open-label sorafenib beyond progression achieved a further 6.7 months of PFS, indicating that sorafenib may continue to slow cancer growth despite radiological evidence of tumour progression.

Lenvatinib

Lenvatinib is the second TKI that has been approved by FDA for the treatment of RAI-R advanced DTC. It is another oral multi-targeted TKI with a different but overlapping mechanism of action to sorafenib, inhibiting VEGFR1-3, FGFR1-4, RET, KIT and platelet-derived growth factor signalling [78, 79]. In a phase II study involving 58 patients with RAI-R advanced DTC treated with lenvatinib, an impressive response rate of 50% and median PFS of 12.6 months were observed [80]. Of note, the response rate for patients who had received previous VEGF therapy was 59%. These results prompted the phase III, randomised, placebo-controlled, multicentre SELECT study where 392 patients with RAI-R locally advanced or metastatic differentiated thyroid cancer that had progressed within the past 12 months were assigned in a 2:1 ratio to lenvatinib (24 mg daily) or placebo [72]. Unlike the DECISION trial, this study included patients with and without prior TKI exposure, and only patients in the placebo group were allowed to receive open-label lenvatinib after protocol-defined progression. The primary end point was PFS as assessed by independent central radiological assessment.

The median PFS was 14.7 months longer in patients treated with lenvatinib than placebo (18.3 vs. 3.6 months; hazard ratio, 0.21; 99% CI, 0.14–0.31), with all pre-specified subgroups (defined according to age, sex, race or ethnic group, prior treatment or no prior treatment with a tyrosine kinase inhibitor, geographic region, histologic subtypes, BRAF or RAS mutation status, and baseline thyrotropin levels) deriving benefit from lenvatinib treatment. An unprecedented response rate of 64.8% was observed with lenvatinib compared to only 1.5% in the placebo group (odds ratio, 28.87; 95% CI, 12.46–66.86). The median time to response in patients treated with lenvatinib was 2 months, which is at the first restaging imaging, suggesting that most responses occurred early during treatment. The median PFS and response rate for patients who entered the open-label phase of the study, i.e. those who received delayed lenvatinib treatment, were 10.1 months and 52.3%, suggesting that patients will still derive benefit from delayed treatment with this agent albeit to a smaller extent compared to those who started treatment earlier.

Management of Common Drug Toxicities

Drug-related toxicities and dose adjustments are common in both the DECISION and SELECT trials. The most frequent drug-related adverse events for sorafenib and lenvatinib in these randomised trials are listed in Table 11.3. Most of the side effects are common to other TKIs, such as diarrhoea, fatigue, anorexia, hand-foot skin reaction and hypertension. The majority of the adverse events are mild to moderate, with severe or life-threatening toxicities occurring in <10% of cases, except for severe hand-foot skin reaction (20.3% of sorafenib-treated patients) and severe hypertension (41.8% of lenvatinib-treated patients). Deaths resulting from drug-related toxicities were rare (0.5% for sorafenib and 2.3% for lenvatinib). Nonetheless, approximately 65% of patients required at least one dose reduction in both trials, highlighting the poor tolerability of these TKIs at the approved starting dose. In light of this, a post-approval open-label, randomised, expanded access programme with lenvatinib at starting doses of 24, 20 or 14 mg is currently underway to evaluate the tolerability and efficacy of lower doses of drug (NCT02211222).

The optimal management of side effects arising from TKI treatment is essential to prevent premature or avoidable dose reduction or drug cessation. Critical to this are patient education and frequent clinical reviews, especially during the first 2 months of treatment. Patients should be encouraged to report any side effects as early as possible so that appropriate supportive care management can be instituted. A dedicated nurse-led symptom management clinic could be utilised to provide early assessment and management of side effects. Whenever possible, side effects should be managed with supportive management or dose interruption, before consideration is given to dose reduction. For prevention of hand-foot skin reaction, patients should be instructed to wear comfortable shoes, avoid direct sun exposure and chemical irritant, and use urea-based moisturiser. Patients should be advised to avoid food that could worsen diarrhoea such as caffeine, dairy and greasy food, and to have antidiarrhoeal medication such as loperamide on hand prior to starting treatment. Blood pressure should be well controlled prior to treatment with lenvatinib or sorafenib, and should be monitored frequently during treatment (every 2 weeks for the first 2 months, then monthly thereafter). TKI should be withheld and antihypertensive therapy optimised if systolic blood pressure is ≥160 mmHg or diastolic blood pressure is ≥100 mmHg. Treatment can be resumed at a reduced dose when systolic blood pressure is ≤150 mmHg and diastolic blood pressure is ≤95 mmHg. As proteinuria is a common adverse event for lenvatinib, patients treated with this TKI should have regular assessment of random urine protein-to-creatinine ratio. However, management of side effects such as fatigue and anorexia can be challenging without resorting to dose reduction.

Selecting Patients for Targeted Therapies

Clinical trial evidence suggested that patients who benefited from TKI treatment were those with radiologically measurable RAI-R progressive disease within the last 12–14 months. Although these criteria are helpful to guide patient selection for systemic TKI treatment in routine practice, they are not sufficient to determine if an individual patient is a good candidate for treatment. When considering a patient with RAI-R DTC for TKI treatment, we have to bear in mind the variable natural history of this disease, the high incidence of treatment-related side effects, and that treatment can improve disease control and potentially survival, but is not curative. A significant proportion of patients with RAI-R DTC can have a relatively long life expectancy with minimal symptoms despite the presence of metastatic disease, underscoring the importance of the timing of treatment initiation in order to achieve the optimum balance of quality and quantity of life. At present, there is no evidence to suggest that earlier treatment offers more clinical benefit than delayed treatment.

Several disease and patient factors should be considered when deciding to initiate systemic treatment [4]. Disease factors to consider include the rate and pattern (focal vs. diffuse) of tumour progression, tumour burden, symptoms, risk of local complications where the tumour is threatening vital structures (e.g. airways, spinal cord, main blood vessels) and whether the progressing tumour can be managed with locally directed therapy (e.g. surgery, radiotherapy) (Table 11.4). Patient factors such as comorbidities (e.g. poorly controlled hypertension, issue with gastrointestinal absorption, recent tracheal radiation), adequacy of baseline performance status and individual wishes are equally important in the decision-making process. Patients who are managed by the "delayed treatment" approach should be monitored regularly with symptom assessment and structural imaging, initially every 3–6 months, until the rate of progression is established. Finally, shared decision-making between the treating clinician and patient regarding the best timing to initiate treatment is critical in ensuring patient's compliance to their surveillance and treatment programme.

Table 11.4 Disease factors to be assessed when considering TKI treatment

Disease factors	Treatment indication
Rate of disease progression	Evidence of RECIST progression in the past 12 months
Pattern of disease progression (diffuse vs. focal)	Evidence of diffuse progression (i.e. multiple lesions enlarging)
Tumour burden	Multiple lesions at least 1 cm in size
Disease-related symptoms	Symptomatic disease that is not amenable to focal therapy (e.g. dyspnoea, diffuse painful bony metastases)
Risk of imminent local complications	Risk of tumour progression threatening vital structures within 6 months (e.g. lung lesions or lymphadenopathy invading airways or main blood vessels, bone lesions causing spinal cord compression)

Other Emerging Systemic Treatment Options for RAI-Refractory Disease

There are ongoing efforts to further improve on current systemic treatment or to develop additional treatment approach in RAI-R advanced DTC. In addition to sorafenib and lenvatinib, other multi-targeted TKIs such as pazopanib, axitinib, motesanib and vandetanib have shown clinical activity in phase II trials with median PFS ranging from 10 to 16.1 months [81–84].

Another personalised approach that has been investigated involves specific targeting of driver mutation in thyroid cancer, such as the use of $BRAF^{V600E}$ inhibitor in $BRAF^{V600E}$ mutant PTC (Fig. 11.2). The first report in the literature of the use of a BRAF inhibitor to treat thyroid cancer was the first-in-man phase I study of vemurafenib [85]. A partial response was seen in one patient with $BRAF^{V600E}$ mutant PTC and stable disease in two other patients. This led to an open-label phase II trial of vemurafenib in patients with RAI-R $BRAF^{V600E}$ mutant PTC [86]. Partial responses were observed in 38.5% of patients who are VEGFR inhibitor naïve, and 27.3% in patients who have been exposed to VEGFR inhibitor. Median PFS was 18.2 months and 8.9 months in the respective cohorts. Another potential target that is druggable is the ALK rearrangement. An interesting case was recently reported of an impressive response to crizotinib in a patient with metastatic anaplastic thyroid cancer harbouring the ALK rearrangement [87]. This treatment strategy could also be explored in advanced PTC with ALK rearrangement.

Finally, immunotherapies with checkpoint inhibitors (e.g. PD-1 or PD-L1), which have shown great promise in other malignancies, are currently being investigated in advanced DTC. The preliminary results from the phase Ib KEYNOTE-028 study, investigating pembrolizumab (anti-PD-1 antibody) in advanced DTC, were presented recently at the 2016 ASCO annual meeting [88]. Of the 22 DTC patients enrolled, partial response was observed in 9.1% and stable disease rate was 54.5%. Median duration of response was not yet reached (range, 35.3–44.1+ week) by the data cut-off. The clinical benefit of pembrolizumab in advanced DTC will be further explored in the phase II KEYNOTE-158 trial (NCT02628067).

Redifferentiation Therapy

A novel approach to treat non-iodine-avid disease is to increase sodium-iodide symporter

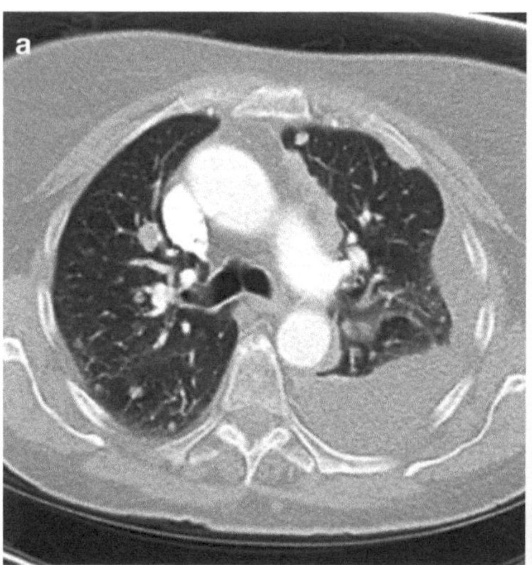

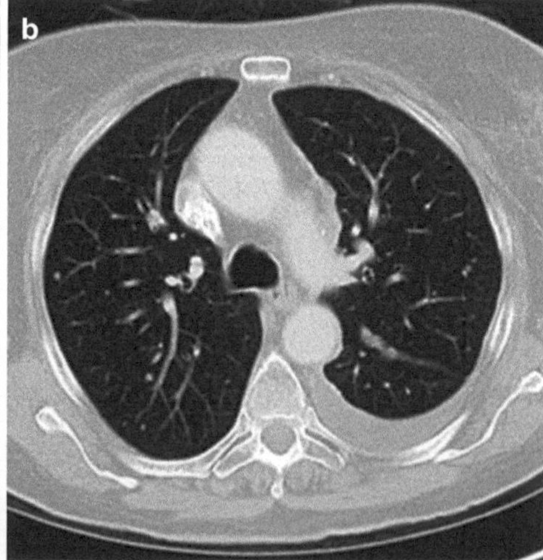

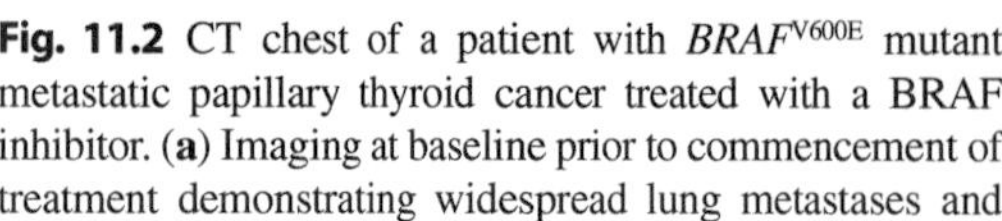

Fig. 11.2 CT chest of a patient with *$BRAF^{V600E}$* mutant metastatic papillary thyroid cancer treated with a BRAF inhibitor. (**a**) Imaging at baseline prior to commencement of treatment demonstrating widespread lung metastases and loculated left-sided pleural effusion. (**b**) Imaging 2 months after commencing treatment showing significant decrease in both number and size of the bilateral pulmonary metastasis and decrease in volume of the left-sided pleural effusion

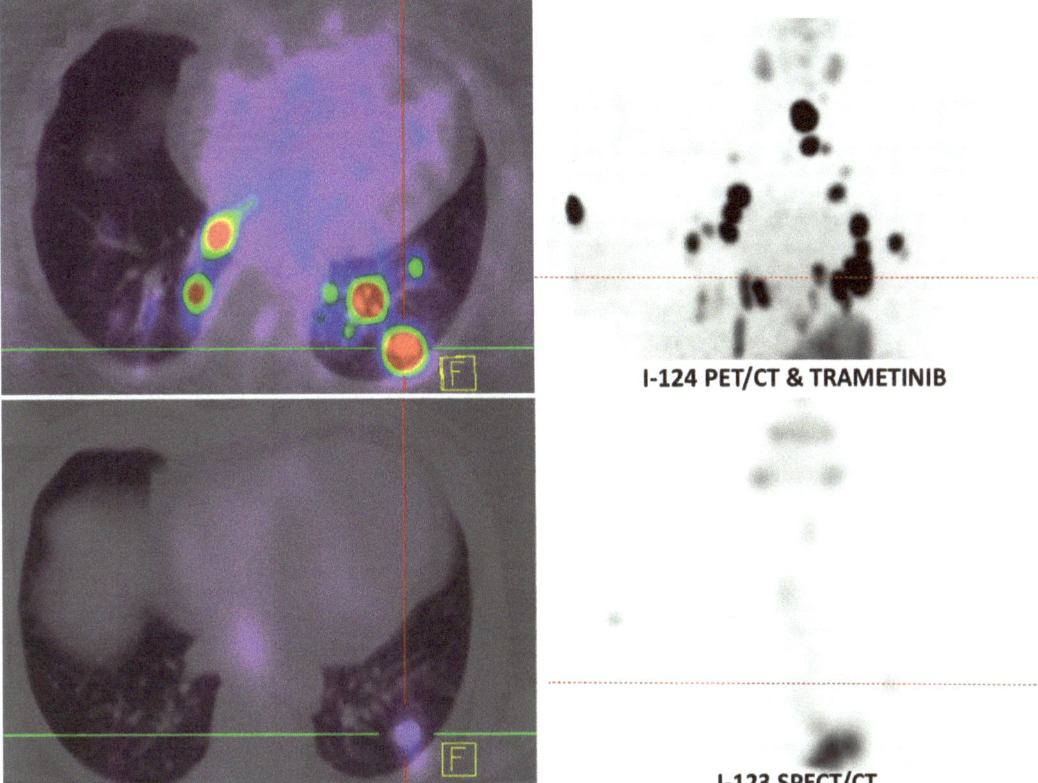

Fig. 11.3 Example of redifferentiation therapy using trametinib. Sixty-year-old woman with RAS-mutant metastatic follicular thyroid carcinoma had iodine refractory metastatic disease, with progressive pulmonary metastases despite repeated I-131 therapy. These are minimally avid on baseline TSH-stimulated I-123 SPECT/CT images (lower images). Repeat TSH-stimulated I-124 PET/CT after 4-week trametinib therapy (upper images) induces very intense uptake associated with multiple morphologically stable pulmonary metastases

expression on thyroid cancer cells to facilitate I-131 therapy (Fig. 11.3). Ho et al. have clearly demonstrated this principle of redifferentiation therapy by administering a 4-week course of selumetinib, a MEK inhibitor, followed by I-124 PET/CT to confirm adequate lesional dosimetry [89]. Eight of 20 patients demonstrated adequate I-124 uptake for treatment, including all 5 patients with NRAS mutations, resulting in a mean reduction in Tg of 89%, and structural response of partial response in 5 cases and stable disease maintained in 3 cases. A similar approach has been used with the BRAF inhibitor dabrafenib in ten patients with BRAF V600E-mutant iodine refractory thyroid cancer, with 60% demonstrating new iodine uptake amenable to treatment with I-131 therapy. Prospective dosimetry using I-124 PET/CT is clearly valuable in this setting to determine response to redifferentiation therapy and determine suitability for I-131.

Conclusion

Patients with metastatic DTC can often look forward to a reasonable life expectancy, and should ideally be managed in an expert multidisciplinary team, with treatment tailored to their individual risk profile. Treatment for metastases may include surgery, radioiodine, external beam radiation or TKIs. Returning to the case outlined in the introduction, urgent surgical decompression and stabilisation of the vertebral metastasis were performed first.

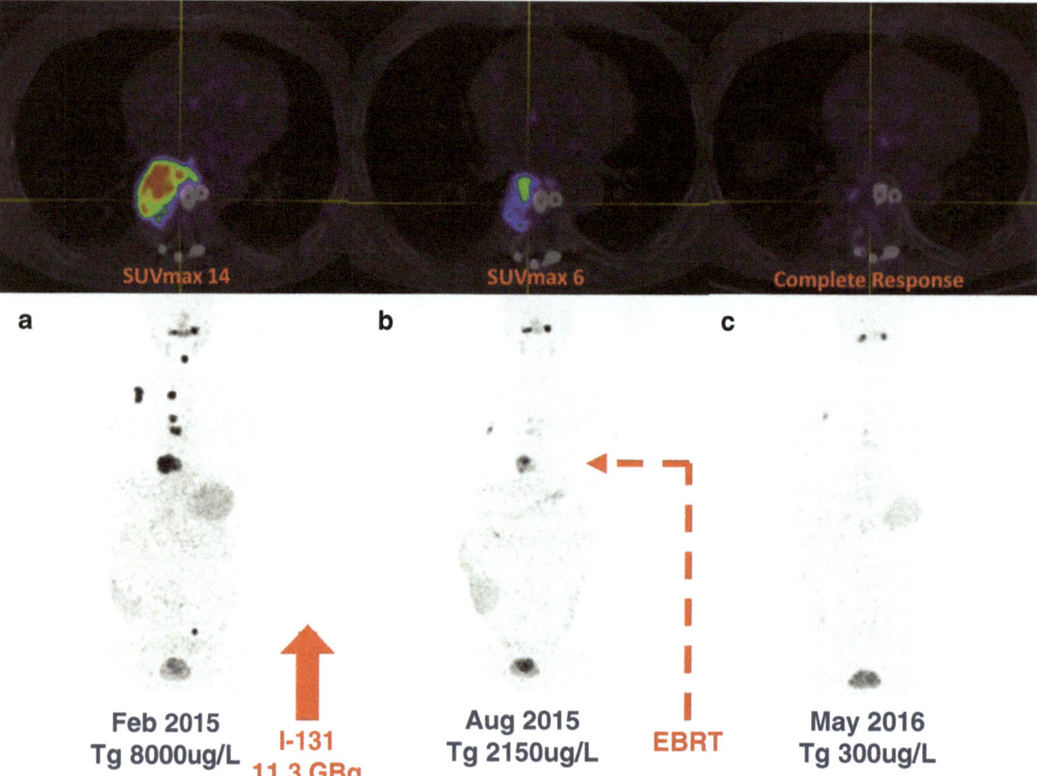

Fig. 11.4 External beam radiotherapy to augment dose from radioactive iodine to critical lesions. Seventy-one-year-old man with a series of I-124 PET/CT fused axial images (upper row) and PET maximum intensity projections (bottom row). Treatment prior to image (**a**) (baseline) involved surgical stabilisation of critical T8 metastasis and total thyroidectomy, with high-dose radioactive iodine therapy (11.3 GBq) administered immediately after image (**a**). Favourable scintigraphic and biochemical response seen on image (**b**) (+6 months), with 75% reduction in Stim Tg. External beam radiotherapy (EBRT) was then administered before image (**c**) (+15 months) confirmed complete response at T8 lesion

Total thyroidectomy was then undertaken to facilitate radioactive iodine therapy, confirming a 35 mm follicular thyroid carcinoma with lymphovascular invasion. I-124 PET/CT imaging was used to guide high-dose treatment with radioactive iodine and to measure response. External beam radiotherapy to the spinal metastasis was subsequently administered to augment the radiation dose to this critical lesion with excellent clinical, biochemical and scintigraphic response (Fig. 11.4). This case highlights the importance of multidisciplinary treatment of metastatic thyroid cancer (surgery, nuclear medicine and radiation oncology) and the role of molecular imaging using FDG and I-124 PET/CT to characterise and assist rational therapeutic decision-making. Other important considerations include the role of pre-therapy I-124 imaging to avoid radioactive iodine when not required, and use of dosimetry to optimise the administered activity in the setting of metastatic disease. In patients with RAI-R DTC, TKI treatment can improve disease control and potentially survival, but has a high incidence of side effects, and is not curative. It should therefore be used only for symptomatic, progressive disease.

References

1. La Vecchia C, Malvezzi M, Bosetti C, et al. Thyroid cancer mortality and incidence: a global overview. Int J Cancer. 2015;136:2187–95.
2. Tuttle RM. Risk-adapted management of thyroid cancer. Endocr Pract. 2008;14:764–74.
3. Ito Y, Miyauchi A, Kihara M, Higashiyama T, Kobayashi K, Miya A. Patient age is significantly related to the progression of papillary microcarcinoma of the thyroid under observation. Thyroid. 2014;24:27–34.
4. Haugen BR, Alexander EK, Bible KC, Doherty GM, Mandel SJ, Nikiforov YE, Pacini F, Randolph GW, Sawka AM, Schlumberger M, Schuff KG, Sherman SI, Sosa JA, Steward DL, Tuttle RM, Wartofsky L. 2015 American Thyroid Association management guidelines for adult patients with thyroid nodules and differentiated thyroid cancer. Thyroid. 2016;26:1–133.
5. Nikiforov YE, Seethala RR, Tallini G, et al. Encapsulated follicular variant of papillary thyroid carcinoma: a paradigm shift to reduce overtreatment of indolent Tumors. JAMA Oncol. 2016;2:1023–9.
6. Kwong N, Marqusee E, Gordon MS, et al. Longterm, treatment-free survival in select patients with distant metastatic papillary thyroid cancer. Endocr Connect. 2014;3:207–14.
7. Durante C, Haddy N, Baudin E, et al. Long-term outcome of 444 patients with distant metastases from papillary and follicular thyroid carcinoma: benefits and limits of radioiodine therapy. J Clin Endocrinol Metab. 2006;91:2892–9.
8. Cohen Y, Xing M, Mambo E, Guo Z, Wu G, Trink B, et al. BRAF mutation in papillary thyroid carcinoma. J Natl Cancer Inst. 2003;95:625–7.
9. Soares P, Trovisco V, Rocha AS, Lima J, Castro P, Preto A, et al. BRAF mutations and RET/PTC rearrangements are alternative events in the etiopathogenesis of PTC. Oncogene. 2003;22:4578–80.
10. Namba H, Nakashima M, Hayashi T, Hayashida N, Maeda S, Rogounovitch TI, et al. Clinical implication of hot spot BRAF mutation, V599E, in papillary thyroid cancers. J Clin Endocrinol Metab. 2003;88:4393–7.
11. Kimura ET, Nikiforova MN, Zhu Z, Knauf JA, Nikiforov YE, Fagin JA. High prevalence of BRAF mutations in thyroid cancer: genetic evidence for constitutive activation of the RET/PTC-RAS-BRAF signaling pathway in papillary thyroid carcinoma. Cancer Res. 2003;63:1454–7.
12. Xing M. BRAF mutation in thyroid cancer. Endocr Relat Cancer. 2005;12:245–62.
13. Lemoine NR, Mayall ES, Wyllie FS, Farr CJ, Hughes D, Padua RA, et al. Activated ras oncogenes in human thyroid cancers. Cancer Res. 1988;48:4459–63.
14. Suarez HG, Du Villard JA, Caillou B, Schlumberger M, Tubiana M, Parmentier C, et al. Detection of activated ras oncogenes in human thyroid carcinomas. Oncogene. 1988;2:403–6.
15. Frattini M, Ferrario C, Bressan P, Balestra D, De Cecco L, Mondellini P, et al. Alternative mutations of BRAF, RET and NTRK1 are associated with similar but distinct gene expression patterns in papillary thyroid cancer. Oncogene. 2004;23:7436–40.
16. Grieco M, Santoro M, Berlingieri MT, Melillo RM, Donghi R, Bongarzone I, et al. PTC is a novel rearranged form of the ret proto-oncogene and is frequently detected in vivo in human thyroid papillary carcinomas. Cell. 1990;60:557–63.
17. Pierotti MA, Bongarzone I, Borrello MG, Mariani C, Miranda C, Sozzi G, et al. Rearrangements of TRK proto-oncogene in papillary thyroid carcinomas. J Endocrinol Investig. 1995;18:130–3.
18. Garraway LA, Lander ES. Lessons from the cancer genome. Cell. 2013;153:17–37.
19. Cancer Genome Atlas Research Network. Integrated genomic characterization of papillary thyroid carcinoma. Cell. 2014;159:676–90.
20. Dinneen SF, Valimaki MJ, Bergstralh EJ, et al. Distant metastases in papillary thyroid carcinoma: 100 cases observed at one institution during 5 decades. J Clin Endocrinol Metab. 1995;80:2041–5.
21. Schlumberger M, Challeton C, De Vathaire F, et al. Radioactive iodine treatment and external radiotherapy for lung and bone metastases from thyroid carcinoma. J Nucl Med. 1996;37:598–605.
22. Mihailovic J, Stefanovic L, Malesevic M. Differentiated thyroid carcinoma with distant metastases: probability of survival and its predicting factors. Cancer Biother Radiopharm. 2007;22:250–5.
23. Lee J, Soh EY. Differentiated thyroid carcinoma presenting with distant metastasis at initial diagnosis. Ann Surg. 2010;251:114–9.
24. Al-Dhahri SF, Al-Amro AS, Al-Shakwer W, et al. Cerebellar mass as a primary presentation of papillary thyroid carcinoma: case report and literature review. Head Neck Oncol. 2009;1:23.
25. Lin JD, Huang MJ, Juang JH, et al. Factors related to the survival of papillary and follicular thyroid carcinoma patients with distant metastases. Thyroid. 1999;9:1227–35.
26. Giovanella L, Clark P, Chiovato L, et al. Thyroglobulin measurement using highly sensitive assays in patients with differentiated thyroid cancer: a clinical position paper. Eur J Endocrinol. 2014;171:R33–46.
27. Giovanella L, Treglia G, Sadeghi R, et al. Unstimulated high-sensitive thyroglobulin in follow-up of differentiated thyroid cancer patients: a metaanalysis. J Clin Endocrinol Metab. 2014;99:440–7.
28. Spencer C, LoPresti J, Fatemi S. How sensitive (second-generation) thyroglobulin measurement is changing paradigms for monitoring patients with differentiated thyroid cancer, in the absence or presence of thyroglobulin autoantibodies. Curr Opin Endocrinol Diabetes Obes. 2014;21:394–404.
29. Robbins RJ, Srivastava S, Shaha A, Ghossein R, Larson SM, Fleisher M, Tuttle RM. Factors influencing the basal and recombinant human thyrotropin-stimulated serum thyroglobulin in patients with

metastatic thyroid carcinoma. J Clin Endocrinol Metab. 2004;89:6010–6.
30. Cherk MH, Francis P, Topliss DJ, et al. Incidence and implications of negative serum thyroglobulin but positive I-131 whole-body scans in patients with well-differentiated thyroid cancer prepared with rhTSH or thyroid hormone withdrawal. Clin Endocrinol. 2012;76:734–40.
31. Ruan M, Shen Y, Chen L, et al. RECIST 1.1 and serum thyroglobulin measurements in the evaluation of responses to sorafenib in patients with radioactive iodine-refractory differentiated thyroid carcinoma. Oncol Lett. 2013;6:480–6.
32. Aide N, Heutte N, Rame JP, et al. Clinical relevance of single-photon emission computed tomography/computed tomography of the neck and thorax in postablation (131)I scintigraphy for thyroid cancer. J Clin Endocrinol Metab. 2009;94:2075–84.
33. Schmidt D, Szikszai A, Linke R, et al. Impact of 131I SPECT/spiral CT on nodal staging of differentiated thyroid carcinoma at the first radioablation. J Nucl Med. 2009;50:18–23.
34. Van Nostrand D, Moreau S, Bandarau VV, et al. (124)I positron emission tomography versus (131) I planar imaging in the identification of residual thyroid tissue and/or metastasis in patients who have well-differentiated thyroid cancer. Thyroid. 2010;20:879–83.
35. Ruhlmann M, Jentzen W, Ruhlmann V, et al. High level of agreement between pretherapeutic 124I PET and intratherapeutic 131I imaging in detecting iodine-positive thyroid cancer metastases. J Nucl Med. 2016;57:1339–42.
36. Warburg O. On the origin of cancer cells. Science. 1956;123:309–14.
37. Pattison DA, Hofman MS. Role of fluorodeoxyglucose PET/computed tomography in targeted radionuclide therapy for endocrine malignancies. PET Clin. 2015;10:461–76.
38. Robbins T, et al. Real-time prognosis for metastatic thyroid carcinoma based on 2-[18F]fluoro-2-deoxy-D-glucose-positron emission tomography scanning. J Clin Endocrinol Metab. 2006;91:498–505.
39. Gasparre G, Porcelli AM, Bonora E, et al. Disruptive mitochondrial DNA mutations in complex I subunits are markers of oncocytic phenotype in thyroid tumours. Proc Natl Acad Sci. 2007;104:9001–6.
40. Deandreis D, Ghuzlan AA, Auperin A, et al. Is 18F-fluorodeoxyglucose-PET/CT useful for the presurgical characterisation of thyroid nodules with indeterminate fine needle aspiration cytology? Thyroid. 2012;22:165–72.
41. Zandieh S, Pokieser W, Knoll P, Sonneck-Koenne C, Kudlacek M, Mirzaei S. Oncocytic adenomas of thyroid-mimicking benign or metastatic disease on 18F-FDG-PET scan. Acta Radiol. 2015;56:709–13.
42. Feine U, Lietzenmayer R, Hanke JP, et al. 18FDG whole-body PET in differentiated thyroid carcinoma. Flipflop in uptake patterns of 18FDG and I131. Nuklearmedizin. 1995;34:127–34.
43. Kelders A, Kennes LN, Krohn T, Behrendt FF, Mottaghy FM, Verburg FA. Relationship between positive thyroglobulin doubling time and 18F-FDG PET/CT positive, 131I-negative lesions. Nucl Med Commun. 2014;35:176–81.
44. Pattison DA, Solomon B, Hicks RJ. A new theranostic paradigm for advanced thyroid carcinoma. J Nucl Med. 2016;57:1493–4.
45. Dong MJ, Liu ZF, Zhao K, et al. Value of 18FDG-PET/PET-CT in differentiated thyroid carcinoma with radioiodine-negative whole-body scan: a meta-analysis. Nucl Med Commun. 2009;30:639–50.
46. McGriff NJ, Csako G, Gourgiotis L, et al. Effects of thyroid hormone suppression therapy on adverse clinical outcomes in thyroid cancer. Ann Med. 2002;34:554–64.
47. Jonklaas J, Sarlis NJ, Litofsky D, et al. Outcomes of patients with differentiated thyroid carcinoma following initial therapy. Thyroid. 2006;16:1229–42.
48. Seidlin S, Oshry E, Yallow AA. Spontaneous and experimentally induced uptake of radioactive iodine in metastases from thyroid carcinoma. J Clin Endocrinol Metab. 1948;8:423–5.
49. Schlumberger M, Catargi B, Borget I, Deandreis D, Zerdoud S, Bridgi B, et al. Strategies of radioiodine ablation in patients with low-risk thyroid cancer. N Engl J Med. 2012;366:1663–73.
50. Freudenberg LS, Jentzen W, Petrich T, et al. Lesion dose in differentiated thyroid carcinoma metastases after rhTSH or thyroid hormone withdrawal: 124I PET/CT dosimetric comparisons. Eur J Nucl Med Mol Imaging. 2010;37:2267–76.
51. Kist JW, de Keizer B, van der Vlies M, et al. 124I PET/CT to predict the outcome of blind 131I treatment in patients with biochemical recurrence of differentiated thyroid cancer: results of a multicenter diagnostic cohort study (THYROPET). J Nucl Med. 2016;57:701–7.
52. Pattison DA, Hicks RJ. Letter: THYROPET Study: is biology or technology the issue? J Nucl Med. 2017;58:354.
53. Maxon HR, Englaro EE, Thomas SR, et al. Radioiodine-131 therapy for well differentiated thyroid cancer: quantitative radiation dosimetric approach—outcome and validation in 85 patients. J Nucl Med. 1992;33:1132–6.
54. Jentzen W, Hoppenbrouwers J, van Leeuwen P, et al. Assessment of lesion response in the initial radioiodine treatment of differentiated thyroid cancer using 124I PET imaging. J Nucl Med. 2014;55:1759–65.
55. Jentzen W, Verschure F, van Zon A, et al. 124I PET assessment of response of bone metastases to initial radioiodine treatment of differentiated thyroid cancer. J Nucl Med. 2016;57:1499–504.
56. Deandreis D, Rubino C, Hernan T, et al. Comparison of empiric versus whole body/blood clearance dosimetry-based approach to radioactive iodine treatment in patients with metastases from differentiated thyroid cancer. J Nucl Med. 2017;58:717.

57. Tuttle RM, Leboeuf R, Robbins RJ, et al. Empiric radioactive iodine dosing regimens frequently exceed maximum tolerated activity levels in elderly patients with thyroid cancer. J Nucl Med. 2006;47:1587–91.
58. Benua RS, Cicale NR, Sonenberg M, Rawson RW. The relation of radioiodine dosimetry to results and complications in the treatment of metastatic thyroid cancer. Am J Roentgenol Radium Ther Nucl Med. 1962;87:171–82.
59. Rubino C, de Vathaire F, Dottorini ME, et al. Second primary malignancies in thyroid cancer patients. Br J Cancer. 2003;89:1638–44.
60. Chiu AC, Delpassand ES, Sherman SI. Prognosis and treatment of brain metastases in thyroid carcinoma. J Clin Endocrinol Metab. 1997;82:3637–42.
61. O'Doherty MJ, Coakley AJ. Drug therapy alternatives in the treatment of thyroid cancer. Drugs. 1998;55:801–12.
62. McWilliams RR, Giannini C, Hay ID, et al. Management of brain metastases from thyroid carcinoma: a study of 16 pathologically confirmed cases over 25 years. Cancer. 2003;98:356–62.
63. Sciubba DM, et al. Diagnosis and management of metastatic spine disease. A review. J Neurosurg Spine. 2010;13:94–108.
64. Harrington KD. Metastatic disease of the spine. J Bone Joint Surg Am. 1986;68A:1110–5.
65. Quan GM, Pointillart V, Palussière J, Bonichon F. Multidisciplinary treatment and survival of patients with vertebral metastases from thyroid carcinoma. Thyroid. 2012;22:125–30.
66. Ramadan S, Ugas MA, Berwick RJ, et al. Spinal metastasis in thyroid cancer. Head Neck Oncol. 2012;4:39.
67. Argiris A, Agarwala SS, Karamouzis MV, Burmeister LA, Carty SE. A phase II trial of doxorubicin and interferon alpha 2b in advanced, non-medullary thyroid cancer. Investig New Drugs. 2008;26:183–8.
68. Shimaoka K, Schoenfeld DA, DeWys WD, Creech RH, DeConti R. A randomized trial of doxorubicin versus doxorubicin plus cisplatin in patients with advanced thyroid carcinoma. Cancer. 1985;56:2155–60.
69. Klein M, Vignaud JM, Hennequin V, Toussaint B, Bresler L, Plenat F, et al. Increased expression of the vascular endothelial growth factor is a pejorative prognosis marker in papillary thyroid carcinoma. J Clin Endocrinol Metab. 2001;86:656–8.
70. Yu XM, Lo CY, Chan WF, Lam KY, Leung P, Luk JM. Increased expression of vascular endothelial growth factor C in papillary thyroid carcinoma correlates with cervical lymph node metastases. Clin Cancer Res. 2005;11:8063–9.
71. Brose MS, Nutting CM, Jarzab B, Elisei R, Siena S, Bastholt L, et al. Sorafenib in radioactive iodine-refractory, locally advanced or metastatic differentiated thyroid cancer: a randomised, double-blind, phase 3 trial. Lancet. 2014;384:319–28.
72. Schlumberger M, Tahara M, Wirth LJ, Robinson B, Brose MS, Elisei R, et al. Lenvatinib versus placebo in radioiodine-refractory thyroid cancer. N Engl J Med. 2015;372:621–30.
73. Wilhelm SM, Carter C, Tang L, Wilkie D, McNabola A, Rong H, et al. BAY 43-9006 exhibits broad spectrum oral antitumor activity and targets the RAF/MEK/ERK pathway and receptor tyrosine kinases involved in tumor progression and angiogenesis. Cancer Res. 2004;64:7099–109.
74. Carlomagno F, Anaganti S, Guida T, Salvatore G, Troncone G, Wilhelm SM, et al. BAY 43-9006 inhibition of oncogenic RET mutants. J Natl Cancer Inst. 2006;98:326–34.
75. Gupta-Abramson V, Troxel AB, Nellore A, Puttaswamy K, Redlinger M, Ransone K, et al. Phase II trial of sorafenib in advanced thyroid cancer. J Clin Oncol. 2008;26:4714–9.
76. Kloos RT, Ringel MD, Knopp MV, Hall NC, King M, Stevens R, et al. Phase II trial of sorafenib in metastatic thyroid cancer. J Clin Oncol. 2009;27:1675–84.
77. Paschke R, Schlumberger M, Nutting C, Jarzab B, Elisei R, Siena S, et al. Exploratory analysis of outcomes for patients with locally advanced or metastatic radioactive iodine-refractory differentiated thyroid cancer (RAI-R DTC) receiving open-label sorafenib post-progression on the phase III DECISION trial. Exp Clin Endocrinol Diabetes 2015;123–P03_05.
78. Matsui J, Funahashi Y, Uenaka T, Watanabe T, Tsuruoka A, Asada M. Multi-kinase inhibitor E7080 suppresses lymph node and lung metastases of human mammary breast tumor MDA-MB-231 via inhibition of vascular endothelial growth factor-receptor (VEGF-R) 2 and VEGF-R3 kinase. Clin Cancer Res. 2008;14:5459–65.
79. Matsui J, Yamamoto Y, Funahashi Y, Tsuruoka A, Watanabe T, Wakabayashi T, et al. E7080, a novel inhibitor that targets multiple kinases, has potent antitumor activities against stem cell factor producing human small cell lung cancer H146, based on angiogenesis inhibition. Int J Cancer. 2008;122:664–71.
80. Cabanillas ME, Schlumberger M, Jarzab B, Martins RG, Pacini F, Robinson B, et al. A phase 2 trial of lenvatinib (E7080) in advanced, progressive, radioiodine-refractory, differentiated thyroid cancer: a clinical outcomes and biomarker assessment. Cancer. 2015;121:2749–56.
81. Locati LD, Licitra L, Agate L, Ou SH, Boucher A, Jarzab B, et al. Treatment of advanced thyroid cancer with axitinib: phase 2 study with pharmacokinetic/pharmacodynamic and quality-of-life assessments. Cancer. 2014;120:2694–703.
82. Sherman SI, Wirth LJ, Droz JP, Hofmann M, Bastholt L, Martins RG, et al. Motesanib diphosphate in progressive differentiated thyroid cancer. N Engl J Med. 2008;359:31–42.
83. Leboulleux S, Bastholt L, Krause T, de la Fouchardiere C, Tennvall J, Awada A, et al. Vandetanib in locally advanced or metastatic differentiated thyroid cancer: a randomised, double-blind, phase 2 trial. Lancet Oncol. 2012;13:897–905.
84. Bible KC, Suman VJ, Molina JR, Smallridge RC, Maples WJ, Menefee ME, et al. Efficacy of pazopanib in progressive, radioiodine-refractory,

metastatic differentiated thyroid cancers: results of a phase 2 consortium study. Lancet Oncol. 2010;11: 962–72.
85. Kim KB, Cabanillas ME, Lazar AJ, Williams MD, Sanders DL, Ilagan JL, et al. Clinical responses to vemurafenib in patients with metastatic papillary thyroid cancer harboring BRAF(V600E) mutation. Thyroid. 2013;23:1277–83.
86. Brose MS, Cabanillas ME, Cohen EE, Wirth LJ, Riehl T, Yue H, et al. Vemurafenib in patients with BRAF(V600E)-positive metastatic or unresectable papillary thyroid cancer refractory to radioactive iodine: a non-randomised, multicentre, open-label, phase 2 trial. Lancet Oncol. 2016;17:1272–82.
87. Godbert Y, Henriques de Figueiredo B, Bonichon F, Chibon F, Hostein I, Perot G, et al. Remarkable response to crizotinib in woman with anaplastic lymphoma kinase-rearranged anaplastic thyroid carcinoma. J Clin Oncol. 2015;33:e84–7.
88. Mehnert J, Varga A, Brose MS, Aggarwal R, Lin C, Prawira A. Pembrolizumab for advanced papillary or follicular thyroid cancer: preliminary results from the phase 1b KEYNOTE-028 study. J Clin Oncol. 2016;34(Suppl) Abstract 6091.
89. Ho AL, Grewal RK, Leboeuf R, Sherman EJ, Pfister DG, Deandreis D, et al. Selumetinib-enhanced radioiodine uptake in advanced thyroid cancer. N Engl J Med. 2013;368:623–32.

12 Medullary Thyroid Carcinoma

Siddhartha Chakravarthy
and Paul Mazhuvanchary Jacob

Introduction

Medullary thyroid carcinoma (MTC) which originates from the parafollicular C cells of the thyroid gland belongs to the group of neuroendocrine tumours, unrelated to the majority of thyroid tumours of follicular cell origin. It was first described as a separate entity with the term 'medullary' by Hazard and colleagues in 1959 as a 'solid, non-follicular histologic pattern, the presence of amyloid in the stroma and a high incidence of lymph node metastasis' [1]. The C cells are neuroectodermal in origin and are concentrated in the junction of upper and middle third of the thyroid lobes. They secrete calcitonin and other substances, including carcinoembryonic antigen (CEA), adrenocortical stimulating hormone (ACTH), histaminases, serotonin and chromogranin [2, 3]. The important secretory products are calcitonin and CEA for use as diagnostic and prognostic tumour markers and their serum concentrations are directly related to the C-cell mass. The discovery of a genetic basis with a strong genotype–phenotype link has revolutionised the management of familial forms of medullary thyroid carcinoma. Improvements in management of familial disease, pathological and surgical expertise and availability of newer modalities of therapy have raised the survival rates in the recent decades.

S. Chakravarthy · P. M. Jacob (✉)
Department of Endocrine Surgery, Christian Medical College and Hospital, Vellore, Tamil Nadu, India
e-mail: mjpaul@cmcvellore.ac.in

Epidemiology and Aetiology

Many sources report that it accounts for 3–5% of thyroid cancers. The current SEER (Surveillance, Epidemiology, and End Results) data report states that MTC constitutes only 1–2% due to the relative increase in the papillary carcinoma of thyroid (PTC) over the last three decades [4]. Majority of the patients (75%) have sporadic MTC and 25% have hereditary MTC. The familial form is transmitted in the autosomal dominant pattern.

Familial medullary thyroid carcinoma is caused by the genetic mutation in 'rearranged during transfection' (RET) proto-oncogene located in chromosome 10q11.2. RET proto-oncogene, discovered by Takahashi and colleagues in 1985, encodes a transmembrane receptor tyrosine kinase that is expressed in derivatives of the neural crest, including neural crest derived tumours such as MTC and pheochromocytoma [5, 6]. The hereditary forms constitute the type 2 multiple endocrine neoplasia syndromes—MEN 2A and B.

1. MEN 2A has four variants:
   (a) Classical MEN 2A—all patients develop MTC, clinically detectable in 25% by age 13 increasing to 70% by age 70; the stimulation test for calcitonin is positive in 95% by age 30. Currently the gene test recommended by age 5 determines all subjects at

R. Parameswaran, A. Agarwal (eds.), *Evidence-Based Endocrine Surgery*,
https://doi.org/10.1007/978-981-10-1124-5_12

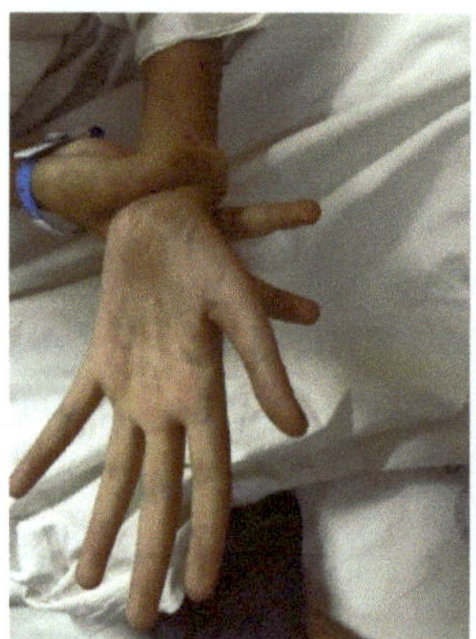
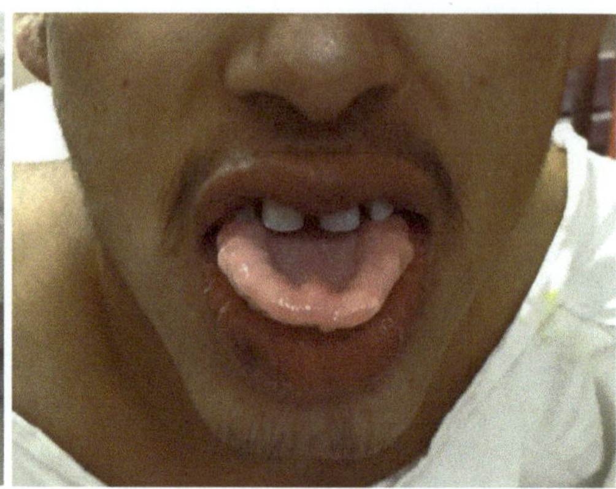

Fig. 12.1 MEN 2B phenotype with marfanoid habitus and oral mucosal neuromas causing thickened lips and tongue

risk. This eliminates the likelihood in 50% of first-degree relatives and obviates the need for close follow-up and fear of the disease. Pheochromocytoma occurs in up to 50% usually after the age of 10 years and occurs more frequently in carriers of exon 10 mutation than exon 11. They are bilateral in up to 50% and mainly produce adrenaline. Hyperparathyroidism is seen in up to 30% usually by the third decade of life; less frequently seen in exon 10 mutation. The disease is commonly caused by parathyroid hyperplasia and develops slowly, mild and asymptomatic.

(b) MEN 2A with cutaneous lichenoid amyloidosis (CLA)—in patients with codon 634 mutations a pruritic, pigmented, papular lesion develops on the upper back early in life preceding the C-cell hyperplasia.

(c) MEN 2A with Hirschsprung's disease (HD)—in patients with exon 10 point mutation, this can be seen in 7% of cases.

(d) Familial MTC—these patients manifest only medullary cancer in all the gene carriers.

2. MEN 2B syndrome is a more aggressive disease with early onset of MTC, with a unique phenotype including skeletal abnormalities (marfanoid habitus, long narrow facies, high arched palate, pectus excavatum, scoliosis, pes cavus and slipped femoral capital epiphysis), generalised ganglioneuromatosis of the entire aerodigestive tract (causing symptoms of bloating, constipation and diarrhoea) and ophthalmological abnormalities (thickened and everted eyelids, mild ptosis and prominent corneal nerves). (See Figs. 12.1 and 12.2). Pheochromocytoma develops in about 50%. The majority of cases present as sporadic disease with de novo mutations causing delayed diagnosis with metastatic disease and poor prognosis.

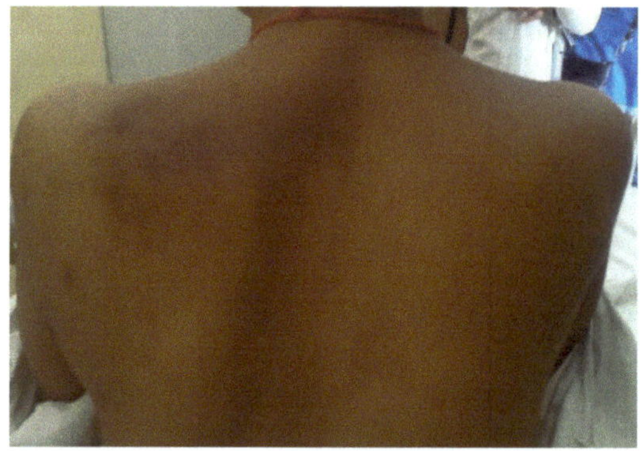

Fig. 12.2 Cutaneous lichenoid amyloidosis in a patient with MEN 2A

Virtually all hereditary patients have RET germline mutations and approximately 50% of sporadic MTCs have somatic RET mutations [7–9]. Other mutations in the HRAS, KRAS and less commonly NRAS genes were found in 18–80% of sporadic MTC lacking RET mutations [10].

Screening for Familial Disease and Recommendations for Intervention

All patients with MTC and first-degree kindred of patients with known mutation should be advised RET germline mutation analysis. In hereditary MTC there is a distinct age-related progression from C-cell hyperplasia (CCH) to MTC and to loco-regional and distant metastasis. This occurs over months to years and depends on the type of RET mutation [11]. The term 'prophylactic thyroidectomy' is removal of thyroid gland before the development of MTC or while it is clinically unapparent and confined to the gland to offer the best chance of cure.

The 2015 ATA guidelines recommend categorising hereditary MTC into three groups based on aggressiveness and age of onset—'moderate risk' (MOD), 'high risk' (H) and 'highest risk' (HST) (Table 12.1). The patients with MEN 2B and RET codon M918T mutation are included in 'highest risk'. The 'high-risk' category includes patients with MEN 2A and RET codon C634 or 883 mutation. The 'moderate-risk' category and includes all patients with hereditary MTC and RET codon mutations other than M918T and C634 [12].

Patients with no special clinical features can be tested in a multi-tiered approach, first for RET mutations in exons 10 and 11 which will help in detecting the five most frequently mutated codons (C634R, C609, C611, C618, C620); if these are negative, then testing is done for exons 8 and 13–16. Once a germline mutation is detected in a patient, RET mutational analysis must be offered to all first-degree relatives who are 'at risk' and RET analysis in the relatives could be limited to screening only the affected codon.

Children with a RET codon M918 (ATA-HST category) should have prophylactic thyroidectomy in the first year of life. Children in ATA-H category should have thyroidectomy at age 5 years, or earlier based on the detection of elevated serum calcitonin levels. Children in the ATA-MOD category are less aggressive and need monitoring with physical examination, ultrasound (USG) of neck and measurement of serum calcitonin. They need thyroidectomy when there is elevation of serum calcitonin or development of nodules on USG [10, 11, 13].

Clinical Features of MTC

The most common clinical presentation of MTC is the appearance of a solitary thyroid nodule; other presentations include a multinodular goitre or incidental finding on neck imaging. Sporadic MTC is the most common form and most patients are asymptomatic, presenting with a solitary thyroid nodule (75–95%) [14, 15] or a multinodular goitre with or without palpable lymph nodes. Neck lymph node enlargement is present in 50% of cases reflecting the aggressive pattern of lymphatic spread. Rarely, diarrhoea can be a paraneoplastic presenting symptom caused by peptide co-secretion from advanced tumour as also Cushing's syndrome when ACTH is produced in excess by the malignant C cells. Some patients present with systemic metastasis with symptoms

Table 12.1 ATA guidelines on timing of prophylactic surgery based on codon mutation

ATA risk level	Moderate (MOD)	High (H)	Highest (HST)
Codon mutation	321, 532, 533, 609, 611, 618, 620, 630, 631, 635, 649, 666, 768, 790, 791, 804, 844, 891, 912	634, 883	918
MTC aggressiveness	A, B	C	D
MTC age of onset	Adult	<5 years	First year of life
Timing of prophylactic surgery	When serum calcitonin becomes elevated/earlier if family chooses	Consider at <5 years. Based on serum calcitonin levels	As early as possible/in the first year of life whichever is earlier

of hormonal excess, i.e. diarrhoea and flushing secondary to increased calcitonin levels. Clinical features of hereditary MTC are described elsewhere.

Diagnosis

The diagnosis of MTC is usually made by fine-needle aspiration cytology (FNAC). The sensitivity of FNAC varies from 50 to 80%. Calcitonin can be measured in the washout fluid of the needle aspirate and these malignant cells are usually positive for immunoreactivity for calcitonin, CEA, chromogranin, synaptophysin and TTF and negative for thyroglobulin [16, 17].

Fine-needle aspiration sample typically shows moderate to marked cellularity. Cells are plasmacytoid, polygonal, round and/or spindle shaped. Nuclei are round and often eccentrically placed, with fine or coarse granular ('salt and pepper') chromatin. Amyloid is seen in 50–80% of cases [18, 19].

In the event FNAC is suspicious, but not diagnostic of MTC, serum calcitonin elevation is sensitive in detecting the disease. Once the diagnosis of MTC is made, serum calcitonin and CEA should be measured. The latest immunochemiluminometric assays for measuring serum calcitonin are highly sensitive and specific. The role of the traditional provocative tests using intravenous calcium and pentagastrin to measure calcitonin levels may not be necessary in the era of widely available testing for genetic mutation [20]. Genetic testing for germline RET mutation is recommended in all patients. In hereditary MTC, 24-h urine metanephrines and normetanephrines or plasma metanephrines and normetanephrines must be done to exclude pheochromocytoma. The presence of hyperparathyroidism is excluded by measuring serum calcium, phosphorus and albumin.

Preoperative Imaging

Ultrasound of the neck is a basic investigation for evaluating a thyroid nodule. It identifies the suspicious thyroid nodule which is hypoechoic and can have smaller hyperechoic foci, which histologically represent microcalcifications in conjunction with amyloid deposits [21]. The USG features of MTC are not much different from PTC and can have a solid internal content, an ovoid to round shape, marked hypoechogenicity and calcifications [22]. Ultrasound also helps in assessing the suspicious central and lateral compartment lymph nodes. Contrast-enhanced computer tomography (CECT) of neck and thorax is done in patients with serum calcitonin >500 pg/mL and in patients with extensive neck disease.

Pathology

Macroscopically, the tumour is firm in consistency and chalky white or red in colour; typically it is located at the junction of upper and middle thirds of the thyroid lobe. Histopathologic appearance shows sheets of spindle, round or polygonal shaped cells separated by fibrous stroma forming a solid trabecular or variable pattern. The cytoplasm is eosinophilic with fine granular appearance and the nuclei are typically uniform with rare mitotic figures. The diagnosis of MTC is confirmed if there is a positive staining for both calcitonin and CEA. C-cell hyperplasia is detected in hereditary MTC on immunostaining as the first histological change. Bilateral CCH is seen in almost all cases of MTC in MEN 2. The current TNM staging is detailed in the table below (Table 12.2).

Treatment of MTC

The differentiation into sporadic and hereditary disease is important in these patients.

In hereditary patients, presence of pheochromocytoma and primary hyperparathyroidism should be looked for prior to surgery by checking the 24-h urinary metanephrines, normetanephrines and serum calcium screening. Due to the risk of hypertensive crisis, pheochromocytoma should be operated first, followed by surgery for MTC. Hyperparathyroidism can be treated surgically along with the thyroidectomy for MTC.

Table 12.2 Staging of MTC by American Joint Committee on cancer TNM classification

Primary tumour (T)[a]			
TX	Primary tumour cannot be assessed		
T0	No evidence of primary tumour		
T1	Tumour 2 cm or less in greatest dimension, limited to the thyroid		
T1a	Tumour 1 cm or less, limited to the thyroid		
T1b	Tumour more than 1 cm, but not more than 2 cm, in greatest dimension, limited to the thyroid		
T2	Tumour more than 2 cm, but not more than 4 cm, in greatest dimension, limited to the thyroid		
T3	Tumour more than 4 cm in greatest dimension limited to the thyroid, or any tumour with minimal extrathyroid extension (e.g. extension to sternothyroid muscle or perithyroid soft tissues)		
T4a	Moderately advanced disease; tumour of any size extending beyond the thyroid capsule to invade subcutaneous soft tissues, larynx, trachea, oesophagus or recurrent laryngeal nerve		
T4b	Very advanced disease; tumour invades prevertebral fascia or encases carotid artery or mediastinal vessels		
Regional lymph nodes (N)[b]			
NX	Regional lymph nodes cannot be assessed		
N0	No regional lymph node metastasis		
N1	Regional lymph node metastasis		
N1a	Metastases to level VI (pretracheal, paratracheal and prelaryngeal/Delphian lymph nodes)		
N1b	Metastasis to unilateral, bilateral or contralateral cervical (levels I, II, III, IV or V) or retropharyngeal or superior mediastinal lymph nodes (level VII)		
Distant metastasis			
M0	No distant metastasis		
M1	Distant metastasis		
Staging			
Stage I	T1	N0	M0
Stage II	T2	N0	M0
	T3	N0	M0
Stage III	T1	N1a	M0
	T2	N1a	M0
	T3	N1a	M0
Stage IVA	T4a	N0	M0
	T4a	N1a	M0
	T1	N1b	M0
	T2	N1b	M0
	T3	N1b	M0
	T4a	N1b	M0
Stage IVB	T4b	Any N	M0
Stage IVC	Any T	Any N	M1

From the 7th Edition of the American Joint Committee on Cancer Staging Manual

[a]All categories may be subdivided: (s) solitary tumour and (m) multifocal tumour (the largest determines the classification)

[b]Regional lymph nodes are the central compartment and the lateral cervical and upper mediastinal lymph node compartments

Surgery offers the only chance of cure in patients with MTC. When the disease is confined to the thyroid gland, total thyroidectomy and central compartmental lymph nodal dissection should be done. If there are significant or suspicious lateral lymph nodes on ultrasound, level II to V nodes should be meticulously dissected. While doing the lateral neck dissection, contralateral lymph nodal dissection can be considered with basal calcitonin levels greater than 200 pg/mL, and tumour greater than 1 cm, or with multiple central compartmental lymph node metastases [23–26]. The rate of lymph nodal metastasis correlates with the size of the primary thyroid tumour (pT1 33%, pT2 53%, pT3 100%, pT4 100%). Mediastinal lymph nodal involvement is found in 50% of pT4 cases [27]. Sternotomy is required in selected patients to remove mediastinal disease (Fig. 12.3). Surgical excision is the only effective form of treatment for lymph nodal metastasis. Dralle has advocated that in node-positive patients a systematic lymphadenectomy has a higher (29.2%) chance of post-operative normalisation of serum calcitonin, and then a selective neck dissection (8.5%) [28].

When medullary carcinoma of thyroid is diagnosed after a lobectomy, completion thyroidectomy may not be required in sporadic patients with normal post-operative calcitonin level and normal lobe on USG because contralateral disease is rare (0–9%) [26]. Completion thyroidectomy with prophylactic central compartment neck dissection is required in patients who have hereditary disease, C-cell hyperplasia, an abnormal remnant lobe on USG or elevated post-operative calcitonin (Fig. 12.2).

In the presence of extensive local disease or systemic disease, less aggressive surgery in the neck is advisable with the focus on preserving speech, swallowing and shoulder mobility functions. It is not possible in most patients with thyroid and lymph nodal disease to cure the patient; however a thorough compartment-based lymph node dissection at surgery is still advisable to prevent local recurrence and attendant functional compromise (Fig. 12.3).

The role of local external beam radiation therapy (EBRT) is to reduce the risk of local recurrence in the neck in the presence of gross residual disease, extrathyroidal invasion and extensive lymph nodal involvement; it does not improve overall survival as noted in the evaluation of the SEER data on use of EBRT in MTC with lymph nodal disease [29].

Systemic treatment should be considered for symptomatic individuals or those with documented significant disease progression (imaging detected progression or calcitonin/CEA doubling time <6 months). Systemic cytotoxic chemotherapy has been associated with low response rates and has reducing relevance; in the absence of more effective therapy, doxorubicin either alone or in combination with 5FU or dacarbazine is the most effective [30, 31]. Isotope ablation techniques using 131I-MIBG or 90Yttrium have been used with low response rates and are utilised in some centres.

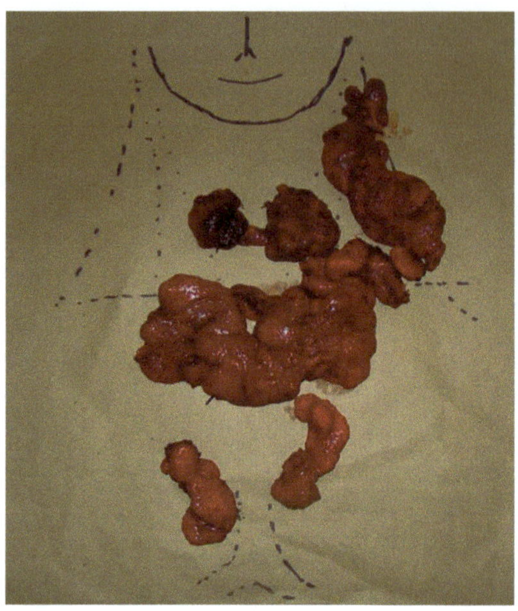

Fig. 12.3 Dissection specimen of locally advanced MTC showing multifocal thyroid primary with multiple central, lateral and mediastinal lymph nodes

Tyrosine kinase inhibitors more recently represent a relevant therapeutic option for treatment of locally advanced or metastatic disease. Currently vandetanib and cabozantinib have FDA approval; additionally other inhibitors like sorafenib, sunitinib, motesanib and axitinib may be considered according to availability and affordability in the local context. These drugs have been shown to increase progression-free survival compared to placebo; however with time the disease becomes resistant; combination therapeutic strategy using TKI drugs against RET and VEGFR targets offers some hope, but metastatic MTC remains a challenging clinical situation and research into new modalities of therapy is required.

Selected metastatic tumours may be treated by surgery, local radiotherapy, radiofrequency ablation and chemoembolisation to control disease progression or to improve the patient's quality of life. Bone lesions when localised and symptomatic can be managed by ablative strategies including surgical resection, palliative focal radiotherapy and intravenous bisphosphonate therapy. Liver metastasis may be treated by surgical resection if focal; radiofrequency ablation or chemoembolisation can be used for multiple lesions.

Diarrhoea is caused by the hyper-secretory and increased motility effects of advanced tumour and hepatic metastasis and can be managed initially with anti-motility agents like loperamide adding somatostatin analogues if required though of doubtful benefit; chemoembolisation of hepatic metastases has been shown to reduce diarrheal symptoms. Cytoreductive surgery may be considered in selected cases of metastatic disease for management of symptoms.

Post-operative Care and Follow-Up

After thyroidectomy, replacement dose of levothyroxine (1.6 mcg/kg ideal body weight in adults, 10–15 mcg/kg in infants and 2–3 mcg/kg in children) should be started [32]. There is no need to suppress TSH as the tumour doesn't arise from the follicular cells and is unresponsive to TSH. Even radioactive iodine doesn't have any role as an adjunct to surgery in the management of MTC [33]. Serum calcium, albumin, phosphorus and parathormone should be measured post-operatively and hypocalcaemia should be corrected with calcium and vitamin D supplements.

Patients in whom serum calcitonin level is below 150 pg/mL should only have a physical examination and ultrasound of the neck; those with values above 150 pg/mL will need regional and systemic assessment for evaluation of metastasis, including USG of the neck, neck and thorax contrast-enhanced CT, contrast-enhanced MRI, and USG of liver, bone scintigraphy, MRI of the spine and pelvis, PET, FDG-PET/CT, and F-DOPA-PET CT [34, 35].

Newer Methods of Prognostication

Dynamic risk stratification—Although the TNM staging provides prognosis regarding mortality, it does not predict the likelihood of recurrence. The risk of recurrence is addressed by modifications of existing staging systems. Dynamic risk stratification was initially proposed for differentiated thyroid cancer risk assessment based on response to therapy and has been validated for medullary cancer using measurement of calcitonin and CEA [36].

Doubling time of serum calcitonin and CEA—Serum calcitonin and CEA should be measured 3 months after surgery due to their prolonged half-life [37, 38]. If the post-operative serum calcitonin and CEA are normal or undetectable, they should be measured every 6 months for 1 year and then yearly thereafter. The measurement of serum levels of calcitonin and CEA at least 6 monthly in the first year will help us in calculating their doubling time for prognostication. Patients with doubling time less than 6 months have poorer prognosis compared to patients with doubling time greater than 24 months [39].

Results and Outcomes

Medullary cancer has been considered of 'intermediate' risk to life between the excellent prognosis of well-differentiated thyroid cancers and dismal outcomes of anaplastic thyroid cancers of follicular cell origin. Although medullary cancer accounts for less than 5% of thyroid cancer, it is responsible for 13% of cancer deaths. A recent study of the SEER database revealed that MTC-specific outcomes over the last three decades have been improving [40]. In the recent decade 2003–2012, the 5- and 10-year disease-specific survival rates for all medullary cancer were 89 and 81%; the disease-specific survival rates for local disease were 99 and 96%, for regional disease they were 91 and 77% and for distant disease the figures were 51% and 44%. The study also noted that the rate of performance of central node dissection at initial surgery had increased. It is likely that multiple factors of improved awareness, counselling, ultrasound detection, availability of expert surgical services and introduction of new targeted therapies will continue to improve outcomes.

Our experience: A review of patients with thyroid cancer managed between January 2008 and December 2016 from the electronic database identified 90 patients with MTC (4.45%) out of 2022 thyroid cancers. All pertinent data was collected and results analysed using STATA (v.10). The mean age of presentation was 40.08 years (range of 14–70) with a slight male preponderance (47 males and 43 females). The clinical presentation was goitre plus cervical lymph nodes seen in 59 patients (65.6%); goitre only in 24 patients (26.7%); pheochromocytoma in 3 patients (3.3%) and screen detected in 4 (4.4%). Systemic metastasis at presentation was seen in 11 patients (12.2%). FNAC was diagnostic in 40/71 (63.4%) while preoperative calcitonin was confirmed to be the best diagnostic test with elevated values in all 75 patients (100%) presenting with thyroid nodules when tested preoperatively. RET testing was performed in 71 patients and relatives at risk and was positive in 25 (35.2%). The mutations among these individuals were seen in the following codons: 634 (12), 804 (8), 790 (3) and 618 (2). Nineteen relatives at risk from the 11 index patients were screened and 12 were RET positive. There was a significant male preponderance noted among the sporadic MTC (M:F = 29:17) compared to a reverse female preponderance 8:17 among the hereditary patients ($p = 0.012$). All 90 patients underwent surgery as the primary modality of treatment. Prophylactic thyroidectomy was performed in three patients while the rest underwent total thyroidectomy with or without lateral neck dissection depending on the nodal status prior to operation. Persistent hypercalcitoninaemia (calcitonin >50 pg/mL) was observed in 62/80 (77.5%) patients. Metaiodobenzylguanidine (MIBG) scan in 40 patients was of limited value in patients with hypercalcitoninaemia, detecting residual disease in 10 (7 in the thyroid bed and 3 in metastatic sites). Recurrent cervical lymph nodes were detected in 18 patients on follow-up, 12 of whom required surgical intervention. The mean duration of follow-up was 32 months; follow-up data was lacking in ten patients. Metastatic disease was detected during follow-up in 16 patients and 8 patients expired. The mean overall survival was over 7 years at 85.75 months (78.7–92.7 95% CI).

Clinical Pearls

1. Suspect MTC in young or middle-aged patients presenting with thyroid nodules and lymph nodes.
2. Calcitonin, though not recommended for routine evaluation of thyroid nodules, should be checked with low threshold whenever there is clinical suspicion of MTC.
3. A complete thyroidectomy and systematic node dissection are the key therapeutic intervention.
4. RET test in all patients will detect hereditary MTC for best chance of cure.
5. The doubling time of calcitonin/CEA reveals more than one elevated value.
6. Think of tyrosine kinase inhibitors or ablative strategies when surgery is not feasible.
7. MTC is best managed by experienced multidisciplinary teams.

Guidelines: Several cancer networks and associations have frequently updated published guidelines for more detailed descriptions of decision-making in clinical situations and can be referred to by practicing clinicians. These are available online from the American Thyroid Association [41], National Comprehensive Cancer Network, European Society for Medical Oncology, British Thyroid Association, Brazilian Society of Endocrinology and Metabolism and the North American Network for Endocrine Tumours.

References

1. Hazard JB, Hawk WA, Crile G. Medullary (solid) carcinoma of the thyroid; a clinicopathologic entity. J Clin Endocrinol Metab. 1959;19(1):152–61.
2. Abe K, Adachi I, Miyakawa S, Tanaka M, Yamaguchi K, Tanaka N, et al. Production of calcitonin, adrenocorticotropic hormone, and beta-melanocyte-stimulating hormone in tumors derived from amine precursor uptake and decarboxylation cells. Cancer Res. 1977;37(11):4190–4.
3. Ishikawa N, Hamada S. Association of medullary carcinoma of the thyroid with carcinoembryonic antigen. Br J Cancer. 1976;34(2):111–5.
4. Cancer of the Thyroid Invasive: Trends in SEER Incidence and U.S. Mortality Using the Joinpoint

Regression Program, 1975–2011(SEER) Stat version 8.1.2 Rate Session. Access the SEER 18 database at www.seer.cancer.gov.
5. Pasini B, Hofstra RM, Yin L, Bocciardi R, Santamaria G, Grootscholten PM, et al. The physical map of the human RET proto-oncogene. Oncogene. 1995;11(9):1737–43.
6. Nakamura T, Ishizaka Y, Nagao M, Hara M, Ishikawa T. Expression of the ret proto-oncogene product in human normal and neoplastic tissues of neural crest origin. J Pathol. 1994;172(3):255–60.
7. Donis-Keller H, Dou S, Chi D, Carlson KM, Toshima K, Lairmore TC, et al. Mutations in the RET proto-oncogene are associated with MEN 2A and FMTC. Hum Mol Genet. 1993;2(7):851–6.
8. Hofstra RM, Landsvater RM, Ceccherini I, Stulp RP, Stelwagen T, Luo Y, et al. A mutation in the RET proto-oncogene associated with multiple endocrine neoplasia type 2B and sporadic medullary thyroid carcinoma. Nature. 1994;367(6461):375–6.
9. Marsh DJ, Learoyd DL, Andrew SD, Krishnan L, Pojer R, Richardson AL, et al. Somatic mutations in the RET proto-oncogene in sporadic medullary thyroid carcinoma. Clin Endocrinol (Oxf). 1996;44(3):249–57.
10. Wells SA, Asa SL, Dralle H, Elisei R, Evans DB, Gagel RF, et al. Revised American Thyroid Association guidelines for the management of medullary thyroid carcinoma. Thyroid. 2015;25(6):567–610.
11. Machens A, Dralle H. Genotype-phenotype based surgical concept of hereditary medullary thyroid carcinoma. World J Surg. 2007;31(5):957–68.
12. American Thyroid Association (ATA) Guidelines Taskforce on Thyroid Nodules and Differentiated Thyroid Cancer, Cooper DS, Doherty GM, Haugen BR, Hauger BR, Kloos RT, et al. Revised American Thyroid Association management guidelines for patients with thyroid nodules and differentiated thyroid cancer. Thyroid. 2009;19(11):1167–214.
13. Leboulleux S, Travagli JP, Caillou B, Laplanche A, Bidart JM, Schlumberger M, et al. Medullary thyroid carcinoma as part of a multiple endocrine neoplasia type 2B syndrome: influence of the stage on the clinical course. Cancer. 2002;94(1):44–50.
14. Saad MF, Ordonez NG, Rashid RK, Guido JJ, Hill CS, Hickey RC, et al. Medullary carcinoma of the thyroid. A study of the clinical features and prognostic factors in 161 patients. Medicine (Baltimore). 1984;63(6):319–42.
15. Kebebew E, Ituarte PH, Siperstein AE, Duh QY, Clark OH. Medullary thyroid carcinoma: clinical characteristics, treatment, prognostic factors, and a comparison of staging systems. Cancer. 2000;88(5):1139–48.
16. Bugalho MJM, Santos JR, Sobrinho L. Preoperative diagnosis of medullary thyroid carcinoma: fine needle aspiration cytology as compared with serum calcitonin measurement. J Surg Oncol. 2005;91(1):56–60.
17. Bhanot P, Yang J, Schnadig VJ, Logroño R. Role of FNA cytology and immunochemistry in the diagnosis and management of medullary thyroid carcinoma: report of six cases and review of the literature. Diagn Cytopathol. 2007;35(5):285–92.
18. Forrest CH, Frost FA, de Boer WB, Spagnolo DV, Whitaker D, Sterrett BF. Medullary carcinoma of the thyroid: accuracy of diagnosis of fine-needle aspiration cytology. Cancer. 1998;84(5):295–302.
19. Green I, Ali SZ, Allen EA, Zakowski MF. A spectrum of cytomorphologic variations in medullary thyroid carcinoma. Fine-needle aspiration findings in 19 cases. Cancer. 1997;81(1):40–4.
20. Mian C, Perrino M, Colombo C, Cavedon E, Pennelli G, Ferrero S, et al. Refining calcium test for the diagnosis of medullary thyroid cancer: cutoffs, procedures, and safety. J Clin Endocrinol Metab. 2014;99(5):1656–64.
21. Gorman B, Charboneau JW, James EM, Reading CC, Wold LE, Grant CS, et al. Medullary thyroid carcinoma: role of high-resolution US. Radiology. 1987;162(1 Pt 1):147–50.
22. Kim S-H, Kim B-S, Jung S-L, Lee J-W, Yang P-S, Kang B-J, et al. Ultrasonographic findings of medullary thyroid carcinoma: a comparison with papillary thyroid carcinoma. Korean J Radiol. 2009;10(2):101–5.
23. Machens A, Hauptmann S, Dralle H. Prediction of lateral lymph node metastases in medullary thyroid cancer. Br J Surg. 2008;95(5):586–91.
24. Machens A, Hauptmann S, Dralle H. Increased risk of lymph node metastasis in multifocal hereditary and sporadic medullary thyroid cancer. World J Surg. 2007;31(10):1960–5.
25. Weber T, Schilling T, Frank-Raue K, Colombo-Benkmann M, Hinz U, Ziegler R, et al. Impact of modified radical neck dissection on biochemical cure in medullary thyroid carcinomas. Surgery. 2001;130(6):1044–9.
26. Miyauchi A, Matsuzuka F, Hirai K, Yokozawa T, Kobayashi K, Ito Y, et al. Prospective trial of unilateral surgery for nonhereditary medullary thyroid carcinoma in patients without germline RET mutations. World J Surg. 2002;26(8):1023–8.
27. Gimm O, Ukkat J, Dralle H. Determinative factors of biochemical cure after primary and reoperative surgery for sporadic medullary thyroid carcinoma. World J Surg. 1998;22(6):562–567-568.
28. Dralle H, Damm I, Scheumann GF, Kotzerke J, Kupsch E, Geerlings H, et al. Compartment-oriented microdissection of regional lymph nodes in medullary thyroid carcinoma. Surg Today. 1994;24(2):112–21.
29. Martinez SR, Beal SH, Chen A, Chen SL, Schneider PD. Adjuvant external beam radiation for medullary thyroid carcinoma. J Surg Oncol. 2010;102(2):175–8.
30. Lorenz K, Brauckhoff M, Behrmann C, Sekulla C, Ukkat J, Brauckhoff K, et al. Selective arterial chemoembolization for hepatic metastases from medullary thyroid carcinoma. Surgery. 2005;138(6):986–93. discussion 993
31. Wertenbroek MWJLAE, Links TP, Prins TR, Plukker JTM, van der Jagt EJ, de Jong KP. Radiofrequency ablation of hepatic metastases from thyroid carcinoma. Thyroid. 2008;18(10):1105–10.

32. Fish LH, Schwartz HL, Cavanaugh J, Steffes MW, Bantle JP, Oppenheimer JH. Replacement dose, metabolism, and bioavailability of levothyroxine in the treatment of hypothyroidism. Role of triiodothyronine in pituitary feedback in humans. N Engl J Med. 1987;316(13):764–70.
33. Saad MF, Guido JJ, Samaan NA. Radioactive iodine in the treatment of medullary carcinoma of the thyroid. J Clin Endocrinol Metab. 1983;57(1):124–8.
34. Ong SC, Schöder H, Patel SG, Tabangay-Lim IM, Doddamane I, Gönen M, et al. Diagnostic accuracy of 18F-FDG PET in restaging patients with medullary thyroid carcinoma and elevated calcitonin levels. J Nucl Med. 2007;48(4):501–7.
35. Giraudet AL, Vanel D, Leboulleux S, Aupérin A, Dromain C, Chami L, et al. Imaging medullary thyroid carcinoma with persistent elevated calcitonin levels. J Clin Endocrinol Metab. 2007;92(11):4185–90.
36. Tuttle RM, Ganly I. Riskstratification in medullary thyroid cancer: moving beyond static anatomic staging. Oral Oncol. 2013;49:695–701.
37. Ismailov SI, Piulatova NR. Postoperative calcitonin study in medullary thyroid carcinoma. Endocr Relat Cancer. 2004;11(2):357–63.
38. Elisei R, Pinchera A. Advances in the follow-up of differentiated or medullary thyroid cancer. Nat Rev Endocrinol. 2012;8(8):466–75.
39. Barbet J, Campion L, Kraeber-Bodéré F, Chatal J-F, GTE Study Group. Prognostic impact of serum calcitonin and carcinoembryonic antigen doubling-times in patients with medullary thyroid carcinoma. J Clin Endocrinol Metab. 2005;90(11):6077–84.
40. Randle RW, Balentine CJ, Leverson GE, Havlena JA, Sippel RS, Schneider DF, Pitt SC. Trends in the presentation, treatment, and survival of patients with medullary thyroid cancer over the past 30 years. Surgery. 2017;161(1):137–46.
41. American Thyroid Association Guidelines Task Force, Kloos RT, Eng C, Evans DB, Francis GL, Gagel RF, et al. Medullary thyroid cancer: management guidelines of the American Thyroid Association. Thyroid. 2009;19(6):565–612.

13 Anaplastic Thyroid Carcinoma

Anish Jacob Cherian and Deepak Abraham

Introduction

Thyroid cancers constitute a varied spectrum of presentation and prognosis. The most common form of thyroid cancer is the well-differentiated thyroid cancers (WDTC) accounting for approximately 80–90%. WDTC generally have an excellent prognosis with multimodality treatment comprising surgery, radioiodine ablation and thyrotropin suppression. On the other end of this spectrum lies the anaplastic thyroid carcinoma (ATC). These are thankfully rare cancers which remain one of the most fatal human cancers. The best modality of treatment for any thyroid cancer is surgical resection, but in ATC upfront surgery is rarely feasible due to rapid local tumour invasion. Majority of patients with ATC succumb to their disease within 6 months to a year as a result of local invasion to the airway or widespread metastasis. Other modalities of treatment such as external radiation and chemotherapy alone have shown poor outcomes. Therefore, the focus of the management of ATC has shifted to understanding the genetic and molecular pathogenesis of these cancers in order to facilitate targeted therapy that may result in improved outcomes for these patients.

A. J. Cherian · D. Abraham (✉)
Department of Endocrine Surgery, Christian Medical College and Hospital, Vellore, Tamil Nadu, India

Epidemiology

The global prevalence of ATC ranges from 1.3 to 9.8% (median—3.6%). In the United States it accounts for less than 2% of all thyroid cancers [1, 2]. The age-adjusted annual incidence is about one to two per million persons per year [3]. A higher incidence of ATC is reported in areas with endemic goitres [4]. Though the incidence of WDTC is on the rise world over, the incidence of ATC has decreased in several countries. Postulated theories for this decrease include increased dietary iodine and better management of WDTC [1, 2, 5–8]. ATC is primarily a disease of the elderly with a median age of presentation at the sixth to seventh decades. Females are more commonly affected than males, 50–70% of affected individuals being females [3, 9–13].

Aetio-Pathogenesis

Where does ATC arise from—de novo or from a pre-existing WDTC? This is an area of controversy. There are reports of WDTC in the background of ATC in histological specimens. It has been suggested that if an extensive sampling is performed, foci of WDTC are eventually found in every ATC specimen. Further evidence from literature shows that up to 80% of ATC arise in goitres of long duration [2, 12]. These facts suggest the possibility of post-malignant

R. Parameswaran, A. Agarwal (eds.), *Evidence-Based Endocrine Surgery*,
https://doi.org/10.1007/978-981-10-1124-5_13

dedifferentiation from WDTC to ATC. On the contrary whole-genomic studies have shown that the chromosomal asset of ATC and WDTC is widely different supporting the hypothesis that some ATC may originate de novo [12]. Hence ATC may arise through both pathways—dedifferentiation from WDTC or de novo.

A number of molecular events have been described in thyroid carcinogenesis and tumour progression. The primary events involve the mitogen-activated kinase (MAPK) signalling pathway and the phosphoinositide-3 kinase PI3 K-Akt-mTor pathway (Fig. 13.1). Dedifferentiation is a dynamic process consisting of a series of mutational events which lead to the progressive accumulation of nuclear instability, derangement of the cell cycle and multiple signal transduction pathways finally resulting in uncontrolled ATC cellular proliferation and genomic instability. Listed below are the factors involved in thyroid carcinogenesis and dedifferentiation [2, 9, 12, 14–17]:

1. RAS: RAS proteins are GTP-binding proteins that regulate cell growth via MAPK and PI3K pathways. Mutation in RAS although significant in diagnosis of follicular carcinoma of the thyroid is seen in up to 60% of ATC. Mutation in RAS results in chromosomal instability which predisposes the cell to genetic and molecular derangements which in turn initiate the dedifferentiation process. Ras mutations have also been found to be important in tumour progression.
2. BRAF: A member of the RAF serine/threonine kinase family. It is a downstream effector of RAS. BRAF mutations activate serine/threonine kinase and have been shown to impede NIS (sodium/iodide symporter) gene expression and NIS membrane localisation, hence promoting dedifferentiation. BRAF is responsible for promoting migration and invasive growth through the activation of MAPK pathway. They do not respond to the negative feedback from ERK. In addition, $BRAF^{V600E}$ mutation increases the expression of vascular endothelial growth factor (VEGF) and hypoxia-inducible factor alpha. Mutations in BRAF are found in up to 35% of ATC.
3. HDAC: This acts as a link between BRAF mutation and NIS silencing. BRAF mutation

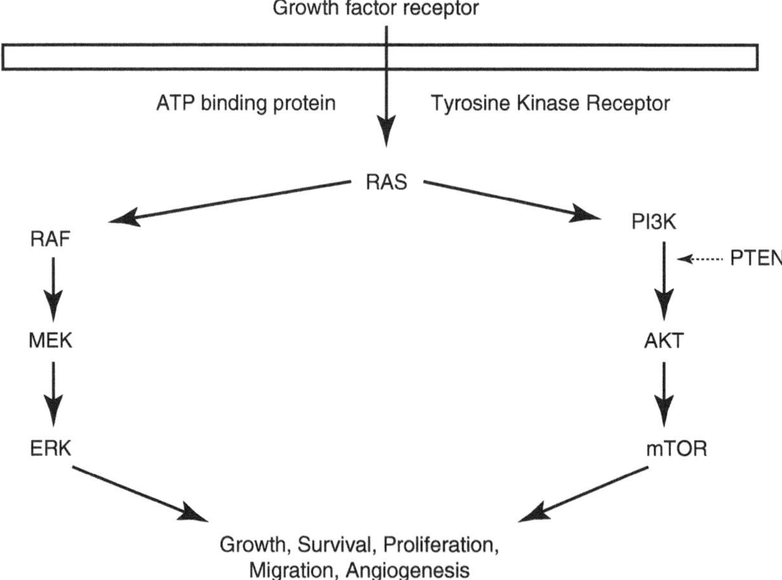

Fig. 13.1 Depicting the mitogen-activated kinase (MAPK) signalling pathway and the phosphoinositide-3 kinase PI3 K-Akt-mTor pathway

upregulates HDAC causing an epigenetic modification via constitution histone acetylation at the NIS promoter site.

4. RET/PTC: This is a chimeric oncogene between RET located on chromosome 10 and the promoter of an unrelated gene resulting in activation of the RET gene. RET/PTC 3 rearrangements found in PTC also have dedifferentiation potential.
5. PIK3CA: This pathway is frequently activated in thyroid carcinomas. Mutation in PIK3CA functions as an oncogene and is believed to play a role in thyroid cancer progression. They promote progression of thyroid adenomas to follicular carcinoma and ATC. These mutations have been detected in more than 50% of ATC.
6. NOTCH 1: This regulates cell proliferation, migration, adhesion and differentiation via transcription regulation. Depending on the cell type Notch can function either as an oncogene or a tumour-suppressor gene. Expression of Notch is decreased in ATC.
7. HES 1: This acts as a downstream effector of Notch 1 and plays a central role in thyrocyte proliferation and differentiation.
8. NF-KB: This belongs to the family of transcription factors that is held inactive in the cytoplasm of resting cells including thyroid cells. They significantly contribute to the establishment and maintenance of pro-tumorigenic microenvironment. Many NFKB target genes are pro-survival genes critical for intrinsic cancer cell resistance to chemotherapy and radiation.
9. Telomerase reverse transcriptase (TERT): It is the catalytic subunit of telomerase, the enzyme responsible for maintaining the length at the end of the chromosome. Two mutations have been reported—C228T and C250T. TERT mutations have been frequently found along with $BRAF^{V600E}$. They were prevalent in aggressive, dedifferentiated thyroid carcinomas. Mutation in TERT causes lengthening of telomerase which helps thyroid cancer cells evade apoptosis and promote cell proliferation through dysfunctional ERK1/2-MEK1/2 signalling. These mutations are seen in up to 50% of ATC.
10. CTNNB1: Dysadhesion is a major feature of aggressive thyroid carcinomas. ß-Catenin is involved in cell adhesion by forming cell membrane complexes with E-cadherin and in signal transduction through the Wnt pathway which activates cell cycle progression genes. Mutations in CTNNB1 gene alter β-catenin phosphorylation sites and prevent its degradation leading to Wnt signalling activation. Decreased membrane β-catenin leads to progressive loss of tumour differentiation. Mutations in CTNNB1 gene have been reported in 25–60% of ATC.
11. PTEN: This is a tumour-suppressor gene. Inactivation of PTEN leads to over-activation of the PI3K-AKT pathway. They occur in 10–20% of ATC.
12. P53: This gene is strongly involved in ATC pathogenesis being identified in up to 80% of ATC. These are also tumour-suppressor genes. Mutations in P53 cause inactivation of apoptosis and cell cycle progression.
13. Anaplastic lymphoma kinase (ALK): A protein involved in the activation of ERK1/2-MEK1/2 and PI3K-AKT pathways. Mutation of this protein results in increased tyrosine kinase activity and over-activation of the above pathways. Mutation of ALK is seen in 11% of ATC.
14. Chromosomal aberrations: A number of mitotic proteins involved in cell cycle checkpoints or engaged in chromosomal assembly and segregation have been shown to be deranged in ATC. One such family is the Aurora kinase family. Aurora kinases are implicated in several aspects of chromosome segregation and cytokinesis. Overexpression of Aurora A has been shown to induce centrosome amplification and to potentiate the oncologic function of RAS.

Pathology/Histological Subtypes

Anaplastic thyroid carcinoma on gross examination is composed of a white, fleshy tumour with extensive areas of necrosis and haemorrhage. These tumours are markedly invasive with a high proliferative index [18, 19]. Microscopically they are composed of anaplastic cells with marked cytological atypia and high mitotic activity (Fig. 13.2a, b). There are five known variants of anaplastic thyroid carcinoma; these include [1, 13, 18, 20–23]:

1. Spindle variant—arranged in fascicles to resemble a sarcoma
2. Pleomorphic giant cell variant—large, pleomorphic giant cells resembling osteoclasts with cellular connective tissue septae
3. Squamoid variant—squamoid cells that are relatively undifferentiated but also appear epithelial with occasional focal keratinisation
4. Paucicellular variant
5. Rhabdoid variant

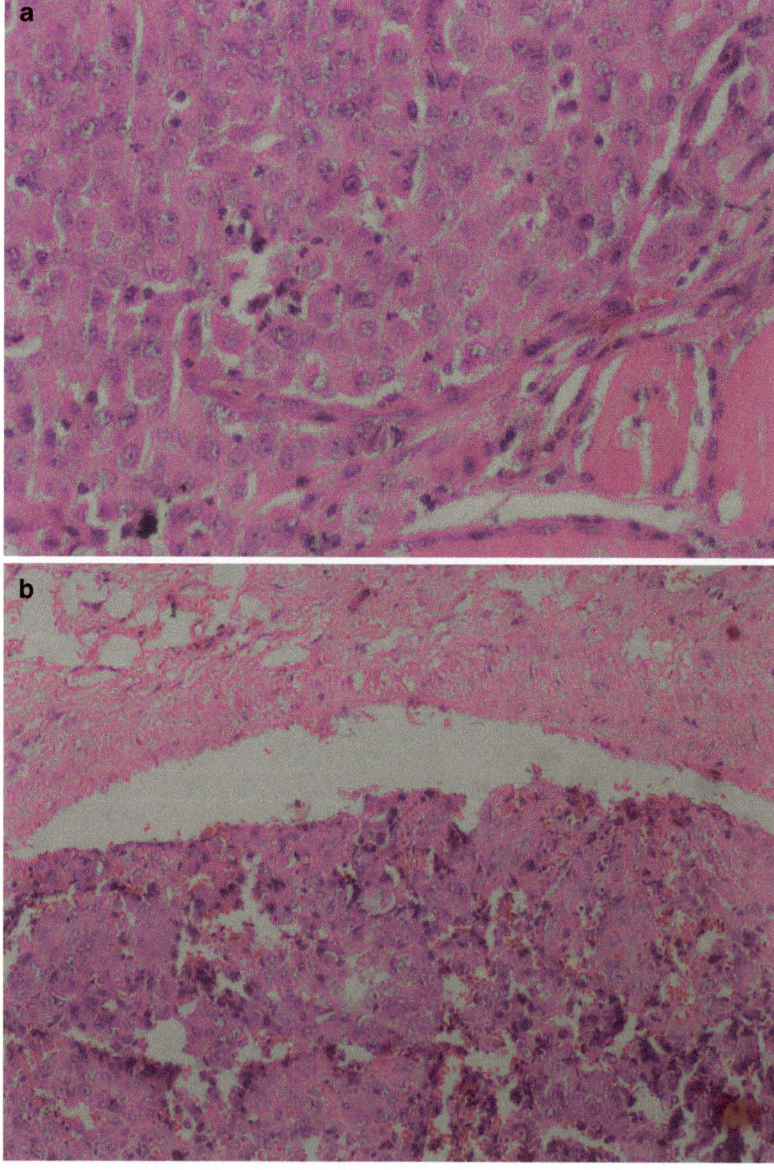

Fig. 13.2 (**a**) Depicting a microscopic picture of ATC: Polygonal tumour cells with vesicular nuclei admixed with neutrophils infiltrating normal thyroid tissue. (**b**) Depicting a tumour in a large-calibre vein

The spindle variant, pleomorphic giant cell variant and squamoid variant are the more common variants seen while the latter two variants are rare. The tumour may be comprised of one of these variants or the tumour may have a mixture of two or more variants. There is no known prognostic significance based on the variants with the exception of paucicellular variant which in some studies was found to affect younger patients and have a more indolent course [22]. Immunohistochemistry can help in differentiating these tumours from other neoplasms. Majority of these tumours are TTF1 and thyroglobulin negative and PAX 8 positive. The prognosis of anaplastic carcinoma may vary depending on the proportion of tumour that is comprised of the anaplastic component.

Clinical Presentation

Anaplastic thyroid carcinoma is a disease of the elderly. The most common mode of presentation is a rapidly enlarging firm to hard fixed neck mass in an elderly person [24–27]. Majority of patients have local invasion of the tumour into the surrounding tissues such as strap muscles, trachea, oesophagus, larynx and prevertebral muscles at presentation and experience pressure symptoms due to this invasion [4]. These pressure symptoms include neck pain, dysphagia, dry cough, voice change and stridor. There may be a history of pre-existing long-standing goitre [28]. Regional lymph node metastasis is seen in up to 40% of patients, while systemic metastasis is seen in 50–60% at presentation [6, 24–26, 29–34]. The most common site of distant metastasis is the lung (80%) followed by bone (5–15%) and brain (5–10%) [5, 6, 35, 36]. Hence patients may also present with symptoms of metastatic disease which include breathlessness on exertion, haemoptysis, bone pain, headache or seizures. Very rarely (<10%) ATC is detected following thyroidectomy as a histologic surprise or with the tumour confined to the thyroid gland.

Investigations

The characteristic mode of presentation generally raises the suspicion of anaplastic thyroid carcinoma. The differential diagnosis to be considered includes the following:

1. Thyroid lymphoma
2. Poorly differentiated thyroid carcinoma
3. Well-differentiated thyroid carcinoma

The investigations in this setting are performed to answer three questions:

1. To confirm the diagnosis
2. To assess the local extent of disease (operability)
3. To look for the presence of systemic metastasis

Fine-needle aspiration cytology (FNAC) is accurate in 90% of cases to diagnose ATC [18, 37]. In situations where FNAC is inconclusive, a core-needle biopsy may be performed to establish the diagnosis. Since lymphoma of the thyroid mimics the presentation of ATC it may be prudent to perform a core biopsy upfront for diagnosis, which is the practice at our institution. Cross-sectional imaging of the neck and thorax in the form of contrast-enhanced computerised tomography (CECT) or magnetic resonance imaging (MRI) is required to assess the local extent of the disease and for the evaluation of operability. Positron emission tomography (PET) scans with concomitant CT scan may be utilised to detect local extent of the tumour as well as systemic metastasis. ATC have a high expression of the glucose transporter Glut-1 and are hence fluorodeoxy-glucose (FDG) avid. Therefore, they are seen on PET scans which may also detect systemic metastasis if present. Hence the additional benefit of performing a PET scan is to differentiate if the metastasis if present is from ATC or from a well-differentiated thyroid carcinoma [38–40].

Staging

Staging of ATC follows the American Joint Committee on Cancer (AJCC) Tumour, Node and Metastasis (TNM) system [1]. All patients presenting with ATC have been classified as stage IV by the AJCC. This stage has been further subclassified based on the extent of disease as depicted in Table 13.1.

Table 13.1 Depicting the AJCC staging for ATC

Stage	T	N	M
IV (a)	Lesions are intra-thyroidal (T4a)	N0	M0
IV (b)	Primary tumour has gross extra-thyroidal extension (T4b)	Any N	M0
IV (c)	Any T	Any N	M1

Treatment

The behaviour of ATC warrants a multidisciplinary approach to its management. The personnel involved in the treatment would include a surgeon, endocrinologist, radiation oncologist, medical oncologist, palliative care physician, gastroenterologist, psychologist or psychiatrist, social worker and a clergy. Therefore, these patients should ideally be managed at a tertiary care centre that has multidisciplinary management teams in place.

Once the diagnosis is confirmed, the next step in the management of ATC is to evaluate for the local extent of the disease and the presence of systemic metastasis. CECT/MRI of the neck and thorax or a PET scan may be performed for the assessment of the same.

A multidisciplinary team meeting along with the patient and relatives should be organised to discuss the options of treatment that can be offered and the expected outcomes and to formulate the goals of care. An algorithm for the management of patients with ATC is depicted in Fig. 13.3.

1. Disease limited to the thyroid (histological surprise):

   Rarely (2–6% cases) ATC is detected as an incidental finding on histopathological examination of a thyroidectomy specimen. These patients present with a goitre and FNAC suggestive of a well-differentiated thyroid carcinoma. They are associated with a better

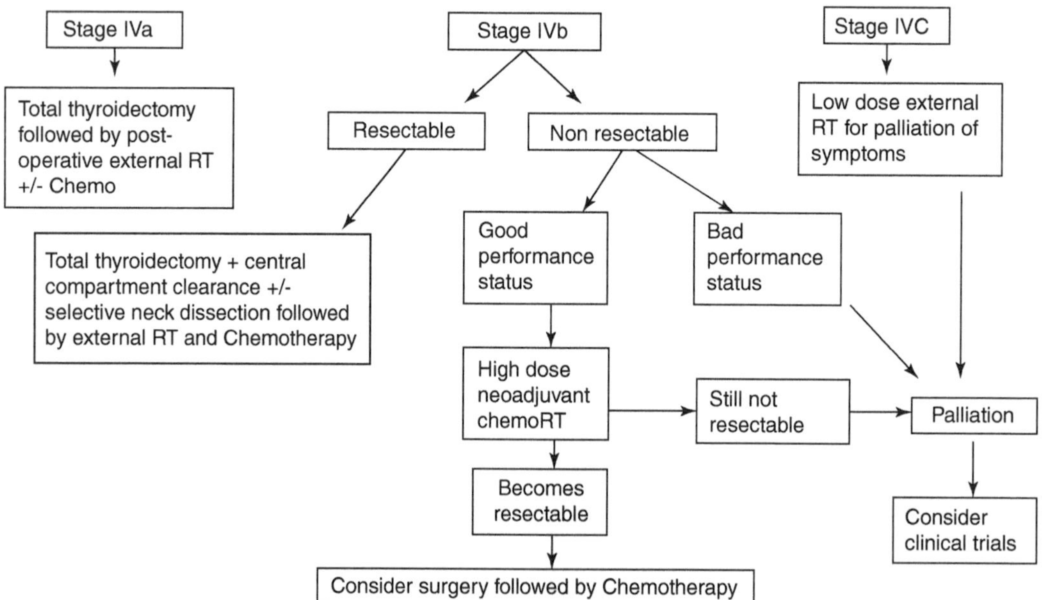

Fig. 13.3 Algorithm for the management of anaplastic thyroid carcinoma

prognosis. The role of completion thyroidectomy if initially only a hemithyroidectomy was performed is based on the characteristics of the non-anaplastic component. The role of adjuvant RT or chemo-RT is controversial though there are recent data to suggest possible improvement in survival from adjuvant chemo-RT in patients with ATC limited to the thyroid [1].

2. Loco-regional disease
   (a) Role of upfront surgery

   The aim of surgery in ATC is gross tumour resection that is R0 or R1 resection (total thyroidectomy with therapeutic cervical lymph node dissection) and not debulking surgery. R0/R1 resection has been shown to be associated with improved loco-regional control resulting in increased median survival [32, 41–45]. Thus, in T4a and b tumours, if curative resection is possible with minimum morbidity, surgery may be offered upfront. This must be followed by adjuvant combination chemo-RT.

   (b) Role of upfront combination chemo-RT

   Unfortunately, more than 80% of patients with ATC present with locally invasive tumours [1]. Assessment of the local extent with CECT/MRI reveals an inoperable disease in the majority. Radical surgery in this setting would result in increased morbidity and a poor quality of life with no survival benefit.

   Previous single-modality treatment regimens with conventional RT or single-agent chemotherapy have shown no improvement in loco-regional disease control or overall survival [46, 47]. In view of disappointing results of the same, multimodality regimes were evaluated.

   Chemotherapeutic agents commonly used in the management of ATC include doxorubicin, bleomycin, cisplatin, paclitaxel and gemcitabine. Doxorubicin was considered the agent of choice until recent studies have shown that combination chemotherapy is more effective [48–50]. Radiation therapy has evolved from high-dose conventional RT to hyperfractionated RT. ATC is a rapidly dividing tumour and hyperfractionated RT minimises the chance for tumour cells to recover between treatments. Hyperfractionated RT in combination with chemotherapy has been shown to increase the tumour response rate making surgery possible in a subset of patients. This results in improved local control and avoids death due to suffocation [47, 51–54]. Hence, in patients with inoperable stage IVb ATC with good performance status neoadjuvant combination chemo-RT may be offered. Patients with a complete or partial response following chemo-RT and in whom the tumour becomes operable may be offered surgery. The relapse rate following chemo-RT alone is high and surgery may decrease this risk of relapse. There is limited data on the improvement in overall and disease-free survival using this approach.

3. Systemic metastasis

   In the presence of systemic metastasis resection of loco-regional disease for palliation may be considered if there is impending airway or oesophageal obstruction. Low-dose external beam RT may be offered for palliation of pain. Patients who desire treatment may be enrolled in clinical trials.

Clinical Trials

Patients who are not candidates for surgery, have not responded to neoadjuvant combination chemo-RT or have metastatic disease may be enrolled in clinical trials. ATC may arise from a pre-existing WDTC or de novo; thus awareness and understanding of the factors involved in this transformation hold the key for potential treatment of this aggressive carcinoma in the years to come. Novel agents under study for treatment in ATC include multikinase inhibitors—gefitinib, sorafenib, axitinib, imatinib and combrestatin, mTOR inhibitors—everolimus, deacetylase inhibitor—panobinostat and valproic acid, and BRAF inhibitor PLX4720 [55].

Tracheostomy

Tracheostomy is associated with secretions that need frequent suctioning. It has its own associated morbidities and decreases the quality of life of the patient. In addition, patients with ATC who require a tracheotomy have a dismal prognosis; hence it is best avoided. On the other hand, it is a lifesaving procedure as it overcomes acute airway distress. This procedure should be reserved for patients in severe airway distress who seek intervention to avoid asphyxia [1].

Allow Natural Death

Patients with ATC usually present at an advanced stage. Despite all modalities of treatment currently available their prognosis is dismal. End-of-life preferences need to be discussed with the patient and relatives regarding intubation, nutrition supplementation, placement of feeding tubes, intravenous access and tracheostomy. Patients who request a limited aggressive care should be counselled regarding allow natural death (AND)—a term that is replacing do not resuscitate (DNR) [1].

Palliative and Hospice Care

Palliative care focuses on pain and symptom management at any time during the patient's treatment whereas hospice care focuses on symptom management for patients who are no longer receiving life-prolonging treatment. Palliative care may be offered to patients undergoing aggressive treatment for ATC and may be useful at any stage of the disease. On the other hand, hospice care is intended for patients who opt for AND as they should be provided dignity and quality of life for the remainder of their illness.

Prognosis

ATC is one of the most aggressive tumours with a grave prognosis. Factors that indicate a worse prognosis include male gender, age >60 years, tumour size >5 cm, extra-thyroidal extension and presence of distant metastasis [10, 33, 56–58]. The estimated median survival is less than 6 months with a 1-year survival witnessed in less than 20% of individuals.

Follow-Up

Being a rare cancer with a very aggressive behaviour, no guidelines for follow-up have been established. It would be prudent to keep these patients on close, short-term follow-up. Patients enrolled in clinical trial or those on chemo-RT would require a CECT/PET scan to assess the response to treatment on follow-up. The interval and intensity of follow-up would depend on the stage at diagnosis and assessment of response to initial therapy.

Conclusion

ATC is a rare form of thyroid carcinoma. It is suspected when an elderly person presents with a rapidly enlarging goitre which is hard in consistency and fixed. FNAC or a core biopsy will help in confirming the diagnosis and this should be followed with imaging to evaluate the local extent of the disease. These tumours are locally aggressive and patients generally have a dismal prognosis. Multimodality treatment regimens involving surgery, hyperfractionated RT and combination chemotherapy have shown to improve local disease control in selected patients. Novel targeted therapies currently being evaluated may provide an improved outcome for these patients in the future.

Personal Review

In our experience in managing 2261 patients with thyroid cancers from 2004 to 2016, 64 patients were diagnosed with anaplastic thyroid carcinoma (2.8%). The mean age of presentation was 61.3 years with 34.4% presenting in the sixth decade of life. The most common presenting symptom was a rapidly enlarging goitre (42.2%) followed by change in voice (31.3%) and stridor (18.8%). Among the 45 patients in whom cross-sectional imaging was performed, 28 (62.2%) had distant metastasis. Majority of patients (48.5%) received only palliation while the remaining patients were managed with surgery, chemotherapy, external beam radiation or tyrosine kinase inhibitors either as a single modality or in combination. Nineteen patients were contactable on follow-up and all had expired. Among them the mean duration of survival was 7.4 months.

Clinical Pearls

1. Suspect ATC in an elderly patient presenting with a rapidly enlarging, hard fixed goitre.
2. Consider a differential diagnosis of lymphoma thyroid and poorly differentiated thyroid carcinoma in this situation.
3. Expedite management:
   (a) Confirm diagnosis—core biopsy
   (b) Evaluate local extent of disease—CECT or PET scan
4. It is important to have a meeting with the immediate family members to explain treatment options, outcomes and formulate treatment goals (curative or palliative intent) upfront.
5. Tracheostomy is reserved for patients who are keen on aggressive treatment and who have severe airway distress to avoid asphyxia.

References

1. Smallridge RC, Ain KB, Asa SL, Bible KC, Brierley JD, Burman KD, et al. American Thyroid Association Guidelines for management of patients with anaplastic thyroid cancer. Thyroid. 2012;22(11):1104–39.
2. O'Neill JP, Shaha AR. Anaplastic thyroid cancer. Oral Oncol. 2013;49(7):702–6.
3. Nagaiah G, Hossain A, Mooney CJ, Parmentier J, Remick SC, Nagaiah G, et al. Anaplastic thyroid cancer: a review of epidemiology, pathogenesis, and treatment. J Oncol. 2011;2011:e542358.
4. Giuffrida D, Gharib H. Anaplastic thyroid carcinoma: current diagnosis and treatment. Ann Oncol. 2000;11(9):1083–9.
5. Tan RK, Finley RK, Driscoll D, Bakamjian V, Hicks WL, Shedd DP. Anaplastic carcinoma of the thyroid: a 24-year experience. Head Neck. 1995;17(1):41–47-48.
6. Ain KB. Anaplastic thyroid carcinoma: behavior, biology, and therapeutic approaches. Thyroid. 1998;8(8):715–26.
7. Demeter JG, De Jong SA, Lawrence AM, Paloyan E. Anaplastic thyroid carcinoma: risk factors and outcome. Surgery. 1991;110(6):956–61. 961-3
8. Bakiri F, Djemli FK, Mokrane LA, Djidel FK. The relative roles of endemic goiter and socioeconomic development status in the prognosis of thyroid carcinoma. Cancer. 1998;82(6):1146–53.
9. Keutgen XM, Sadowski SM, Kebebew E. Management of anaplastic thyroid cancer. Gland Surg. 2015;4(1):44–51.
10. Sun C, Li Q, Hu Z, He J, Li C, Li G, et al. Treatment and prognosis of anaplastic thyroid carcinoma: experience from a single institution in China. PLoS One. 2013;8(11):e80011.
11. Parenti R, Salvatorelli L, Magro G. Anaplastic thyroid carcinoma: current treatments and potential new therapeutic options with emphasis on TfR1/CD71. Int J Endocrinol. 2014;2014:685396.
12. Ragazzi M, Ciarrocchi A, Sancisi V, Gandolfi G, Bisagni A, Piana S. Update on anaplastic thyroid carcinoma: morphological, molecular, and genetic features of the most aggressive thyroid cancer. Int J Endocrinol. 2014;2014:790834.
13. Patel KN, Shaha AR. Poorly differentiated and anaplastic thyroid cancer. Cancer Control. 2006;13(2):119–28.
14. Papp S, Asa SL. When thyroid carcinoma goes bad: a morphological and molecular analysis. Head Neck Pathol. 2015;9(1):16–23.
15. Smith N, Nucera C. Personalized therapy in patients with anaplastic thyroid cancer: targeting genetic and epigenetic alterations. J Clin Endocrinol Metab. 2015;100(1):35–42.
16. Hsu K-T, Yu X-M, Audhya AW, Jaume JC, Lloyd RV, Miyamoto S, et al. Novel approaches in anaplastic thyroid cancer therapy. Oncologist. 2014;19(11):1148–55.
17. Viola D, Valerio L, Molinaro E, Agate L, Bottici V, Biagini A, et al. Treatment of advanced thyroid cancer with targeted therapies: ten years of experience. Endocr Relat Cancer. 2016;23(4):R185–205.
18. Are C, Shaha AR. Anaplastic thyroid carcinoma: biology, pathogenesis, prognostic factors, and treatment approaches. Ann Surg Oncol. 2006;13(4):453–64.
19. Basolo F, Pollina L, Fontanini G, Fiore L, Pacini F, Baldanzi A. Apoptosis and proliferation in thyroid carcinoma: correlation with bcl-2 and p53 protein expression. Br J Cancer. 1997;75(4):537–41.

20. Albores-Saavedra J, Sharma S. Poorly differentiated follicular thyroid carcinoma with rhabdoid phenotype: a clinicopathologic, immunohistochemical and electron microscopic study of two cases. Mod Pathol. 2001;14(2):98–104.
21. Lai ML, Faa G, Serra S, Senes G, Daniele GM, Boi F, et al. Rhabdoid tumor of the thyroid gland: a variant of anaplastic carcinoma. Arch Pathol Lab Med. 2005;129(3):e55–7.
22. Canos JC, Serrano A, Matias-Guiu X. Paucicellular variant of anaplastic thyroid carcinoma: report of two cases. Endocr Pathol. 2001;12(2):157–61.
23. Feng G, Laskin WB, Chou PM, Lin X. Anaplastic thyroid carcinoma with rhabdoid features. Diagn Cytopathol. 2015;43(5):416–20.
24. Nel CJ, van Heerden JA, Goellner JR, Gharib H, McConahey WM, Taylor WF, et al. Anaplastic carcinoma of the thyroid: a clinicopathologic study of 82 cases. Mayo Clin Proc. 1985;60(1):51–8.
25. Venkatesh YS, Ordonez NG, Schultz PN, Hickey RC, Goepfert H, Samaan NA. Anaplastic carcinoma of the thyroid. A clinicopathologic study of 121 cases. Cancer. 1990;66(2):321–30.
26. Hadar T, Mor C, Shvero J, Levy R, Segal K. Anaplastic carcinoma of the thyroid. Eur J Surg Oncol. 1993;19(6):511–6.
27. Ain KB. Anaplastic thyroid carcinoma: a therapeutic challenge. Semin Surg Oncol. 1999;16(1):64–9.
28. Aldinger KA, Samaan NA, Ibanez M, Hill CS. Anaplastic carcinoma of the thyroid: a review of 84 cases of spindle and giant cell carcinoma of the thyroid. Cancer. 1978;41(6):2267–75.
29. Biganzoli L, Gebbia V, Maiorino L, Caraci P, Iirillo A. Thyroid cancer: different outcomes to chemotherapy according to tumour histology. Eur J Cancer. 1995;31A(13–14):2423–4.
30. Lo CY, Lam KY, Wan KY. Anaplastic carcinoma of the thyroid. Am J Surg. 1999;177(4):337–9.
31. Passler C, Scheuba C, Prager G, Kaserer K, Flores JA, Vierhapper H, et al. Anaplastic (undifferentiated) thyroid carcinoma (ATC). Langenbeck's Arch Surg. 1999;384(3):284–93.
32. Pierie J-PEN, Muzikansky A, Gaz RD, Faquin WC, Ott MJ. The effect of surgery and radiotherapy on outcome of anaplastic thyroid carcinoma. Ann Surg Oncol. 2002;9(1):57–64.
33. Kebebew E, Greenspan FS, Clark OH, Woeber KA, McMillan A. Anaplastic thyroid carcinoma. Cancer. 2005;103(7):1330–5.
34. Agrawal S, Rao RS, Parikh DM, Parikh HK, Borges AM, Sampat MB. Histologic trends in thyroid cancer 1969-1993: a clinico-pathologic analysis of the relative proportion of anaplastic carcinoma of the thyroid. J Surg Oncol. 1996;63(4):251–5.
35. Besic N, Auersperg M, Us-Krasovec M, Golouh R, Frkovic-Grazio S, Vodnik A. Effect of primary treatment on survival in anaplastic thyroid carcinoma. Eur J Surg Oncol. 2001;27(3):260–4.
36. McIver B, Hay ID, Giuffrida DF, Dvorak CE, Grant CS, Thompson GB, et al. Anaplastic thyroid carcinoma: a 50-year experience at a single institution. Surgery. 2001;130(6):1028–34.
37. Lang BH-H, Lo C-Y. Surgical options in undifferentiated thyroid carcinoma. World J Surg. 2007;31(5):969–77.
38. Poisson T, Deandreis D, Leboulleux S, Bidault F, Bonniaud G, Baillot S, et al. 18F-fluorodeoxyglucose positron emission tomography and computed tomography in anaplastic thyroid cancer. Eur J Nucl Med Mol Imaging. 2010;37(12):2277–85.
39. Nguyen BD, Ram PC. PET/CT staging and posttherapeutic monitoring of anaplastic thyroid carcinoma. Clin Nucl Med. 2007;32(2):145–9.
40. Samih N, Hovsepian S, Notel F, Prorok M, Zattara-Cannoni H, Mathieu S, et al. The impact of N- and O-glycosylation on the functions of Glut-1 transporter in human thyroid anaplastic cells. Biochim Biophys Acta. 2003;1621(1):92–101.
41. Swaak-Kragten AT, de Wilt JHW, Schmitz PIM, Bontenbal M, Levendag PC. Multimodality treatment for anaplastic thyroid carcinoma—treatment outcome in 75 patients. Radiother Oncol. 2009;92(1):100–4.
42. Haigh PI, Ituarte PH, Wu HS, Treseler PA, Posner MD, Quivey JM, et al. Completely resected anaplastic thyroid carcinoma combined with adjuvant chemotherapy and irradiation is associated with prolonged survival. Cancer. 2001;91(12):2335–42.
43. Goutsouliak V, Hay JH. Anaplastic thyroid cancer in British Columbia 1985-1999: a population-based study. Clin Oncol (R Coll Radiol). 2005;17(2):75–8.
44. Brignardello E, Gallo M, Baldi I, Palestini N, Piovesan A, Grossi E, et al. Anaplastic thyroid carcinoma: clinical outcome of 30 consecutive patients referred to a single institution in the past 5 years. Eur J Endocrinol. 2007;156(4):425–30.
45. Kihara M, Miyauchi A, Yamauchi A, Yokomise H. Prognostic factors of anaplastic thyroid carcinoma. Surg Today. 2004;34(5):394–8.
46. Veness MJ, Porter GS, Morgan GJ. Anaplastic thyroid carcinoma: dismal outcome despite current treatment approach. ANZ J Surg. 2004;74(7):559–62.
47. Derbel O, Limem S, Ségura-Ferlay C, Lifante J-C, Carrie C, Peix J-L, et al. Results of combined treatment of anaplastic thyroid carcinoma (ATC). BMC Cancer. 2011;11(1):469.
48. De Besi P, Busnardo B, Toso S, Girelli ME, Nacamulli D, Simioni N, et al. Combined chemotherapy with bleomycin, adriamycin, and platinum in advanced thyroid cancer. J Endocrinol Investig. 1991;14(6):475–80.
49. Voigt W, Kegel T, Weiss M, Mueller T, Simon H, Schmoll HJ. Potential activity of paclitaxel, vinorelbine and gemcitabine in anaplastic thyroid carcinoma. J Cancer Res Clin Oncol. 2005;131(9):585–90.
50. Shimaoka K, Schoenfeld DA, DeWys WD, Creech RH, DeConti R. A randomized trial of doxorubicin versus doxorubicin plus cisplatin in patients with advanced thyroid carcinoma. Cancer. 1985;56(9):2155–60.
51. Segerhammar I, Larsson C, Nilsson I-L, Bäckdahl M, Höög A, Wallin G, et al. Anaplastic carcinoma of the

thyroid gland: treatment and outcome over 13 years at one institution. J Surg Oncol. 2012;106(8):981–6.
52. Tennvall J, Lundell G, Wahlberg P, Bergenfelz A, Grimelius L, Akerman M, et al. Anaplastic thyroid carcinoma: three protocols combining doxorubicin, hyperfractionated radiotherapy and surgery. Br J Cancer. 2002;86(12):1848–53.
53. Tennvall J, Lundell G, Hallquist A, Wahlberg P, Wallin G, Tibblin S. Combined doxorubicin, hyperfractionated radiotherapy, and surgery in anaplastic thyroid carcinoma. Report on two protocols. The Swedish Anaplastic Thyroid Cancer Group. Cancer. 1994;74(4):1348–54.
54. De Crevoisier R, Baudin E, Bachelot A, Leboulleux S, Travagli J-P, Caillou B, et al. Combined treatment of anaplastic thyroid carcinoma with surgery, chemotherapy, and hyperfractionated accelerated external radiotherapy. Int J Radiat Oncol Biol Phys. 2004;60(4):1137–43.
55. Denaro N, Nigro CL, Russi EG, Merlano MC. The role of chemotherapy and latest emerging target therapies in anaplastic thyroid cancer. Onco Targets Ther. 2013;9:1231–41.
56. Gilliland FD, Hunt WC, Morris DM, Key CR. Prognostic factors for thyroid carcinoma. A population-based study of 15,698 cases from the Surveillance, Epidemiology and End Results (SEER) program 1973–1991. Cancer. 1997;79(3):564–73.
57. Kim TY, Kim KW, Jung TS, Kim JM, Kim SW, Chung K-W, et al. Prognostic factors for Korean patients with anaplastic thyroid carcinoma. Head Neck. 2007;29(8):765–72.
58. Sugitani I, Kasai N, Fujimoto Y, Yanagisawa A. Prognostic factors and therapeutic strategy for anaplastic carcinoma of the thyroid. World J Surg. 2001;25(5):617–22.

14 Inherited Thyroid Cancer

Joycelyn Lee and Joanne Ngeow

Introduction

Thyroid cancer is common and has a steadily rising incidence [1]. Papillary thyroid cancer (PTC) is the most common histologic subtype, accounting for more than 90% of all thyroid cancers. Over 90% of thyroid cancers are sporadic, with less than 10% being familial [2]. Familial thyroid cancers can be divided into familial non-medullary thyroid cancers (FNMTC), or familial medullary thyroid cancers (FMTC) according to their cell of origin. Among FNMTC, about 5% are associated with defined syndromes and occur with a preponderance of non-thyroidal tumours [3] (see Diagram 14.1). The majority however are non-syndromic FNMTC. FMTC, on the other hand, is most commonly associated with multiple endocrine neoplasia (MEN). The presence of certain histological subtypes should also prompt consideration of familial thyroid cancer.

J. Lee
Cancer Genetics Service, Division of Medical Oncology, National Cancer Centre Singapore, Singapore, Singapore

J. Ngeow (✉)
Cancer Genetics Service, Division of Medical Oncology, National Cancer Centre Singapore, Singapore, Singapore

Lee Kong Chian School of Medicine, Nanyang Technological University, Singapore, Singapore
e-mail: joanne.ngeow.y.y@singhealth.com.sg

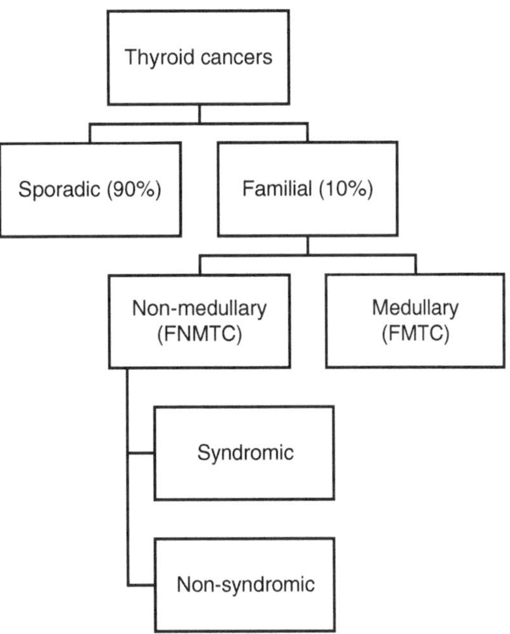

Diagram 14.1 Approach to familial thyroid cancers

Background/Aetiology

Recognising familial thyroid cancers is important as they generally tend to be more aggressive than sporadic thyroid cancers. Recognition also allows for the physician to screen the patient and his or her family members for the need for genetic counselling and testing, and allows for the implementation of surveillance and an opportunity for intervention. Several red flags that should draw the clinician's attention to the possibility of famil-

R. Parameswaran, A. Agarwal (eds.), *Evidence-Based Endocrine Surgery*,
https://doi.org/10.1007/978-981-10-1124-5_14

ial disease include the presence of a personal or family history of thyroid or other cancers, a diagnosis of thyroid cancer before the age of 45 years old, the presence of multifocal disease and aggressive disease with local invasion [4], and a diagnosis of specific histological subtypes, such as medullary thyroid cancer and cribriform-morular variant of papillary thyroid cancer.

Familial Non Medullary Thyroid Cancer (FNMTC)

Syndromic FNMTC

PTC is the most common histological subtype in both familial and non-familial non-medullary thyroid cancer. As previously mentioned, about 5% of FNMTC occur in defined syndromes. This includes Cowden syndrome, familial adenomatous polyposis, Gardner syndrome, Carney complex, Werner syndrome and DICER1 syndrome. Although uncommon, recognising syndromic FNMTC is important as their corresponding germline mutations are often highly penetrant and actionable. Recognition also allows for intervention in the form of counselling and organisation of necessary surveillance and screening for probands and their families.

Some of the more common syndromes associated with FNMTC are presented below, and summarised in Table 14.1.

Cowden Syndrome

Cowden syndrome (CS) is an autosomal dominant disorder characterised by the hamartomatous changes and epithelial tumours of multiple organs most commonly associated with germline inactivating mutations of the *PTEN* tumour-suppressor gene (TSG). It is part of the PTEN hamartoma tumour syndrome (PHTS), which also includes subsets of Bannayan-Riley-Ruvalcaba syndrome (BRRS), Proteus syndrome (PS) and Proteus-like syndrome [5]. PHTS is defined as the presence of a germline *PTEN* mutation irrespective of clinical syndrome. BRRS is characterised by macrocephaly, intestinal polyposis, lipomas and pigmented macules of the glans penis, while PS is highly variable and

Table 14.1 Summary of syndromic non-medullary thyroid cancers (adapted from Vriens et al. [49])

Syndrome	Associated germline mutations	Thyroid cancer subtype	Extrathyroidal clinical features
Cowden syndrome	*PTEN* mutation	Papillary thyroid cancer	Hamartomas
	SDHB-D mutation	Follicular thyroid cancer	Mucocutaneous lesions
	KLLN promoter methylation		Macrocephaly
Familial adenomatous polyposis	*APC* mutation	Papillary thyroid cancer, including cribriform-morular variant	Multiple adenomatous polyps of gastrointestinal tract, especially colon
Garder's syndrome			In Gardner syndrome, additional extra-colonic manifestations may be seen including osteomas, desmoid tumours, hypertrophic retinal pigment epithelium and supernumerary teeth
Carney complex	*PRKAR1A* mutation	Papillary thyroid cancer	Myxomas of soft tissues; skin and mucosal pigmentation, adrenal tumours
		Follicular thyroid cancer	
		Follicular adenoma	
Werner syndrome	*WRN* mutation	Follicular thyroid cancer	Premature ageing; scleroderma-like skin changes, cataracts, short stature, premature greying and/or hair thinning
		Papillary thyroid cancer	
		Anaplastic thyroid cancer	
DICER1 syndrome	*DICER1* mutation	Papillary thyroid cancer	Ovarian Sertoli-Leydig cell tumours, cystic nephroma
		Multinodular goitre	

involves congenital malformations and overgrowth of multiple tissues. Proteus-like syndrome describes individuals with clinical features of PS yet who do not meet its diagnostic criteria. The International Cowden Consortium criteria for the diagnosis of Cowden syndrome include pathognomonic, major and minor criteria (Table 14.2) [6]. Of note however, many of the clinical features associated with CS are also present and common in the general population, such as that of fibrocystic breast disease and uterine fibroids.

CS is a highly penetrant genetic disorder. More than 90% of individuals with *PTEN* mutations are believed to manifest some features of the syndrome (although rarely cancer) by age 20, and by age 30 nearly 100% of mutation carriers are believed to have developed at least some of the mucocutaneous signs. As many as 45% of patients with Cowden syndrome may be due to de novo *PTEN* mutations [7]. The Cleveland Clinic score is a risk predictor tool based on clinical manifestations, with a score of 10 or more associated with a pretest probability of 3%, and can be used to help decide who to refer to the geneticist for counselling and germline *PTEN* mutation testing [8].

Thyroid disease is the most common extracutaneous manifestation of Cowden syndrome, occurring in more than 50% of affected individuals, and may include both benign thyroid abnormalities and thyroid cancers [9], with an overrepresentation of follicular thyroid cancers, especially among those with *PTEN* germline mutations. Follicular adenomas are very common and often multiple in this syndrome. Individuals with Cowden syndrome have an approximately 70-fold increased risk of FNMTC compared to the general population, with most being multicentric and evolving from a pre-existing follicular adenoma. Most of these cancers belong to the papillary subtype, though follicular thyroid cancer is disproportionately common in patients with positive germline *PTEN* mutations [10] and the diagnosis of follicular thyroid carcinoma is a major criterion for the clinical diagnosis of the syndrome. The average age of thyroid cancer onset in Cowden syndrome is in the 30s–40s [10], though germline *PTEN* mutations are also associated with paediatric-onset thyroid cancers [11].

Children positive for germline *PTEN* mutations hence are recommended to undergo a baseline surveillance thyroid ultrasound from the age

Table 14.2 International Cowden Consortium operation criteria for the diagnosis of Cowden syndrome (revised 2000)

Pathognomonic criteria	Mucocutaneous lesion
	Facial trichilemmomas
	Acral keratosis
	Papillomatous lesions
	Mucosal lesions
Major criteria	Breast cancer
	Thyroid cancer, especially follicular thyroid cancer
	Macrocephaly (occipital-frontal circumference ≥97th percentile)
	Lhermitte-Duclos disease (presence of a cerebellar dysplastic gangliocytoma)
	Endometrial carcinoma
Minor criteria	Other thyroid lesions (e.g. goitre)
	Mental retardation (IQ ≤75)
	Hamartomatous intestinal polyps
	Fibrocystic disease of the breast
	Lipomas
	Fibromas
	Genitourinary tumours or genitourinary malformations
An operational diagnosis of Cowden syndrome is made if:	
An individual meets any of the following criteria	• Pathognomonic mucocutaneous lesions alone if there are – ≥6 facial papules, of which ≥3 are trichilemmomas – Cutaneous facial papules and oral mucosal papillomatosis – Oral mucosal papillomatosis and acral keratoses, or six or more palmo-plantar keratosis • Two or more major criteria of which one is either macrocephaly or Lhermitte-Duclos disease • One major and three minor criteria Four minor criteria
In the presence of a family member who meets diagnostic criteria for Cowden syndrome	• A pathognomonic mucocutaneous lesion • Any one major criterion with or without minor criteria • Two minor criteria

of 6. Patients negative for *PTEN* mutations, but who meet the clinical diagnostic criteria for Cowden syndrome, may be positive for other genetic abnormalities like *SDHB-D* variant genes [12] and *KILLIN* promoter methylation [13], both which are associated with late age of onset of manifestations. These patients hence are only recommended to start thyroid ultrasound surveillance from the age of 18 (or 5 years before earliest age of onset in a family member) [10]. Germline *PIK3CA* and *AKT1* mutations have also been implicated [14].

In addition to thyroid ultrasounds, CS patients should also have formal dermatologic and breast examinations in view of the other manifestations of CS.

Familial Adenomatous Polyposis and Gardner Syndrome

Familial adenomatous polyposis (FAP) is an autosomal dominant disorder due to inactivation mutations of the adenomatous polyposis colic (*APC*) tumour-suppressor gene on chromosome 5q21. The APC protein is part of the beta-catenin complex in the Wnt/beta-catenin pathway; mutations in APC lead to loss of the beta-catenin destruction complex, increasing nuclear translocation of beta-catenin and so increasing gene transcription and cellular proliferation [15].

FAP is characterised by the early presence of multiple colonic adenomatous polyps with malignant potential. Gardner syndrome is a variant of FAP in which patients develop colonic manifestations as well as osteomas and other soft-tissue lesions. Other extra-colonic manifestations in FAP and its variants include desmoid tumours, congenital hypertrophy of the retinal pigmented epithelium (CHRPE) and thyroid tumours. Penetrance is nearly complete for the colonic polyps but is variable for extra-colonic manifestations, and may be dependent to some extent on the specific *APC* mutation [16]. A genotype-phenotype correlation has been suggested as well for the thyroid manifestations with patients with mutations at the 5′ end proximal to codon 528 as well as in codon 1061 implicated at being at increased risk for thyroid cancer [16].

The risk of developing thyroid cancer in FAP patients is estimated to be around 2% [17], with most of them being papillary in histological subtype. Histologically, there is often a characteristic cribriform pattern with solid areas and a spindle cell component, with marked fibrosis [18]. The rare cribriform-morular histological variant is observed in <1% of all PTC cases, but is seen in 20–40% of FAP-associated thyroid cancers. This variant occurs most commonly in females aged under 30 [19, 20], with a female predominance ratio of as high as 10—17:1 [21], even higher than the typical 3—4:1 female-to-male ratio seen in sporadic PTC. In up to one-third of FAP cases, PTC may be the first clinical manifestation of FAP [22] and the diagnosis of a cribriform-morular patterned thyroid carcinoma, even in the absence of colonic manifestations, should prompt clinicians to screen the patient and family members for FAP. The cribriform-morular variant is generally associated with a better prognosis than other papillary thyroid carcinomas [23]. Most female patients with FAP and papillary thyroid cancer have an additional *RET/PTC* somatic mutation in addition to the *APC* germline mutation.

Yearly thyroid clinical examination and ultrasound are recommended for all patients with FAP [24].

Carney Complex

Carney complex is a rare autosomal dominant disease. It is characterised by mucocutaneous pigmentation in a typical distribution involving the lips, conjunctiva and genital mucosal area, in addition to a variety of non-endocrine and endocrine tumours [25] including that of primary pigmented nodular adrenocortical disease (PPNAD), growth hormone (GH)-producing adenoma and testicular tumours. It is associated with inactivating mutations or large deletions of the *PRKAR1A* tumour-suppressor gene with a high penetrance of >95% by age 50 years [26]. A patient is diagnosed with Carney complex if he or she has two major criteria or one major criterion and a first-degree relative with Carney complex or an inactivating *PRKAR1A* mutation. The *PRKAR1A* gene encodes for the type 1A regulatory subunit of protein kinase A (PKA).

In patients with Carney complex, the thyroid is usually multinodular with multiple adenomas appearing from early in life [27]. Both PTC and FTC can be present in up to 15% of patients [28]. Patients with a clinical phenotype of Carney complex can be tested for the presence of germline *PRKAR1A* mutation and should be screened for thyroid cancer.

Werner Syndrome

Werner syndrome is an autosomal recessive disease characterised by a phenotype of premature ageing with grey hair, scleroderma-like skin changes and bilateral cataracts, as well as other manifestations including diabetes mellitus, premature atherosclerosis and hypogonadism. It is caused by the inheritance of biallelic pathogenic variants in the *WRN* gene on chromosome 8p.

In the syndrome, there is an increased risk of both benign thyroid lesions and papillary thyroid cancers. Other histological subtypes of thyroid cancer, including the follicular subtype and the anaplastic subtype, are more commonly seen in the Asian population.

Patients with the clinical phenotype of Werner syndrome can be tested for the presence of germline *WRN* gene mutation and should be screened for thyroid cancer.

DICER1 Syndrome

The *DICER1* gene on chromosome 14q is involved in the regulation of miRNA and its mutation increases the risk of familial pleuropulmonary blastoma (FPB), cystic nephroma and ovarian Sertoli-Leydig cell tumours (SLCT) [29]. It has been associated with familial multinodular goitre and both somatic and germline mutations in the gene have been associated with differentiated thyroid cancer, the former usually in the setting of prior radiation or chemotherapy exposure for malignancy [30].

Overall though, the prevalence of thyroid cancer in DICER1 syndrome is low and evaluation should be clinically guided. The utility of ultrasound for surveillance is unknown.

Non-syndromic FNMTC

In the absence of syndromes, FNMTC is defined as the presence of non-medullary thyroid cancer in two or more first-degree relatives, in the absence of predisposing environmental factors. Non-syndromic FNMTC often displays a pattern of autosomal dominant inheritance with incomplete penetrance and variable expressivity. Although the exact causative genes have not been identified, linkage analyses have found at least two different chromosomal regions that may harbour putative susceptibility genes, namely the *forkhead box E1 (FOXE1)* gene at chromosome 9q, the *hyaluronan-binding protein 2 (HABP2)* gene located on chromosome 10q, the *SRGAP1* gene on chromosome 12q and the *TITF-1/NKX2.1* gene on 14q, of which only the first two have been validated by multiple study groups. The candidate genes at these loci however are as yet unknown and seem to account for only a minority of FNMTC. Hence, if no clinical signs of syndromic FNMTC are observed there is currently no need to proceed with germline genetic testing as the candidate genes for FNMTC are not yet well characterised.

The *FOXE1* gene encodes *FOXE1* transcription factor, or thyroid transcription factor 2 (*TTF-2*), and plays a role in the migration of thyroid precursor cells from the pharynx to the neck [31]. In a genome-wide association study (GWAS) of an Icelandic, Columbus and Spanish cohort, two single-nucleotide polymorphisms (SNP) were found to be associated with increased risk of PTC, namely rs965513 located on chromosome 9q near *FOXE1* and rs944289 on chromosome 14q near *NKX2-1* [32].

It is controversial whether patients with non-syndromic FNMTC tend to have more aggressive tumours compared to those with sporadic NMTC with some series reporting higher recurrence rates and lower disease-free survival, and others reporting no increase in disease aggressiveness. They are often diagnosed at a younger age, and have a higher incidence of multifocal tumours, extrathyroidal invasion, bilateral disease and lymph node metastases at presentation [33, 34]. The phenomenon of anticipation can also occur in FNMTC, with earlier age of disease onset and increased severity in successive generations [35].

In FNMTC, first-degree relative 10 years or older, including the generation anterior to the index case, should have thyroid ultrasound screening, which can result in earlier diagnosis with a lower rate of extrathyroidal invasion [36]. Total or near-total thyroidectomy, with a central neck lymph node dissection, is the recommended surgical treatment in these patients, to minimise residual tissue left behind and because of the high incidence of multicentric disease. A therapeutic lateral neck node dissection should also be performed if there is lymph node involvement preoperatively by imaging or clinical examination. High-dose radioiodine ablation with I-131 after thyroidectomy is also recommended. Despite the aggressive treatment approach used in most cases of FNMTC, up to 12% will have persistent disease after an operation and 44% will have recurrent disease requiring further operations [37]. The role of prophylactic thyroidectomy, unlike that practiced in FMTC, is controversial.

Familial Medullary Thyroid Carcinoma

The histopathological features of patients with familial medullary thyroid carcinoma (FMTC) are similar to those seen in sporadic medullary thyroid cancer, except that they tend to be bilateral and multiple. While medullary thyroid carcinoma represents only 10% of all thyroid cancers, an estimated 25% of medullary thyroid carcinomas (MTCs) occur in hereditary forms, as part of the MEN2 syndrome or as the MTC-only syndrome.

MEN2 syndrome consists of three variants, MEN2A, MEN 2B and FMTC (also known as inherited medullary carcinoma without associated endocrinopathies), with all three subtypes involving high risk of developing MTC.

Nearly all MEN2 syndromes (including MEN2A, MEN2B and FMTC) are caused by germline-activating mutations in the *RET* (*RE*-arranged during *T*ransfection) proto-oncogene, located on chromosome 10q, which are inherited as autosomal dominant traits with a high penetrance but variable expression. The *RET* proto-oncogene encodes for a transmembrane receptor of the tyrosine kinase family and is expressed in cells of the neural crest, branchial arches and urogenital origin. Somatic *RET* mutations are also implicated in up to 50% of sporadic MTCs [38], and interestingly chromosomal translocations causing RET activation also occur in 20–30% of patients with PTC [39]. In non-*RET*-mutated cases of FMTC, mutations in the *NTRK1* gene have also been implicated [40].

MEN2A is characterised by the triad of medullary thyroid carcinoma (MTC), phaeochromocytoma and parathyroid adenoma. In classical MEN2A, 95% of the *RET* germline mutations occur in codons 609, 611, 618 or 620 of exon 10, or codon 634 of exon 11 [41]. Almost all patients develop MTC, with variable frequencies of development of phaeochromocytomas and parathyroid adenomas depending on the specific *RET* mutation.

MEN2B patients share the same features as those with MEN2A, with additional neuroendocrine associations of mucosal ganglioneuromas and Marfanoid skeletal features. MTC in MEN2B often presents in infancy, is highly aggressive and metastasises early. Approximately 95% of patients have *RET* germline mutations in exon 16. Less than 5% have a *RET* germline mutation in exon 15 and these patients tend to have a less aggressive MTC.

The syndrome of FMTC is characterised by the presence of a *RET* germline mutation in families with medullary thyroid carcinoma alone without accompanying evidence of phaeochromocytoma or other tumours [42].

In addition, there are several histopathological findings that differentiate familial MTC from sporadic MTC [43], namely that FMTC tumours tend to be bilateral, multicentric and associated with neoplastic C-cell hyperplasia (CCH) and show early lymph node metastases. The presence of these features should prompt further family history taking and consideration for referral for clinical cancer genetics risk assessment.

Almost all patients with MEN IIB develop MTC, with a clinical course that is more aggressive than in MEN-IIA, and for MEN-IIB patients prophylactic thyroidectomy is often preferred in the first year of life. In contrast, the aggressiveness and age of onset of FMTC can vary depending on the specific type of *RET* mutation present [44]. For example, mutations in codons 918, 883 and 634 are associated with the highest penetrance and predispose to MEN 2B and 2A; on the contrary, germline V804 mutations have a lower penetrance and later age of onset [44]. This genotype-phenotype correlation means that different timing and extent of surgery may be recommended depending on the specific germline mutation identified, with the American Thyroid Association (ATA) having published codon-specific guidelines [45] (Table 14.3). In general though, prophylactic total thyroidectomy and central cervical lymph node dissection are recommended to most patients with a family history of MTC and who are RET positive by age 6, if there are thyroid nodules or the patient has a raised blood calcitonin level [46]. Children in the highest risk category, such as those with a *RET* codon M918T mutation, should have a thyroidectomy in the first month to first year of life.

Table 14.3 American Thyroid Association (ATA) risk level and timing of prophylactic thyroidectomy in MEN-IIA syndrome

ATA risk level	*RET* codon affected	Timing of prophylactic thyroidectomy
Level A	Codons 768, 790, 791, 804, 891	• Total thyr • Can consider delay operative resection if: – Normal annual serum calcitonin – Normal annual neck ultrasound (no lesions >5 mm and no concerning adenopathy) – Less aggressive family history – Family preference
Level B	Codons 609, 611, 618, 620, 630	
Level C	Codon 634	• Total thyroidectomy by age 5
Level D	Codons 883, 918 Tandem mutations (804–805, 804–806, 804–904)	• Total thyroidectomy with central compartment lymph node dissection, with sampling of level II–V by 6 months

Due to the relatively high incidence of familial disease in patients with MTC, all newly diagnosed patients and their first-degree relatives should be screened for the presence of a *RET* mutation. The diagnostic criteria for MEN 2A are the presence of MTC, phaeochromocytoma, hyperparathyroidism and a germline *RET* gene mutation. The mutation frequency is >98%; thus few families present a diagnostic dilemma when fewer than three clinical features are present. In cases in which only one or two clinical features are present, the diagnosis can be made either when a first-degree relative shows MEN 2A features or a *RET* mutation is identified. At a minimum, the diagnosis can be made when two clinical features are present, even when an autosomal dominant pattern is not evident and a *RET* mutation has not been demonstrated [45].

All MEN-II syndrome patients or *RET*-mutated patients should be screened annually for medullary thyroid cancer by basal or stimulated calcitonin. Screening for MTC coupled with early prophylactic thyroidectomy has been shown to confer survival benefit [47]. Patients diagnosed with MTC confined to the neck and cervical lymph nodes should have a total thyroidectomy with dissection of the central lymph node compartment and of any involved lateral neck compartments. In patients diagnosed with MTC after a hemithyroidectomy, a completion thyroidectomy is recommended for patients with hereditary MTC.

The risks and complication rates tend to be higher in children than adults when performing a thyroidectomy and surgery should be carried out in specialised centres. Complications which may occur include recurrent laryngeal nerve palsies and hypocalcaemia from hypoparathyroidism. Patients with MTC should also be preoperatively screened for a possible undiagnosed phaeochromocytoma through the measurement of plasma or 24-h urine normetanephrine and metanephrine levels [48]. If a phaeochromocytoma is detected, it should be removed prior to surgery for the MTC.

Clinical Pearls

- Beware of the red flags suggesting a familial thyroid cancer: bilaterality, multifocality, positive family history, medullary thyroid cancer, cribriform-morular variant of papillary cancer.
- In suspected familial non-medullary thyroid cancers, look out for syndromic features:
  - If syndrome features are present, consider targeted genetic testing and referral to a genetic counsellor for appropriate counselling and surveillance implementation.
  - If syndromic features are not present, no evidence for genetic testing currently.

References

1. Davies L, Welch HG. Current thyroid cancer trends in the United States. JAMA Otolaryngol Head Neck Surg. 2014;140(4):317–22.
2. Xing M. Molecular pathogenesis and mechanisms of thyroid cancer. Nat Rev Cancer. 2013;13(3):184–99.
3. Nose V. Familial non-medullary thyroid carcinoma: an update. Endocr Pathol. 2008;19(4):226–40.
4. Zhang Q, et al. Clinical analysis of familial nonmedullary thyroid carcinoma. World J Surg. 2016;40(3):570–3.
5. Waite KA, Eng C. Protean PTEN: form and function. Am J Hum Genet. 2002;70(4):829–44.
6. Pilarski R, et al. Cowden syndrome and the PTEN hamartoma tumor syndrome: systematic review and revised diagnostic criteria. J Natl Cancer Inst. 2013;105(21):1607–16.
7. Mester J, Eng C. Estimate of de novo mutation frequency in probands with PTEN hamartoma tumor syndrome. Genet Med. 2012;14(9):819–22.
8. Tan MH, et al. A clinical scoring system for selection of patients for PTEN mutation testing is proposed on the basis of a prospective study of 3042 probands. Am J Hum Genet. 2011;88(1):42–56.
9. Hall JE, Abdollahian DJ, Sinard RJ. Thyroid disease associated with Cowden syndrome: a meta-analysis. Head Neck. 2013;35(8):1189–94.
10. Ngeow J, et al. Incidence and clinical characteristics of thyroid cancer in prospective series of individuals with Cowden and Cowden-like syndrome characterized by germline PTEN, SDH, or KLLN alterations. J Clin Endocrinol Metab. 2011;96(12):E2063–71.
11. Smith JR, et al. Thyroid nodules and cancer in children with PTEN hamartoma tumor syndrome. J Clin Endocrinol Metab. 2011;96(1):34–7.
12. Ni Y, et al. Germline SDHx variants modify breast and thyroid cancer risks in Cowden and Cowden-like syndrome via FAD/NAD-dependant destabilization of p53. Hum Mol Genet. 2012;21(2):300–10.
13. Bennett KL, Mester J, Eng C. Germline epigenetic regulation of KILLIN in Cowden and Cowden-like syndrome. JAMA. 2010;304(24):2724–31.
14. Orloff MS, et al. Germline PIK3CA and AKT1 mutations in Cowden and Cowden-like syndromes. Am J Hum Genet. 2013;92(1):76–80.
15. Veeman MT, Axelrod JD, Moon RT. A second canon. Functions and mechanisms of beta-catenin-independent Wnt signaling. Dev Cell. 2003;5(3):367–77.
16. Septer S, et al. Thyroid cancer complicating familial adenomatous polyposis: mutation spectrum of at-risk individuals. Hered Cancer Clin Pract. 2013;11(1):13.
17. Houlston RS, Stratton MR. Genetics of non-medullary thyroid cancer. QJM. 1995;88(10):685–93.
18. Son EJ, Nose V. Familial follicular cell-derived thyroid carcinoma. Front Endocrinol (Lausanne). 2012;3:61.
19. Levy RA, et al. Cribriform-morular variant of papillary thyroid carcinoma: an indication to screen for occult FAP. Familial Cancer. 2014;13(4):547–51.
20. Uchino S, et al. Age- and gender-specific risk of thyroid cancer in patients with familial adenomatous polyposis. J Clin Endocrinol Metab. 2016;101(12):4611–7.
21. Groen EJ, et al. Extra-intestinal manifestations of familial adenomatous polyposis. Ann Surg Oncol. 2008;15(9):2439–50.
22. Cetta F, et al. Germline mutations of the APC gene in patients with familial adenomatous polyposis-associated thyroid carcinoma: results from a European cooperative study. J Clin Endocrinol Metab. 2000;85(1):286–92.
23. Pradhan D, Sharma A, Mohanty SK. Cribriform-morular variant of papillary thyroid carcinoma. Pathol Res Pract. 2015;211(10):712–6.
24. Jarrar AM, et al. Screening for thyroid cancer in patients with familial adenomatous polyposis. Ann Surg. 2011;253(3):515–21.
25. Correa R, Salpea P, Stratakis CA. Carney complex: an update. Eur J Endocrinol. 2015;173(4):M85–97.
26. Stratakis CA. Carney complex: a familial lentiginosis predisposing to a variety of tumors. Rev Endocr Metab Disord. 2016;17(3):367–71.
27. Rothenbuhler A, Stratakis CA. Clinical and molecular genetics of carney complex. Best Pract Res Clin Endocrinol Metab. 2010;24(3):389–99.
28. Stratakis CA, Kirschner LS, Carney JA. Clinical and molecular features of the carney complex: diagnostic criteria and recommendations for patient evaluation. J Clin Endocrinol Metab. 2001;86(9):4041–6.
29. Slade I, et al. DICER1 syndrome: clarifying the diagnosis, clinical features and management implications of a pleiotropic tumour predisposition syndrome. J Med Genet. 2011;48(4):273–8.
30. de Kock L, et al. Exploring the association between DICER1 mutations and differentiated thyroid carcinoma. J Clin Endocrinol Metab. 2014;99(6):E1072–7.

31. De Felice M, et al. A mouse model for hereditary thyroid dysgenesis and cleft palate. Nat Genet. 1998;19(4):395–8.
32. Gudmundsson J, et al. Common variants on 9q22.33 and 14q13.3 predispose to thyroid cancer in European populations. Nat Genet. 2009;41(4):460–4.
33. Uchino S, et al. Familial nonmedullary thyroid carcinoma characterized by multifocality and a high recurrence rate in a large study population. World J Surg. 2002;26(8):897–902.
34. Wang X, et al. Endocrine tumours: familial nonmedullary thyroid carcinoma is a more aggressive disease: a systematic review and meta-analysis. Eur J Endocrinol. 2015;172(6):R253–62.
35. Capezzone M, et al. Familial non-medullary thyroid carcinoma displays the features of clinical anticipation suggestive of a distinct biological entity. Endocr Relat Cancer. 2008;15(4):1075–81.
36. Sadowski SM, et al. Prospective screening in familial nonmedullary thyroid cancer. Surgery. 2013;154(6):1194–8.
37. Alsanea O, Clark OH. Familial thyroid cancer. Curr Opin Oncol. 2001;13(1):44–51.
38. Marsh DJ, et al. Somatic mutations in the RET protooncogene in sporadic medullary thyroid carcinoma. Clin Endocrinol. 1996;44(3):249–57.
39. Santoro M, Melillo RM, Fusco A. RET/PTC activation in papillary thyroid carcinoma: European journal of endocrinology prize lecture. Eur J Endocrinol. 2006;155(5):645–53.
40. Gimm O, et al. Mutation analysis reveals novel sequence variants in NTRK1 in sporadic human medullary thyroid carcinoma. J Clin Endocrinol Metab. 1999;84(8):2784–7.
41. Raue F, Frank-Raue K. Genotype-phenotype correlation in multiple endocrine neoplasia type 2. Clinics (Sao Paulo). 2012;67(Suppl 1):69–75.
42. Morrison PJ, Atkinson AB. Genetic aspects of familial thyroid cancer. Oncologist. 2009;14(6):571–7.
43. Nose V. Familial thyroid cancer: a review. Mod Pathol. 2011;24(Suppl 2):S19–33.
44. Eng C, et al. The relationship between specific RET proto-oncogene mutations and disease phenotype in multiple endocrine neoplasia type 2. International RET mutation consortium analysis. JAMA. 1996;276(19):1575–9.
45. American Thyroid Association Guidelines Task Force, et al. Medullary thyroid cancer: management guidelines of the American Thyroid Association. Thyroid. 2009;19(6):565–612.
46. Clark OH. Controversies in familial thyroid cancer 2014. Ulus Cerrahi Derg. 2014;30(2):62–6.
47. Kebebew E, et al. Medullary thyroid carcinoma: clinical characteristics, treatment, prognostic factors, and a comparison of staging systems. Cancer. 2000;88(5):1139–48.
48. Salehian B, Samoa R. RET gene abnormalities and thyroid disease: who should be screened and when. J Clin Res Pediatr Endocrinol. 2013;5(Suppl 1):70–8.
49. Vriens MR, et al. Clinical features and genetic predisposition to hereditary nonmedullary thyroid cancer. Thyroid. 2009;19(12):1343–9.

15 Neuromonitoring in Thyroid Surgery

Dipti Kamani, Selen Soylu, and Gregory W. Randolph

Introduction

Recurrent laryngeal nerve (RLN) injury is one of the most fearful complications of thyroid surgery. In an effort to minimize the risk of RLN injury, intraoperative nerve monitoring (IONM) is increasingly becoming popular as a useful adjunct to visual identification, adding a new functional dynamic during thyroid surgery. This chapter presents the principles and application of monitoring techniques for RLN, utility of intraoperative neuromonitoring in thyroid surgery, as well as new advances in the technique.

> **I am convinced the best management of RLN injuries is of a preventative character.**
>
> —Lahey (1938)

D. Kamani · S. Soylu
Massachusetts Eye and Ear Infirmary, Division of Thyroid and Parathyroid Surgery, Department of Otolaryngology, Harvard Medical School, Boston, MA, USA

G. W. Randolph (✉)
Massachusetts Eye and Ear Infirmary, Division of Thyroid and Parathyroid Surgery, Department of Otolaryngology, Harvard Medical School, Boston, MA, USA

Division of Surgical Oncology, Endocrine Surgical Service, Massachusetts General Hospital, Harvard Medical School, Boston, MA, USA
e-mail: Gregory_Randolph@meei.harvard.edu

Background

Over the years, thyroid surgery has evolved into a graceful modern-day operation focused on surgical outcomes. Indeed, injury to the recurrent laryngeal nerve (RLN) is one of the most feared complications of thyroid surgery. Lahey introduced the routine dissection and demonstration of the RLN during thyroid surgery [1]. The role of RLN identification in prevention of injury to the RLN during thyroid surgery is long established [2]. While visual identification of RLN is the gold standard for prevention of RLN injury, the development of intraoperative neuromonitoring (IONM) in thyroid surgery has added a functional dynamic by demonstrating that a structurally intact RLN may not necessarily equate a functionally intact nerve [3]. The central dogma of neural monitoring is that a visually identified, surgically preserved, and morphologically intact nerve may not necessarily function normally. In thermal, traction, and compression injuries, RLN may structurally remain intact; a functional assessment of the nerve is required in order to identify the injury.

Iatrogenic RLN Injury

While bilateral vocal cord paralysis (VCP) can be particularly devastating, often resulting in tracheotomy, unilateral VCP is also detrimental and may

R. Parameswaran, A. Agarwal (eds.), *Evidence-Based Endocrine Surgery*,
https://doi.org/10.1007/978-981-10-1124-5_15

be associated with aspiration and voice changes that are sufficient to affect vocation, and furthermore can have significant economic as well as medicolegal consequences [4]. Rates of permanent RLN paralysis in expert hands are reported in the range of 1–2% [5]. A recent review of 27 articles that analyzed over 25,000 thyroidectomy patients found that the average postoperative VCP rate was 9.8% and ranged from 0 to 18.6% [6]. It should be noted that the rates of RLN paralysis following thyroidectomy in the literature are likely underestimated due to difficulty in recognizing many of the intraoperative RLN injuries, lower inclination of surgical units with unfavorable data to report their findings, variability in related symptoms, and inconsistency in performing postoperative laryngeal examination by various surgical units [7]. The Scandinavian Quality Register states that RLN paralysis rate doubles when all patients undergo postoperative laryngeal exam routinely [8]. In order to appreciate the true rate of RLN injury, preoperative and postoperative laryngeal examinations are essential in all patients.

Preoperative and Postoperative Laryngeal Exam

Preoperative laryngeal exam can detect asymptomatic VCP, raise the suspicion of invasive disease, influence the intraoperative management of invaded nerve, avoid wrong indictment of postoperative paralysis, and provide a documented information to compare postoperative vocal cord function. Postoperative laryngeal exam is the only obtainable precise outcome measure for postoperative RLN function, voice changes, and VCP that can occur in isolation [9]. Additionally, it allows for postoperative patient safety and planning of contralateral surgery. Routine performance of preoperative and postoperative laryngeal exam in thyroidectomy patients is recommended by the British Association of Endocrine and Thyroid Surgeons, the German Association of Endocrine Surgery, and the International Neural Monitoring Study Group [10–12]. The recommendations for preoperative and postoperative voice assessment are provided in the American Academy of Otolaryngology Head and Neck Surgery (AAOHNS) voice guidelines [4]. Preoperative laryngeal exam is recommended in all thyroid cancer patients in the American Thyroid Association Goiter Surgery Guidelines and the American Thyroid Association Anaplastic Cancer Guidelines [13]. The American Head and Neck Society Invasive Thyroid Cancer Guidelines and NCCN both recommend preoperative laryngeal exam in all thyroid cancer patients [14].

IONM Technique, Standards, and Setup

Variation in IONM application across multiple centers is noticeable, and may be due to the use of diverse electrodes, techniques, and output recordings leading to diversified and incomparable results. Consequently, this heterogeneity may limit the overall utility and applicability of the IONM technology. To promote uniformity in IONM application and to avoid common setup and technical errors, the International Nerve Monitoring Study Group (INMSG) has published guidelines for IONM application [10]. Additionally, it should be noted that a successful IONM requires a multidisciplinary approach with collaborative work between the anesthesiologist and surgeon. Macias et al. have outlined an up-to-date algorithm and a monitoring protocol particularly focused on anesthesia parameters that are necessary for successful IONM [15].

Technique

Various neural monitoring methods include glottic observation, laryngeal palpation, endotracheal tube (ETT)-based surface electrodes, and postcricoid surface electrodes [10, 16, 17]. The monitoring systems offer either audio feedback or both audio feedback and visual waveform information. The audio-only systems have a few important pitfalls: (1) The differentiation between the signal and the artifact may not be possible; (2) distinct features of a waveform such as amplitude, latency, and morphology cannot be seen and documented; and (3) quantification of the response is not possible leading to issues in detection of impending RLN injury and pathological states of the RLN.

The most preferred neural monitoring equipment is an ETT-based system that includes both audio feedback and a visual graphic documentation of the electromyography (EMG) waveform elicited from thyroarytenoid muscle. Both needle-based electrodes and surface electrodes may be used. Manufactured ETT with paired stainless steel electrodes exposed at the level of the glottis or a standard ETT with thin electrodes secured over the tube with adhesive pads can be used.

The Setup

A basic setup of the neural monitoring equipment is shown in Fig. 15.1.

Following a standard setup algorithm minimizes intraoperative problems related to IONM system. The electrocautery unit should be kept at least 10 ft. away from the neural monitoring unit to avoid electrical interference. Ground electrodes are adhered to the shoulder or the sternum. After the equipment is set up, it is confirmed that the recording-side and the stimulation-side circuitry is complete.

Muscle relaxants used during anesthesia may temper with EMG response and lead to inaccurate quantitative analysis during IONM. Thus, use of muscle relaxants or paralytic agents to maintain anesthesia should be avoided. Short-acting muscle relaxants at the time of induction can be used. The endotracheal tube should be inserted without the use of any lubricant jelly or any other coating. It is recommended to use suction and possibly a drying agent to avoid pooling of saliva, which may obscure the EMG signals. The largest possible size tube should be used to ensure that the electrodes abut closely to the vocal cords. Since the tube displacement of up to 6 cm can occur during final positioning of the patient, especially with neck extension, it is imperative that tube placement checks are performed once the patient is in the final position [18]. Presence of respiratory variations can help establish proper tube placement; alternatively repeat direct laryngoscopy can be performed. Respiratory variations are small waveforms with amplitudes of 30–70 μV that cause coarsening of the baseline EMG. Respiratory variation can be seen during a small window of time when the effect of the muscle relaxant given at the time of induction wears off and the patient is in a lighter plane of anesthesia just before the patient starts to move spontaneously or "buck" [19] (Fig. 15.2). At final positioning, the impedance

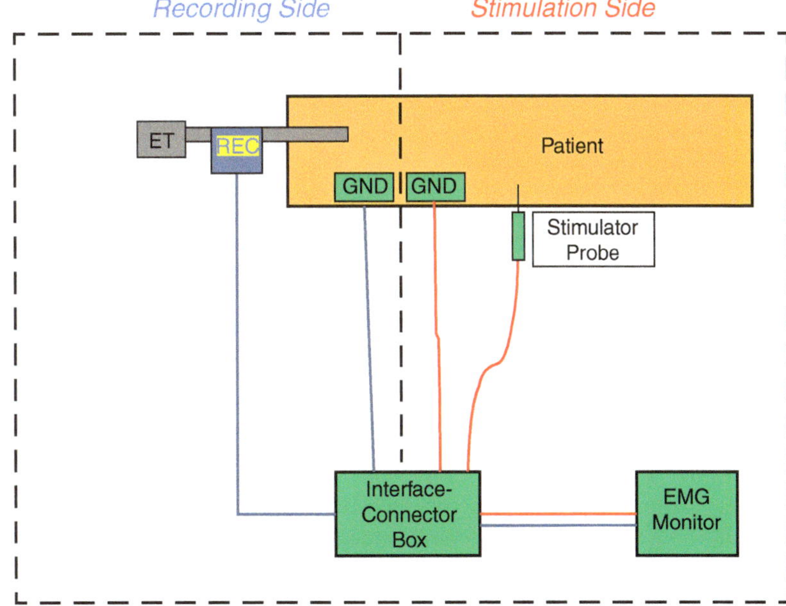

Fig. 15.1 Basic IONM equipment setup. *ET* endotracheal tube, *REC* recording electrodes, and *GND* ground electrodes

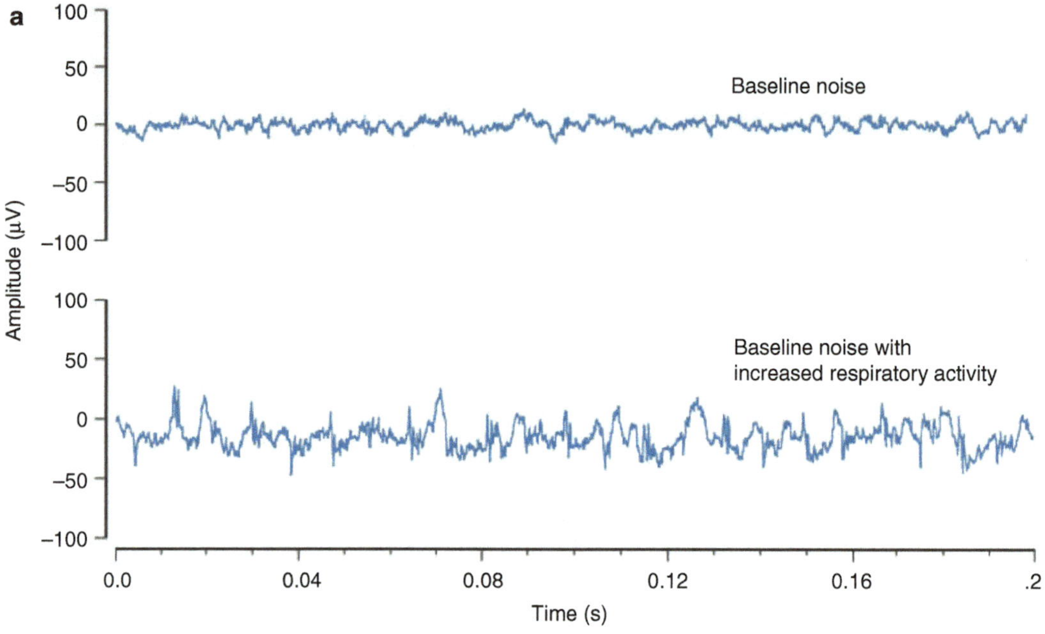

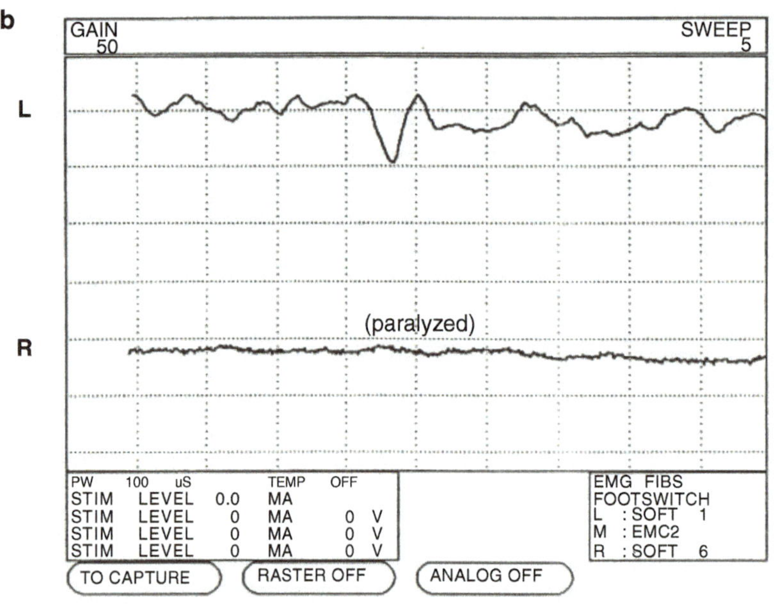

Fig. 15.2 Respiratory variation. Left and right baseline tracings in a patient—the left vocal cord demonstrates normal respiratory variation (30–70 μV). The right vocal cord is electrically silent (patient had preoperatively diagnosed right vocal cord paralysis)

of the electrodes should be less than 5 Ω and the imbalance between the two sides should be less than 1 Ω. Higher impedance imbalance may suggest inappropriate tube placement requiring repositioning whereas if the overall impedance is high then the ground electrodes require a check or replacement. Once the setup is complete, it is important to set the monitor event threshold at 100 μV and the stimulator probe to a pulsatile output of 4 per second. At the initiation of surgery, the stimulation of strap muscles resulting into a gross muscle twitch can be performed to confirm absence of paralytic agents as well as intact stimulatory pathway.

For each patient, essential data pertaining to IONM include preoperative laryngeal exam L1, an initial intraoperative suprathreshold vagal nerve stimulation V1, and an initial intraoperative RLN stimulation R1 that are recorded at the beginning. A similar set of events that include R2 and V2 need to be recorded at the end of the surgery, followed by a postoperative laryngeal exam L2 [20, 21]. A suprathreshold current of 2 mA is useful for neural mapping, whereas once the RLN has been visualized the current can be reduced to 1 mA for further testing and end-of-surgery prognostication.

EMG Waveform

The amplitude of a monitoring waveform is defined in the International Guidelines as the vertical height of the apex of the positive initial waveform deflection to the lowest point in the net subsequent opposite polarity phase of the waveform (Fig. 15.3). Caragacianu et al. found that no statistically significant difference exists between the amplitude when the nerve is stimulated by suprathreshold levels at 1 or 2 mA. Normative values were thus defined at 1 mA. The study established a clinically useful normative range of amplitude that can be useful for surgical decision-making [22]. Latency definition in the IONM literature is inconsistent; the INMSG defines latency as the time from the stimulation spike to the appearance of the first evoked waveform peak (Fig. 15.3). Latency recordings are distinctive and can not only differentiate artifacts from neural stimulated structures and but also distinguish RLN, superior laryngeal nerve, and vagus nerve and differentiate left from right vagus nerve easily. Threshold is defined as the current that, applied to the nerve, first starts to trigger minimal EMG activity. Normative EMG data and graphical waveforms generated from RLN, SLN, and left and right vagus nerve have been described and are depicted in Fig. 15.4 [23].

Passive EMG Activity During IONM

A frequently occurring passive EMG activity implies mechanical nerve injury or cautery stress; evaluation of surgical maneuvers is imperative at the time. Several researchers have reported that such bursts of passive activity correlate with some degree of nerve injury [24–26]. But, till date, their relationship to frank VCP is not proven.

IONM Application

Use of IONM is increasing lately and is evident through the recent surgical survey data demonstrating the use of IONM during thyroid surgeries by almost 80% head and neck surgeons and by 65% of general surgeons in the USA with a significant increase in just past few years [27, 28]. Noticeably, over 95% of endocrine surgical fellows who had an exposure to nerve monitoring

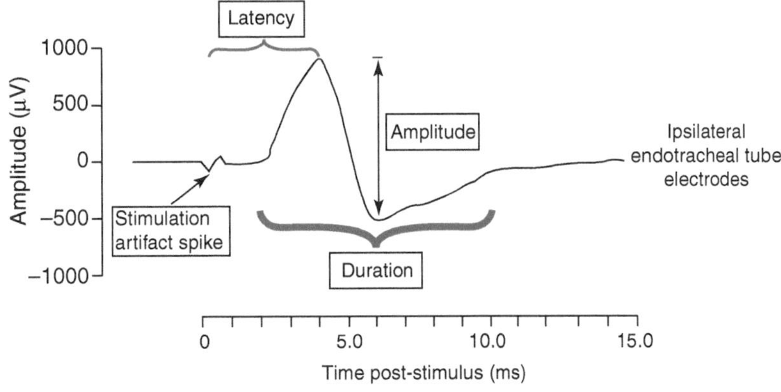

Fig. 15.3 EMG recording showing amplitude and latency measurements of unilateral recurrent laryngeal nerve stimulation recorded by ipsilateral endotracheal tube electrodes

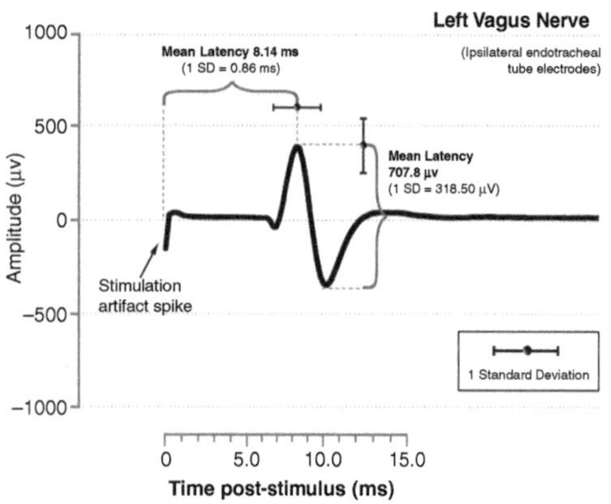

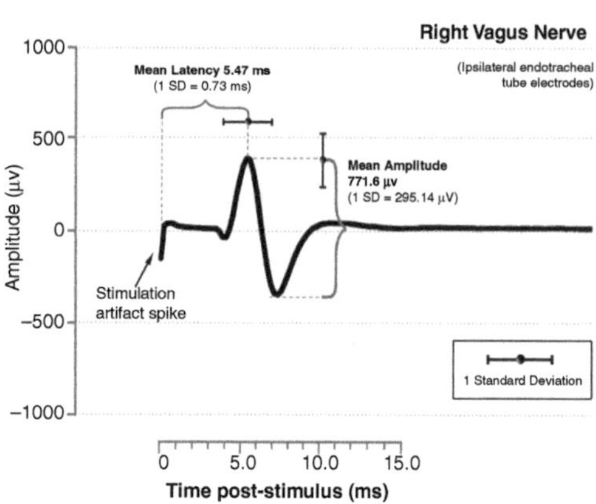

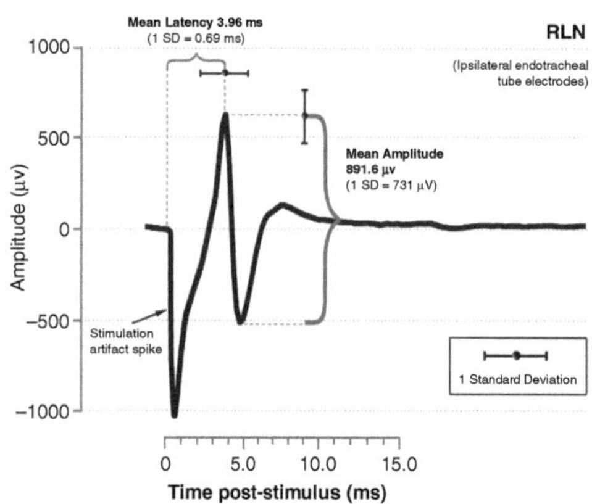

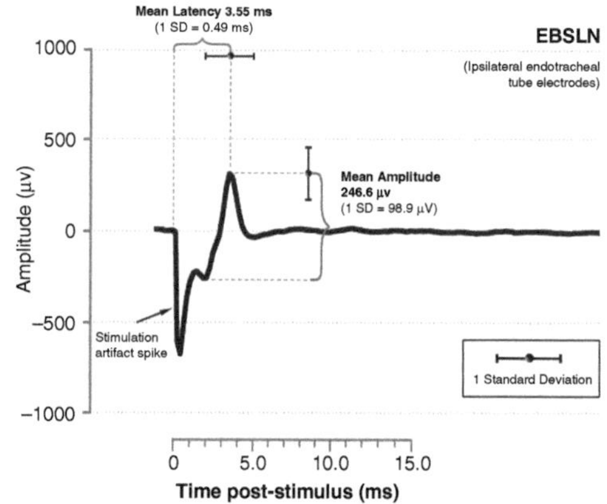

Fig. 15.4 Ipsilateral endotracheal electrode recording for the left and right vagus nerve, pooled recurrent laryngeal nerve (RLN), and pooled external branch of superior laryngeal nerve (EBSLN) illustrating normative waveform morphology, latency, and amplitude

during their endocrine fellowship training implemented its use in some or all of their cases in their surgical practice [29]. Literature reported on patterns of use of IONM suggest that surgeons who most commonly employ neural monitoring are higher volume surgeons [30].

Benefits of IONM Can Be Characterized into Following Categories

1. *Neural Mapping and Identification*:
   IONM aids in visualization of nerve, and the speed of RLN identification is improved with IONM as compared to visual identification alone [31]. Linear electrical stimulation in the paratracheal region assists in mapping the course of the RLN. This neural map can be used for further dissection for nerve visualization. IONM is especially valuable in revision surgeries as in such situations scar tissue makes nerve identification difficult, as well as in large goiters and invasive malignancies where anatomy is distorted.
2. *Insight into Pathologic States of the RLN*:
   Even when a nerve is invaded by malignancy, it can demonstrate significant residual EMG response upon stimulation of a nerve. Further, residual EMG can be present in the setting of preoperative VCP. In a study by our unit, we found that about a third of the patients with VCP due to nerve invasion revealed significant EMG activity [9]. When

such a nerve is resected, the surgeon needs to be aware of the consequent functional issues attributable to the residual electrophysiologic activity in the nerve. The patient may experience additional dysphagia and aspiration to some extent. Hence, presence of intraoperative EMG activity should be considered during surgical management of invaded nerve. Notably, IONM can provide important insights into the functioning of invaded nerves which are not obtainable with visual identification alone.

3. *Detection of Intraoperative Injury and Prognostication of Nerve Function*:
   The ability to predict the functional status of RLN with reasonable accuracy is one of the most important applications of IONM, as it assists the surgeon in avoiding bilateral VCP. Visual identification alone is insufficient to prognosticate postoperative RLN function. A nerve injured by blunt trauma or stretching may appear visually intact, and in such situations structural integrity does not necessarily translate into a normal postoperative functionality. A study of more than 3600 cases from the Scandinavian endocrine quality register reported that only 11.3% injuries were predicted by the surgeons, and only 16% (1 out of 6) bilateral injuries were identified intraoperatively [32]. Thus, close to 90% of the injuries are not visually identifiable. In contrast, IONM is a highly precise neural function test and has >95% negative predictive value [33–37]. The positive predictive value of IONM is lower and can be variable; this is related to the use of accurate definition of loss of signal (LOS) and implementation of equipment troubleshooting. Universal and accurate definition of LOS and a better knowledge of normative neural monitoring parameters can greatly augment prognostic function of IONM. This is one of the focuses of upcoming INMSG guidelines. After confirming that the LOS is due to neural injury, injured nerve segment can be identified by performing retrograde testing of the affected RLN, starting from the laryngeal entry point and progressing proximally. This can allow for treatment of the injury as well as present learning opportunities for the surgeon. In the setting of LOS, bilateral VCP can be avoided by postponing contralateral surgery; this concept of postponing contralateral surgery in the setting of nerve-related LOS is possibly the utmost extension of neural prognostication function of IONM. The cost-effectiveness of neural monitoring as it relates to LOS and staged thyroidectomy has recently been evaluated by Al-Qurayshi et al., utilizing a Markov chain model subjected to Monte Carlo simulation cost modeling in the US population. Using rates of contralateral RLN palsy ranging from 1 to 17%, they found that nerve monitoring with LOS incorporation into the surgical strategy is the most cost-effective algorithm [38].

Interpretation of LOS During IONM

LOS (LOS) during IONM could be encountered due to several reasons; first and foremost equipment/setup-related LOS should be ruled out before considering true LOS. The laryngeal twitch response to ipsilateral and contralateral vagal stimulation should be assessed to evaluate the integrity of the IONM setup. Presence of laryngeal twitch confirms proper functioning of the stimulating side of equipment. Recording-side equipment issues usually result from improper tube positioning, inadequacy of current, and use of paralytic agents that should also be deliberated. An event must satisfy three conditions to be categorized as true LOS:

1. Presence of a satisfactory EMG (amplitude >500 μV) at the beginning of IONM
2. No or low response (i.e., 250 μV or lower) with stimulation at 1–2 mA in a dry field
3. Absence of laryngeal twitch and/or glottis twitch on ipsilateral vagal stimulation

Presence of a true LOS should prompt the surgeon to identify the site of injury and to abort the associated maneuver if possible. LOS may also impact the surgical plan and may lead to postponement of surgery on the contralateral side [39] (Fig. 15.5). There is significant clinical evidence

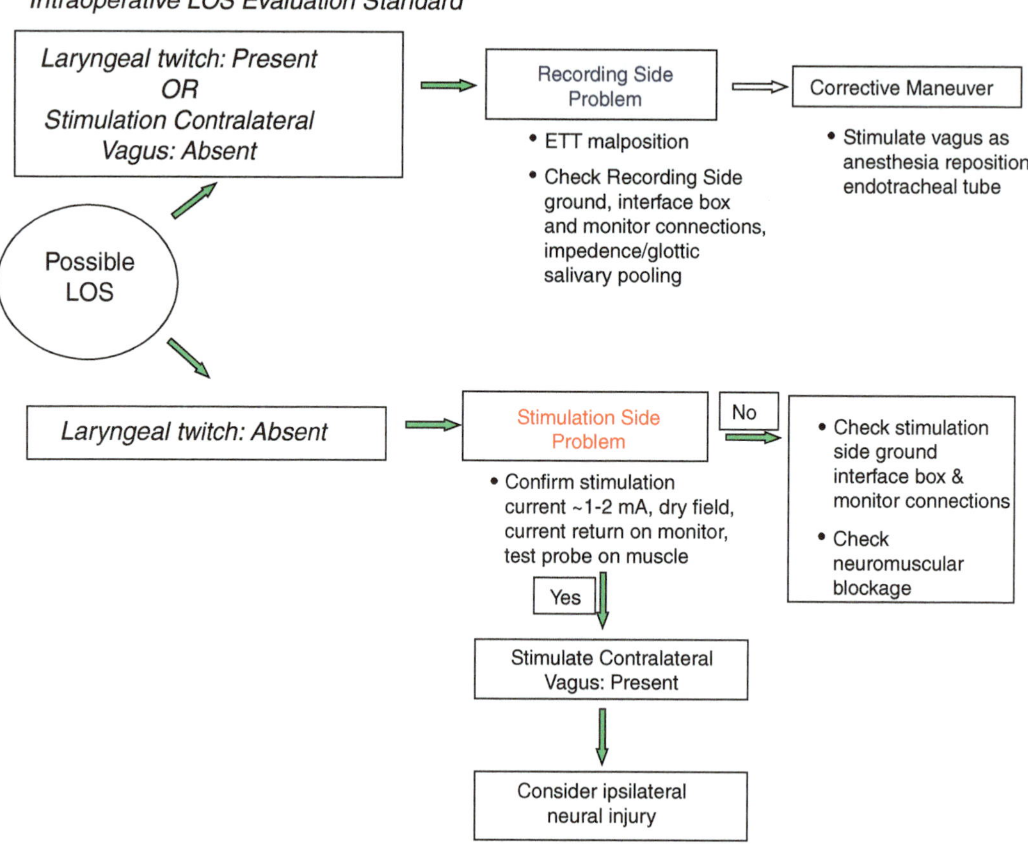

Fig. 15.5 Intraoperative evaluation of loss of signal (LOS) algorithm

in support of staging of contralateral surgery in the event of LOS [40–43]. LOS definition, interpretation, and staged surgery are discussed in detail in the upcoming INMSG guidelines.

Prognostic Testing Errors

False-positive error (when LOS is noted intraoperatively, but the nerve function is intact postoperatively): False-positive errors can result from:

1. Stimulation of the nerve in a wet bloody surgical field
2. Equipment errors on the recording side (displacement of endotracheal tube, improper grounding of electrodes)
3. Use of improper neuromuscular blockade
4. Early neuronal recovery especially if there is delay in performing postoperative laryngoscopy by a few days

False-negative error (when positive EMG response is present at RLN stimulation at the end of the surgery but there is absence of nerve function postoperatively): This type of error is infrequent, particularly when IONM is performed in a systematic manner.

False-negative error can result from the following:

1. Stimulation of the nerve distal to the site of injury: This can be avoided by routinely performing post-dissection vagal stimulation (V2).
2. Trauma related to endotracheal tube leading to laryngeal edema, and dislocation of the arytenoid cartilage.
3. Injury to the nerve after the final stimulation, e.g., during wound closure.
4. In the setting of extralaryngeal branching of the RLN, a posterior branch injury may not be detected by IONM.

Evidence-Based Discussion on Impact of Neuromonitoring on Rate of RLN Injury

While analyzing the literature to assess the impact of neuromonitoring on the rate of postoperative VCP, it is important to keep in mind that (1) to achieve an adequate statistical power, very large sample size is needed because of extremely low incidence of the end points—transient and permanent RLN injury. Dralle et al. have shown that an adequately powered study to obtain a statistically significant difference would need nine million patients per arm for benign goiter surgery and 40,000 patients per arm for thyroid malignancy surgery [44]. (2) There is significant heterogeneity in the available literature. (3) There are several, hard-to-isolate confounding factors, e.g., surgeon's expertise, the nature of the disease, and the type and extent of the surgical procedure. (4) Additionally, use of preoperative and postoperative laryngoscopy to document vocal cord status is not enforced in all research studies, thus missing a documented measure of vocal cord status.

A brief discussion of the available significant relevant literature with level 1 (meta-analysis and randomized trials), level 2 (outcome research and systematic review), and level 5 (case series) evidence is presented here. A meta-analysis by Zheng et al. found statistically significant differences in the incidences of overall and transient RLN palsy with the use of IONM versus visual RLN identification alone during thyroidectomy but did not find statistically significant difference for the incidence of persistent RLN palsy between these two groups [45]. Higgins et al. in their meta-analysis showed no statistically significant difference in the true VCP rate with the use of IONM versus visual RLN identification alone during thyroidectomy [46]. Meta-analysis by Pisanu et al. did not demonstrate any statistically significant difference in the incidence of RLN palsy in IONM versus visual identification alone during thyroidectomy. Notably, they advised researchers to interpret these results with caution, as they were largely based on non-randomized observational studies and suggested that multicenter, prospective, randomized trials based on strict criteria of standardization followed by clustered meta-analysis are required [47]. Recently, Lombardi et al. in their meta-analysis found that the use of IONM did not demonstrate significant benefit over visualization alone in decreasing RLN injury rates [48]. However, bulk of the studies included in their review were non-randomized studies. Many studies reviewing RLN paralysis rate with and without monitoring in select populations such as high-risk surgeries, surgeries for thyroid cancer, and surgeries performed by low-volume surgeons showed improved rates of RLN paralysis [49–51]. Barczynski in their randomized study comparing nerve monitoring with visualization alone showed significantly lower rates of temporary paralysis but not in permanent paralysis, specifically in high-risk surgeries [52]. Lower rates of permanent RLN paralysis with neural monitoring are noted in a study based on endocrine surgery quality data from the Scandinavian Endocrine Surgical Quality Registry [32]. Barczynski et al. in their retrospective study of 850 patients with revision surgeries concluded that IONM statistically significantly reduces the rate of transient RLN paralysis in revision surgeries [53].

Current Advances in IONM

1. *Continuous Vagal Monitoring*:
While intermittent IONM is extremely useful in assisting a surgeon, its greatest limitation lies in its intermittent evaluation of the RLN, thereby allowing the risk of neural injury in between stimulations [32, 44, 54]. This could underlie the reports that suggest that the intermittent IONM (most commonly used format of IONM) may be limited in its ability to prevent neural injury [32, 55–58]. Continuous IONM (CIONM) with vagal nerve electrode is a new format of IONM in which constant, real-time intraoperative EMG data is obtained from vagus and RLN circuitry. The reports of adverse effects of continuous vagal stimulation are rare [59, 60]. There are several reports of intermittent (IONM) and continuous monitoring series with hundreds of patients receiving thousands of nerve stimulations without any associated significant neural, cardiac, pulmonary, or gastrointestinal vagal side effects [49, 61–65]. The real-time EMG information obtained by CIONM can help overcome the limitation of the traditional intermittent IONM by its ability to detect impending RLN injury. The adverse EMG changes picked up by CIONM can indicate an impending neural injury and enable the surgeons to prompt a corrective action such as aborting associated maneuvers that may have led to adverse EMG changes, thus likely avoiding permanent injury. However, it is prudent that a surgeon can identify and differentiate true adverse events from artifacts. Our unit has studied EMG adverse events and defined mild combined events (mCE) and severe combined events (sCE) by using a combination of decrease in amplitude with increase in latency. Mild combined events (mCE) were defined as amplitude decrease of 50–70% with a concordant latency increase of 5–10% and severe combined events (sCE) were defined as amplitude decrease of >70% with a concordant latency increase of >10%.

   We noted that mCE as well as isolated amplitude or latency changes were not associated with VCP. However, sCE were more significant events that were potentially reversible if the related maneuver was aborted, but if allowed to continue sCE could progress to LOS (typically much less reversible) and to likely postoperative VCP. One should keep in mind that IONM in general is more useful for preventing impeding stretch or compression neural injury than a transactional nerve injury [64].
2. *Superior Laryngeal Nerve (SLN) Monitoring*:
Injury to external branch of the SLN (EBSLN) leads to cricothyroid muscle dysfunction that impacts vocal projection and the ability to produce higher registers of the voice. Although subtle, these voice changes can affect professional voice users significantly. EBSLN is at risk of injury during superior pole dissection and ligation of superior thyroid vessels. Intraoperative detection of EBSLN injury is challenging. Up to 20% of EBSLNs run a subfascial course; thus intraoperative visual identification of EBSLN is not possible in all cases [66]. Postoperatively, EBSLN injury is often missed due to absence of associated identifiable changes in vocal cords. EBSLN injury is reported in up to 58% of patients undergoing thyroid surgery [67].

   IONM of EBSLN allows for stimulation and identification of all EBSLNs including the subfascial EBLNs [68]. The laryngeal head of the sternothyroid is used as a landmark for EBSLN identification; the tissue parallel and underneath the laryngeal head of the sternothyroid muscle is stimulated to delineate distal course of EBSLN before it pierces the cricothyroid muscle. A cricothyroid muscle twitch elicited by this stimulation is currently used for EBSLN localization. The EBSLN monitoring guidelines by INMSG provide detailed report on its application and utility [69].
3. *Intraoperative Identification of Nonrecurrent Laryngeal Nerve*:
The nonrecurrent laryngeal nerve (NRLN), a rare anatomical variant of RLN, is more commonly found on the right side (0.5–1% of all RLNs). Left NRLN is rare (0.04%) and is associated with situs inversus. NRLN does not affect RLN function in any way but surgically it makes the nerve more vulnerable to injury, especially when a surgeon is unaware of its

presence. The preoperative identification of NRLN by imaging modalities remains challenging. An inadvertent injury to NRLN can be avoided if the surgeon is aware of its presence prior to dissecting in related cervical region. An IONM electrophysiologic algorithm can help identify NRLN before commencing dissection in the related area. The presence of positive EMG response to proximal stimulation of vagus at the superior border of thyroid cartilage and absence of EMG response to distal stimulation of vagus below the inferior border of fourth tracheal ring can reliably identify all NRLNs [70]. Brauckhoff et al. demonstrated successful NRLN identification by similar vagal stimulation technique [56]. The electrophysiological parameters such as amplitude, latency, and threshold of right NRLN are similar to those of right RLN. Some reports have explored the latency values of NRLN and suggest that a latency of less than 3.5 ms strongly favors suspicion of NRLN [71]. Further studies are necessary to establish this latency cutoff as a conclusive indicator of NRLN.

Clinical Pearls

1. The benefits of IONM are perceived when the electrophysiological data and functional dynamic obtained by IONM are used to complement visual nerve identification.
2. Following proper standards of IONM is vital in reducing errors in its interpretation.
3. Neural monitoring requires a completely bloodless field and has a learning curve.
4. The additional cost of IONM provides valuable supplementary information that can help the surgeon in nerve identification, in making surgical decisions regarding nerve management, in avoiding bilateral VCP by postponing contralateral surgery in the setting of neural related LOS, and in predicting postoperative nerve function.

References

1. Lahey F. Exposure of the recurrent laryngeal nerves in thyroid operations: further experience. Surg Gynecol Obstet. 1938;194:239.
2. Lahey FH, Hoover WB. Injuries to the recurrent laryngeal nerve in thyroid operations: their management and avoidance. Ann Surg. 1938;108:545–62.
3. Riddell V. Thyroidectomy: prevention of bilateral recurrent nerve palsy. Results of identification of the nerve over 23 consecutive years (1946–69) with a description of an additional safety measure. Br J Surg. 1970;57:1–11.
4. Chandrasekhar SS, Randolph GW, Seidman MD, et al. Clinical practice guideline: improving voice outcomes after thyroid surgery. Otolaryngol Head Neck Surg. 2013;148:S1–37.
5. Kern KA. Medicolegal analysis of errors in diagnosis and treatment of surgical endocrine disease. Surgery. 1993;114:1167–73; discussion 1173–4.
6. Jeannon JP, Orabi AA, Bruch GA, Abdalsalam HA, Simo R. Diagnosis of recurrent laryngeal nerve palsy after thyroidectomy: a systematic review. Int J Clin Pract. 2009;63:624–9.
7. Lo CY, Kwok KF, Yuen PW. A prospective evaluation of recurrent laryngeal nerve paralysis during thyroidectomy. Arch Surg. 2000;135:204–7.
8. Bergenfelz A, Jansson S, Mårtensson H, et al. Scandinavian quality register for thyroid and parathyroid surgery: audit of surgery for primary hyperparathyroidism. Langenbeck's Arch Surg. 2007;392:445–51.
9. Kamani D, Darr EA, Randolph GW. Electrophysiologic monitoring characteristics of the recurrent laryngeal nerve preoperatively paralyzed or invaded with malignancy. Otolaryngol Head Neck Surg. 2013;149:682–8.
10. Randolph GW, Dralle H. Abdullah Het al. Electrophysiologic recurrent laryngeal nerve monitoring during thyroid and parathyroid surgery: international standards guideline statement. Laryngoscope. 2011;121(Suppl 1):S1–16.
11. The British Association of Endocrine and Thyroid Surgeons Third National Audit Report. 2009.
12. Musholt TJ, Clerici T, Dralle H, et al. German Association of Endocrine Surgeons practice guidelines for the surgical treatment of benign thyroid disease. Langenbeck's Arch Surg. 2011;396:639–49.
13. Chen AY, Bernet VJ, Carty SE, et al. American thyroid association statement on optimal surgical management of goiter. Thyroid. 2014;24:181–9.
14. Phelan E, Potenza A, Slough C, Zurakowski D, Kamani D, Randolph G. Recurrent laryngeal nerve monitoring during thyroid surgery: normative vagal and recurrent laryngeal nerve electrophysiological data. Otolaryngol Head Neck Surg. 2012;147:640–6.
15. Macias AA, Eappen S, Malikin I, Goldfarb J, Kujawa S, Konowitz PM, Kamani D, Randolph GW. Intraoperative electrophysiologic monitoring of the recurrent laryngeal nerve during thyroid and parathyroid surgery : the Massachusetts eye and ear infirmary monitoring protocol with collab-

orative experience in over 3000 cases. Head Neck. 2016;38(10):1487–94.
16. Randolph GW, Kobler JB, Wilkins J. Recurrent laryngeal nerve identification and assessment during thyroid surgery: laryngeal palpation. World J Surg. 2004;28:755–60.
17. Rea JL. Postcricoid surface laryngeal electrode. Ear Nose Throat J. 1992;71:267–9.
18. Yap SJ, Morris RW, Pybus DA. Alterations in endotracheal tube position during general anaesthesia. Anaesth Intensive Care. 1994;22:586–8.
19. Chambers KJ, Pearse A, Coveney J, et al. Respiratory variation predicts optimal endotracheal tube placement for intra-operative nerve monitoring in thyroid and parathyroid surgery. World J Surg. 2015;39:393–9.
20. Chiang FY, Lee KW, Chen HC, et al. Standardization of intraoperative neuromonitoring of recurrent laryngeal nerve in thyroid operation. World J Surg. 2010;34:223–9.
21. Randolph G. Surgical anatomy of recurrent laryngeal nerve. In: Randolph GW, editor. Surgery of the thyroid and parathyroid glands. Philadelphia: Saunders; 2013.
22. Caragacianu D, Kamani D, Randolph GW. Intraoperative monitoring: normative range associated with normal postoperative glottic function. Laryngoscope. 2013;123:3026–31.
23. Sritharan N, Chase M, Kamani D, Randolph M, Randolph GW. The vagus nerve, recurrent laryngeal nerve, and external branch of the superior laryngeal nerve have unique latencies allowing for intraoperative documentation of intact neural function during thyroid surgery. Laryngoscope. 2015;125:E84–9.
24. Dong CC, Macdonald DB. Akagami ret al. Intraoperative facial motor evoked potential monitoring with transcranial electrical stimulation during skull base surgery. Clin Neurophysiol. 2005;116:588–96.
25. Prass RL. Iatrogenic facial nerve injury: the role of facial nerve monitoring. Otolaryngol Clin N Am. 1996;29:265–75.
26. Pearlman RC, Isley MR, Ruben GD, et al. Intraoperative monitoring of the recurrent laryngeal nerve using acoustic, free-run, and evoked electromyography. J Clin Neurophysiol. 2005;22:148–52.
27. Singer MC, Rosenfeld RM, Sundaram K. Laryngeal nerve monitoring: current utilization among head and neck surgeons. Otolaryngol Head Neck Surg. 2012;146:895–9.
28. Ho Y, Carr MM, Goldenberg D. Trends in intraoperative neural monitoring for thyroid and parathyroid surgery amongst otolaryngologists and general surgeons. Eur Arch Otorhinolaryngol. 2013;270:2525–30.
29. Marti JL, Holm T, Randolph G. Universal use of intraoperative nerve monitoring by recently fellowship-trained thyroid surgeons is common, associated with higher surgical volume, and impacts intraoperative decision-making. World J Surg. 2016;40:337–43.
30. Sturgeon C, Sturgeon T, Angelos P. Neuromonitoring in thyroid surgery: attitudes, usage patterns, and predictors of use among endocrine surgeons. World J Surg. 2009;33:417–25.
31. Sari S, Erbil Y, Sumer A, et al. Evaluation of recurrent laryngeal nerve monitoring in thyroid surgery. Int J Surg (London England). 2010;8:474–8.
32. Bergenfelz A, Jansson S, Kristoffersson A, et al. Complications to thyroid surgery: results as reported in a database from a multicenter audit comprising 3,660 patients. Langenbeck's Arch Surg. 2008;393:667–73.
33. Hamelmann WH, Meyer T, Timm S, Timmermann W. A critical estimation of intraoperative neuromonitoring (IONM) in thyroid surgery. Zentralbl Chir. 2002;127:409–13.
34. Tomoda C, Hirokawa Y, Uruno T, et al. Sensitivity and specificity of intraoperative recurrent laryngeal nerve stimulation test for predicting vocal cord palsy after thyroid surgery. World J Surg. 2006;30:1230–3.
35. Dralle H, Sekulla C, Lorenz K, Brauckhoff M, Machens A. Intraoperative monitoring of the recurrent laryngeal nerve in thyroid surgery. World J Surg. 2008;32:1358–66.
36. Thomusch O, Sekulla C, Machens A, Neumann HJ, Timmermann W, Dralle H. Validity of intraoperative neuromonitoring signals in thyroid surgery. Langenbeck's Arch Surg. 2004;389:499–503.
37. Chan WF, Lo CY. Pitfalls of intraoperative neuromonitoring for predicting postoperative recurrent laryngeal nerve function during thyroidectomy. World J Surg. 2006;30:806–12.
38. Al-Qurayshi Z, Randolph GW, Alshehri M, Kandil E. Analysis of variations in the use of intraoperative nerve monitoring in thyroid surgery. JAMA Otolaryngol Head Neck Surg. 2016;142:584.
39. Goretzki PE, Schwarz K, Brinkmann J, Wirowski D, Lammers BJ. The impact of intraoperative neuromonitoring (IONM) on surgical strategy in bilateral thyroid diseases: is it worth the effort? World J Surg. 2010;34:1274–84.
40. Melin M, Schwarz K, Lammers BJ, Goretzki PE. IONM-guided goiter surgery leading to two-stage thyroidectomy—indication and results. Langenbeck's Arch Surg. 2013;398:411–8.
41. Melin M, Schwarz K, Pearson MD, Lammers BJ, Goretzki PE. Postoperative vocal cord dysfunction despite normal intraoperative neuromonitoring: an unexpected complication with the risk of bilateral palsy. World J Surg. 2014;38:2597–602.
42. Sarkis LM, Zaidi N, Norlen O, Delbridge LW, Sywak MS, Sidhu SB. Bilateral recurrent laryngeal nerve injury in a specialized thyroid surgery unit: would routine intraoperative neuromonitoring alter outcomes? ANZ J Surg. 2017;87:364–7.
43. Sadowski SM, Soardo P, Leuchter I, Robert JH, Triponez F. Systematic use of recurrent laryngeal nerve neuromonitoring changes the operative strategy in planned bilateral thyroidectomy. Thyroid. 2013;23:329–33.
44. Dralle H, Sekulla C, Haerting J, et al. Risk factors of paralysis and functional outcome after recurrent laryngeal nerve monitoring in thyroid surgery. Surgery. 2004;136:1310–22.
45. Zheng S, Xu Z, Wei Y, Zeng M, He J. Effect of intraoperative neuromonitoring on recurrent laryngeal nerve

palsy rates after thyroid surgery—a meta-analysis. J Formos Med Assoc. 2013;112:463–72.
46. Higgins TS, Gupta R, Ketcham AS, Sataloff RT, Wadsworth JT, Sinacori JT. Recurrent laryngeal nerve monitoring versus identification alone on post-thyroidectomy true vocal fold palsy: a meta-analysis. Laryngoscope. 2011;121:1009–17.
47. Pisanu A, Porceddu G, Podda M, Cois A, Uccheddu A. Systematic review with meta-analysis of studies comparing intraoperative neuromonitoring of recurrent laryngeal nerves versus visualization alone during thyroidectomy. J Surg Res. 2014;188:152–61.
48. Lombardi CP, Carnassale G, Damiani G, et al. "The final countdown": is intraoperative, intermittent neuromonitoring really useful in preventing permanent nerve palsy? Evidence from a meta-analysis. Surgery. 2016;160:1693–706.
49. Schneider R, Randolph GW, Barczynski M, et al. Continuous intraoperative neural monitoring of the recurrent nerves in thyroid surgery: a quantum leap in technology. Gland Surg. 2016;5:607–16.
50. Wong KP, Mak KL, Wong CK, Lang BH. Systematic review and meta-analysis on intra-operative neuromonitoring in high-risk thyroidectomy. Int J Surg (London, England). 2017;38:21–30.
51. Thomusch O, Sekulla C, Walls G, Machens A, Dralle H. Intraoperative neuromonitoring of surgery for benign goiter. Am J Surg. 2002;183:673–8.
52. Barczynski M, Konturek A, Cichon S. Randomized clinical trial of visualization versus neuromonitoring of recurrent laryngeal nerves during thyroidectomy. Br J Surg. 2009;96:240–6.
53. Barczynski M, Konturek A, Pragacz K, Papier A, Stopa M, Nowak W. Intraoperative nerve monitoring can reduce prevalence of recurrent laryngeal nerve injury in thyroid reoperations: results of a retrospective cohort study. World J Surg. 2014;38:599–606.
54. Dackiw AP, Rotstein LE, Clark OH. Computer-assisted evoked electromyography with stimulating surgical instruments for recurrent/external laryngeal nerve identification and preservation in thyroid and parathyroid operation. Surgery. 2002;132:1100–6; discussion 1107–8.
55. Echeverri A, Flexon PB. Electrophysiologic nerve stimulation for identifying the recurrent laryngeal nerve in thyroid surgery: review of 70 consecutive thyroid surgeries. Am Surg. 1998;64:328–33.
56. Brauckhoff M, Walls G, Brauckhoff K, Thanh PN, Thomusch O, Dralle H. Identification of the non-recurrent inferior laryngeal nerve using intraoperative neurostimulation. Langenbeck's Arch Surg. 2002;386:482–7.
57. Chan WF, Lang BH, Lo CY. The role of intraoperative neuromonitoring of recurrent laryngeal nerve during thyroidectomy: a comparative study on 1000 nerves at risk. Surgery. 2006;140:866–72. ' discussion 872–3
58. Beldi G, Kinsbergen T, Schlumpf R. Evaluation of intraoperative recurrent nerve monitoring in thyroid surgery. World J Surg. 2004;28:589–91.
59. Terris DJ, Chaung K, Duke WS. Continuous vagal nerve monitoring is dangerous and should not routinely be done during thyroid surgery. World J Surg. 2015;39:2471–6.
60. Almquist M, Thier M, Salem F. Cardiac arrest with vagal stimulation during intraoperative nerve monitoring. Head Neck. 2016;38:E2419.
61. Brennan J, Moore EJ, Shuler KJ. Prospective analysis of the efficacy of continuous intraoperative nerve monitoring during thyroidectomy, parathyroidectomy, and parotidectomy. Otolaryngol Head Neck Surg. 2001;124:537–43.
62. Hemmerling TM, Schmidt J, Bosert C, Jacobi KE, Klein P. Intraoperative monitoring of the recurrent laryngeal nerve in 151 consecutive patients undergoing thyroid surgery. Anesth Analg. 2001;93:396–9, 393rd contents page
63. Lamade W, Meyding-Lamade U, Buchhold C, et al. [First continuous nerve monitoring in thyroid gland surgery]. Chirurg. 2000;71:551–7.
64. Phelan E, Schneider R, Lorenz K, et al. Continuous vagal IONM prevents recurrent laryngeal nerve paralysis by revealing initial EMG changes of impending neuropraxic injury: a prospective, multicenter study. Laryngoscope. 2014;124:1498–505.
65. Schneider R, Randolph GW, Sekulla C, et al. Continuous intraoperative vagus nerve stimulation for identification of imminent recurrent laryngeal nerve injury. Head Neck. 2013;35:1591–8.
66. Lennquist S, Cahlin C, Smeds S. The superior laryngeal nerve in thyroid surgery. Surgery. 1987;102:999–1008.
67. Jansson S, Tisell LE, Hagne I, Sanner E, Stenborg R, Svensson P. Partial superior laryngeal nerve (SLN) lesions before and after thyroid surgery. World J Surg. 1988;12:522–7.
68. Darr AE, Tufano R, Ozdemir S, Kamani D, Hurwitz S, Randolph GW. Superior laryngeal nerve quantitative intraoperative monitoring is possible in all thyroid surgeries. Laryngoscope. 2014;124(4):1035–41.
69. Barczynski M, Randolph GW, Cernea CR, et al. External branch of the superior laryngeal nerve monitoring during thyroid and parathyroid surgery: International neural monitoring study group standards guideline statement. Laryngoscope. 2013;123(Suppl 4):S1–14.
70. Kamani D, Potenza AS, Cernea CR, Kamani YV, Randolph GW. The nonrecurrent laryngeal nerve: anatomic and electrophysiologic algorithm for reliable identification. Laryngoscope. 2015;125:503–8.
71. Brauckhoff M, Machens A, Sekulla C, Lorenz K, Dralle H. Latencies shorter than 3.5 ms after vagus nerve stimulation signify a nonrecurrent inferior laryngeal nerve before dissection. Ann Surg. 2011;253:1172–7.

Complications in Thyroid Surgery

16

Radan Dzodic, Nada Santrac, Ivan Markovic, Marko Buta, and Merima Goran

Introduction

William Stewart Halsted said: *"The extirpation of the thyroid gland for goiter typifies, perhaps, better than any operation, the supreme triumph of the surgeon's art"* [1].

From ancient times, attempts to treat goiter were recorded; however they were rare and related to large goiters with threat to suffocation [2]. The first typical partial thyroidectomy was successfully performed in 1791 by French surgeon Pierre Joseph Desault [3]. However, number of lethal outcomes after thyroid surgery led many great surgeons of that time, such as Robert Liston and Samuel Gross, to think that thyroid surgery is not justified in any case [2]. The great breakthrough in thyroid surgery happened in the second half of the nineteenth century. There were three important events that changed the course of surgery drastically: introduction of general anesthesia in 1846 by Boston dentist William Morton [4], Lister's discovery of antisepsis in 1867 [5], and development of hemostatic forceps in European clinics (around 1870) [2]. The central role among thyroid surgery giants remains reserved for Swiss surgeon Emil Theodor Kocher (1841–1917), acclaimed as the father of thyroid surgery. He was the first "high-volume" endocrine surgeon who showed that surgical training and meticulous technique reduce complications in thyroid surgery. By the end of his life, he managed to reduce perioperative mortality rate during thyroid operations from 40 to 0.5% after over 5000 operations [2]. He is acclaimed not only for mastering the surgical technique, but also for his contributions in physiology and pathology of thyroid gland, for which he was awarded with the Nobel Prize in 1909 [2].

Background

From the very beginnings of thyroid surgery to modern times, the significance of a surgeon remains of the same importance. Surgeon is thought to be an important prognostic factor, not only for the outcome and survival, but also for the complications rate [6]. However, regardless of the improvements in surgical technique and technical support, complications still occur.

Thyroid surgery is the surgery of parathyroid glands and recurrent laryngeal nerves. Injuries to these structures are severe. Other major complications include bleeding, infection, superior laryn-

R. Dzodic (✉) · N. Santrac · I. Markovic · M. Buta · M. Goran
Faculty of Medicine, Department of Surgery, University of Belgrade, Belgrade, Serbia

Department of Endocrine and Head and Neck Surgery, Surgical Oncology Clinic, Institute for Oncology and Radiology of Serbia, Belgrade, Serbia

R. Parameswaran, A. Agarwal (eds.), *Evidence-Based Endocrine Surgery*,
https://doi.org/10.1007/978-981-10-1124-5_16

geal nerve injury, thoracic duct injury, as well as injury of the lateral neck nerves, arteries, and veins. Some minor complications include pain, paresthesia, neck and shoulder stiffness, seroma, poor scaring, granuloma, sinus (fistula), and wound dehiscence. Some of the complications are life threatening, like carotid artery injury or invasion by tumor or infection, skin necrosis, dysphagia, fistulas between organs and skin, chyle leakage and pneumothorax, as well as injuries to the organs (esophagus, larynx, trachea). Tracheomalacia is a dangerous complication, with diverse etiology. Potential causes related to thyroid surgery are trauma by intubation and tracheotomy, external compression of trachea by large thyroid tumors, or locally advanced thyroid malignancy, especially anaplastic carcinoma. Thyrotoxic crisis, as a life-threatening complication of thyroid surgery, can be prevented by good preoperative preparation of patients with hyperthyreosis. Hypothyroidism in patients with total thyroidectomy should not be considered as a complication of the treatment, yet as a malpractice. All patients must have adequate levothyroxine replacement (partial or full), or suppression (in malignant disease), depending on the body weight and the desired serum thyrotropin (TSH) levels.

Bleeding

Bleeding in thyroid surgery can occur during the surgical procedure (intraoperative) or during postoperative course, and it can be arterial, venous, capillary, or combined. It can be dramatic and potentially fatal surgical complication. Life-threatening intraoperative bleedings (IB) are very uncommon nowadays, especially if surgery is performed by a high-volume surgeon. This may be attributed to the fact that most of the patients are treated in specialized centers where the surgical technique is established at the highest level.

Bleeding in the early postoperative course is not frequent and according to the literature its incidence ranges from 0.6 to 2.9% [7]. The critical time for postoperative bleeding (PB) is the initial 6-hours period, but it was also observed during the second postoperative day. Most common causes of PB are loss of an arterial ligature and collapsed veins which were not ligated during surgery. Any effort, cough, vomiting, or blood pressure elevation, can cause hemorrhage.

Risk factors. Increased risk for IB is observed in patients with prolonged systemic anticoagulation treatment, coagulopathies, acetylsalicylic acid use, and low doses of heparin application [8]. Capillary bleeding *ex vacuo* from large surfaces is observed after removing large goiters (400–500 g or more). Patients undergoing reoperations are with increased risk of IB and PB due to fibrosis and disturbed anatomic landmarks. External beam radiotherapy (EBRT) of the neck causes sclerotic changes of capillaries, other vascular structures, and tissues. Thyroid surgery in patients with previous EBRT carries increased risk of IB, even from large arteries (brachiocephalic trunk, common carotid artery). The most severe, even fatal, are injuries of vital blood vessels in the mediastinal region while performing sternotomy or mediastinal dissection after preoperative EBRT.

Presentation. The most dramatic IB in thyroid surgery origins from thyroid arteries and branches, especially in large goiters, or hyperthyreosis, where the caliber of the vessels is very large. Rather severe bleeding is caused by transection of inferior laryngeal artery, and reckless placement of the pens, with ligation or suture, may easily lead to another major complication: accidental injury of the recurrent laryngeal nerve.

The main clinical symptoms of PB include neck swelling, changes of skin color around the wound edges, voice hoarseness, shortness of breath, hematoma formation, or bleeding directly between wound edges [7]. If not recognized on time, growing hematoma can lead to mechanical asphyxia by laryngeal edema or tracheal compression, or even to refractory cardiac and respiratory arrest by irritation of vagal nerves. The amount of blood in the vacuum drainage during the early postoperative course is often unreliable for assessment of PB, since drains are often nonfunctional due to coagulum.

Evaluation. In IB, it is important to identify the injured blood vessel and the leakage point, as well as to assess best options for stopping it. The necessary level of blood vessel ligation should be defined in order to prevent, for example, parathyroid gland ischemia. Close wound observation for signs, as well as monitoring of the drainage, is mandatory in postoperative course for timely verification of the bleeding.

Prevention. Adequate preoperative preparation is important for patients with high risk for IB. Prevention of IB is assured by meticulous surgical technique. Intraoperative hemostasis can be accomplished by ligating, suturing, or clipping, using thermocautery or with different vessel-sealing systems. Intraoperative wound washing and Valsalva maneuver can be useful to identify potential venous bleedings [7]. Intraoperative control of major blood vessels during lateral neck dissection might be difficult in patients who had EBRT and previous surgeries. In these circumstances, bleeding is potentially lethal, and presence of vascular surgeon in the team is strongly advised. Capillary bleeding from large wound surfaces can be prevented by topical hemostatic agents or tissue adhesive application, along with Redon drainage. In patients who had several surgeries or previous EBRT, it is advised to apply Mikulicz's tamponade, along with Redon drainage [9] (Fig. 16.1).

Treatment. Patients with IB require immediate, but careful, ligation, suture, or clip placement. Prior to this, it is necessary to obtain visual control on the parathyroid glands and recurrent laryngeal nerves. In case that transected superior thyroid artery (branches) retracts in the soft tissues, it is possible to control the bleeding by approaching part where it arises from the external carotid artery.

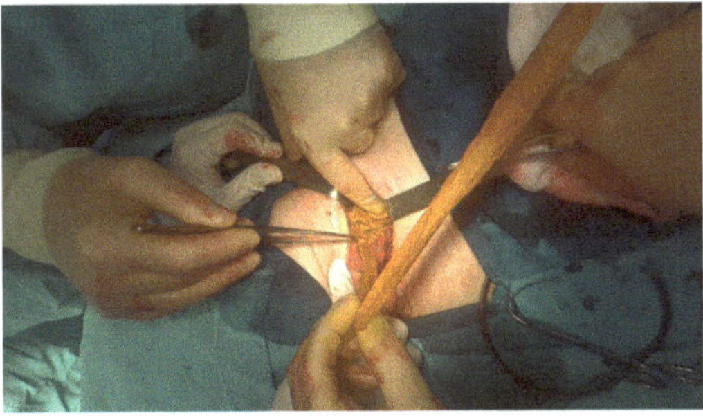

Fig. 16.1 Placing of Mikulicz's tamponade in the central neck region after thyroid carcinoma surgery

In mild PB clinical symptoms and signs, a placement of the Mikulicz's tamponade in thyroid bed should be attempted in sterile conditions, as well as the replacement of the drains. In more severe clinical presentation, urgent in-bed hematoma evacuation is mandatory, followed by urgent intubation in the operating theatre, wound exploration, and definite hemostasis in sterile conditions, with drainage [9, 10]. Mikulicz's tamponade must be removed within 24 h to prevent infection, while Redon drainage is usually kept for 24–48 h.

Infection

Although postoperative wound infection and bleeding accounted for the majority of lethal outcomes after thyroid surgery in the nineteenth century, nowadays these complications are rare. Surgical site infections (SSI) after thyroidectomy are reported between 0.5 and 3% in literature [11–14], being very rare. They occur as a result of an inadequate sterile surgical technique, with skin saprophytes as the most common causes [15]. Many risk factors, preoperative or surgery related (intraoperative), were recognized as important for SSI in thyroid surgery. Although routine antibiotic prophylaxis is not recommended for "clean surgeries" [16], the use of antibiotics in prevention of SSI is rather common [17].

SSI presentation can be mild to severe, even life threatening. The most important is timely diagnosis, providing prompt and adequate treatment, whether conservative or invasive (drainage, surgical re-exploration).

Risk factors. Many perioperative risk factors were recognized as important for development of SSI in thyroid surgery. Some of the significant preoperative factors are obesity, body mass index, American Society of Anesthesiology (ASA) class, weight loss, chronic steroid use, diabetes, chronic obstructive pulmonary disease, congestive heart failure, pneumonia, smoking, and alcohol use [18]. Most important intraoperative factors for SSI are operative time and wound classification, which are directly related to surgical technique, surgery extent, locally advanced tumors, and reoperations. Operative time is prolonged by more extensive thyroid resection, lymph node dissections and reoperations, especially in obese patients [12, 13, 19], which indirectly increases the risk for SSI.

Presentation. SSI in thyroid surgery may manifest as superficial (skin and subcutaneous tissue affected) and deep (deep soft tissues affected, i.e. muscles and fascia) [7]. Mildest form of SSI is cellulitis that manifests with erythema, warmth and tenderness of the skin around the surgical incision, without suppuration. Phlegmon is a more severe, suppurative form of diffuse SSI, affecting neck subcutaneous tissue, with a potential to spread to the mouth floor or mediastinal region, being life threatening. Abscess is a localized SSI, characterized by local inflammation signs and pus. If superficial, it may be fluctuant during palpation, with tenderness. If deep (internal), it may be difficult to diagnose, since the only local manifestation is pain; but the presence of general symptoms like fever, tachycardia and leukocytosis must be an alarm for it [7]. If not recognized on time, it can be manifested as suffocation due to laryngeal edema or tracheal compression.

Evaluation. Close wound observation on regular postoperative checkups is mandatory for local signs of infection (erythema, warmth, swelling, tenderness, pain, loss of function). Pus expressed from the superficial abscess or drained surgically should be analyzed by Gram stain and bacterial culture in order to choose the most adequate antibiotics [7]. Ultrasound evaluation of abscess is useful, as well as computed tomography and endoscopy in deep abscess localization, to exclude organ lesions [7].

Prevention. The key to prevention of SSI is good, anatomic, nonaggressive surgical technique, following rules of asepsis and antisepsis. Routine antibiotic prophylaxis has not been proven beneficial in the literature. The patients with certain risk of SSI should be closely monitored, even discharged form hospital with antibiotic coverage [13]. Intraoperative factors are not always predictable, thus cannot be used for selecting the high-risk patients for prophylactic antibiotic use. However, these patients can be administered antibiotics during surgery or postoperatively, to reduce the possibility for SSI, although these data are not well documented in literature.

Treatment. The most important step in SSI is timely diagnosis, providing prompt and adequate treatment, whether conservative or invasive (drainage, surgical re-exploration). A conservative approach may be considered in patients with superficial SSI and no evident progression [13]. Cellulitis should be treated with antibiotics against gram-positive organisms, according to antibiogram. For deep-neck abscesses, broad-spectrum antibiotics should be used (e.g., cefuroxime, clindamycin) until receiving definitive bacterial culture results [7]. Abscess should be drained, with direct antibiotic coverage according to culture finding. Sometimes, in order to treat severe, life-threatening deep-neck abscess, a surgical re-exploration is necessary.

Hypoparathyroidism

Hypoparathyroidism (HPT) is one of the most frequent and most severe complications of thyroid surgery. Postoperative HPT is caused by intraoperative damage of the parathyroid glands (PTG) or their devascularization, or by accidental removal of unrecognized PTGs. Its prevalence ranges from 19 to 38% in transient, and 0–3% in permanent HPT, although it is probably underestimated [20]. It varies in relation to surgeon's skill and thyroid surgery extent, underlying that the surgeon is a factor of prognosis [6]. HPT treatment consists of alleviating the symptoms, since there is no adequate substitute for parathyroid hormone (PTH). Therefore, preservation of PTG vein and arterial supply is crucial in thyroid surgery [21].

Risk factors. The most important risk factors for HPT are lack of surgeon's experience and traumatic surgical technique [6]. Inexperienced surgeons can remove the PTGs with thyroid gland and lymph nodes, or disrupt their blood supply. "Rough" surgical technique can cause soft-tissue edema and venous stasis, which results in PTG infarction. The incidence of postoperative HPT is directly proportional to surgery extent, being highest in patients with Graves' disease or malignancy, reaching 25% [22]. Reoperations or locally advanced thyroid carcinomas carry significantly higher risk for HPT.

Presentation. Symptoms and signs of hypocalcemia include perioral and digital paresthesia, tetany, carpopedal spasm, positive Trousseau's and Chvostek's sign, mental status changes, laryngospasm, seizures, prolonged QT interval on ECG, and cardiac arrest. Most patients are initially asymptomatic. Symptoms typically develop when adjusted serum calcium levels fall below 1.9 mmol/L, but this is not a rule [7, 23].

Evaluation. All patients with bilateral central neck exploration are at risk for injury of PTGs and should be screened for HPT. PTG function can be assessed by measuring ionized calcium adjusted for albumin and PTH levels, before and after surgery, for comparison. In hypocalcemic patients, normal postoperative PTH level predicts normalization of calcemia [7]. Low PTH levels, with hypocalcemia, select patients at risk for prompt calcium replacement therapy. Some authors recommend introducing therapy if immediate postoperative PTH levels decrease under 1.5 pmol/L and morning serum calcium falls under 2.0 mmol/L [24]. Recent studies [25] suggest measurement of intact PTH on the first postoperative day as an efficient predictor of parathyroid function and a cost-effective way to select patients for calcium and vitamin D supplementation.

Prevention. Prevention of HPT can be achieved either by preservation of PTGs *in situ* on adequate vascular pedicles (venous and arterial) [21, 26–29] or by performing autotransplantation if their blood supply is compromised [30–32]. *Surgical technique of preservation of PTGs in situ* (with intact capsule) includes extracapsular thyroidectomy and meticulous, atraumatic surgery, while maintaining bloodless surgical field [27]. After identification and de-attachment of PTGs from thyroid capsule, and preservation of their arteries, branches of thyroid arteries can be ligated. Preservation of inferior thyroid artery branches is considered a key step in prevention of HPT, since it provides 90% of PTG blood supply; thus ligating the main artery would lead to PTG devascularization [33, 34]. Preservation of venous blood vessels is as equally important as preservation of arterial blood supply, but more technically challenging. Disruption of venous drainage causes venous stasis and PTG infraction, and superior PTGs are at higher risk [35]. It is of great importance to avoid ligation of middle thyroid, i.e. Kocher's vein, because it drains 30% of PTG venous blood. Ligating its branches, instead, avoids venous infraction [21]. Preservation of PTGs is particularly difficult in extracapsular thyroid tumor spread, presence of central lymph node metastases and reoperations. Sometimes PTG needs to be removed, or partially resected, due to its proximity to the thyroid carcinoma. Nowadays, preservation of PTGs is facilitated by utilization of Harmonic scalpel, Ligasure, or bipolar pincette. Dissection is safer using 2.5–3.5 magnification lenses, as well as laryngeal and vagal nerve neuromonitoring. Properly vascularized PTGs have shiny capsule and typical yellowish-brown color. If ischemia is suspected, needle or scalper puncturing, with bleeding as a result, can suggest that PTGs are with good vascularization [21]. Otherwise, if their vascularization is compromised, or they cannot be preserved on vascular pedicles, *autotransplantation of PTGs* should be performed as a standard surgical procedure for preventing HPT [30–32, 36, 37]. Whether reasons for autotransplantation are vascular or oncologic, frozen section analysis needs to be performed to confirm the origin of the tissue. PTG tissue is then sliced into millimeter pieces to ensure good vascularization through passive diffusion. Autotransplantation is most commonly orthotopic (sternocleidomastoid muscle) [31], but it can be heterotopic, as well (different anatomical position, such as brachioradial muscle). Both types of autotransplantation have clear indications, advantages and disadvantages.

Treatment. Management of hypocalcemia depends on the severity of symptoms. Asymptomatic, hypocalcemic patients should not receive calcium supplementation since it may suppress parathyroid function. In patients with acute symptomatology, intravenous calcium gluconate is the preferred therapy. Protocol consists of intravenous administration of 10–20 mL of 10% calcium gluconate in 50–100 mL of 5% dextrose over 10 min, with mandatory ECG monitoring [23]. Chronic hypocalcemia is treated with oral calcium (1–2 g per day in several doses) and vitamin D supplements (calcitriol 0.25–1 mcg per day) [7]. This can be repeated until the patient is asymptomatic. In 1–2 months, serum calcium analysis should be performed, and if findings are satisfactory, oral calcium supplementation can be ceased. If there is no improvement for longer than 6 months, this usually indicates permanent hypoparathyroidism [7]. However, there is no adequate substitute for PTH.

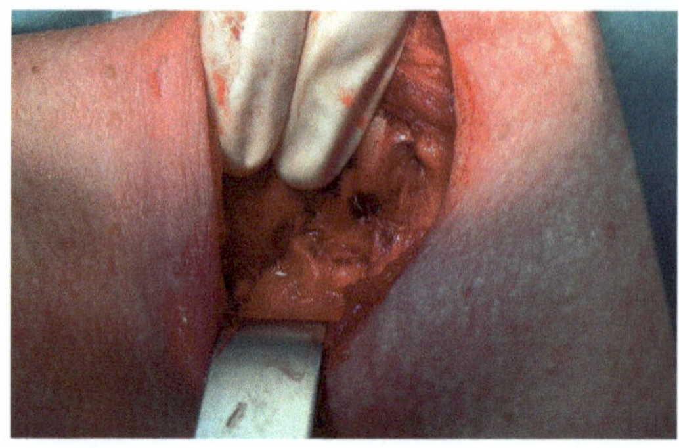

Fig. 16.2 Nonrecurrent course of the inferior laryngeal nerve on the right side of the neck

Recurrent Laryngeal Nerve Injury

Recurrent laryngeal nerve (RLN) injury rates vary in the relevant literature from 0.5 to 10%, reaching up to 20% in more extensive thyroid cancer surgery [38]. Injury mechanisms are various, including compromised blood supply, contusion, traction, thermal damage, misplaced ligation, and complete or partial transection. Prevention of this injury is crucial for good quality of life. Prerequisite for visual identification and RLN preservation is fine surgical technique, with good hemostasis and meticulous dissection, but, above all, an excellent knowledge of RLN anatomy and important thyroid bed landmarks. Treatment of this major, even life-threatening, complication of thyroid surgery is possible and depends on the injury type. Improvement can be rather significant, even complete voice recovery with restoring of vocal cord movement.

Risk factors. Some anatomical landmarks can be very useful for the RLN identification, but there are also great pitfalls in its preservation [38, 39]. These include variations of RLN course on both sides, extralaryngeal terminal RLN branching [40], nonrecurrent course of the inferior laryngeal nerve [41] (Fig. 16.2), variable relations between inferior thyroid artery and RLN [42], Zuckerkandl's tubercle [43], and Berry's ligament. RLN injuries are more common in large hypervascular goiters, adhesions in thyroiditis, thyroid carcinoma surgery, reoperations, or patients with previous EBRT [38, 44]. Extrathyroid tumor extension, malignant RLN infiltration and gross central lymphonodal metastases interfere with RLN identification and adequate preservation. In some cases, it is necessary to "shave off" the tumor from the nerve, performing partial layer resection, which carries risk of certain damage of the RLN function. When RLN transection is inevitable in curative thyroid carcinoma surgery, immediate reconstruction must be performed [45]. Important risk factor for RLN injury is, certainly, the lack of surgeon's experience [46, 47].

Presentation. RLN injuries can be transient or permanent, as well as unilateral or bilateral. The consequence of any RLN injury is a vocal cord paresis or paralysis. Quality of life in patients with RLN palsy, especially permanent, is severely reduced. Symptomatology of RLN palsies varies from mild voice quality changes and breathiness, to dysphagia, aspiration, severe hoarseness, stridor and respiratory distress. Patients with unilateral vocal cord paralysis present with hoarseness or breathiness days to weeks after surgery; further atrophy of the nerve causes worsening of the symptoms [7]. Patients with bilateral vocal cord paralysis usually have acute manifestation after extubation, with stridor, respiratory distress, or both. On occasion, these symptoms are less severe postoperatively, with dyspnea or stridor on exertion at follow-up [7].

Evaluation. Vocal cord mobility should be routinely assessed preoperatively in all patients undergoing thyroid surgery. Techniques of evaluation include indirect and fiber-optic laryngoscopy [7]. Postoperative assessment should also be performed [7], if not immediately after surgery, at least in patients that experience some symptomatology. Laryngeal electromyography should be used to distinguish vocal cord paralysis from injury to the cricoarytenoid joint during intubation, as well as to gather information on prognosis of patients with RLN palsy [48].

Prevention. Palpation and visual identification of RLNs present a "gold standard" in thyroid surgery. It is reported that the RLN injury rate is higher if the nerve is not identified (4–6.6%), compared to the clear visualization (0–2.1%) [7]. Intraoperative nerve monitoring (IONM), if available, can minimize the risk of RLN injury, especially in reoperations [49].

Excellent knowledge of anatomic landmarks and RLN position variations is highly significant for its preservation [7, 46]. Most frequent RLN injuries are misplaced ligations or RLN transections in the vicinity of the crossing point with inferior thyroid artery (branches) [42]. It is very important not to ligate/suture one of the nerve branches if bleeding from inferior thyroid artery occurs. Also, it is advisable to preserve a minimum amount of thyroid tissue at the RLN laryngeal entry point to be sure that the nerve is intact. Fine, meticulous surgical technique enables good control of the hemostasis. Gentle dissection of the nerve, without traction or use of thermocautery in its vicinity, reduces possibility of the iatrogenic nerve damage. Approaches to RLNs should also be modified depending on the pathoanatomic settings. In large mediastinal goiters, RLN position can be anterior to or lateralized by the enlarged lobe. The nerve can be dissected safely from the large goiter back to the tracheoesophageal groove, which prevents its transection during luxation of the goiter. In central neck dissection, it is mandatory to always have visual control over the RLN, especially if metastases are gross or confluent around the nerve circumference. In reoperations, it is more convenient to identify the nerve somewhat lower in the paratracheal region, since there is less scar tissue, or to approach "backdoor" to the tracheoesophageal groove.

In patients with preoperative unilateral vocal cord paralysis, the use of IONM is absolutely indicated. Surgery of benign disease should be sparing in these cases, since there is more damage than benefit of it. In malignant disease, however, depending on the risk for the patient, the surgery extent should be debated. If the risk is low, it would be probably safer to limit surgery to hemithyroidectomy with lymph node staging. On the opposite, oncological treatment should be completed, given the low RLN injury rates in experienced surgeons, the reliability of IONM, and the benefit of complete thyroid removal [7].

Treatment. Complications in thyroid surgery occur even in highly experienced teams [50]. It is, however, important to possess knowledge and skills to diagnose and treat each one of them. Some interventions have to be prompt, and acute, while others can be planned safely. In cases of bilateral RLN injury, presented with complete airway obstruction after extubation, re-intubation has to be performed, sometimes even urgent tracheotomy [7]. Cordotomy and arytenoidectomy are the most common procedures in these patients, with the aim to enlarge the airway and the airflow, which enables patients to be decannulated. In other circumstances, when symptomatology is not life threatening, no corrective procedures are necessary in the first 6 months after total thyroidectomy, since there can be improvement in reversible injuries [7]. In permanent RLN injuries, it is possible to perform medialization, reinnervation, or liberation.

1. Medialization is the most common treatment, performed by ENT specialists, with the goal to improve contact between the vocal cords. The use of absorbable gelatin sponge is a temporary solution, while an implant made of silicone or polytetrafluoroethylene is a permanent one [7].
2. Reinnervation procedures are performed by thyroid surgeons in patients with complete or partial RLN transection. They intend to maintain, or restore, the tonus of the intrinsic laryngeal musculature, which prevents the atrophy of the vocal cords and improves the symptoms [7]. However, they do not restore the vocal cord movement. Nerve reconstruction depends on surgeon's skills and experience [50]. *The primary neurorrhaphy*, or direct suture, provides best outcome in

patients in whom immediate repair is performed after accidental or intentional transection (due to RLN infiltration). In personal series, all patients with immediate direct suture had better phonation 1 month after the procedure, with occasional vocal fatigue that was completely lost 6 months after the repair. On the other hand, one female patient that was given a delayed reconstruction by direct anastomosis 23 years after injury had a full symptoms recovery and small amplitudes of vocal cord movement on laryngoscopy [50]. If end-to-end anastomosis is not possible, reinnervation may be performed by anastomosing the RLN *with ansa cervicalis, phrenic nerve, or preganglionic sympathetic neurons*. Based on personal experience [50], Miyauchi's technique with ansa cervicalis is safe and feasible; it provides good outcome for patients, with no morbidity. Better results are observed in cases of immediate reconstruction. Improved phonation was observed in over 40% of patients 2–6 months after the repair, while it was evident in all patients a year after the reconstruction. Miyauchi's technique is also useful in bilateral RLN paralysis and severe symptomatology, since unilateral reconstruction provides loss of stridorous breathing and dysphonia [50].

3. Liberation is an original technique of Prof. Radan Dzodic [50] that consists of meticulous removal of the misplaced ligation (i.e. granuloma) on the RLN of preserved integrity (Fig. 16.3). Visual identification of RLN is achieved via "backdoor" approach. In personal experience, one patient with RLN paralysis and liberation performed 16 years after the injury had a complete voice recovery, normal vocal cord position and movements on laryngoscopy [50]. Liberation technique is very comfortable and provides complete voice recovery within a few weeks from operation. It is a useful method which enables patients with RLN paresis/paralysis a significant improvement of phonation, being especially beneficial for patients with severe symptomatology and poor quality of life. This procedure should be indicated in all cases when misplaced ligation is verified intraoperatively.

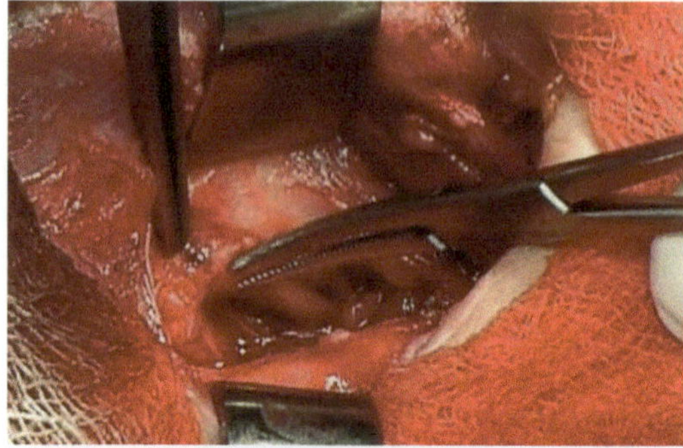

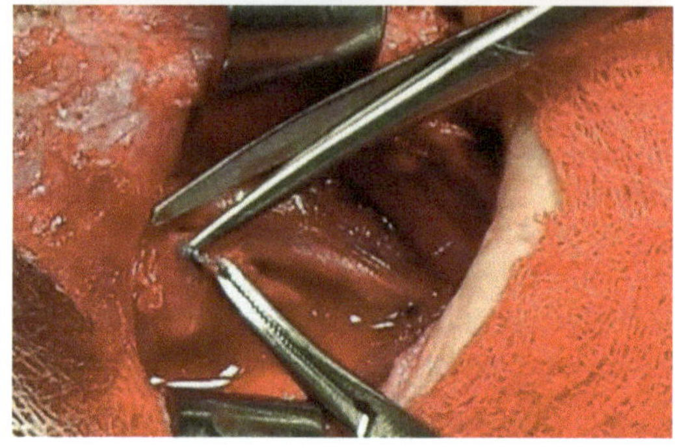

Fig. 16.3 Technique of liberation of recurrent laryngeal nerve from misplaced ligation. On the upper photo, tip of the tweezer is showing a misplaced ligation on the right recurrent laryngeal nerve, at its laryngeal entry point. On the lower photo, misplaced ligation is retracted by the Mosquito forceps, while the ligation is being meticulously removed by scissors. Photos were originally taken during one of the reoperations of thyroid carcinoma, performed in our institution

All procedures that alleviate symptoms of RLN injury have to be accompanied by phoniatric rehabilitation in order for results to be improved and lasting.

External Branch of the Superior Laryngeal Nerve Injury

The external branch of the superior laryngeal nerve (EBSLN) is highly susceptible to damage in thyroid surgery, with injury rates estimated up to 25% [7]. EBSLN trauma results in an inability to create a high-pitched sound. However, the symptoms can be inapparent. Prevention of this injury is of extreme importance, given that the only treatment, so far, is a speech therapy.

Risk factors. The most important risk factors for EBSLN injury are inexperienced surgeon and insufficient knowledge on anatomy. Large hypervascular goiters, high position of the thyroid in the neck, as well as scar tissue from previous surgery, interfere with EBSLN preservation. Locally advanced thyroid carcinoma with cricothyroid muscle infiltration (T4a stage) is a clinicopathological setting that almost certainly will lead to EBSLN dysfunction. Excessive use of thermocautery in the EBSLN vicinity or placing the suture on soft tissues of the upper pole of the lobe can lead to the EBSLN injury. In addition, direct trauma to the cricothyroid muscle with thermocautery can cause muscle dysfunction and presentation similar to EBSLN injury [7].

Presentation. In majority of patients, EBSLN injury is completely inapparent. Sometimes they present with mild hoarseness, decreased vocal stamina, or loss of the upper register [7]. In people who professionally rely on their voice, EBSLN injury has the strongest presentation.

Evaluation. Diagnosis of EBSLN injury is very difficult. On laryngoscopy, posterior glottic rotation toward the paretic side and bowing of the vocal fold on the weak side may be noted; the affected vocal fold may be lower than the normal one. Videostroboscopy demonstrates an asymmetric, mucosal traveling wave. Laryngeal electromyography demonstrates cricothyroid muscle denervation [7].

Prevention. EBSLN, on its course toward cricothyroid muscle [51], lays over lateral surface of the inferior constrictor of the pharynx and it is closely related to the superior thyroid artery (STA) and upper pole of the thyroid lobe. Most commonly, EBSLN crosses STA 1 cm above the upper pole, but it can also cross STA less than 1 cm above, or, rarely, under the upper pole (type 2b nerve) [52]. A critical area where EBSLN gets injured is 1.5–2 cm away from the thyroid capsule [7]. Preventive measures for EBSLN preservation include meticulous dissection and ligation of the STA terminal branches as close to the thyroid capsule as possible, and restricted thermocautery use near the expected anatomical projection of EBSLN. EBSLN should not be visualized and dissected at all costs, but a surgeon must bear in mind its position and vicinity to upper pole of the lobe. Also, dissection near cricothyroid muscle should be safe, and noninvasive, in order to avoid direct muscular damage.

Treatment. In half of the patients with this complication, the EBSLN dysfunction is irreversible [53]. There is no effective treatment for EBSLN injury other than a speech therapy; thus prevention of this complication is an imperative for all surgeons with interest in thyroid. Authors' personal choice is implantation of ansa cervicalis branch into cricothyroid muscle, for it is known that reinnervation affects muscle's structure and function [54], which might alleviate symptomatology.

Thoracic Duct Lesion

Thoracic duct lesion (TDL) is a rare, but severe, complication of thyroid surgery, with an incidence of 1–3% [55]. It manifests with chyle leakage from neck fistula or chylothorax, and is potentially lethal. This injury may occur on the right side of the neck, as well.

Risk factors. TDL in thyroid surgery usually occurs after lateral neck dissections, especially in gross lymph node metastases, or after diagnostic lymph node biopsy of fifth neck region. Anatomical variations [56], reoperations, as well as previous EBRT of the neck [57], increase the risk of TDL.

Presentation. Intraoperative TDL can be recognized immediately. In the postoperative course, patients with TDL usually have milky-white drainage, rarely clear, yellowish (if on fat-free diet). Fistulas can be small (less than 500 mL per day) or large (more than 500 mL, even 2–3 L per day). Consequences of chyle leakage are metabolic, nutritional, and immunological. Severe electrolyte disbalance and hypoproteinemia in prolonged chyle leakage can be lethal. Local wound complications, such as skin damage and wound infection, can also progress to septic complications and death [58].

Evaluation. Patients should be closely monitored for quantity and quality of the wound drainage, along with biochemical analyses.

Prevention. Meticulous surgical technique, surgeon's experience, and anatomy knowledge can prevent TDL. However, if TDL occurs, it is an imperative to recognize this complication intraoperatively and immediately repair, in order to prevent serious consequences.

Treatment. If TDL is recognized during surgery, it is mandatory to try surgical repair with 3-0 or 4-0 nonabsorbable sutures. Soft tissues and surrounding fascia should also be engaged in the sutures to cover the defect in duct wall, but also to reduce the potential space for chyle leakage. Further, muscle flap can be used, mesh, as well as fibrin glue or sclerosing agents (talc or doxycycline). If TDL is recognized postoperatively, first-line treatment is conservative, focusing on reducing the chyle leakage and spontaneous closure of the fistula. These measures include pressure dressing, medium-chain triglyceride enteral diet or total parenteral nutrition, fluid and electrolyte correction, and antibiotic prophylaxis. If drainage is removed, sometimes repeated percutaneous aspirations are necessary [58]. Other conservative measures include negative-pressure wound therapy [58], use of somatostatin and somatostatin analogues (octreotide) [59], or injection of *Pseudomonas aeruginosa* [60]. In case of the conservative treatment failure (drainage >500 mL per day prolonged over a week, or small fistula persistent over a longer period), or occurrence of other complications, treatment approach should be more invasive. One of the options is percutaneous embolization of the thoracic duct performed by intervention radiologist. Other option is surgical exploration, with TDL repair by suture, local tissue flaps, mesh, microsurgical lymphovenous anastomosis, or ligation of thoracic duct [58, 59]. "Redo surgery" is of less success, compared to one-time TDL reparation during initial surgery, due to changes on tissue caused by chyle leakage.

Spinal Accessory Nerve Injury

Spinal accessory nerve (SAN) is usually damaged during lateral neck dissections or cervical lymph node biopsies, in case of posterior triangle lymphadenopathy, especially after previous EBRT or previous operations in this region [61]. This injury leads to isolated trapezius muscle dysfunction, which presents by shoulder drop, displaced scapula, and difficult abduction of the arm. Meticulous surgical technique, knowledge on anatomy and variations, restricted use of thermocautery in the SAN vicinity, and avoiding of excessive nerve traction are prerequisites for good functional and oncological outcome of thyroid surgery [61]. Visual identification of SAN during neck dissection is mandatory for its preservation, and nerve stimulator may be helpful [62]. If SAN has to be sacrificed to achieve clear margins, the sural nerve may be used for reconstruction, or simple direct suture [61].

Horner's Syndrome

Horner's syndrome is a lesion of the neck sympathetic chain, characterized by ptosis, miosis, enophthalmos, and anhidrosis on the side of the injury. It is a very rare complication (0.2%), usually described in literature as case reports. It can occur after thyroid cancer surgery with lateral neck dissections or lymph node biopsy, especially in reoperations or previous EBRT [63, 64]. Injury mechanisms include traction, transection, ischemia, or thermal damage with thermocautery. Depending on the injury mechanism, it can be permanent or transitory (when symptoms persist from several days to several months) [63, 64]. If lesion occurs, vitamin B complex is typically administered.

Minor Complications

Minor complications of thyroid surgery include events related to surgical site like pain, paresthesia, seroma, poor scaring, granuloma, sinus (fistula), and wound dehiscence. These can significantly reduce quality of life due to prolonged hospitalizations or repeated surgeries.

Majority of patients have some type of discomfort at the surgical site. Paresthesia is probably the most common minor complication of thyroid surgery, with underestimated influence on the quality of life. Sometimes numbness of skin up to the submental region is present. Pain is usually acute in over 80% of patients, but it can persist 3 months after surgery or more (chronic in 5%).

Surgical site seromas are a common postoperative complication. If they are small, spontaneous resorption in a few days is possible. Large seromas may be aspirated under sterile conditions, sometimes in a repeated manner. It is debatable in the relevant literature whether there is usefulness in draining of the wound postoperatively and for how long [7]. However, drain may suggest increased wound discharge, and keeping it longer prevents seroma formation.

Poor scar formation can refer to keloids on skin incision or skin "sticking" to underlying structures, producing a tension while swallowing. It is frequent after wound infection and in darker skin tone. Also, presternal drainage most commonly results in keloid scarring. Prevention of poor scarring consists of placing incision in a natural skin crease over the thyroid gland, to provide adequate exposure, while minimizing retraction trauma of the incision edges. However, if the damage to the skin edges is significant, they can be resected prior to wound closure [7]. Keloid scar treatment is complex and prolonged. Treatment modalities include radiotherapy, corticosteroid application, or redo surgeries for excision.

Granulomas form around surgical suture, commonly around nonabsorbable materials. Sometimes, they result in a small abscess around the suture that discharges through skin, forming a tract or fistula called sinus [7]. Prevention of these complications consists of placing a reasonable number of ligatures during surgery. Treatment is surgical excision of granulomas or fistulas.

Wound dehiscence usually occurs if surgical sutures are removed too soon, or in patients that had EBRT of the neck, and can be prevented.

Sometimes, minor complications can take chronic course, reducing the quality of patient's life. The most difficult are deformities on the neck region as a result of mutilation and extensive scars.

Conclusion

Thyroid surgery is the surgery of PTGs and RLNs. Injuries to these structures are severe, but preventable, as well as other complications. The key to prevention is meticulous surgical technique, with excellent knowledge on anatomic landmarks and variations in the neck. This reduces intraoperative and postoperative bleeding rates, as well as the risk for SSI and occurrence of minor complications. Palpation and visual identification of RLN are a gold standard for its preservation, bearing in mind that it can have nonrecurrent course. PTGs should be gently handled to avoid their injury. It is as equally important to preserve their venous drainage, not only their arterial blood supply. Timely diagnosis and adequate treatment of every complication are mandatory. Hypoparathyroidism requires calcium and PTH monitoring, with calcium substitution for as much time as necessary. It is possible to alleviate symptoms of injured RLNs by one of these surgical techniques: medialization, reinnervation, or nerve liberation. Surgeon is the most important prognostic factor, not only for the outcome and survival, but also for the complications rate.

Clinical Pearls

1. There are two key steps in PTG preservation *in situ*: (a) avoid ligation of inferior thyroid artery (it provides 90% of PTG blood supply) - instead ligate its branches; and (b) avoid ligation of Kocher's vein (it drains 30% of PTG venous blood) - instead ligate its branches close to thyroid capsule.
2. It is imperative to visualize RLN and meticulously preserve it up to the laryngeal entry point, without traction or use of thermocautery in its vicinity. Prior to identification, it is possible to palpate it.
3. Reinnervation procedures do not restore the vocal cord movement; however, they restore the tonus of the intrinsic laryngeal musculature, which prevents the atrophy of the vocal cords and alleviate symptomatology.
4. RLN liberation by removal of the misplaced ligation (i.e. granuloma) on the RLN of preserved integrity is a very comfortable technique that provides complete voice recovery within a few weeks from operation.

References

1. Halsted WS. The operative history of goiter: the author's operation. Johns Hopkins Hosp Rep. 1920;19:71–257.
2. Becker WF. Presidential address: pioneers in thyroid surgery. Ann Surg. 1977;185(5):493–504.
3. Desault PJ. Giraud. J Chir (Paris) 1792; 3:3.
4. History of Anaesthesia Society. 2017. http://www.histansoc.org.uk/timeline.html. Accessed 20 Jan 2017.
5. Pitt D, Aubin JM. Joseph Lister: father of modern surgery. Can J Surg. 2012;55(5):E8–9.
6. Pasieka JL. The surgeon as a prognostic factor in endocrine surgical diseases. Surg Oncol Clin N Am. 2000;9(1):13–20.
7. Sharma PK. Complications of thyroid surgery. 2016. http://emedicine.medscape.com/article/852184-overview#a1. Accessed 20 Dec 2016.
8. Promberger R, Ott J, Kober F, et al. Risk factors for postoperative bleeding after thyroid surgery. Br J Surg. 2012;99(3):373–9.
9. Orsoni JL, Charleux H. Rehabilitation of Mikulicz's drain. An irreplaceable procedure in difficult drainage [Article in French]. Presse Med. 1983;12(12):757–9.
10. Rosenbaum MA, Haridas M, McHenry CR. Life-threatening neck hematoma complicating thyroid and parathyroid surgery. Am J Surg. 2008;195(3):339–43.
11. Rosato L, Avenia N, Bernante P, et al. Complications of thyroid surgery: analysis of a multicentric study on 14,934 patients operated on in Italy over 5 years. World J Surg. 2004;28:271.
12. Bergenfelz A, Jansson S, Kristoffersson A, et al. Complications to thyroid surgery: results as reported in a database from a multicenter audit comprising 3,660 patients. Langenbeck's Arch Surg. 2008;393:667.
13. Dionigi G, Rovera F, Boni L, Dionigi R. Surveillance of surgical site infections after thyroidectomy in a one-day surgery setting. Int J Surg. 2008;6(l):S13–5.
14. De Palma M, Grillo M, Borgia G, et al. Antibiotic prophylaxis and risk of infections in thyroid surgery: results from a national study (UEC-Italian Endocrine Surgery Units Association). Updates Surg. 2013;65:213–6.
15. Dionigi G, Rovera F, Boni L, Castano P, Dionigi R. Surgical site infections after thyroidectomy. Surg Infect. 2006;7(2):S117–20.
16. Mangram AJ, Horan TC, Pearson ML, et al. Guideline for prevention of surgical site infection, 1999. Centers for Disease Control and Prevention (CDC) Hospital Infection Control Practices Advisory Committee. Am J Infect Control. 1999;27(2):97–132.
17. Moalem J, Ruan DT, Farkas RL, et al. Patterns of antibiotic prophylaxis use for thyroidectomy and parathyroidectomy: results of an international survey of endocrine surgeons. J Am Coll Surg. 2010;210(6):949–56.
18. Elfenbein DM, Schneider DF, Chen H, Sippel RS. Surgical site infection after thyroidectomy: a rare but significant complication. J Surg Res. 2014;190(1):170–6.
19. Buerba R, Roman SA, Sosa JA. Thyroidectomy and parathyroidectomy in patients with high body mass index are safe overall: analysis of 26,864 patients. Surgery. 2011;150(5):950–8.
20. Edafe O, Antakia R, Laskar N, Uttley L, Balasubramanian SP. Systematic review and meta-analysis of predictors of post-thyroidectomy hypocalcaemia. Br J Surg. 2014;101(4):307–20.
21. Dzodic RR. Prevention of hypoparathyroidism in total thyroidectomies. Doctoral dissertation. Belgrade: Medical Faculty, University of Belgrade; 1994.
22. Shaha AF, Burnett C, Jaffe B. Parathyroide autotransplantation during thyroid surgery. J Surg Oncol. 1991;46(1):21–4.
23. Turner J, Gittoes N, Selby P. Society for Endocrinology Clinical Committee. Emergency management of acute hypocalcaemia in adult patients. Endocr Connect. 2016;5(5):G7–8.
24. Wong C, Price S, Scott-Coombes D. Hypocalcaemia and parathyroid hormone assay following total thyroidectomy: predicting the future. World J Surg. 2006;30(5):825–32.
25. Selberherr A, Scheuba C, Riss P, Niederle B. Postoperative hypoparathyroidism after thyroidectomy: efficient and cost-effective diagnosis and treatment. Surgery. 2015;157(2):349–53.
26. Halsted WS, Evans HM. The parathyroid glandules. Their blood supply and their preservation in operation upon the thyroid gland. Ann Surg. 1907;46(4):489–506.
27. Attie JN, Khafif RA. Preservation of parathyroid glands during total thyreoidectomy. Improved technique utilizing microsurgery. Am J Surg. 1975;130(4):399–404.
28. Dunlop DAB, Papapoulos SE, Lodge RW, Fulton AJ, Kendall BE, O'Riordan JLH. Parathyroid venous sampling: anatomic considerations and results in 95 patients with primary hyperparathyroidism. Br J Radiol. 1980;53:183–91.
29. Schwartz AE, Friedman EW. Preservation of the parathyroid glands in total thyroidectomy. Surg Gynecol Obstet. 1987;165:327–32.
30. Alveryd A. Parathyroid glands in thyroid surgery. Acta Chir Scand (Suppl). 1968;389:1–120.
31. Wells SA Jr, Gunnells JC, Shelburne JD, Schneider AB, Sherwood LM. Transplantation of the parathyroid glands in man: clinical indications and results. Surgery. 1975;78(1):34–44.
32. Paloyan E, Lawrence AM, Paloyan D. Successful autotransplantation of the parathyroid glands during total thyreoidectomy for carcinoma. Surg Gynecol Obstet. 1977;145(3):364–8.
33. Wang C. The anatomic basis of parathyroid surgery. Ann Surg. 1976;183(3):271–5.
34. Delattre JF, Flament JB, Palot JP, Pluot M. Les variations des parathyroids. J Chir (Paris). 1982;119(11):633–41.
35. Cannoni M, Pech A, Tiziano JP, Thomassin JM, Goubert JL, Zanaret M, Abdoul S. Le risque parathyroidien dans les thyroidectomies. Ann Otolaryngol Chir Cervicofac. 1982;99:237–44.

36. Matsuura H, Sako K, Marchetta FC. Successful reimplantation of autogenous parathyroids tissue. Am J Surg. 1969;118(5):779–82.
37. Hickey RC, Samaan NA. Human parathyroid autotransplantation: proved function by radioimmunoassay of plasma parathyroid hormone. Arch Surg. 1975;110(8):892–5.
38. Calò PG, Pisano G, Medas F, Tatti A, Tuveri M, Nicolosi A. Risk factors in reoperative thyroid surgery for recurrent goitre: our experience. G Chir. 2012;33(10):335–8.
39. Gurleyik E. Surgical anatomy of bilateral extralaryngeal bifurcation of the recurrent laryngeal nerve: similarities and differences between both sides. N Am J Med Sci. 2014;6(9):445–9.
40. Pradeep PV, Jayashree B, Harshita SS. A closer look at laryngeal nerves during thyroid surgery: a descriptive study of 584 nerves. Anat Res Int. 2012;2012:490390.
41. Donatini G, Carnaille B, Dionigi G. Increased detection of non-recurrent inferior laryngeal nerve (NRLN) during thyroid surgery using systematic intraoperative neuromonitoring (IONM). World J Surg. 2013;37(1):91–3.
42. Yalçin B. Anatomic configurations of the recurrent laryngeal nerve and inferior thyroid artery. Surgery. 2006;139(2):181–7.
43. Gurleyik E, Gurleyik G. Incidence and surgical importance of Zuckerkandl's tubercle of the thyroid and its relations with recurrent laryngeal nerve. ISRN Surg. 2012;2012:450589.
44. Hayward NJ, Grodski S, Yeung M, Johnson WR, Serpell J. Recurrent laryngeal nerve injury in thyroid surgery: a review. ANZ J Surg. 2013; 83(1–2):15–21.
45. Feng Y, Yang D, Liu D, Chen J, Bi Q, Luo K. Immediate recurrent laryngeal nerve reconstruction in the treatment of thyroid cancer invading the recurrent laryngeal nerve. Zhonghua Zhong Liu Za Zhi. 2014;36(8):621–5.
46. Randolph GW. Surgical anatomy of the recurrent laryngeal nerve. In: Randolph GW, editor. Surgery of the thyroid and parathyroid glands. Philadelphia: Saunders-Elsevier; 2003. p. 300–42.
47. Miyauchi A, Ishikawa H, Matsusaka K, et al. Treatment of recurrent laryngeal nerve paralysis by several types of nerve suture. Nihon Geka Gakkai Zasshi. 1993;94(6):550–5.
48. Parnes SM, Satya-Murti S. Predictive value of laryngeal electromyography in patients with vocal cord paralysis of neurogenic origin. Laryngoscope. 1985;95(11):1323–6.
49. Barczyński M, Konturek A, Pragacz K, Papier A, Stopa M, Nowak W. Intraoperative nerve monitoring can reduce prevalence of recurrent laryngeal nerve injury in thyroid reoperations: results of a retrospective cohort study. World J Surg. 2014;38(3):599–606.
50. Dzodic R, Markovic I, Santrac N, Buta M, Djurisic I, Lukic S. Recurrent laryngeal nerve liberations and reconstructions: a single institution experience. World J Surg. 2016;40(3):644–51.
51. Cernea CR, Ferraz AR, Cordeiro AC. Surgical anatomy of the superior laryngeal nerve. In: Randolph GW, editor. Surgery of the thyroid and parathyroid glands. Philadelphia: Saunders-Elsevier; 2003. p. 293–9.
52. Cernea CR, Dedivitis RA, Ferraz AR, Brandão LG. How to avoid injury of the external branch of superior laryngeal nerve. In: Cernea CR, Dias FL, Fliss D, Lima RA, Myers EN, Wei WI, editors. Pearls and pitfalls in head and neck surgery. Basel: Karger; 2012. p. 4–5.
53. Cernea CR, Ferraz AR, Furlani J, et al. Identification of the external branch of the superior laryngeal nerve during thyroidectomy. Am J Surg. 1992;164(6):634–9.
54. Steindler A. Direct neurotization of paralyzed muscles: further study of the question of direction nerve implantation. Am J Orthop Surg. 1916;14:707–19.
55. Shimada K, Sato I. Morphological and histological analysis of the thoracic duct at the jugulo-subclavian junction in Japanese cadavers. Clin Anat. 1997;10(3):163–72.
56. Santaolalla F, Anta JA, Zabala A, Del Rey Sanchez A, Martinez A, Sanchez JM. Management of chylous fistula as a complication of neck dissection: a 10-year retrospective review. Eur J Cancer Care (Engl). 2010;19(4):510–5.
57. Zapanta PE. Chylous fistula of the neck. 2016. http://emedicine.medscape.com/article/1418727-overview. Accessed 20 Dec 2016.
58. Polistena A, Vannucci J, Monacelli M, et al. Thoracic duct lesions in thyroid surgery: An update on diagnosis, treatment and prevention based on a cohort study. Int J Surg. 2016;28(Suppl 1):S33–7.
59. Barili F, Polvani G, Topkara VK, et al. Administration of octreotide for management of postoperative high-flow chylothorax. Ann Vasc Surg. 2007;21(1):90–2.
60. Wei T, Liu F, Li Z, Gong Y, Zhu J. Novel management of intractable cervical chylous fistula with local application of Pseudomonas aeruginosa injection. Otolaryngol Head Neck Surg. 2015;153(4):561–5.
61. Oxford LE, O'Brien JC Jr. How to manage the XI nerve in neck dissections. In: Cernea CR, Dias FL, Fliss D, Lima RA, Myers EN, Wei WI, editors. Pearls and pitfalls in head and neck surgery. Basel: Karger; 2012. p. 44–5.
62. Müller-Vahl H. Iatrogenic spinal accessory nerve injury. Ann R Coll Surg Engl. 1983;65(4):276–7.
63. González-Aguado R, Morales-Angulo C, Obeso-Agüera S, Longarela-Herrero Y, García-Zornoza R, Acle Cervera L. Horner's syndrome after neck surgery. Acta Otorrinolaringol Esp. 2012;63(4):299–302.
64. Giannaccare G, Gizzi C, Fresina M. Horner syndrome following thyroid surgery: the clinical and pharmacological presentations. J Ophthalmic Vis Res. 2016;11(4):442–4.

17 Endoscopic and Robotic Thyroidectomy: An Evidence Approach

Xueying Goh and Chwee Ming Lim

Introduction

Thyroidectomy performed via the midline transverse incision remains the standard thyroidectomy approach ever since Theodor Kocher revolutionised thyroid surgery with his technique in the 1800s. With enhanced optics and development of energy devices capable of sealing moderate-calibre (5–8 mm) vessels, the ability to perform thyroidectomy through small midline incisions or via remote access incisions is made possible. Moreover, the desire of some patients to avoid conspicuous midline neck scars led to the push for alternate approaches to the thyroid through remote-access incisions.

In this chapter, we will review the evidence in the use of endoscopic and robotic thyroidectomy in the management of thyroid diseases.

X. Goh
Department of Otolaryngology—Head and Neck Surgery, National University Health System, Singapore, Singapore

C. M. Lim (✉)
Department of Otolaryngology—Head and Neck Surgery, National University Health System, Singapore, Singapore

Department of Otolaryngology, National University of Singapore, Singapore, Singapore
e-mail: chwee_ming_lim@nuhs.edu.sg

Background of Endoscopic/Robotic Thyroidectomy Development

The first use of endoscopic system in thyroidectomy was first described by Miccoli where he pioneered the minimally invasive video-assisted thyroidectomy (MIVAT) technique, utilising a small 2 cm midline skin crease incision. Thyroidectomy was performed in the usual fashion through the midline, but with the aid of endoscope visualisation and energy devices, the ability to perform thyroidectomy was made possible via this small mini skin crease incision. This technique not only resulted in a better cosmetic outcome, but also reduced hospital stay by negating the possible need for surgical drains [1, 2].

In an Asian patient cohort, where there is a predisposition to hypertrophic scar or where there is a cultural bias of not having a surgical midline neck scar, remote-access thyroidectomy is an attractive technique in managing this group of patients. Ohgami in 2000 first described a remote-access thyroidectomy technique performed using endoscope through the breast approach, and this was sequentially reported by Ikeda who described the transaxillary endoscopic thyroidectomy in 2001 [3, 4]. Subsequently, other endoscopic remote-access approaches have been developed and performed safely and effectively, when compared to standard midline thyroidectomy.

In 2009, Kang et al. from South Korea popularised the transaxillary robotic assisted

R. Parameswaran, A. Agarwal (eds.), *Evidence-Based Endocrine Surgery*,
https://doi.org/10.1007/978-981-10-1124-5_17

thyroidectomy using the da Vinci robot (Intuitive Surgical Inc., Sunnyvale California, USA) [5]. With this success, other groups have established a viable alternative of remote-access robotic assisted thyroidectomy via the retroauricular approach [6].

Recently, following the success of the remote-access thyroidectomy techniques, a truly 'scar-less' thyroid surgery performed using the natural orifice transluminal endoscopic surgery (NOTES) philosophy was established via the transoral approach. Wilhelm first described transoral endoscopic thyroid surgery in humans in 2010 via sublingual approach, while Wang and Nakajo modified this to the oral vestibule approach [7–9]. A recent case series by Anuwong et al. presented the largest series of transoral thyroidectomy of 60 cases demonstrating its feasibility and efficacy, and thus offering another viable remote-access approach in thyroidectomy [10].

Candidacy for Endoscopic or Robotic Thyroidectomy

The selection criteria and contraindications for endoscopic or robotic thyroidectomy vary between institutions, and correlate with the centre's experience and volume. The American Thyroid Association (ATA) statement on remote-access thyroidectomy recommends the following factors for patient selection [11]:

Patient factors

1. Thin body habitus (body mass index (BMI) <35 kg/m^2)[1]
2. Absence of excessive body fat along flap trajectory

Disease factors

1. Well circumscribed <3 cm nodule on ultrasound
2. Thyroid lobe <5–6 cm in largest dimension
3. No ultrasound features of thyroiditis

Absolute contraindications

1. Thyroid cancer with gross extrathyroidal extension
2. Thyroid cancer with lymph node involvement
3. Retrosternal extension
4. Graves' disease
5. Previous neck surgery

However, these candidacy criteria are evolving as many high-volume thyroidectomy centres have reported good safety and oncologic results even in cancers requiring either central and/or lateral neck dissections [6, 14–17].

Surgical Techniques

Surgical approaches for endoscopic and robotic thyroidectomies can be broadly classified into transcervical approach and remote-access approach. Remote-access approaches are further classified according to the midline approaches and the lateral approaches to the thyroid bed. Table 17.1 summarises the endoscopic and robotic assisted thyroidectomy.

Table 17.1 Endoscopic and robotic thyroidectomy approaches

Transcervical approaches
1. Minimally invasive video-assisted thyroidectomy (MIVAT)
Remote-access approaches
1. Midline approaches
(a) Breast approach
(b) Combined breast-axillary approach
Axillo-bilateral breast approach (ABBA)
Bilateral axillo-breast approach (BABA)
(c) Natural orifice/transoral thyroidectomy
Sublingual approach
Vestibular approach
2. Lateral approaches
(a) Transaxillary approach
(b) Retroauricular/modified facelift approach

[1]The ATA statement did not qualify the definition of thin habitus, but many authors have used an arbitrary BMI cut-off of less than 35–40 in transaxillary and retroauricular thyroidectomies [12, 13].

Transcervical Approaches [18, 19]

Minimally invasive video-assisted thyroidectomy (MIVAT) is the commonest endoscopic assisted transcervical midline approach to the thyroid. This is performed by placing a 2 cm midline skin crease incision. Subplatysmal flaps are not typically raised, and the dissection is deepened till the strap muscles. At this point, the strap muscles are separated in the midline and the thyroid gland is exposed. A specially- designed mini right-angle 'Miccoli' retractor is used to retract the strap muscles and blunt dissection is performed to free the thyroid off the strap muscles. The 30° angled endoscopes is then introduced and using an energy device, the superior thyroid vessels are dissected and divided. The endoscope affords magnified high-definition view of the surgical bed allowing the external branch of the superior laryngeal nerve (EBSLN) to be typically identified and preserved. The thyroid gland is then rotated medially and delivered out of the wound to expose the tracheoesophageal groove. The recurrent laryngeal nerve (RLN) is then identified and the gland dissected off the Berry's ligament. After hemostasis, the straps are tagged loosely with a single suture and wound is closed like in a conventional thyroidectomy. Surgical drains are not typically placed because the area of dissection is fairly limited. The main drawback is that this approach is reserved for small nodules (usually less than 2 cm).

Remote-Access Thyroidectomy

1. **Midline** [4, 10, 14, 17, 20–23]
   Breast
   The first remote-access thyroidectomy was the endoscopic breast approach reported by Ohgami et al. [4]. This approach was subsequently modified to combined breast and axillary approaches such as the endoscopic axillo-bilateral breast approach (ABBA) first described by Shimazu in 2002 [20], and the endoscopic and robotic bilateral axillo-breast approach (BABA) described by Choi et al. in 2007 [17]. These midline approaches have their surgical ports inserted at the periareolar creases, parasternal as well as axilla for endoscopic or robotic instruments to be inserted. Carbon dioxide insufflation is needed to create the surgical working space. Each technique uses different variations of ports and instrument placement to approach the thyroid and is beyond the scope of this chapter.
   Transoral
   Transoral thyroidectomy is performed either via the vestibule or via trans-floor of mouth approach with the former gaining more popularity as it does not crease a fistula into the neck. However, the mental nerve is at risk of injury with the trans-vestibule approach and care is needed to avoid the expected direction of the mental nerve during the port placement. The working space is created typically using carbon dioxide insufflation with the endoscope camera positioned in the midline through a subplatysmal tunnel. Once the working space is created, two separate instruments (energy device and a grasper forceps) are placed at 30–45 angles to the midline port. This surgical field afforded by this approach is similar to open thyroidectomy and therefore can be learned fairly quickly by thyroid surgeons. In a similar fashion, the midline raphe of the strap muscle is divided and the thyroid gland is exposed. The superior thyroid artery is ligated between the energy devices before the gland is retracted medially to expose the tracheoesophageal groove. A main difference in this approach is that the RLN is typically identified near the cricothyroid joint when it enters the larynx. Both parathyroid glands are usually well visualised during the dissection and can be safely preserved. One of the drawbacks in this approach is the need to morselize the thyroid gland in order to deliver the gland through the midline 1 cm incision. This is done via an Endo Catch bag (Covidien-Medtronic, Minnesota, USA) to avoid spillage during the delivery process.
2. **The lateral approaches** [3, 5, 12, 13, 24, 25]
   Transaxillary
   Transaxillary thyroidectomy is one of the commonest remote-access approaches which was first described as an endoscopic technique by Ikeda et al. and subsequently popularised

by Chung et al. using the Da Vinci robot [3, 26]. The patient is laid supine with mild head extension with the arm adducted and flexed at the shoulder in order to expose the axilla. This positioning can cause brachial plexopathy and hence some centres advocate intraoperative somatosensory evoked potential (SSEP) monitoring of the median and ulnar nerve to prevent this complication. In our experience, using a modified arm position with lesser shoulder extension and abduction has not resulted in brachial plexopathy due to less traction of these nerves during surgery. This approach can be done either with carbon dioxide (CO_2) insufflation or with a gasless approach. In the insufflation technique, trocars are placed in the axillary region as well as an optional working port inferomedial to the main axillary port. The plane is dissected superficial to the pectoralis major (PM) around the clavicle and towards the sternocleidomastoid (SCM), before dissecting beneath the strap muscles laterally and identifying the omohyoid muscle. Once the omohyoid is retracted, the thyroid gland is usually well visualised. In the gasless technique, a 5–6 cm incision is made in the axilla around 5–8 mm inferior to the anterior axillary fold. This is followed raising a subcutaneous flap towards the clavicle superficial to the PM, and subsequently in the subplatysmal plane over the strap muscle. The strap muscles are raised off the gland and a Chung retractor (Marina Medical, Sunrise, Florida, USA) is placed to retract the strap muscles to expose the thyroid gland from the lateral approach. The robot may be docked subsequently to perform the thyroidectomy.

Several centres have reported concurrent robot-assisted central neck dissection with total thyroidectomies utilising the same transaxillary incision. However, visualisation of the contralateral RLN through the ipsilateral incision is limited, and this surgery should be reserved for thyroid surgeons conversant and experienced with robotic thyroidectomy.

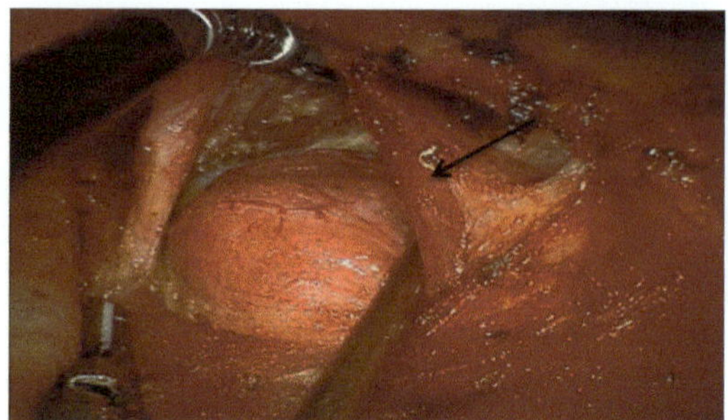

Fig. 17.1 Retroauricular robotic assisted left thyroidectomy. The omohyoid (black arrow) is retracted exposing the left thyroid lobe

Retroauricular

Retroauricular or modified 'facelift' approach was first described by Terris et al. in 2011 as a robotic approach [12, 25]. This approach was initially developed to address the shortcomings of the transaxillary approach through an easier positioning of patient, avoidance of brachial plexopathy and a shorter dissection distance to the thyroid bed from the retroauricular incision. This technique is performed using a gasless technique and uses a rhytidectomy incision that is raised superficial to the SCM. The thyroid is then approached laterally under the strap muscles after retraction of the omohyoid muscle, as in a lateral approach to the thyroid (Fig. 17.1). A modified 'Chung' retractor is then used to retract the strap muscle and the thyroid gland is exposed. Due to its versatility and the familiarity with head and neck surgeons, the retroauricular approach is quickly developing into the 'workhorse' approach for robotic head and neck surgery in some centres, where total thyroidectomies, submandibular gland excision, lateral neck dissections, Sistrunk procedures and neck mass excisions have been described [6].

Evidence-Based Data

Despite the emerging use of these alternate approaches, it is important to be cognizant of their possible drawbacks, since the morbidity of the conventional open thyroidectomy surgery is low.

Although there are numerous studies that report superior outcomes for these alternative approaches, such as reduced inpatient stay, reduced post-operative pain and reduced need for drains (for MIVAT), the main benefit of these alternative approach over the traditional approach is the superior cosmetic outcomes. Not surprisingly, these approaches, especially the remote-access approaches, have not gained worldwide endorsement in thyroidectomy given the familiarity, safety and effectiveness of the traditional midline approach, and the increased costs and learning curves required to master these techniques. Most published data are limited to large-volume case series reports in high-volume thyroidectomy centres and several meta-analyses have also been performed to evaluate the safety, efficacy, complication rate and clinical outcome of these alternative techniques. The evidence for performing endoscopic/robotic thyroidectomies is summarised as follows, and presented in Table 17.3.

Cosmesis and Patient Satisfaction

Compared with conventional thyroidectomy (CT), many studies have showed better visual numeric scale or verbal scaled response perception of cosmetic results in favour of MIVAT [2, 27]. Similarly many studies have shown superior patient-reported cosmetic outcome for remote-access robotic or endoscopic thyroidectomies compared to open thyroidectomies [9, 28–32].

Given the minimally invasive nature of the MIVAT, apart from better cosmesis, lower post-operative pain scores have been seen compared to open thyroidectomy [2, 27]. Ikeda similarly reported improved swallowing functions following after endoscopic transaxillary thyroidectomy compared with the open technique [26].

Operative Time and Learning Curve

These remote-access thyroidectomies are intuitively more time consuming, due to a more extensive dissection, difficulty in manipulation of the rigid endoscopic instruments and docking time of the surgical robot. This aspect has been borne out with the literature favouring a shorter operative time with CT. Lang et al. in a meta-analysis comparing robotic and endoscopic techniques found no significant difference in the operative time between endoscopic and robotic approaches when analysed according to the extent of surgery [33]. However it is reported that robotic thyroidectomy has a shorter learning curve compared to endoscopic thyroidectomy, with surgeons requiring 35–45 robotic cases and 55–70 endoscopic cases to reach a plateau of operating time [15]. Interestingly, the operating times seem to continue to decline for endoscopic surgery compared to robotic surgery, with endoscopic thyroidectomy reaching a shorter 'steady-state' operative time in the long run [34].

Oncological Outcomes

As experience increases in several centres with these alternative approaches, indications have been extended to concurrent lateral and/or central neck dissection, in addition to total thyroidectomy. Using serum thyroglobulin (Tg) as a surrogate indicator of surgical completeness in thyroid cancer, Miccoli reported in his experience with MIVAT that after total thyroidectomy, 85.2% had undetectable Tg levels post-surgery, with the remaining having a low mean Tg value of 0.47 ng/mL. Lee et al. similarly studied the surgical completeness of robotic gasless transaxillary thyroidectomy versus open thyroidectomy, and found similar stimulated Tg levels post-total thyroidectomy, but the post-surgical radioactive iodine (RAI) uptake was significantly higher ($p = 0.004$) in the robotic thyroidectomy group. This is attributed to the fact that the contralateral lobectomy was performed using the same axillary incision for the robotic group and consequently a small remnant thyroid tissue near the contralateral Berry's ligament may be left behind due to difficult visualisation and also to minimise thermal injury to the RLN from the ultrasonic sealing device [35]. However, there was no significant difference in the radioiodine nuclide update following RAI ablation. In a more recent meta-analysis by Son et al., pooled data from five studies did not find any significant difference in the post-operative stimulated Tg levels between open and robotic thyroidectomy [31]. This may be due to the increased expertise and experience coming from the more recent publications in these high-volume thyroidectomy centres. With respect to neck dissection done for thyroid cancers, Son et al. reported significantly fewer retrieved neck nodes in the robotic thyroidectomy group compared to the open thyroidectomy group. This finding holds true in both central neck dissection and modified radical neck dissection specimen performed for thyroid cancers [31].

The concept of cancer seeding from these remote-access approaches is rare although a case of suprapectoral track recurrence of a 6 cm follicular variant of papillary thyroid cancer has been reported after robotic assisted transaxillary total thyroidectomy. Therefore, prevention of tumour spillage from these remote sites is paramount in order to prevent this rare occurrence of track seeding [36].

Our opinion is that remote-access thyroidectomy can be performed safely with excellent oncologic results in patients with T1–T2 thyroid cancer and select T3 cancer) (without any gross extrathyroidal extension) in high-volume thyroid units. These results have been validated in large comparative case series of the oncologic outcomes between open thyroidectomy and remote-access thyroidectomy [31, 35, 37]. This is especially relevant in patients who are young and may desire a "scarless" neck for treating these small thyroid cancers.

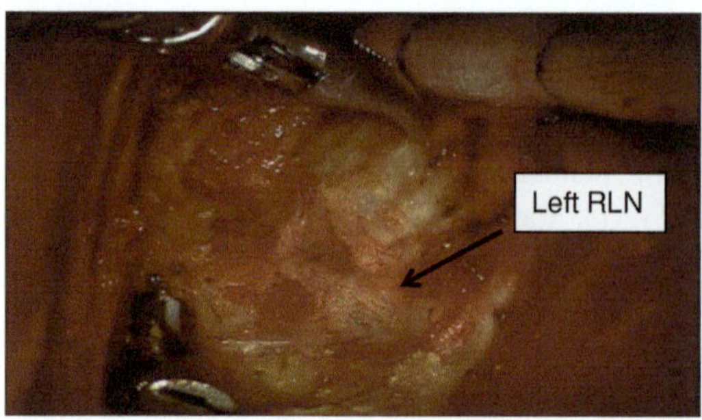

Fig. 17.2 Left recurrent laryngeal nerve (black arrow) in the tracheo-oesophageal groove following robotic assisted retroauricular thyroidectomy

Complications

Recurrent Laryngeal Nerve Palsy

Recurrent laryngeal nerve (RLN) palsy is the most reported complication following thyroidectomy and the key to preventing injury is proper identification of the nerve and meticulous atraumatic dissection of the nerve from the thyroid gland. A meta-analysis by Lang et al. comparing robotic thyroidectomy and CT found that robotic thyroidectomy is associated with a significantly higher rate of transient RLN palsy ($p = 0.016$), though rates of permanent palsy are similar between the two groups [38]. However this is not contrary to other published reports where most case-controlled studies and some meta-analyses, reported no significant differences in risk of RLN palsy (both transient and permanent) for robotic/endoscopic thyroidectomy versus CT. Many authors feel that the visualisation of the RLN is superior in endoscopic or robotic thyroidectomy compared to CT (Fig. 17.2). However, the initial unfamiliarity of these remote-access approaches plus the lack of tactile feedback may place the nerve at risk. Ban et al. showed in his series of 3000 robotic thyroidectomies that though not significant, the incidence of transient RLN palsy was reduced after the first 1000 cases [39]. In a meta-analysis comparing robotic and endoscopic approaches, there was a higher rate of temporary RLN palsy in endoscopic compared to robotic thyroidectomies, and these RLN palsy rates were independent of surgical numbers [33].

Post-operative Hypoparathyroidism/Hypocalcaemia

The risks of hypoparathyroidism/hypocalcaemia vary across the literature, with most large studies showing no statistically significant differences between the rates of hypocalcaemia for these alternative approaches when compared to CT. However, Jackson et al. in his meta-analysis found a significant difference in transient hypocalcaemia rates favouring CT compared to robotic thyroidectomy [29]. On the contrary, Kim et al. found that the patients who had endoscopic ABBA thyroidectomy were less likely to have transient hypocalcaemia post-surgery compared to CT [40].

Haematoma/Seroma

With more extensive dissection, and the push for drainless/outpatient surgery, there is a theoretical increased risk of haematoma and seroma for these new thyroidectomy approaches. However, this fear of an increased risk of seroma or haematoma formation post-thyroidectomy has not been borne out in the literature [2, 38, 40, 41].

Other Complications

Although the magnified surgical field in endoscopic and robotic surgery allows better identification and preservation of vital structures, this overmagnified view can result in a narrower surgical field, which paradoxically may lead to other complications rarely seen with the conventional thyroidectomy. Major complications such as chyle leaks, tracheal injuries, Horner's syndrome, carotid injury, brachiocephalic vein injury, oesophageal injury and even oesophageal transections have been reported with these alternative approaches [12, 17, 39]. On the other hand, many centres have reported good results and low complication rates for these procedures, and improvement is likely anticipated as the surgeon's experience increases. Therefore, careful patient selection and surgeon's continual training and initial proctorship are important for the novice in gaining confidence and good clinical outcomes in performing this more technically demanding thyroidectomy from the remote-access sites.

Endoscopic Versus Robotic Thyroidectomy

While both robotic and endoscopic systems give magnified visualisation of the surgical field, endoscope visualisation is two-dimensional compared to the three-dimensional view in the robotic system. Additionally, these long instruments, pivoted at remote trocar site, tend to amplify the tremors and may reduce the dexterity of the dissection further. Endoscopic thyroidectomy also requires a good endoscopic assistant to hold the camera steadily and to follow the dissection process with the operating surgeon seamlessly. The Da Vinci robot, the only Food and Drug Administration (FDA)-approved surgical robot, addresses some of the drawbacks of endoscopic system. It has a non-assistant-dependent three-dimensional camera system with excellent appreciation of the surgical field. Its wristed instruments and fine motion scaling of movements also reduce physiologic tremors and facilitate improved dexterity in dissection. However these benefits are at the expense of increased cost and operative time. A summary of the pros and cons of each system is appended in Table 17.2.

Table 17.2 Comparison between endoscopic and robotic thyroidectomy

Endoscopic thyroidectomy	Robotic thyroidectomy
Advantages	*Advantages*
– Less cost – Shorter set-up time – More easily available	– Three-dimensional visualisation – Non-assistant-dependent camera view – Wristed instruments – Modulated movements to reduce physiologic tremor – Shorter learning curve
Disadvantages	*Disadvantages*
– Two-dimensional visualisation – Assistant-dependent camera view – Rigid, non-articulated instruments	– Higher cost – Longer set-up time – Not available in all institutions

Future Surgical Robot Technology for Robotic Thyroidectomy

In 2014, Intuitive Surgical launched the Da Vinci Xi robot, which superseded the previous Da Vinci Si system. The Xi platform enhances the Si system by having a camera that can be mounted in any of the surgical arms and hence improved manoeuvrability of the operating arms. The instrument arms also boast a larger range of

Table 17.3 Summary of selected evidence comparing outcomes between endoscopic, robotic and conventional thyroidectomy

Studies	Operating time (min)	Blood loss	RLN injury	Hypocalcaemia	Hematoma/ seroma	Cosmesis	Oncological outcomes	Other outcomes
Lee 2012 [15] (*n* = 2612) Multicentre study RT—1769 ET—843 Thyroid cancer patients	**Favours RT vs. ET for total thyroidectomy** (*p* = 0.001) No difference between RT and ET for subtotal thyroidectomy Learning curve: RT—Time required for RT decreased after 35–50 pts ET—55–70 pts	NR	**No difference** Transient: RT: 3.8% ET: 4.9 (*p* = NS) Permanent RT: 0.5% ET: 0.1% (*p* = NS)	**No difference** Transient: RT: 39.1% ET: 36.7% (*p* = NS) Permanent RT: 0% ET: 0.2% (*p* = NS)	**No difference** Haematoma Observation RT: 0.5% ET: 0.6% (*p* = NS) Reoperation RT: 0.1% ET: 0.4% (*p* = NS)	NR	NR	No difference for chyle leak, tracheal injury, brachial plexus injury, oesophageal injury, seroma
Jackson 2013 [29] (Meta-analysis) 794 Open 965 ET 1112 RT – 69 BABA – 1054 TA	**Favours CT** *Robotic vs. open* Increased mean difference: 42.05 min more in robotic (95% CI, 29.23–54.87) *Robotic vs. endoscopic* Robotic 20.99 min shorter (95%CI: -59.03 to 17.05, NS)	NR	**No difference for transient or permanent RLN palsy** Robot vs. CT Transient: *p* = 0.83 Permanent: *p* = 0.99 Robot vs. endoscopic Transient: *p* = 0.96 Permanent: *p* = 0.22	**Favours CT** *Robot vs. open* Increased risk of transient hypocalcaemia in robot RR: 0.39 (*p* = 0.001) No difference in permanent hypocalcaemia *Robot vs. endoscopic* No difference in permanent or transient hypocalcaemia	**No difference** *Robot vs. CT* Haematoma *p* = 0.94 Seroma *p* = 0.99 *Robot vs. endoscopic* Haematoma *p* = 0.34 Seroma *p* = 0.62	**Favours RT** Pooled net mean difference of −1.35 (95%CI: −0.169,-1.09)	**No difference** No difference in post-op Tg levels between robot and CT, robot and endoscopic	Chyle leak: No difference between robot and CT and robot and Endoscopic voice
Lang 2014 [33] (Meta-analysis) (*n* = 2375) RT—839 CT—1536	**Favours CT vs. RT** CT had reduced OR time of 55.8 min (53.1–58.5) (*p* < 0.001)	No difference between RT and CT	**Favours CT vs. RT for transient RLN palsy** Transient: RT more likely OR 2.44 (*p* = 0.016) Permanent: OR 1.64 (*p* = NS)	**No difference between RT and CT for transient or permanent hypocalcaemia**	**No difference between RT and CT**	Favours RT vs. CT	NR	RT has less swallowing complaints

Lang 2014 [33] (Meta-analysis) ($n = 3510$) RT—2167 ET—1343	**No difference between RT and ET** Lobectomy: – No significant difference Total thyroidectomy – No significant difference	NR	**Favours RT vs. ET** Transient: RT: 2.6% ET: 3.3% ($p = 0.035$)	**No difference between RT and ET** Transient: RT: 35.6% ET: 31.3% (p = NS) Permanent RT: 0.1% ET: 1.6% (p = NS)	**No difference between RT and ET** Haematoma RT: 0.6% ET: 1.0% (p = NS) Seroma (p = NS)	NR	**No difference between RT and ET** No significant difference in no. of retrieved central lymph nodes and post-operative TG	Seroma, wound infection, skin burn, tracheal injury, brachial plexus injury and chyle leak similar between RT and ET
Sun 2014 (Meta-analysis) ($n = 1931$) RT—726 CT—1205	**Favours CT vs. RT RT exceeded CT by 76.6 min**	NR	**No difference between RT and CT**	**No difference between RT and CT**	**No difference between RT and CT**	No meta-analysis done	No meta-analysis done	No difference in rate of chyle leak
Son 2015 [31] (Meta-analysis) ($n = 3136$) 9 studies robotic TA 5 studies BABA RT—1066 CT—2070 Thyroid cancer patients	**Favours CT vs. RT** Transaxillary Robotic vs. CT WMD 39.77 (total thyroid) (p = <0.00001) WMD 30.05 No difference between BABA total thyroidectomy, transaxillary partial thyroidectomy and CT	**Favours Robotic TA vs. CT** Standardised mean difference: –0.28 p = 0.04	**No difference**	**No difference**	**No difference**	**Favours robotic TA vs. CT** $p < 0.0001$	**No difference for post-op Tg between RT and CT** More retrieved LNs in CT vs. RT in MRND and CCND	

(continued)

Table 17.3 (continued)

Studies	Operating time (min)	Blood loss	RLN injury	Hypocalcaemia	Hematoma/ seroma	Cosmesis	Oncological outcomes	Other outcomes
Kandil 2016 (Meta-analysis) ($n = 4878$) RT—1902 ET—1100 CT—1876	RT: 166.58 ± 58.3 min CT: 130.4 ± 48.3 min ET: 140.9 ± 34.8 min	**Favours RT vs. CT** – Less blood loss in RT vs. CT	**No difference between RT and CT or RT and ET** ET vs. RT Transient: NS Permanent: NS	**Favour CT vs. RT for transient hypocalcaemia** ET vs. RT Transient ($p = 0.014$) Permanent ($p =$ NS) CT vs. RT Transient ($p < 0.001$) Permanent ($p = 0.658$)	**No difference**	NR	CT vs. RT **No difference in Tg**	No difference in seroma/ haematoma/ chyle leak/ tracheal injury Pain at 4 and 24 h CT vs. RT – Favour RT

RT robotic thyroidectomy, *ET* endoscopic thyroidectomy, *CT* conventional thyroidectomy, *Tg* thyroglobulin, *WMD* weight mean difference, *TA* transaxillary, *BABA* bilateral axillo-breast approach, *NR* not reported, *NS* not significant, *CI* confidence interval

Table 17.4 Comparison between the Da Vinci Si and the Da Vinci Xi surgical robot

	Da Vinci Si	Da Vinci Xi
Camera-endoscope system	• 8.5 and 12 mm • ~60 degrees field of view • No autofocus/auto-white balance • 3D calibration required • Camera-endoscope can only be placed on camera arm • Draping required	• 8 mm • ~80 degrees field of view • Autofocus and auto-white balance • 3D calibration not required • Camera-endoscope can be placed on any of the 4 robotic arms • No draping required
Docking of arms	• No overhead boom rotation docking system • Unassisted surgeon-dependent docking • Arm spar width: 2.9 in.	• Overhead boom-mounted system for docking of arms • Computer LASER-assisted docking which automatically positions the overhead boom based on anatomical site • Arm spar width: 1.7 in.
Instruments	• 5 mm and 8 mm • Lower range of motion (ROM) compared to Xi • Able to support the Erbe Endowrist vessel sealer	• 8 mm • Additional ~1.75 in. of additional reach • Larger ROM • Able to support the Erbe Endowrist vessel sealer
Cautery generator	• No integrated cautery generator	• Integrated Erbe Vio dV cautery generator system
Other technology		• Integrated operating table • Development of Da Vinci single-port (SP) robotic surgical system

movement as well as a computer-assisted overhead docking system that allows more ease in docking, thereby reducing docking time. The smaller and thinner robotic arms are also useful to prevent collision of the arms in tight confined operating spaces. Although the experience with the Xi is at its infancy, early studies have shown faster docking times and operative time in abdominal surgeries performed with Xi when compared to the Si platform, with equivalent perioperative outcomes [42, 43]. Table 17.4 summarises the differences between the two platforms at the time of writing.

Conclusion

Open conventional thyroidectomy is a standard surgical technique with excellent safety and outcomes. Changing societal and cultural preferences and improving endoscopic and surgical technology have led to the rapid development of alternative endoscopic and robotic approaches in order to improve the aesthetic outcomes of thyroidectomy. High-volume centres around the world have demonstrated equivalency in safety, oncological effectiveness and long-term complication rates for these alternative approaches compared with the conventional thyroidectomy. Nevertheless, appropriate patient selection and overcoming the initial learning curve are crucial in order to ensure excellent surgical and cosmetic outcomes.

References

1. Miccoli P, Berti P, Marco R, Massimo C, Materazzi G, Galleri D. Minimally invasive video-assisted thyroidectomy. Am J Surg. 2001;181:567–70. https://doi.org/10.1097/MLG.0b013e318162cad6.
2. Pisanu A, Podda M, Reccia I, Porceddu G, Uccheddu A. Systematic review with meta-analysis of prospective randomized trials comparing minimally invasive video-assisted thyroidectomy (MIVAT) and conventional thyroidectomy (CT). Langenbeck's Arch Surg. 2013;398(8):1057–68. https://doi.org/10.1007/s00423-013-1125-y.

3. Ikeda Y, Takami H, Niimi M, Kan S, Sasaki Y, Takayama J. Endoscopic thyroidectomy by the axillary approach. Surg Endosc. 2001;15(11):1362–4. https://doi.org/10.1007/s004640080139.
4. Ohgami M, Ishii S, Arisawa Y, et al. Scarless endoscopic thyroidectomy: breast approach for better cosmesis. Surg Laparosc Endosc. 2000;10(1):1–4. http://www.scopus.com/inward/record.url?eid=2-s2.0-0033967740&partnerID=tZOtx3y1.
5. Kang SW, Lee SC, Lee SH, et al. Robotic thyroid surgery using a gasless, transaxillary approach and the da Vinci S system: the operative outcomes of 338 consecutive patients. Surgery. 2009;146(6):1048–55. https://doi.org/10.1016/j.surg.2009.09.007.
6. Byeon HK, Kim DH, Chang JW, et al. Comprehensive application of robotic retroauricular thyroidectomy: the evolution of robotic thyroidectomy. Laryngoscope. 2016;126(8):1952–7. https://doi.org/10.1002/lary.25763.
7. Wilhelm T, Metzig A. Endoscopic minimally invasive thyroidectomy (eMIT): a prospective proof-of-concept study in humans. World J Surg. 2011;35(3):543–51. https://doi.org/10.1007/s00268-010-0846-0.
8. Nakajo A, Arima H, Hirata M, et al. Trans-oral video-assisted neck surgery (TOVANS). A new transoral technique of endoscopic thyroidectomy with gasless premandible approach. Surg Endosc. 2013;27(4):1105–10. https://doi.org/10.1007/s00464-012-2588-6.
9. Wang C, Zhai H, Liu W, et al. Thyroidectomy: a novel endoscopic oral vestibular approach. Surgery (United States). 2014;155(1):33–8. https://doi.org/10.1016/j.surg.2013.06.010.
10. Anuwong A. Transoral endoscopic thyroidectomy vestibular approach: a series of the first 60 human cases. World J Surg. 2016;40(3):491–7. https://doi.org/10.1007/s00268-015-3320-1.
11. Berber E, Bernet V, Fahey T 3rd, et al. American Thyroid Association statement on remote access thyroid surgery. Thyroid. 2016;26(3):331–7. https://doi.org/10.1089/thy.2015.0407.
12. Terris DJ, Singer MC, Seybt MW. Robotic facelift thyroidectomy: II. Clinical feasibility and safety. Laryngoscope. 2011;121(8):1636–41. https://doi.org/10.1002/lary.21832.
13. Holsinger FC, Chung WY. Robotic thyroidectomy. Otolaryngol Clin N Am. 2014;47(3):373–8. https://doi.org/10.1016/j.otc.2014.03.001.
14. Lee KE, Kim E, Koo DH, Choi JY, Kim KH, Youn YK. Robotic thyroidectomy by bilateral axillo-breast approach: review of 1026 cases and surgical completeness. Surg Endosc. 2013;27(8):2955–62. https://doi.org/10.1007/s00464-013-2863-1.
15. Lee J, Yun JH, Choi UJ, Kang SW, Jeong JJ, Chung WY. Robotic versus endoscopic thyroidectomy for thyroid cancers: a multi-institutional analysis of early postoperative outcomes and surgical learning curves. J Oncol. 2012;2012:1. https://doi.org/10.1155/2012/734541.
16. Byeon HK, Holsinger FC, Tufano RP, et al. Endoscopic retroauricular thyroidectomy: preliminary results. Surg Endosc. 2016;30(1):355–65. https://doi.org/10.1007/s00464-015-4202-1.
17. Choi JY, Lee KE, Chung KW, et al. Endoscopic thyroidectomy via bilateral axillo-breast approach (BABA): review of 512 cases in a single institute. Surg Endosc. 2012;26(4):948–55. https://doi.org/10.1007/s00464-011-1973-x.
18. Bakkar S, Materazzi G, Biricotti M, et al. Minimally invasive video-assisted thyroidectomy (MIVAT) from A to Z. Surg Today. 2016;46(2):255–9. https://doi.org/10.1007/s00595-015-1241-0.
19. Miccoli P, Biricotti M, Matteucci V, Ambrosini CE, Wu J, Materazzi G. Minimally invasive video-assisted thyroidectomy: reflections after more than 2400 cases performed. Surg Endosc. 2015;30:2489–95. https://doi.org/10.1007/s00464-015-4503-4.
20. Shimazu K, Shiba E, Tamaki Y, et al. Endoscopic thyroid surgery through the axillo-bilateral-breast approach. Surg Laparosc Endosc Percutan Tech. 2003;13(3):196–201. https://doi.org/10.1097/00129689-200306000-00011.
21. Lee HY, You JY, Woo SU, et al. Transoral periosteal thyroidectomy: cadaver to human. Surg Endosc. 2015;29(4):898–904. https://doi.org/10.1007/s00464-014-3749-6.
22. Witzel K, Von Rahden BHA, Kaminski C, Stein HJ. Transoral access for endoscopic thyroid resection. Surg Endosc. 2008;22(8):1871–5. https://doi.org/10.1007/s00464-007-9734-6.
23. Clark JH, Kim HY, Richmon JD. Transoral robotic thyroid surgery. Gland Surg. 2015;4(5):429–34. https://doi.org/10.3978/j.issn.2227-684X.2015.02.02.
24. Holsinger FC, Terris DJ, Kuppersmith RB. Robotic thyroidectomy: operative technique using a transaxillary endoscopic approach without CO2 insufflation. Otolaryngol Clin N Am. 2010;43(2):381–8. https://doi.org/10.1016/j.otc.2010.01.007.
25. Singer MC, Terris DJ. Robotic facelift thyroidectomy. Otolaryngol Clin N Am. 2014;47(3):425–31. https://doi.org/10.1016/j.otc.2014.02.001.
26. Ikeda Y, Takami H, Sasaki Y, Takayama J, Niimi M, Kan S. Comparative study of thyroidectomies: endoscopic surgery vs conventional open surgery. Surg Endosc. 2002;16(12):1741–5. https://doi.org/10.1007/s00464-002-8830-x.
27. Zhang P, Zhang HW, Han XD, Di JZ, Zheng Q. Meta-analysis of comparison between minimally invasive video-assisted thyroidectomy and conventional thyroidectomy. Eur Rev Med Pharmacol Sci. 2015;19(8):1381–7.
28. Lee J, Nah KY, Kim RM, Ahn YH, Soh EY, Chung WY. Differences in postoperative outcomes, function, and cosmesis: open versus robotic thyroidectomy. Surg Endosc. 2010;24(12):3186–94. https://doi.org/10.1007/s00464-010-1113-z.
29. Jackson N, Yao L, Tufano RP, Kandil E. Safety of robotic thyroidectomy approaches: meta-analysis and

systematic review. Head Neck. 2014;10(1002):137–43. https://doi.org/10.1002/hed.

30. Choi SH, Baek JH, Lee JH, et al. Initial clinical experience with BRAF ^{V600E} mutation analysis of core-needle biopsy specimens from thyroid nodules. Clin Endocrinol (Oxf). 2016;84(4):607–13. https://doi.org/10.1111/cen.12866.
31. Son SK, Kim JH, Bae JS, Lee SH. Surgical safety and oncologic effectiveness in robotic versus conventional open thyroidectomy in thyroid cancer: a systematic review and meta-analysis. Ann Surg Oncol. 2015;22:3022–32. https://doi.org/10.1245/s10434-015-4375-9.
32. Chung E-J, Park M-W, Cho J-G, et al. A prospective 1-year comparative study of endoscopic thyroidectomy via a retroauricular approach versus conventional open thyroidectomy at a single institution. Ann Surg Oncol. 2015;22(9):3014–21. https://doi.org/10.1245/s10434-014-4361-7.
33. Lang BHH, Wong CKH, Tsang JS, Wong KP. A systematic review and meta-analysis comparing outcomes between robotic-assisted thyroidectomy and non-robotic endoscopic thyroidectomy. J Surg Res. 2014;191(2):389–98. https://doi.org/10.1016/j.jss.2014.04.023.
34. Kiong KL, Iyer NG, Skanthakumar T, et al. Transaxillary thyroidectomies: a comparative learning experience of robotic vs endoscopic thyroidectomies. Otolaryngol Head Neck Surg. 2015;152(5):820–6. https://doi.org/10.1177/0194599815573003.
35. Lee S, Lee CR, Lee SC, et al. Surgical completeness of robotic thyroidectomy: a prospective comparison with conventional open thyroidectomy in papillary thyroid carcinoma patients. Surg Endosc. 2014;28(4):1068–75. https://doi.org/10.1007/s00464-013-3303-y.
36. Bakkar S, Frustaci G, Papini P, et al. Track recurrence after robotic transaxillary thyroidectomy: a case report highlighting the importance of controlled surgical indications and addressing unprecedented complications. Thyroid. 2016;26(4):559–61. https://doi.org/10.1089/thy.2015.0561.
37. Lee SG, Lee J, Kim MJ, et al. Long-term oncologic outcome of robotic versus open total thyroidectomy in PTC: a case-matched retrospective study. Surg Endosc. 2016;30(8):3474–9. https://doi.org/10.1007/s00464-015-4632-9.
38. Lang BH-H, Wong CKH, Tsang JS, Wong KP, Wan KY. A systematic review and meta-analysis comparing surgically-related complications between robotic-assisted thyroidectomy and conventional open thyroidectomy. Ann Surg Oncol. 2014;21(3):850–61. https://doi.org/10.1245/s10434-013-3406-7.
39. Ban EJ, Yoo JY, Kim WW, et al. Surgical complications after robotic thyroidectomy for thyroid carcinoma: a single center experience with 3,000 patients. Surg Endosc. 2014;28(9):2555–63. https://doi.org/10.1007/s00464-014-3502-1.
40. Kim SK, Kang SY, Youn HJ, Jung SH. Comparison of conventional thyroidectomy and endoscopic thyroidectomy via axillo-bilateral breast approach in papillary thyroid carcinoma patients. Surg Endosc. 2016;30(8):3419–25. https://doi.org/10.1007/s00464-015-4624-9.
41. Kwon H, Yi JW, Song R-Y, et al. Comparison of bilateral axillo-breast approach robotic thyroidectomy with open thyroidectomy for graves' disease. World J Surg. 2016;40(3):498–504. https://doi.org/10.1007/s00268-016-3403-7.
42. Abdel Raheem A, Sheikh A, Kim DK, et al. Da Vinci Xi and Si platforms have equivalent perioperative outcomes during robot-assisted partial nephrectomy: preliminary experience. J Robot Surg. 2016;11:1–9. https://doi.org/10.1007/s11701-016-0612-x.
43. Morelli L, Guadagni S, Di Franco G, et al. Use of the new da Vinci Xi® during robotic rectal resection for cancer: a pilot matched-case comparison with the da Vinci Si®. Int J Med Robot. 2016;7(April):375–92. https://doi.org/10.1002/rcs.1728.

Part II

Parathyroid

18 Primary Hyperparathyroidism

Manju Chandran

Case Vignette

A 43-year-old Chinese man, working in information technology as a consultant, with no significant past medical history underwent a corporate health screening that detected the following abnormalities:

Serum calcium 3.10 mmol/L (2.09–2.46 mmol/L)
Serum phosphate 0.74 mmol/L (0.94–1.50 mmol/L
Intact PTH: 57.9 pmol/L (0.9–6.2 pmol/L)

He was referred to the endocrinologist by his company GP.

He states that he is in good health and does not have any complaints of note. He is not on any over-the-counter supplements. He is puzzled by the abnormal blood tests and wonders what should be done for it.

Introduction

Primary hyperparathyroidism is an endocrine disorder, the classic hallmark features of which are elevated or inappropriately normal parathyroid hormone levels in the presence of hypercalcaemia. A distinction has to be made in mild, relatively asymptomatic cases between primary hyperparathyroidism and a rare, autosomal dominant condition; familial hypocalciuric hypercalcaemia (FHH) in which an inactivating mutation of the calcium-sensing receptor gene leads to an increase in the set point for suppression of PTH secretion by serum calcium suppression [1]. A subtype of primary hyperparathyroidism that has recently gained recognition and acceptance is normocalcaemic primary hyperparathyroidism. In this condition both total and ionised calcium levels are normal in the presence of a persistently elevated parathyroid hormone level and all causes of secondary hyperparathyroidism including vitamin D insufficiency, renal failure and idiopathic hypercalciuria have been excluded.

Epidemiology and Pathology

Primary hyperparathyroidism is one of the commonest endocrine disorders. Its age-adjusted prevalence is reported to be 232.7 cases per 100,000 amongst women and 85.2 per 100,000 men [2]. The peak incidence is in the 5–6th decades of life and there appears to be a female-to-male ratio of

M. Chandran
Osteoporosis and Bone Metabolism Unit, Department of Endocrinology, Singapore General Hospital, Singapore, Singapore
e-mail: manju.chandran@singhealth.com.sg

R. Parameswaran, A. Agarwal (eds.), *Evidence-Based Endocrine Surgery*,
https://doi.org/10.1007/978-981-10-1124-5_18

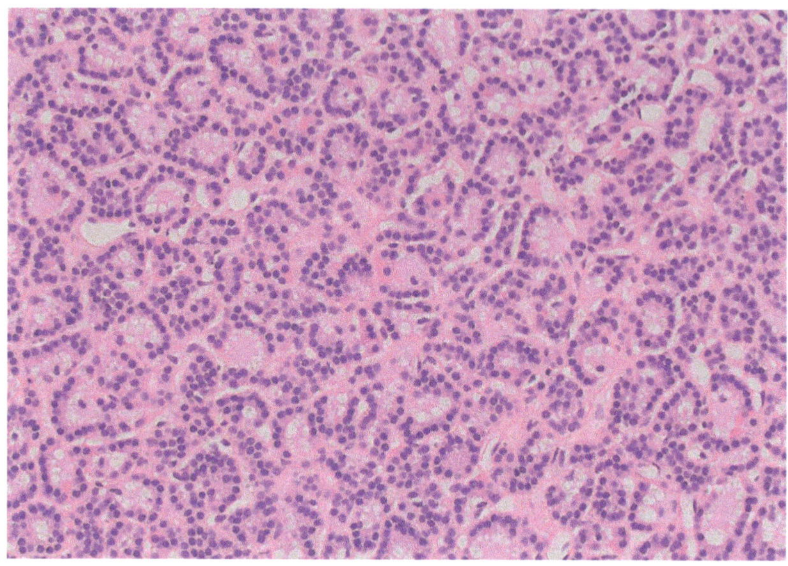

Fig. 18.1 High-power view of the centre of chief cell adenoma. Cells are nearly uniform

3–4:1 [3]. The prevalence is likely to be more in sub-populations such as patients with osteoporosis [4]. The widespread use of the autoanalyser to perform multichannel screening with routine determinations of serum calcium coincided with a dramatic increase in the incidence of primary hyperparathyroidism in the 1970s [5]. A second peak in the late 1990s was reported in the USA that coincided with the introduction of national guidelines for osteoporosis with an increase in targeted screening for hyperparathyroidism as part of evaluation for osteoporosis [5].

A solitary, benign parathyroid adenoma is responsible in the majority of cases (~80–90%) of surgically proven PHPT. Less commonly, it is due to four-gland hyperplasia (~10–15%) and the remainder are secondary to multiple adenomas (~4%) [6]. Very rarely it is due to parathyroid carcinoma (<1%) [7]. Due to the embryonic origin and migration pattern during intrauterine development of the inferior and superior parathyroid glands, the gland(s) may not be located in the neck, posterior to the thyroid, but may be found in several possible ectopic sites including the superior mediastinum, retro-oesophageally, within the thymus and also intra-thyroidally [8].

There are no clear clinical predictors to differentiate single-gland adenoma from multi-gland hyperplasia except perhaps in patients with familial syndromes like multiple endocrine neoplasia types 1 and 2A where it should be presumed that the disease involves multi-gland hyperplasia [9].

Grossly, a parathyroid adenoma weighs between 300 milligrams to several grams. The overall size can range anywhere from smaller than 1 cm to larger than 3 cm. Histologically, parathyroid adenomas are composed of sheets of cells interspersed with a delicate capillary network (Fig. 18.1). A rim of normal or atrophic parathyroid tissue beyond the adenoma capsule with a distinct interface (Fig. 18.2) may be seen if the adenoma is not very large [10]. While most adenomas are composed of chief cells, a small percentage may be composed of more than 90% oxyphilic cells.

In parathyroid hyperplasia, all four glands are enlarged. Microscopically, two major patterns are identified. In diffuse chief cell hyperplasia, solid cellular masses comprised of mainly chief cells are present with minimal or absent stromal fat. Nodular or adenomatous hyperplasia consists of circumscribed nodules of chief or oxyphil cells. The nodules are devoid of fat and little fat is found in the intervening stroma [11].

The tumours in parathyroid carcinomas are larger than adenomas with an average weight of 12 g. Microscopically, parathyroid carcinomas are characterised by a trabecular arrangement of tumour cells that are divided by fibrous

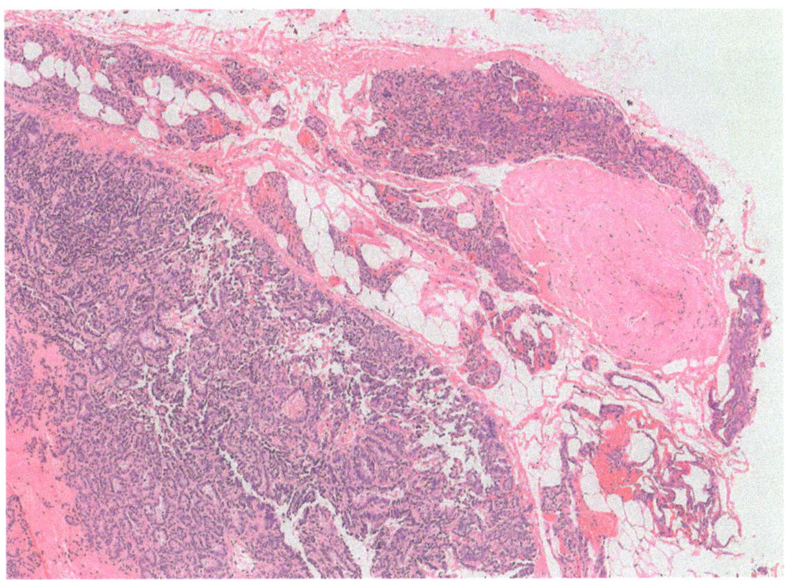

Fig. 18.2 Portion of parathyroid adenoma abutting "normal" rim. Distinct interface between the adenoma (right) and residual normal parathyroid tissue with fat at the edge (left)

bands. Capsular and vessel wall invasion is seen and mitotic figures are found within the tumour cells [10].

Immunohistochemistry analysis may be useful in the identification of parathyroid lesions. In addition to the cytoplasmic staining for PTH in chief cells that is easily identifiable, low-molecular-weight cytokeratins, chromogranin A, vimentin and glial fibrillary acidic protein may be immunoreactive [10]. It has been suggested that an immunohistochemical signature composed of loss of expression of parafibromin, retinoblastoma protein (Rb), p27, Bcl-2a, mdm-2 and APC, along with positivity for galectin-3, overexpression of p53 and increased MIB-I (Ki67) proliferation index more than 5%, be identified to confirm a diagnosis of parathyroid cancer in a parathyroid lesion with suspicious histological features [7].

Aetiology

The mechanisms underlying the neoplastic transformation of parathyroid tissue in primary hyperparathyroidism are still unclear. Patients with prior history of radiation exposure to the head and neck may be at risk for the development of primary hyperparathyroidism years later [12]. Primary hyperparathyroidism associated with familial syndromes has a clear genetic origin [13, 14]. Molecular studies have suggested that parathyroid adenomas are monoclonal in origin [15] and these studies have focused on the genetic rearrangement that places the PRAD1 (parathyroid adenomatosis 1) oncogene in juxtaposition to the 5′ regulatory region of the PTH gene, with resultant activation of the PRAD1 oncogene under the influence of the PTH regulatory apparatus as a cause for the parathyroid cell growth in primary hyperparathyroidism [16]. However, it must be noted that this gene rearrangement has been found in only a small percentage of parathyroid adenomas.

Clinical Presentation

The classic hallmarks of primary hyperparathyroidism used to be the literal manifestations of "Stones, bones, groans and psychiatric overtones". However, the clinical presentation of this disorder has changed dramatically especially in countries where biochemical screening is routinely performed; with most patients being diagnosed with the disorder following incidental discovery of hypercalcaemia either during workup of other conditions or more commonly during health screening [3]. Though symptomatic disease continues to be the predominant form in countries such as India [17] and Saudi Arabia [18], recent publications from some of these countries appear to suggest that the presentation may be shifting towards a milder phenotype and that the disease is being diagnosed earlier [19]. This is likely a function of surveillance and screening and does not reflect a true change in the phenotypic variability of primary hyperparathyroidism. Another point that may influence the clinical presentation of symptomatic versus asymptomatic disease may relate to the prevalence of vitamin D deficiency in the population [19].

Although PTH stimulates distal tubular reabsorption of calcium, the increased filtered load of calcium caused by hypercalcaemia may lead to increased renal calcium excretion. The nephrolithiasis that may be seen in primary hyperparathyroidism can be attributed at least partially to the presence of hypercalciuria and the result of diffuse deposition of calcium salts in the renal parenchyma. Though older studies have demonstrated that as many as 40% of patients had stone disease [20], the incidence of overt nephrolithiasis has diminished with the changing clinical profile of the disease. Primary hyperparathyroidism is also associated with reduction of renal function [21]. Polyuria, considered a classic presentation of symptomatic hyperparathyroidism, is driven largely by hypercalcaemia leading to alteration of the renal concentrating mechanism at the renal medulla [22]. Less commonly, coexisting nephrogenic diabetes insipidus secondary to hypercalcaemia may account for the polyuria and polydipsia observed [23].

Skeletal involvement classically presents as osteitis fibrosa cystica, the result of excessive osteoclast activity. The spectrum of the radiological findings in osteitis fibrosa cystica can vary from subperiosteal resorption of the phalanges to "salt-and-pepper" appearance of the skull and to tapering of the distal clavicles. Brown tumours, collections of osteoclasts intermixed with poorly mineralised woven bone, may be seen in the long bones. These may be associated with bone pain and even fractures [24]. Another important effect of the prolonged bone resorption caused by the elevated levels of PTH is osteopenia and osteoporosis [25].

Gastrointestinal manifestations of symptomatic primary hyperparathyroidism include abdominal pain, nausea and anorexia [26, 27]. Acute pancreatitis likely secondary to hypercalcaemia has also been reported [28]. This presentation is unlikely to be a common one however with a large series from Rochester, Minnesota, suggesting that no more than a 1.5% of primary hyperparathyroid patients have coexistent pancreatitis [29]. Peptic ulcer disease may be more common in patients with primary hyperparathyroidism particularly in patients with multiple endocrine neoplasia 1 with coexisting Zollinger-Ellison syndrome [6].

The neuropsychiatric manifestations reported in primary hyperparathyroidsm may be difficult to identify as the features are usually vague and non-specific. The symptoms include depression, cognitive dysfunction, psychosis and fatigue [30]. These symptoms have not consistently shown to improve after curative parathyroidectomy and the scanty data that does exist regarding improvement following parathyroidectomy is difficult to evaluate because of the lack of accurate quantitative tools for assessing these symptoms in primary hyperparathyroidism [31].

Other non-classical manifestations that may be related to primary hyperparathyroidism include involvement of the cardiovascular system, with hypertension, left ventricular hypertrophy and higher mean carotid intima-media thickness on carotid ultrasound [32–34] being observed more commonly in patients with primary hyperparathyroidism compared to controls. As with neuropsychiatric manifestations, no strong data exist to demonstrate consistent reversal of these cardiovascular features with parathyroidectomy.

Asymptomatic PHPT

Although overt bone disease is no longer a common occurrence in PHPT, skeletal involvement is frequently observed using sophisticated radiological and imaging techniques. The DXA signature of PHPT has been the classical pattern of cortical bone loss seen in the distal 1/3rd radius giving rise to the notion that PTH in primary hyperparathyroidism is protective against trabecular bone loss [35]. This perception needs to be corrected in view of recent studies that identify trabecular bone involvement through the application of new imaging and analytical approaches. Studies using high-resolution peripheral quantitative computed tomography (HRpQCT), an imaging modality that can differentiate between trabecular and cortical components of peripheral skeletal sites such as the tibia and the radius, have shown that patients with PHPT have decreased volumetric densities at both trabecular and cortical compartments compared to controls. These changes were more pronounced at the radius than at the tibia [36, 37]. Trabecular bone score (TBS) is a grey-level textural indexing score that provides an indirect index of trabecular microarchitecture through its application on DXA images of the lumbar spine [38]. A high TBS value reflects a dense homogenous trabecular network associated with greater bone strength whereas a low TBS value reflects a more porous heterogenous trabecular network. In a cross-sectional study conducted on 22 postmenopausal women with PHPT, the L1–L4 T-score assessed by DXA was well above the WHO osteoporosis threshold (T-score $\leq$2.5) in the clear majority of subjects. Only 3 (14%) patients were classified as osteoporotic and 7 (32%) as osteopenic. In marked contrast, TBS at the lumbar spine showed degraded (TBS $\leq$1.20) in 8 (36%) patients, and partially degraded (TBS >1.20 and <1.35) microarchitecture in an additional 8 patients (36%), Normal values (TBS $\geq$1.35) were found in only 6 (27%) subjects. The mean TBS of the whole group was 1.24, markedly below the normal threshold ($\geq$1.35) [39]. Epidemiological data for years that have shown an increased fracture risk at vertebral (composed mainly of trabecular bone) sites [40] despite the paradox of relatively normal lumbar spine BMD by DXA now has an explanation. This new knowledge has influenced the most recent guidelines that recommend an evaluation of the trabecular compartment of the bone. Vertebral X-ray/Vertebral Fracture Analysis (VFA) and/or trabecular bone score (TBS) are now recommended in the routine evaluation of primary hyperparathyroidism.

About 7% of patients with asymptomatic primary hyperparathyroidism have been reported to have renal calculi when imaging studies are conducted [41]. This is much higher compared to the 1.6% prevalence noted in individuals without primary hyperparathyroidism.

Normocalcaemic primary hyperparathyroidism (NPHPT) is an entity that is being increasingly recognised. It is characterised by elevated PTH levels in the presence of a normal serum calcium. This entity was first formally recognised in 2008 at the 3rd International Workshop on the Management of Asymptomatic Hyperparathyroidism [42]. The prevalence rates amongst community-based populations have been reported to range from 0.44 [43] to 11% [44] when different cut-off values for PTH and 25 OH D levels were used. Thus, methodological differences in identification may play a role in the different prevalence rates reported. Patients with NPHPT usually come to medical attention during the process of evaluation for low bone mineral density. This condition must be distinguished from secondary hyperparathyroidism wherein the parathyroid gland over activity has a non-parathyroid cause such as renal insufficiency or gastrointestinal tract disorders associated with malabsorption of vitamin D, calcium or both. The parathyroid glands in secondary hyperparathyroidism respond to the hypocalcaemic stimulus with hypersecretion of PTH which returns the serum calcium to normal levels. Other conditions that must be excluded before making the diagnosis of NPHPT since they may be associated with elevations of PTH are idiopathic hypercalciuria and use of medications such as bisphosphonates, the RANK ligand inhibitor denosumab, thiazide diuretics and lithium.

Though the potential selection bias of significantly more skeletal involvement being identified from those cases of NPHPT diagnosed at specialised bone metabolic centres has to be considered, it does appear that there is a high prevalence of osteoporosis, fragility fractures and nephrolithiasis with prevalence rates of 57%, 11% and 14%, respectively, noted in one study of patients with proven NPHPT [42].

The natural history of NPHPT is reportedly variable and no clear-cut features are present that will predict who amongst these patients will have disease progression. Of 37 patients followed up for a median duration of 3 years in one study, 40% were shown to progress to overt primary hyperparathyroidism with 7/37 patients demonstrating hypercalcaemia, 1/37 developing kidney stone and fracture, respectively, and two demonstrating marked hypercalciuria. Six out of the 37 patients had >10% BMD loss at one or more sites during the follow-up period [42]. On the contrary, another study in 277 vitamin D-sufficient individuals with proven NPHPT did not show progression to overt disease despite a 17-year follow-up [44].

Diagnosis

The diagnosis of primary hyperparathyroidism depends on biochemical tests. The sine qua non of the disease, viz. hypercalcaemia, in association with frankly elevated or inappropriately normal PTH levels is seen in most patients with primary hyperparathyroidism. Though measuring ionised calcium adds little to the routine diagnostic assessment of primary hyperparathyroidism its measurement is important in patients with presumed normocalcaemic PHPT. In order to make the diagnosis of NPHPT, ionised calcium levels should be normal [45].

Circulating PTH levels can be measured by radioimmuno- or immuno-radiometric assays. Either second-generation assays referred to as intact PTH assays that measure the full-length 1–84 PTH or third-generation assays commonly referred to as bio-intact PTH assays that measure only the intact PTH molecule and not the C-terminal or 7–84 fragments of PTH can be used for diagnosis [46].

Measurement of 24-h urinary calcium excretion is not always required for the diagnosis of primary hyperparathyroidism but estimating the ratios of calcium to creatinine clearance in a 24-h urine collection is important to help differentiate familial hypocalciuric hypercalcaemia (FHH) from mild primary hyperparathyroidism. The former, an autosomal dominant disorder caused by an inactivating mutation in the calcium-sensing receptor (CASR) gene in the parathyroid glands and the kidneys, is characterised by mild elevations of serum PTH and calcium levels with very low urinary calcium excretion. It is important to distinguish it from primary hyperparathyroidism since it neither requires parathyroidectomy nor is cured by it. The ratio is calculated from 24-h urinary calcium and creatinine and serum calcium and creatinine concentrations using the following formula:

$$\begin{aligned}&\text{Urine Ca / Cr clearance ratio}\left(\text{UCCR}\right)\\&=\left(24-\text{h urine calcium}\times\text{serum creatinine}\right)\\&\div\left(\text{Serum calcium}\times 24-\text{h urine creatinine}\right)\end{aligned}$$

A value less than 0.01 in an individual who is not vitamin D deficient is highly suggestive of FHH. However, as many as two-thirds of PHPT patients may have CCCR below 0·02 because of milder primary hyperparathyroidism [47] or concomitant vitamin D insufficiency [48]. It has been suggested that a two-step approach be used to discriminate FHH from primary hyperparathyroidism [49]. The first step involves estimating the UCCR with a level of <0.02 identifying 98% of patients with FHH. This cut-off will still include around 35% of patients with PHPT. The second step is to perform a CASR mutation analysis in the group with a CCCR <0.02, to separate patients with FHH from patients with primary hyperparathyroidism.

Though not essential to clinch the diagnosis, other biochemical findings that may be seen in primary hyperparathyroidism include mild hyperchloraemic acidosis and hypophosphataemia.

Role of Genetic Testing

The majority of patients with PHPT do not require genetic testing. Approximately 10% of patients with PHPT will have a mutation in 1 out of 11 genes [50]. Genetic testing if available should be performed in select patients in whom a familial form of PHPT is suspected including young patients and those with a family history of

Table 18.1 Genetic disorders associated with primary hyperparathyroidism and familial hypocalciuric hypercalcaemia

Disorder	Gene(s) affected	Organ(s) involved and characteristics
Multiple Endocrine Neoplasia (MEN) 1	Menin	– Parathyroid gland in ~90% (in affected individuals, hypercalcaemia manifests in almost all by age 50 years) – Neuroendocrine tumours of the pancreas and GIT in 60% – Pituitary tumours in 30% – Other rarer entities: Neuroendocrine tumours of the thymus and bronchus, adrenal hyperplasia and adenomas, lipomas, leiomyomas and angiofibromas
Multiple Endocrine Neoplasia (MEN) 2 A	RET	Parathyroid gland in ~30%, medullary thyroid cancer, and adrenal pheochromocytomas
MEN 4	CDKN1B	Parathyroid Gland in ~80%, Pituitary tumours in ~40%, Pancreatic Neuroendocrine Tumours, Carcinoids, Adrenocortical tumours, Thyroid and Reproductive Organ tumours, Renal Angiomyolipomas
Hyperparathyroidism—jaw tumour syndrome	CDC73	Parathyroid Glands (Cystic Adenomas) and Fibro-Osseus lesions of the jaw. Risk of Parathyroid Cancer is 10-15%
Familial isolated hyperparathyroidism	Mutations of Menin, Fibromin, CASR, Cyclin Dependent Kinase Inhibitors-CDKN1A, CDKN2B	Parathyroid Gland
Neonatal severe hyperparathyroidism	CASR	Parathyroid Gland
Familial Hypocalciuric Hypercalcemia (FHH) 1	CASR	Parathyroid Gland
Familial Hypocalciuric Hypercalcemia (FHH) 2	GNA11	Parathyroid Gland
Familial Hypocalciuric Hypercalcemia (FHH) 3	AP2S1	Parathyroid Gland
Sporadic Primary Hyperparathyroidism	Somatic alterations in MEN1, CCND1/PRAD1, Cyclin Dependent Kinase Inhibitors-CDKN1B, CDKN1A, CDKN2B, CDKN2C	Parathyroid Gland

PHPT, multi-gland involvement or clinical findings suspicious for multiple endocrine neoplasia type 1 (MEN1) [50]. Hypercalcaemia is manifest in virtually all patients with MEN-1 by the age of 50 (Table 18.1).

Imaging and Methods of Localisation of the Parathyroid Lesion(s)

Imaging studies are not used to make the diagnosis of primary hyperparathyroidism (this is based on biochemical data) or to decide about whether to pursue surgical therapy (this is based on clinical criteria). Imaging studies are used to guide the operative approach once surgery has been decided upon as the treatment modality that will be employed. Advances in imaging modalities in the last two decades along with changes in institutional practices with respect to diagnostic workup for primary hyperparathyroidism and a shift towards minimally invasive surgery have resulted in a greater reliance on preoperative imaging and localisation in primary hyperparathyroidism [51]. Several imaging modalities have been found to be useful to image and locate the

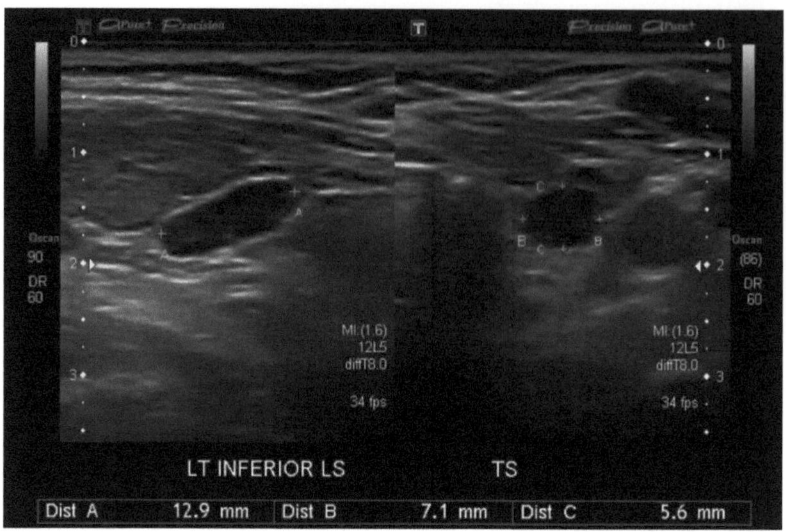

Fig. 18.3 USS of left inferior parathyroid adenoma: Longitudinal and transverse views of left thyroid lobe and parathyroid adenoma. The parathyroid nodule is located inferior to the left thyroid lobe

affected gland(s) in primary hyperparathyroidism. The ability of these preoperative localisation methods to correctly identify pathologic parathyroid glands has been very variable depending on the patient population studied (single-adenoma versus multiple-gland disease), technique employed and experience of the operator and centre [52].

In sonography (USS), enlarged parathyroid glands appear as round or oval-shaped homogenous hypoechoic nodules situated in the extrathyroidal region of the central neck compartment, and are separated from the thyroid lobes by an echogenic capsule fascia plane (Fig. 18.3). The sensitivity of USS in preoperative localisation in primary hyperparathyroidism has been shown to range from 48.3 to 96.2% [53].

Parathyroid scintigraphy is most commonly performed now with Tc99m methoxyisobutylisonitrile (Tc99mMIBI or sestamibi), a cationic lipophilic derivative of technetium. This is taken up by both the thyroid and parathyroid glands but is retained longer in the more mitochondrial rich parathyroid tissue [54]. Either the dual-tracer (MIBI-pertechnetate) subtraction technique based on the principle that Tc-99m pertechnetate is taken up only by the thyroid gland or the MIBI dual-phase (early-delayed) technique based on the longer retention in the parathyroid is used (Fig. 18.4). The images are acquired in 5-min static views from an anterior view of the neck including the upper part of the thorax up to 30 min after the administration of 15–20 millicurie of Tc99m sestamibi. In the subtraction technique, 5 millicurie of Tc99m per technetate is then administered intravenously and subsequent static imaging is performed over another 30 min. The images acquired in the MIBI phase and in the MIBI-pertechnetate phases are digitally subtracted. In the dual-phase MIBI technique, further MIBI imaging is performed at 60 and 120 min. The scintigraphic scan is considered to be positive for parathyroid lesions when focal abnormal increased uptake is detected in the initial and delayed MIBI images in the dual-phase technique or increased uptake is noted in the initial MIBI images without concordant pertechnetate uptake in the dual-tracer techniques, respectively. Sensitivity of MIBI scintigraphy in identifying the diseased parathyroid gland ranges from 61.4 to 94% [53]. The presence of oxyphil cells within the parathyroid adenoma is considered essential for a positive sestamibi scan. An oxyphil content more than 20% quadruples the rate of obtaining a positive sestamibi scan and small adenomas less than 600 mg in weight with less than 20% of oxyphil cells may be associated with a negative scan [55]. Sensitivity is also lower in multi-gland disease and in concomitant thyroid disease [56]. It has been suggested that the use of sestamibi scanning and ultrasonography is complementary and that most adenomatous lesions will be picked up by one or both modality.

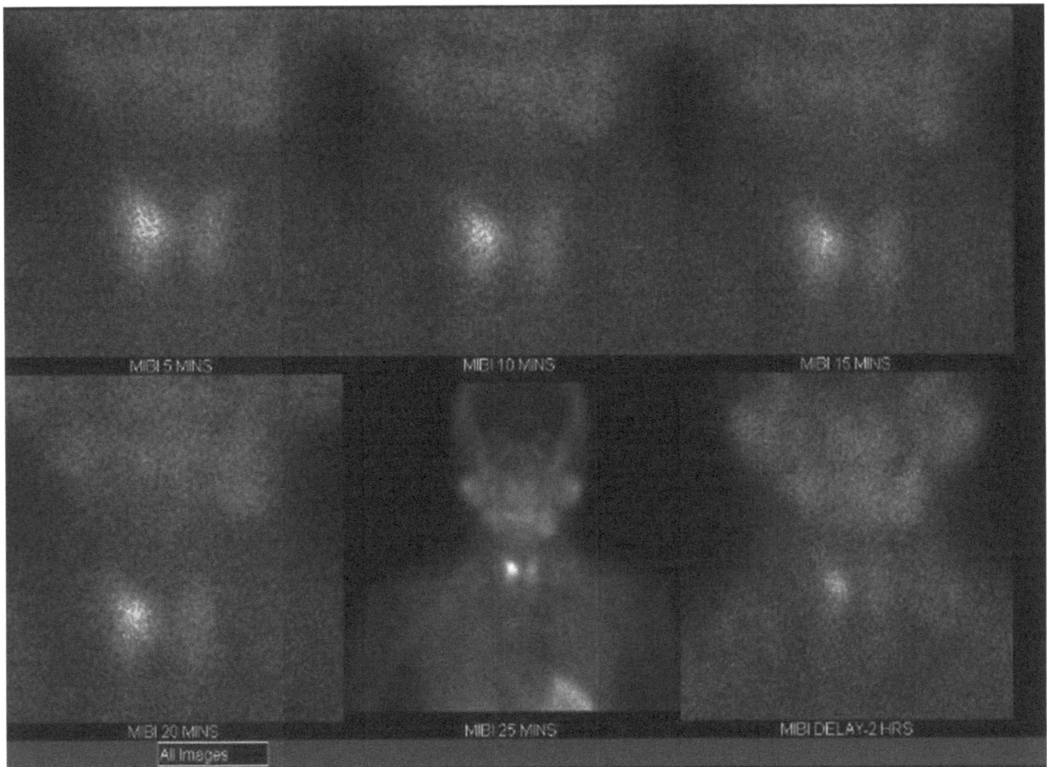

Fig. 18.4 Dual-phase 99m Tc-sestamibi scintigraphy of a patient with raised serum parathyroid level showing differential tracer washout at the lower pole of the right thyroid lobe indicative of a right inferior parathyroid adenoma

The sensitivity of dual-phase technetium 99m sestamibi can be enhanced by combining it with single-photon emission computed tomography/CT (SPECT/CT). It helps to demonstrate lesions in all three dimensions and allows visualisation of posterior adenomas in the retro-oesophageal position that would be otherwise masked by thyroid tracer uptake. This technique has been shown to have incremental diagnostic value in identifying parathyroid adenomas especially in patients with concurrent autoimmune thyroiditis [57] or multinodular goitre [58].

Concordant localisation findings by both sestamibi and ultrasound is in general needed in cases where minimal invasive or limited exploration surgery is entertained. In cases where sestamibi and/or ultrasound are negative or equivocal, four-dimensional computed tomography (4D CT) has shown promising results in localising elusive parathyroid adenoma(s) and facilitating minimally invasive or limited exploration surgery [59, 60].

4D CT is a relatively new multiphase imaging modality in which the first three "dimensions" are multiplanar CT axial acquisitions with coronal and sagittal reformations. The fourth "dimension" of 4D CT is change in enhancement over time in arterial, and delayed (venous) phase imaging. On 4D CT, parathyroid adenomas typically demonstrate low attenuation in the non-contrast phase, intense enhancement on arterial phase and washout of contrast on delayed phase [61] (Fig. 18.5). These uptake characteristics help differentiate parathyroid lesions from lymph nodes and thyroid nodules. Unlike conventional CT that has not been shown to be helpful in differentiating superior from inferior parathyroid glands, the overall accuracy of 4D CT for the localisation of a single hyperfunctional parathyroid gland to a quadrant in the neck is 73–97% [62]. 4D CT also appears to have good accuracy in identifying hyperplastic parathyroid glands and in the reoperative setting [63]. Though 4D CT may have value as a pri-

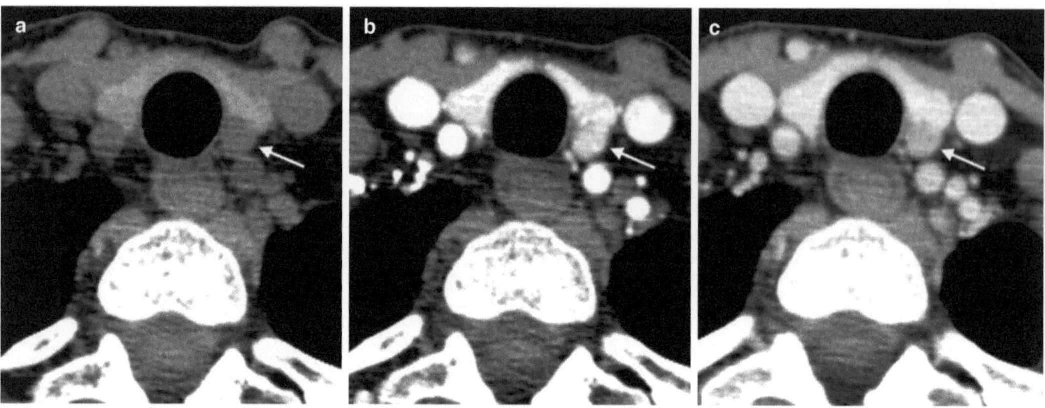

Fig. 18.5 4D CT scan showing a hypodense nodule contiguous with the left posterior thyroid gland that demonstrates low attenuation in non-contrast phase (**a**), intense enhancement in arterial phase (**b**) and rapid washout in delayed phase

mary imaging modality also [64], it has to be noted that the thyroid-specific radiation dose associated with 4D CT is 50 times that of MIBI [65]. MIBI and USS hence probably should remain the primary imaging modality in the workup of primary hyperparathyroidism and this appears to be the favoured approach by most practicing surgeons currently [66]. Concomitant use of MIBI and USS has been shown through several studies to give a combined sensitivity of more than 90% in detecting parathyroid adenoma [67]. Using more than one imaging technique has also been shown to be more cost effective because it decreases the likelihood of a bilateral exploration [68].

Invasive methods of localisation like arteriography and selective venous sampling have also been employed in specialised centres for challenging cases as well as prior to reoperations where the source of hyperparathyroidism remains elusive.

Management

In clearly symptomatic individuals, surgery is indicated barring strong medical contraindications [69]. Non-classic symptoms such as neuropsychiatric or cardiovascular manifestations are not surgical indications per se since these symptoms and manifestations have not been shown to consistently improve after parathyroidectomy [70, 71].

Management of Asymptomatic Disease

How to deal with a disease that is brought to clinical attention by a test and not necessarily by symptoms is a vexing problem. The decision to operate on patients with asymptomatic hyperparathyroidism is challenging, especially since the natural history of most asymptomatic cases appears to be indolent, with PHPT shown to progress only in 1/3rd of individuals over a 15-year follow-up period [72].

Guidelines for the management of asymptomatic primary hyperparathyroidism: The summary statement from the Fourth International Workshop in 2014 suggests the following criteria as indication for parathyroidectomy [69]:

(Presence of one or more of the following)

(a) Serum calcium concentration of 1.0 mg/dL (0.25 mmol/L) or more above the upper limit of normal.
(b) Estimated glomerular filtration rate (eGFR) <60 mL/min.
(c) Peri- or postmenopausal women and men at least 50 years old who have a bone density at the hip, lumbar spine or distal radius that is more than 2.5 standard deviations below peak bone mass (T-score <−2.5) (in premenopausal women and men younger than 50 years, a Z-score of <−2.5 at any of these sites is recommended as a cut-off point) and/

or presence of skeletal involvement as assessed by X-ray, vertebral fracture assessment (VFA), TBS or HRpQCT. Substantial trabecular disease as manifested by low TBS as well as the presence of a vertebral fracture would support a decision for surgery.
(d) Twenty-four-hour urinary calcium >400 mg/day (>10 mmol/day) and increased stone risk by biochemical stone risk profile.
(e) Nephrolithiasis or nephrocalcinosis by radiograph, ultrasound or CT.
(f) Age less than 50 years.

In the absence of any of the above, asymptomatic patients can be offered the option of being monitored for the development of symptomatic disease or for the manifestation of any of the criteria that would meet the guidelines for surgery. This includes annual reassessment of serum calcium, serum creatinine and estimated glomerular filtration rate and annual to 2-yearly reassessment of the bone mineral density by DXA, with X-ray or VFA of the spine if clinically indicated. These guidelines must be interpreted and applied as per different individual practices, considering not only each patient's concerns and expectations but also the availability of local surgical expertise. This also means that it may be reasonable to consider surgery in the asymptomatic hyperparathyroid patient without any of the prespecified criteria within the guidelines for surgery if the patient does not wish to take the risk of disease progression with observation alone.

The 2014 guidelines also provide for an approach to the management of NPHPT. The above criteria for surgery should be applied to those patients who become hypercalcaemic on annual follow-up. If the patient continues to be normocalcaemic but there is disease-associated progression with fractures, continued bone loss, nephrolithiasis or nephrocalcinosis, surgery should be offered [69].

Surgery for Primary Hyperparathyroidism

The definitive treatment for primary hyperparathyroidism is surgery and most surgical data suggest a cure rate of 95–98% in experienced hands with low complication rates [73]. The traditional operative approach involved bilateral neck exploration with identification of all four glands to identify and remove the pathological gland(s). With the understanding that single-gland disease is the major cause of primary hyperparathyroidism, and with the advent of sensitive preoperative localisation imaging and intraoperative adjuncts such as intraoperative parathyroid hormone monitoring, the landscape of surgery for PHPT has changed significantly in the last two decades with a shift towards minimally invasive surgeries [59, 66].

Though an assortment of diverse parathyroidectomy procedures is often described as "minimally invasive" the precise surgical technique that qualifies for the term is controversial. The term theoretically refers to any operative approach be it open or endoscopic by which the diseased gland is removed with minimum invasion of or disruption to the surrounding tissues. In general, however it might be preferable to refer to parathyroid surgeries as limited exploration or bilateral exploration surgeries. Limited exploration surgeries may include focal exploration which involves examination and excision of one parathyroid gland only or a unilateral exploration that examines the two parathyroid glands located on one side of the neck. Bilateral exploration (BE) examines all four parathyroid glands [59]. It must be noted that the outcome of a preoperative localisation procedure should not influence the decision to operate but should simply direct whether to perform a limited or bilateral exploration. The objective of surgery is to remove the culprit adenoma in single-gland disease and in cases of multi-gland adenomas, hyperplasia and syndromic conditions to perform a subtotal or total parathyroidectomy with autotransplantation. Because of the increased risk for morbidity and failure in reoperation, the current consensus calls for two concordant imaging studies localising the hyperfunctioning parathyroid adenoma in primary hyperparathyroidism before a limited exploration is considered [74]. Be it minimally invasive parathyroidectomy or limited exploration or classical bilateral neck exploration surgery, operative success is highly dependent on surgical volume [75, 76] and expertise [75].

Intraoperative use of iPTH (IOPTH) monitoring with a post-resection drop in venous levels by more than 50% indicative of successful operation has been proposed as a useful tool to guide surgeons in performing minimally invasive surgery and also in reducing the risk of missing additional hyperfunctioning parathyroid glands that may have been missed on preoperative imaging [77]. However literature also exists to show that intraoperative use of parathyroid hormone monitoring may not significantly add value and that surgical success of minimal invasive parathyroidectomy is not significantly increased with its use [78].

Benefits of successful parathyroidectomy include normalisation of biochemical indices (serum calcium, parathyroid hormone level), improvement of bone mineral density [79], bone microarchitecture [80] and reduction of bone turnover [81] and fracture risk [82]. A reduction in the risk of recurrent nephrolithiasis has also been noted [83]. Recent data also appears to suggest that surgical treatment may retard progression of the renal dysfunction associated with primary hyperparathyroidism [84, 85]. Curative parathyroidectomy may also lead to improvements in quality of life [86].

Medical Management of Primary Hyperparathyroidism

As described earlier, asymptomatic patients without clear indications for surgery can be carefully monitored. Calcium intake should follow established guidelines for the general population. There is no indication to restrict calcium intake in patients with PHPT [69]. It is recommended that all patients with PHPT have their serum 25 D levels measured [69] and a serum level of at least 20–30 ng/dL should be achieved with careful vitamin D supplementation. Specific dosing regimens are unfortunately not available from clinical trial data. This practice appears to be safe in patients with mild hyperparathyroidism and has been shown to lead to a reduction in PTH levels without exacerbation of hypercalcaemia [87, 88]. It must be noted however that the hypercalcaemia was mild in the patients studied, with serum calcium levels not exceeding 10 mg/dL (3 mmol/L), and that it was observed that some patients given vitamin D replacement experienced an increase in urinary calcium excretion [88].

Medical treatment can be considered in patients who are symptomatic but are poor candidates for surgery or in those who refuse surgery. Oral bisphosphonates have been shown to improve bone mineral density at the lumbar spine and femoral neck [89, 90] in patients with primary hyperparathyroidism but have not shown efficacy in reducing serum calcium, PTH or urinary calcium levels. There is no data to show that they reduce fracture rates in PHPT.

Intravenous bisphosphonates have been shown to help with control of hypercalcaemia in PHPT [91, 92].

Cinacalcet belongs to a class of medications known as calcimimetics that can alter the function of the calcium-sensing receptor and interfere directly with the production of parathyroid hormone. Treatment of primary hyperparathyroidism with cinacalcet was associated with normalisation of the serum calcium and maintenance of the normocalcaemia over a 3–5-year period [93, 94]. Cinacalcet however has not been shown to improve bone mineral density. When a group of patients with PHPT receiving cinacalcet alone was compared to a matched group receiving both cinacalcet and alendronate, though there was normalisation of serum calcium and lowering of PTH levels in both groups, there was a significant improvement in BMD only in those patients who received both alendronate and cinacalcet [95]. Though strong evidence for efficacy is lacking, combining the two medications in those in whom it is desirable to control hypercalcaemia as well as improve BMD holds considerable appeal.

The RANK ligand inhibitor denosumab has also been shown to be particularly effective in normalising calcium in some cases of bisphosphonate and cinacalcet-refractory hypercalcaemia from hyperparathyroidism secondary to parathyroid cancer [96].

Special Situations

Primary Hyperparathyroidism in Pregnancy

Primary hyperparathyroidism though uncommonly reported in pregnancy may carry significant maternal and foetal risks. Maternal presentations have included pancreatitis, severe vomiting, nephrolithiasis and recurrent urinary tract infections [97, 98]. Hypocalcaemia with attendant tetany due to suppression of foetal parathyroid hormone, premature birth, low birth weight and even foetal death have been reported [98]. During the diagnostic evaluation, it must be noted that though ionised calcium levels do not change significantly during the three trimesters, total serum calcium declines across the gestational period, likely secondary to plasma volume expansion and so the upper limit of normal for total serum calcium is lower than in the non-pregnant state. Surgery during the second trimester, preferably minimally invasive parathyroidectomy if preoperative localisation with USS is successful in localising the tumour, is the preferred treatment option for symptomatic patients [99]. However, for asymptomatic patients or in those with only mild hypercalcaemia, just careful observation may be warranted though the newborn should be carefully monitored for hypocalcaemia in such a situation [99].

Conclusion

Despite being recognised for more than 100 years, primary hyperparathyroidism remains a disorder that is incompletely understood. The change in its clinical presentation from a severely symptomatic disease to a predominantly asymptomatic one is a reflection of increasingly conducted routine surveillances and health screenings rather than a true change in phenotype of the disease. It has come to light that, to identify to the full extent the involvement of the skeleton and kidneys in this disease, more sophisticated and thorough imaging modalities need to be employed. This holds true even for asymptomatic disease. Recent advances in preoperative localising modalities and the use of laboratory techniques such as intraoperative PTH assays and the demand for more cost-effective and shorter hospitalisations have led to a change in the landscape of surgery for primary hyperparathyroidism with a shift and proclivity to more minimally invasive surgeries. The release of periodic consensus guidelines reflects the need for updated information with regard to evaluation and management of this disorder. More work needs to be done to tease out the natural history of the entity of normocalcaemic primary hyperparathyroidism as well as the pathogenesis behind the non-classical manifestations such as involvement of the cardiovascular system in primary hyperparathyroidism.

Follow-Up of Case Vignette

24-Hour urine calcium showed hypercalciuria of 11.23 mmol/day. Fractional excretion of calcium was 2.1%. DXA scan was performed and showed Z-score of −1.5, −1.1, −0.7 and −1.9 over the left femoral neck, left total hip, lumbar spine and distal third of left forearm, respectively.

Given the unequivocally high serum calcium and parathyroid hormone with marked hypercalciuria, the diagnosis of primary hyperparathyroidism was made. Despite absence of symptoms, the young age (<50 years), high serum calcium and marked hypercalciuria were strong indications to recommend parathyroidectomy.

Ultrasound and sestamibi scan showed a sestamibi-avid parathyroid adenoma measuring 0.6 × 0.8 × 0.7 cm postero-inferior to the left lobe of the thyroid.

Successful minimal invasive parathyroidectomy of the left inferior parathyroid adenoma was performed with resolution of hypercalcaemia and hyperparathyroidism.

A repeat DXA scan 1 year after surgery showed improvement in BMD of 12.9%, 17.0% and 20.5% over the left total hip, left femoral neck and lumbar spine, respectively. BMD at the distal third of left forearm remained unchanged.

Acknowledgements The author would like to gratefully acknowledge the help of Dr. Leow Wei Qiang and Dr. Lau Kah Weng, Associate Consultants in the Department of Anatomical Pathology, Singapore General Hospital, for providing the histopathological slides and to Dr Matthew Tan, Consultant Endocrinologist for helping to coordinate the inclusion of the slides and the case vignette in the manuscript.

References

1. Dahir K, Broome J, Shinall MC. Differentiating familial hypocalciuric hypercalcemia from primary hyperparathyroidism. Endocr Pract. 2003;19(4):697–702.
2. Yeh MW, Ituarte PHG, Zhou HC, Nishimoto S, Liu ILA, Harari A, et al. Incidence and prevalence of primary hyperparathyroidism in a racially mixed population. J Clin Endocrinol Metab. 2013;98(3):1122–9.
3. Oliveira UEM, Ohe MN, Santos RO, Cervantes O, Abrahão M, Lazaretti-Castro M, et al. Analysis of the diagnostic presentation profile, parathyroidectomy indication and bone mineral density follow-up of Brazilian patients with primary hyperparathyroidism. Braz J Med Biol Res. 2007;40(4):519–26.
4. Yung CK, Fook-Chong S, Chandran M. The prevalence of recognized contributors to secondary osteoporosis in South East Asian men and post-menopausal women. Are Z score diagnostic thresholds useful predictors of their presence? Arch Osteoporos. 2012;7:49–56.
5. Griebeler ML, Kearns AE, Ryu E, Hathcock MA, Melton LJ, Wermers RA, et al. Secular trends in the incidence of primary hyperparathyroidism over five decades (1965–2010). Bone. 2014;73C:1–7.
6. Lee NC, Norton JA. Multiple-gland disease in primary hyperparathyroidism: a function of operative approach? Arch Surg. 2002;137(8):896–9; discussion 899
7. Duan K, Mete Ö. Parathyroid carcinoma: diagnosis and clinical implications. Turk Patoloji Derg. 2015;31(Suppl 1):80–97.
8. Roy M, Mazeh H, Chen H, Sippel RS. Incidence and localization of ectopic parathyroid adenomas in previously unexplored patients. World J Surg. 2013;37(1):102–6.
9. Eller-Vainicher C, Chiodini I, Battista C, Viti R, Mascia ML, Massironi S, et al. Sporadic and MEN1-related primary hyperparathyroidism: differences in clinical expression and severity. J Bone Miner Res. 2009;24(8):1404–10.
10. Carlson D. Parathyroid pathology: hyperparathyroidism and parathyroid tumors. Arch Pathol Lab Med. 2010;134(11):1639–44.
11. Grimelius L, Akerström G, Johansson H, Bergström R. Anatomy and histopathology of human parathyroid glands. Pathol Annu. 1981;16(Pt 2):1–24.
12. Beard CM, Heath H, O'Fallon WM, Anderson JA, Earle JD, Melton LJ, et al. Therapeutic radiation and hyperparathyroidism. A case-control study in Rochester, Minn. Arch Intern Med. 1989;149(8):1887–90.
13. Larsson C, Friedman E. Localization and identification of the multiple endocrine neoplasia type 1 disease gene. Endocrinol Metab Clin N Am. 1994;23(1):67–79.
14. Villablanca A, Wassif WS, Smith T, Höög A, Vierimaa O, Kassem M, et al. Involvement of the MEN1 gene locus in familial isolated hyperparathyroidism. Eur J Endocrinol. 2002;147(3):313–22.
15. Fialkow PJ, Jackson CE, Block MA, Greenawald KA. Multicellular origin of parathyroid "adenomas". N Engl J Med. 1977;297(13):696–8.
16. Arnold A. Genetic basis of endocrine disease 5. Molecular genetics of parathyroid gland neoplasia. J Clin Endocrinol Metab. 1993;77(5):1108–12.
17. Pradeep PV, Jayashree B, Mishra A, Mishra SK. Systematic review of primary hyperparathyroidism in India: the past, present, and the future trends. Int J Endocrinol. 2011;2011: Article ID: 921814, 9 p.
18. Malabu UH, Founda MA. Primary hyperparathyroidism in Saudi Arabia: a review of 46 cases. Med J Malaysia. 2007;62(5):394–7.
19. Jha S, Jayaraman M, Jha A, Jha R, Modi KD, Kelwadee JV, et al. Primary hyperparathyroidism: a changing scenario in India. Indian J Endocrinol Metab. 2016;20(1):80–3.
20. Mallette LE, Bilezikian JP, Heath DA, Aurbach GD. Primary hyperparathyroidism: clinical and biochemical features. Medicine (Baltimore). 1974;53(2):127–46.
21. Yu N, Donnan PT, Leese GP. A record linkage study of outcomes in patients with mild primary hyperparathyroidism: the Parathyroid Epidemiology and Audit Research Study (PEARS). Clin Endocrinol. 2011;75(2):169–76.
22. Goldfarb S, Agus ZS. Mechanism of the polyuria of hypercalcemia. Am J Nephrol. 1984;4(2):69–76.
23. Ellis G, Spirtos G, Polsky F, Med J. Primary hyperparathyroidism and coexisting nephrogenic diabetes insipidus: rapid postoperative correction. South Med J. 1991;84(8):1019–22.
24. Bandeira F, Cusano NE, Silva BC, Cassibba S, Almeida CB, Machado VCC, et al. Bone disease in primary hyperparathyroidism. Arq Bras Endocrinol Metabol. 2014;58(5):553–61.
25. Mosekilde L. Primary hyperparathyroidism and the skeleton. Clin Endocrinol. 2008;69(1):1–19.
26. Gardner E, Hersh T, Med J. Primary hyperparathyroidism and the gastrointestinal tract. Southerly. 1981;74:197–9.
27. Chan AK, Duh QY, Katz MH, Siperstein AE, Clark OH. Clinical manifestations of primary hyperparathyroidism before and after parathyroidectomy. A case-control study. Ann Surg. 1995;222(3):402–12; discussion 412
28. Carnaille B, Oudar C, Pattou F, Combemale F, Rocha J, Proye C, et al. Pancreatitis and primary hyperparathyroidism: forty cases. Aust N Z J Surg. 1998;68:117–9.

29. Khoo TK, Vege SS, Abu-Lebdeh HS, Ryu E, Nadeem S, Wermers RA, et al. Acute pancreatitis in primary hyperparathyroidism: a population-based study. J Clin Endocrinol Metab. 2009;94(6):2115–8.
30. Coker LH, Rorie K, Cantley L, Kirkland K, Stump D, Burbank N, et al. Primary hyperparathyroidism, cognition, and health-related quality of life. Ann Surg. 2005;242(5):642–50.
31. Solomon BL, Schaaf M, Smallridge RC. Psychologic symptoms before and after parathyroid surgery. Am J Med. 1994;96(2):101–6.
32. Lind L, Hvarfner A, Palmér M, Grimelius L, Akerström G, Ljunghall S, et al. Hypertension in primary hyperparathyroidism in relation to histopathology. Eur J Surg. 1991;157(8):457–9.
33. Smith J, Page M, John R. Augmentation of central arterial pressure in mild primary hyperparathyroidism. Endocrinol Metab. 2000;85:3515.
34. Rubin MR, Maurer MS, McMahon DJ, Bilezikian JP, Silverberg SJ. Arterial stiffness in mild primary hyperparathyroidism. J Clin Endocrinol Metab. 2005;90(6):3326–30.
35. Parisien M, Silverberg SJ, Shane E, Dempster DW, Bilezikian JP. Bone disease in primary hyperparathyroidism. Endocrinol Metab Clin N Am. 1990;19(1):19–34.
36. Stein EM, Silva BC, Boutroy S, Zhou B, Wang J, Udesky J, et al. Primary hyperparathyroidism is associated with abnormal cortical and trabecular microstructure and reduced bone stiffness in postmenopausal women. J Bone Miner Res. 2013;28(5):1029–40.
37. Hansen S, Beck Jensen JE, Rasmussen L, Hauge EM, Brixen K. Effects on bone geometry, density, and microarchitecture in the distal radius but not the tibia in women with primary hyperparathyroidism: a case-control study using HR-pQCT. J Bone Miner Res. 2010;25(9):1941–7.
38. Silva BC, Bilezikian JP. Trabecular bone score: perspectives of an imaging technology coming of age. Arq Bras Endocrinol Metabol. 2014;58(5):493–503.
39. Silva BC, Boutroy S, Zhang C, McMahon DJ, Zhou B, Wang J, et al. Trabecular bone score (TBS)—a novel method to evaluate bone microarchitectural texture in patients with primary hyperparathyroidism. J Clin Endocrinol Metab. 2013;98(5):1963–70.
40. Vignali E, Viccica G, Diacinti D, Cetani F, Cianferotti L, Ambrogini E, et al. Morphometric vertebral fractures in postmenopausal women with primary hyperparathyroidism. J Clin Endocrinol Metab. 2009;94(7):2306–12.
41. Rejnmark L, Vestergaard P, Mosekilde L. Nephrolithiasis and renal calcifications in primary hyperparathyroidism. J Clin Endocrinol Metab. 2011;96(8):2377–85.
42. Lowe H, McMahon D, Rubin M, Bilezikian J, Silverberg S. Normocalcemic primary hyperparathyroidism: further characterization of a new clinical phenotype. Endocrinol Metab. 2007;92(8):3001–5.
43. Vignali E, Cetani F, Chiavistelli S, Meola A, Saponaro F, Centoni R, et al. Normocalcemic primary hyperparathyroidism: a survey in a small village of Southern Italy. Endocr Connect. 2015;4(3):172–8.
44. Kontogeorgos G, Trimpou P, Laine CM, Oleröd G, Lindahl A, Landin-Wilhelmsen K, et al. Normocalcaemic, vitamin D-sufficient hyperparathyroidism - high prevalence and low morbidity in the general population: a long-term follow-up study, the WHO MONICA project, Gothenburg, Sweden. Clin Endocrinol. 2015;83(2):277–84.
45. Glendenning P, Gutteridge DH, Retallack RW, Stuckey BG, Kermode DG, Kent GN, et al. High prevalence of normal total calcium and intact PTH in 60 patients with proven primary hyperparathyroidism: a challenge to current diagnostic criteria. Aust NZ J Med. 1998;28(2):173–8.
46. Rodgers SE, Lew JI. The parathyroid hormone assay. Endocr Pract. 2011;17(Suppl 1):2–6.
47. Glendenning P. Diagnosis of primary hyperparathyroidism: controversies, practical issues and the need for Australian guidelines. Intern Med J. 2003;33(12):598–603.
48. Moosgaard B, Vestergaard P, Heickendorff L, Melsen F, Christiansen P, Mosekilde L, et al. Vitamin D status, seasonal variations, parathyroid adenoma weight and bone mineral density in primary hyperparathyroidism. Clin Endocrinol. 2005;63(5):506–13.
49. Christensen SE, Nissen PH, Vestergaard P, Heickendorff L, Brixen K, Mosekilde L, et al. Discriminative power of three indices of renal calcium excretion for the distinction between familial hypocalciuric hypercalcaemia and primary hyperparathyroidism: a follow-up study on methods. Clin Endocrinol. 2008;69(5):713–20.
50. Eastell R, Brandi ML, Costa AG, D'Amour P, Shoback DM, Thakker RV, et al. Diagnosis of asymptomatic primary hyperparathyroidism: proceedings of the Fourth International Workshop. J Clin Endocrinol Metab. 2014;99(10):3570–9.
51. Kunstman JW, Kirsch JD, Mahajan A, Udelsman R. Clinical review parathyroid localization and implications for clinical management. J Clin Endocrinol Metab. 2013;98(3):902–12.
52. Mihai R, Simon D, Hellman P. Imaging for primary hyperparathyroidism—an evidence-based analysis. Langenbeck's Arch Surg. 2009;394(5):765–84.
53. Cheung K, Wang TS, khyar FF, Roman SA, Sosa JA. A meta-analysis o f preoperative localization techniques for patients with primary hyperparathyroidism. Ann Surg Oncol. 2012;19(2):577–83.
54. Palestro CJ, Tomas MB, Tronco GG. Radionuclide imaging of the parathyroid glands. Semin Nucl Med. 2005;35(4):266–76.
55. Erbil Y, Kapran Y, Işsever H, Barbaros U, Adalet I, Dizdaroğlu F, et al. The positive effect of adenoma weight and oxyphil cell content on preoperative localization with 99mTc-sestamibi scanning for primary hyperparathyroidism. Am J Surg. 2008;195(1):34–9.
56. Lal A, Chen H. The negative sestamibi scan: is a minimally invasive parathyroidectomy still possible? Ann Surg Oncol. 2007;14(8):2363–6.

57. Hwang SH, Rhee Y, Yun M, Yoon JH, Lee JW, Cho A, et al. Usefulness of SPECT/CT in parathyroid lesion detection in patients with thyroid parenchymal 99mTc-sestamibi retention. Nucl Med Mol Imaging. 2017;51(1):32–9.
58. Lorberboym M, Ezri T, Schachter PP. Preoperative technetium Tc 99m sestamibi SPECT imaging in the management of primary hyperparathyroidism in patients with concomitant multinodular goiter. Arch Surg. 2005;140(7):656–60.
59. Tan M, Ng J, Eisman J, Ng D, Hansen L, Chandran M, et al. Review of imaging and operative modalities performed in patients with primary hyperparathyroidism at a mid-volume surgical Centre in Southeast Asia. Ann Acad Med Singap. 2016;45(5):191–7.
60. Lundstroem A, Trolle W, Soerensen C, Myschetzky P. Preoperative localization of hyperfunctioning parathyroid glands with 4D-CT. Eur Arch Otorhinolaryngol. 2015;273(5):1253–9.
61. Hoang JK, Sung WK, Bahl M, Phillips CD. How to perform parathyroid 4D CT: tips and traps for technique and interpretation. Radiology. 2014;270(1):15–24.
62. Kelly HR, Hamberg LM, Hunter GJ. 4D-CT for preoperative localization of abnormal parathyroid glands in patients with hyperparathyroidism: accuracy and ability to stratify patients by unilateral versus bilateral disease in surgery-naive and re-exploration patients. AJNR Am J Neuroradiol. 2014;35(1):176–81.
63. Cham S, Sepahdari AR, Hall KE, Yeh MW, Harari A. Dynamic parathyroid computed tomography (4DCT) facilitates reoperative parathyroidectomy and enables cure of missed hyperplasia. Ann Surg Oncol. 2015;22:3537.
64. Eichhorn-Wharry LI, Carlin AM, Talpos GB. Mild hypercalcemia: an indication to select 4-dimensional computed tomography scan for preoperative localization of parathyroid adenomas. Am J Surg. 2011;201(3):334–8; discussion 338
65. Mahajan A, Starker LF, Ghita M, Udelsman R, Brink JA, Carling T, et al. Parathyroid four-dimensional computed tomography: evaluation of radiation dose exposure during preoperative localization of parathyroid tumors in primary hyper parathyroidism. World J Surg. 2012;36(6):1335–9.
66. Greene AB, Butler RS, McIntyre S, Barbosa GF, Mitchell J, Berber E, et al. National trends in parathyroid surgery from 1998 to 2008: a decade of change. J Am Coll Surg. 2009;209(3):332–43.
67. Lumachi F, Ermani M, Basso S, Zucchetta P, Borsato N, Favia G, et al. Localization of parathyroid tumours in the minimally invasive era: which technique should be chosen? Population-based analysis of 253 patients undergoing parathyroidectomy and factors affecting parathyroid gland detection. Endocr Relat Cancer. 2001;8(1):63–9.
68. Wang TS, Cheung K, Farrokhyar F, Roman SA, Sosa JA. Would scan, but which scan? A cost-utility analysis to optimize preoperative imaging for primary hyperparathyroidism. Surgery. 2011;150(6):1286–94.
69. Bilezikian JP, Brandi ML, Eastell R, Silverberg SJ, Udelsman R, Marcocci C, et al. Guidelines for the management of asymptomatic primary hyperparathyroidism: summary statement from the Fourth International Workshop. J Clin Endocrinol Metab. 2014;99(10):3561–9.
70. Walker MD, Silverberg SJ. Parathyroidectomy in asymptomatic primary hyperparathyroidism: improves "bones" but not "psychic moans". J Clin Endocrinol Metab. 2007;92(5):1613–5.
71. Silverberg SJ, Clarke BL, Peacock M, Bandeira F, Boutroy S, Cusano NE, et al. Current issues in the presentation of asymptomatic primary hyperparathyroidism: proceedings of the Fourth International Workshop. J Clin Endocrinol Metab. 2014;99(10):3580–94.
72. Rubin MR, Bilezikian JP, McMahon DJ, Jacobs T, Shane E, Siris E, et al. The natural history of primary hyperparathyroidism with or without parathyroid surgery after 15 years. J Clin Endocrinol Metab. 2008;93(9):3462–70.
73. Livingston CD. Radioguided parathyroidectomy is successful in 98.7% of selected patients. Endocr Pract. 2014;20(4):305–9.
74. Henry JF. Minimally invasive thyroid and parathyroid surgery is not a question of length of the incision. Langenbeck's Arch Surg. 2008;393(5):621–6.
75. Udelsman R, Lin Z, Donovan P. The superiority of minimally invasive parathyroidectomy based on 1650 consecutive patients with primary hyperparathyroidism. Ann Surg. 2011;253(3):585–91.
76. Chen H, Wang TS, Yen TWF, Doffek K, Krzywda E, Schaefer S, et al. Operative failures after parathyroidectomy for hyperparathyroidism: the influence of surgical volume. Ann Surg. 2010;252(4):691–5.
77. Stalberg P, Sidhu S, Sywak M, Robinson B, Wilkinson M, Delbridge L, et al. Intraoperative parathyroid hormone measurement during minimally invasive parathyroidectomy: does it "value-add" to decision-making? J Am Coll Surg. 2006;203(1):1–6.
78. Rajeev P, Stechman MJ, Kirk H, Gleeson FV, Mihai R, Sadler GP, et al. Safety and efficacy of minimally-invasive parathyroidectomy MIP under local anaesthesia without intra-operative PTH measurement. Int J Surg. 2013;11(3):275–7.
79. Tournis S, Fakidari E, Dontas I, Liakou C, Antoniou J, Galanos A, et al. Effect of parathyroidectomy versus risedronate on volumetric bone mineral density and bone geometry at the tibia in postmenopausal women with primary hyperparathyroidism. J Bone Miner Metab. 2014;32(2):151–8.
80. Hansen S, Hauge EM, Rasmussen L, Jensen JEB, Brixen K. Parathyroidectomy improves bone geometry and microarchitecture in female patients with primary hyperparathyroidism: a one-year prospective controlled study using high-resolution peripheral quantitative computed tomography. J Bone Miner Res. 2012;27(5):1150–8.
81. Alonso S, Ferrero E, Donat M, Martínez G, Vargas C, Hidalgo M, et al. The usefulness of high pre-operative

levels of serum type I collagen bone markers for the prediction of changes in bone mineral density after parathyroidectomy. J Endocrinol Investig. 2012;35(7):640–4.
82. VanderWalde LH, Liu ILA, O'Connell TX, Haigh PI. The effect of parathyroidectomy on bone fracture risk in patients with primary hyperparathyroidism. Arch Surg. 2006;141(9):885–9; discussion 889
83. Rowlands C, Zyada A, Zouwail S, Joshi H, Stechman MJ, Scott-Coombes DM, et al. Recurrent urolithiasis following parathyroidectomy for primary hyperparathyroidism. Ann R Coll Surg Engl. 2013;95(7):523–8.
84. Tassone F, Guarnieri A, Castellano E, Baffoni C, Attanasio R, Borretta G, et al. Parathyroidectomy halts the deterioration of renal function in primary hyperparathyroidism. J Clin Endocrinol Metab. 2015;100(8):3069–73.
85. Tay YKD, Khoo J, Chandran M. Surgery or no surgery: what works best for the kidneys in primary hyperparathyroidism? A study in a multi-ethnic Asian population. Indian J Endocrinol Metab. 2016;20(1):55–61.
86. Murray SE, Pathak PR, Schaefer SC, Chen H, Sippel RS. Improvement of sleep disturbance and insomnia following parathyroidectomy for primary hyperparathyroidism. World J Surg. 2014;38(3):542–8.
87. Das G, Eligar V, Govindan J, Bondugulapati LNR, Okosieme O, Davies S, et al. Impact of vitamin D replacement in patients with normocalcaemic and hypercalcaemic primary hyperparathyroidism and coexisting vitamin D deficiency. Ann Clin Biochem. 2015;52(Pt 4):462–9.
88. Grey A, Lucas J, Horne A, Gamble G, Davidson JS, Reid IR, et al. Vitamin D repletion in patients with primary hyperparathyroidism and coexistent vitamin D insufficiency. J Clin Endocrinol Metab. 2005;90(4):2122–6.
89. Khan AA, Bilezikian JP, Kung AWC, Ahmed MM, Dubois SJ, Ho AYY, et al. Alendronate in primary hyperparathyroidism: a double-blind, randomized, placebo-controlled trial. J Clin Endocrinol Metab. 2004;89(7):3319–25.
90. Misiorowski W. [Alendronate increases bone mineral density in patients with symptomatic primary hyperparathyroidism]. Endokrynol Pol. 2005;56(6):871–5.
91. Tal A, Graves L. Intravenous pamidronate for hypercalcemia of primary hyperparathyroidism. South Med J. 1996;89(6):637–40.
92. Pecherstorfer M, Brenner K, Zojer N. Current management strategies for hypercalcemia. Treat Endocrinol. 2003;2(4):273–92.
93. Peacock M, Bilezikian JP, Bolognese MA, Borofsky M, Scumpia S, Sterling LR, et al. Cinacalcet HCl reduces hypercalcemia in primary hyperparathyroidism across a wide spectrum of disease severity. J Clin Endocrinol Metab. 2011;96(1):E9–18.
94. Marcocci C, Chanson P, Shoback D, Bilezikian J, Fernandez-Cruz L, Orgiazzi J, et al. Cinacalcet reduces serum calcium concentrations in patients with intractable primary hyperparathyroidism. J Clin Endocrinol Metab. 2009;94(8):2766–72.
95. Faggiano A, Di Somma C, Ramundo V, Severino R, Vuolo L, Coppola A, et al. Cinacalcet hydrochloride in combination with alendronate normalizes hypercalcemia and improves bone mineral density in patients with primary hyperparathyroidism. Endocrine. 2011;39(3):283–7.
96. Vellanki P, Lange K, Elaraj D, Kopp PA, El Muayed M. Denosumab for management of parathyroid carcinoma-mediated hypercalcemia. J Clin Endocrinol Metab. 2014;99(2):387–90.
97. Pachydakis A, Koutroumanis P, Geyushi B, Hanna L. Primary hyperparathyroidism in pregnancy presenting as intractable hyperemesis complicating psychogenic anorexia: a case report. J Reprod Med. 2008;53(9):714–6.
98. Truong MT, Lalakea ML, Robbins P, Friduss M. Primary hyperparathyroidism in pregnancy: a case series and review. Laryngoscope. 2008;118(11):1966–9.
99. Schnatz PF, Curry SL. Primary hyperparathyroidism in pregnancy: evidence-based management. Obstet Gynecol Surv. 2002;57(6):365–76.

Parathyroid Imaging

19

Nani H. Md. Latar, George S. Petrides, and Sebastian Aspinall

Introduction

Thirty years ago the interventional radiologist John Doppman wrote in his paper on re-operative parathyroid surgery, "In my opinion, the only localizing study indicated in a patient with untreated primary hyperparathyroidism (PHPT) is to localize an experienced surgeon". Since that time, parathyroid imaging and surgery have undergone major changes including improvement in scintigraphy with planar and tomographic (3-dimensional) images, fusion of tomograms with anatomical information from conventional computed tomography (CT), advances in radiopharmaceuticals, high-resolution ultrasonography (US) and 4-dimensional CT (4D CT), and the emergence of targeted parathyroidectomy, made possible by the development of sensitive preoperative imaging modalities and intraoperative parathyroid hormone (ioPTH) assays.

Despite the advances in parathyroid imaging since that time, every experienced parathyroid surgeon knows that enlarged, hyper-functioning parathyroid glands found at surgery for PHPT are still missed on preoperative imaging scans, and this occurs particularly in multi-gland disease (MGD). Therefore John Doppman's often-quoted words are still very relevant today despite the plethora of parathyroid imaging investigations that have now been developed.

Indications

Why do we do parathyroid imaging? The traditional approach to parathyroid surgery is bilateral neck exploration (BNE) in first-time patients with primary hyperparathyroidism, once the diagnosis has been confirmed biochemically. In experienced hands this approach has a success rate of up to 95%. Nowadays parathyroid localisation imaging is generally considered a mandatory part of the workup to parathyroid surgery. There are two main reasons for this. Firstly it can identify major ectopia of the parathyroid glands that occurs in 1–2% of the population, for which a different surgical approach is needed to achieve operative success (e.g. sternotomy for mediastinal parathyroid glands). Secondly it identifies those patients that are suitable for targeted parathyroidectomy.

N. H. Md. Latar
Department of Surgery, Universiti Kebangsaan Malaysia Medical Centre, Kuala Lumpur, Malaysia

Newcastle University, Newcastle upon Tyne, UK

G. S. Petrides
Newcastle upon Tyne Hospitals, NHS Foundation Trust, Newcastle upon Tyne, UK

S. Aspinall (✉)
North Tyneside General Hospital, Newcastle upon Tyne, UK
e-mail: Sebastian.Aspinall@northumbria-healthcare.nhs.uk

R. Parameswaran, A. Agarwal (eds.), *Evidence-Based Endocrine Surgery*, https://doi.org/10.1007/978-981-10-1124-5_19

Surgical Approaches to the Parathyroid Glands

Bilateral neck exploration (BNE), focused unilateral neck exploration (UNE) and minimally invasive parathyroidectomy (MIP) are the commonest surgical approaches to the parathyroid glands. The latter two operations are considered targeted or focussed approaches.

The advantages of focussed-approach parathyroidectomy include reduced operating time, costs and morbidity, including post-operative hypocalcaemia and vocal cord palsy, without compromising cure rate [1–4]. Given that the majority (>80%) of patients with PHPT have a single parathyroid adenoma, which is suitable for the focussed approach, the advancement in this surgical strategy over the past 25 years is understandable. However recent doubt has emerged regarding the durability of the focussed approach [5] showing lower long-term cure rates for PHPT following focussed-approach parathyroidectomy [6, 7].

It has also been shown that if all the parathyroid glands are inspected at parathyroidectomy, more abnormal parathyroid glands are found [8], i.e. focussed approaches may be missing abnormal parathyroid glands in a proportion of patients that are responsible for late recurrence. It is with this in mind that we consider the role of parathyroid imaging.

Anatomy and Embryology of Parathyroid Glands

Knowledge of parathyroid embryology and anatomy is essential for those involved in interpreting parathyroid imaging. The two paired parathyroid glands are derived from the third and fourth pharyngeal pouches around the fifth week of gestation. The superior glands arise from the fourth pharyngeal pouch and descend in close relation to the developing thyroid gland before settling at their final position posterolateral to the mid-portion of the thyroid gland. This is usually at the level of cricoid cartilage (>90%) within a 1 cm radius of the intersection between the inferior thyroid artery and recurrent laryngeal nerve. The inferior parathyroid glands arise from the third pharyngeal pouch along the thymus. Their final positions are often posterior or lateral to the inferior pole of the thyroid (69%) or lying within the thyrothymic ligament (12–39%) [9]. Due to their longer course of descent, the final position of the inferior glands is more variable than the superior parathyroid glands.

The size of a normal parathyroid gland is approximately 5–6 mm (length), 3–4 mm (width) and 2 mm (depth) and weigh between 30 and 60 mg [10]. Typically there are four parathyroid glands, though the number can vary.

Parathyroid glands are located in ectopic locations in 2–43% in anatomical series [11] and 16–20% of clinical studies in PHPT [12, 13]. Common ectopic locations include the tracheo-oesophageal groove (17.3%) [14]; retro-oesophageal (3.2%) [14]; thymus (17%) [15]; intra-thyroidal (4%) [16]; and mediastinum as low as the aorto-pulmonary window [17] or within the carotid sheath [18]. Major ectopia of the parathyroid gland (e.g. mediastinal) necessitating a surgical approach via the chest is present in 1–2%.

Imaging Modalities

There are multiple parathyroid imaging methods that are available, which include ultrasonography (US), scintigraphy, computed tomography (CT), magnetic resonance imaging (MRI), positron emission tomography (PET), combined modalities such as single-photon emission computed tomography (SPECT-CT) and venous sampling. Each has its own advantages and disadvantages, and there is variability in the imaging modality and techniques used across endocrine centres, depending on local expertise and preference.

Ultrasonography (US)

US is quick, inexpensive, convenient and non-invasive. It doesn't expose the patient to ionising radiation and provides information on concurrent

Table 19.1 Diagnostic performance of US in preoperative parathyroid localisation in primary hyperparathyroidism

Author year	Sensitivity (%)	PPV	Specificity (%)	Accuracy	Number of cases	Lateralise or localise	Patient- or parathyroid-based outcome
Koslin 1998	84	90			37	Localise	
Kebapci 2004	84	92			52	Localise	
Gilat 2004	89	98	33		77	Localise	
Solorzano 2006	76	90	97	91	226	Localise	
Erbil 2008	80	97			80	Localise	
Whitson 2008	67	82	33	61	226	Localise	
Abboud 2008	96.2	98.3	75		253	Localise	
Aspinall 2012	64	88	96	86	65	Localise	
Brown 2015	64	89			89	Lateralise	
Starker 2011	71	87			87	Lateralise	
	48	81.6			87	Localise	
Rodgers 2006	57		94		75	Lateralise	
	29		89		75	Localise	
Lindqvist 2009	82	95	96		264	Lateralise	Parathyroid
	66	79	94		264	Localise	Parathyroid
	83	93	27		264	Lateralise	Patient
	81	81	12		264	Localise	Patient

thyroid pathology and facilitates biopsy of incidental thyroid nodules if indicated. The position of surgical incision and direction of anatomical dissection can be directed by performing ultrasound intraoperatively. Parathyroid US is performed with a high-resolution transducer of 5–15 MHz in a supine patient with neck extended. Abnormal parathyroid glands appear as hypoechoic, ovoid structures on US, whereas normal parathyroid glands which are generally below the size limit of resolution of US are not visible.

When comparing the outcomes of studies of parathyroid US in patients undergoing first-time surgery for PHPT the definition of what constitutes a positive scan needs to be borne in mind. Outcomes may be considered positive if they localise an adenoma to a quadrant of the neck, lateralise to a side of the neck or correctly differentiate superior from inferior parathyroid glands anatomically. Sensitivities and specificities of parathyroid US may be quoted on a patient- or parathyroid-based basis. This is illustrated in the paper by Lindqvist et al. [19] (Table 19.1), though in general studies reporting patient-based or lateralisation outcomes show higher sensitivities but lower specificities [20, 21].

The accuracy of US for parathyroid localisation is comparable to scintigraphy with a pooled sensitivity of 76.1% and positive predictive value of 93.2% from a recent meta-analysis [22].

Operator Factors

The results of ultrasonography are operator dependent, so limiting parathyroid ultrasonography to experienced, dedicated clinicians or sonographers is preferred [23]. There is now a wealth of studies showing excellent outcomes from surgeon-based parathyroid localisation [24–27]. Parathyroid surgeons should learn and perform their own ultrasonography, as this concentrates experience, and in addition perioperative neck ultrasonography facilitates incision placement and anatomical dissection. The surgeon who carries out perioperative neck ultrasonography also benefits from instant feedback from the operative findings, which results in a steep learning curve (Fig. 19.1 and Table 19.1).

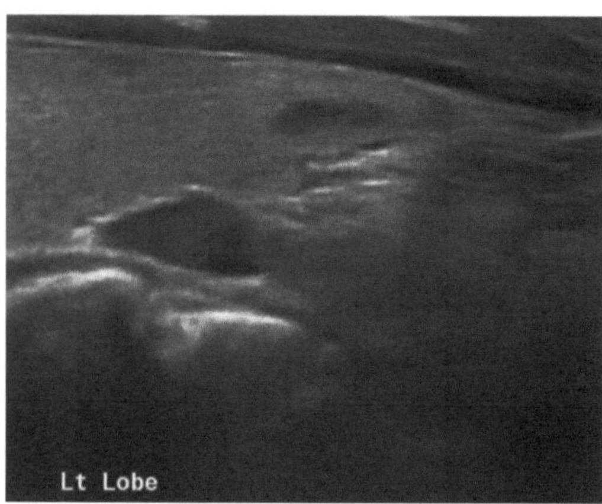

Fig. 19.1 Sagittal plane showing parathyroid adenoma posterior and inferior to left lobe of thyroid gland on ultrasonography

Limitations (Patient factors):

- Multi-gland disease (MGD)
- Posteriorly located upper gland (PLUGs)
- Parathyroid gland size/volume
- Body mass index (BMI)
- Thyroid nodules
- Ectopic gland(s)

Scintigraphy

Scintigraphy is a type of diagnostic molecular imaging which involves the administration of a radiopharmaceutical that is concentrated in an organ of interest, where an image of its distribution is captured by a camera system in two (planar) or three (tomographic) dimensions. Radiopharmaceuticals comprise a carrier biological molecule (e.g. methoxyisobutylisonitrile), and a radionuclide or tracer isotope (e.g. 99m technetium) to give the radiopharmaceutical 99m technetium methoxyisobutylisonitrile (^{99m}Tc-MIBI) used commonly in parathyroid scintigraphy.

In parathyroid scintigraphy ^{99m}Tc-MIBI, concentrated in the mitochondria of parathyroid adenoma, emits γ-rays that are filtered through a collaminator, to produce an image. In tomographic scintigraphy images are acquired with gamma cameras mounted on a rotating gantry and manipulated by a computer to generate 3-dimensional tomograms known as single-photon emission tomography (SPECT). The functional SPECT images can then be fused with anatomical images from conventional computed tomography (SPECT-CT).

Accuracy of Parathyroid Scintigraphy

In comparing the results of parathyroid localisation scintigraphy studies, it is important to consider that different protocols are used in these studies: using various radiopharmaceuticals; single- or dual-radiopharmaceutical techniques (dual-tracer techniques use subtraction thyroid scintigraphy with pertechnetate (^{99m}Tc-O4) or iodine-123 (^{123}I)); different image acquisition methods (pinhole or parallel-hole collaminator); timing of image acquisition (single versus dual phase); planar or tomographic imaging; and more recently fused hybrid imaging with SPECT-CT. The wide variation in reported sensitivity of parathyroid scintigraphy in PHPT of 39% to >90% [28] can be accountable to the different techniques used between studies. Several excellent reviews and meta-analyses of parathyroid imaging in PHPT with scintigraphy have now been published [22, 29].

Interpretation of Outcomes of Parathyroid Scintigraphy

The sensitivity of ^{99m}Tc-MIBI-SPECT is reported by Lindqvist et al. [19] as 92% for patient based on correct side, 91% patient-based correct quadrant, 84% parathyroid-based correct side and 73% parathyroid-based correct quadrant (the respective specificities for these outcomes being 12, 8, 94 and 91%). Ectopically located parathyroid glands are located more often on scintigraphy than US, though in a study of 80 patients with PHPT by Erbil et al. ectopic location did not significantly affect the accuracy of ^{99m}Tc-MIBI [30].

Limitations:

- Parathyroid weight/volume/size
- Content of oxyphil cells
- Position: superiorly located gland difficult to see
- Severity of hyperparathyroidism
- Thyroid nodules
- Lymph nodes
- Brown adipose tissue

Severity of disease has also been shown to affect the accuracy of scintigraphy; Bandeira et al. [31] in a study of 64 patients with PHPT showed that ^{99m}Tc-MIBI was positive in 64% with asymptomatic disease, 83% with nephrolithiasis and 100% with severe bone disease. False-positive scintigraphy results, due to uptake in thyroid nodules, lymph nodes [32] and brown adipose tissue [33], also reduces the specificity of ^{99m}Tc-MIBI but these false positives can be reduced with the use of SPECT-CT [34] (Table 19.2).

Technique-Related Factors

(a) Pinhole versus parallel-hole collaminators

The greater spatial resolution capabilities of pinhole versus parallel-hole collaminators, which is particularly suited to imaging small structures in the neck, has been shown to improve the sensitivity of parathyroid scintigraphy using single (^{99m}Tc-MIBI)-tracer, dual-phase protocol [35, 36] and dual (^{99m}Tc-MIBI ^{123}I)-tracer, single-phase protocol [36, 37].

(b) Planar imaging

In the single-tracer, dual-phase technique images are taken 10 min and 90–120 min after injection of ^{99m}Tc-MIBI, prolonged retention of which in the parathyroid enables parathyroid localisation. In the dual-tracer subtraction method, thyroid scintigraphy is also undertaken with ^{99m}Tc-pertechnetate [38, 39] or ^{123}I [40] and the images digitally subtracted to identify the parathyroid adenoma. The superiority of dual-tracer (^{123}I or ^{99m}Tc-pertechnetate) over single-tracer scintigraphy has been reported in some studies [36, 41, 42] although the reduced radiation dose from dual-phase imaging also has benefits.

(c) Planar imaging versus single-photon emission computed tomography (SPECT)

The addition of SPECT acquisition to planar scintigraphy has been shown to increase the accuracy of parathyroid localisation [43–47] and should ideally be used routinely for parathyroid localisation prior to surgery for PHPT [48]. A recent meta-analysis has shown a pooled sensitivity and positive predictive value of 78.9 and 90.7% for ^{99m}Tc-MIBI-SPECT, which is comparable to ultrasound [22].

(d) ^{99m}Tc-MIBI-SPECT has the advantage of localising ectopic and posteriorly placed adenomas that are often missed on US [42]. Some studies have failed to find a significant benefit of SPECT over planar acquisition [49]. Planar images are commonly undertaken as well as tomographic ones during parathyroid localisation imaging.

Hybrid Single-Photon Emission Computed Tomography-CT (SPECT-CT)

Fusion of sestamibi SPECT images with conventional CT provides information on the anatomical location of the parathyroid adenoma and is widely known as SPECT-CT. A recent meta-analysis by Wei et al. [50] looked at 18 studies and found the sensitivity of SPECT-CT to be much greater than that of SPECT or planar imaging alone (SPECT-CT 84%, SPECT 6%, planar 63%). The same meta-analysis also demonstrated that the positive predictive value of SPECT-CT exceeded that of scintigraphic methods alone. This is likely due to the anatomical correlation which not only increases the specificity by reducing false-positive scans due to ^{99m}Tc-MIBI uptake in cervical lymph nodes and thyroid nodules but is also useful for operative planning. A further meta-analysis by Treglia et al. [51] demonstrated a similar detection rate of 88% for SPECT-CT on both a per-patient- and per-lesion-based analysis. Diagnostic confidence also

Table 19.2 Diagnostic performance of ^{99m}Tc-MIBI either as single modality or in combination with image subtraction acquired using planar, SPECT or SPECT-CT

	Tracer	Thyroid scintigraphy subtraction	Image acquisition	Sensitivity (%)	Specificity (%)	Accuracy	PPV	Number of patients	Detection parameter
Sharma 2006	^{99m}Tc-MIBI	No	Planar	62			95.3	138	
	^{99m}Tc-MIBI	No	SPECT	73			91.7	165	
	^{99m}Tc-MIBI	^{123}I	SPECT	96			89	350	
	^{99m}Tc-MIBI	No	SPECT-CT	83			91	131	
Freudenberg 2006	^{99m}Tc-MIBI	No	Planar	74	96		89	84	
	^{99m}Tc-MIBI	No	Planar + SPECT	81	96		89	84	
	^{99m}Tc-MIBI	99mTcO4	Planar + SPECT	87	97		92	84	
Lavely 2007	^{99m}Tc-MIBI	No	Parallel-hole planar	56.5	98.7		79.0	110	
	^{99m}Tc-MIBI	No	SPECT	61.5	98.7		79.4	110	
	^{99m}Tc-MIBI	No	SPECT-CT	72	99.1		87.3	110	
Nichols 2008	^{99m}Tc-MIBI	99mTcO4	Pinhole planar	88	88	88	89	462	
	^{99m}Tc-MIBI	99mTcO4	SPECT	83	84	83	85	462	
Tunninen 2013	^{99m}Tc-MIBI	^{123}I	Parallel planar	63.3–80	93.9–97	86.5–89.6		51	
	^{99m}Tc-MIBI	^{123}I	Pinhole planar	76.7–80	92.4–95.5	88.5–89.6		51	
	^{99m}Tc-MIBI	^{123}I	SPECT-CT	63.3-76.7	92.4–98.5	85.4–89.6		51	
	^{99m}Tc-MIBI	No	Parallel-hole planar	15.8–31.6	93.9–100	75–76.5		51	
	^{99m}Tc-MIBI	No	SPECT-CT	10-16.7	100	71.9–74		51	
Lindqvist 2009	^{99m}Tc-MIBI		Parallel-hole SPECT	84	91	91		264	Lateralise
	^{99m}Tc-MIBI		Parallel-hole SPECT	73	94	81		264	Localise
Starker 2011	^{99m}Tc-MIBI	No	Planar + SPECT	61.6			84.2	52	Lateralise
	^{99m}Tc-MIBI	No	Planar + SPECT	40			78.9	52	Localise
Brown 2015	^{99m}Tc-MIBI	^{99m}TO4-	Pinhole planar + SPECT-CT	74			87	89	Lateralise
Tomas 2008	^{99m}Tc-MIBI	No	Pinhole planar	89	93	91	88	49	
	^{99m}Tc-MIBI	No	Parallel-hole planar	56	96	74	94	49	
Klingensmith 2013	^{99m}Tc-MIBI	No	Pinhole planar	66.2				33	
	^{99m}Tc-MIBI	No	Parallel planar	43.2				33	
	^{99m}Tc-MIBI	^{123}I	Pinhole planar	83.8				33	
	^{99m}Tc-MIBI	^{123}I	Parallel planar	62.2				33	
Hindie 1998	^{99m}Tc-MIBI	No	Pinhole planar	79	95	77		30	
	^{99m}Tc-MIBI	^{123}I single phase	Pinhole planar	94	98	93		30	
Caveny 2012	^{99m}Tc-MIBI	No	Pinhole planar	66				37	
	^{99m}Tc-MIBI	^{123}I single phase	Pinhole planar	94				37	
	^{99m}Tc-MIBI	^{123}I dual phase	Pinhole planar	90				37	

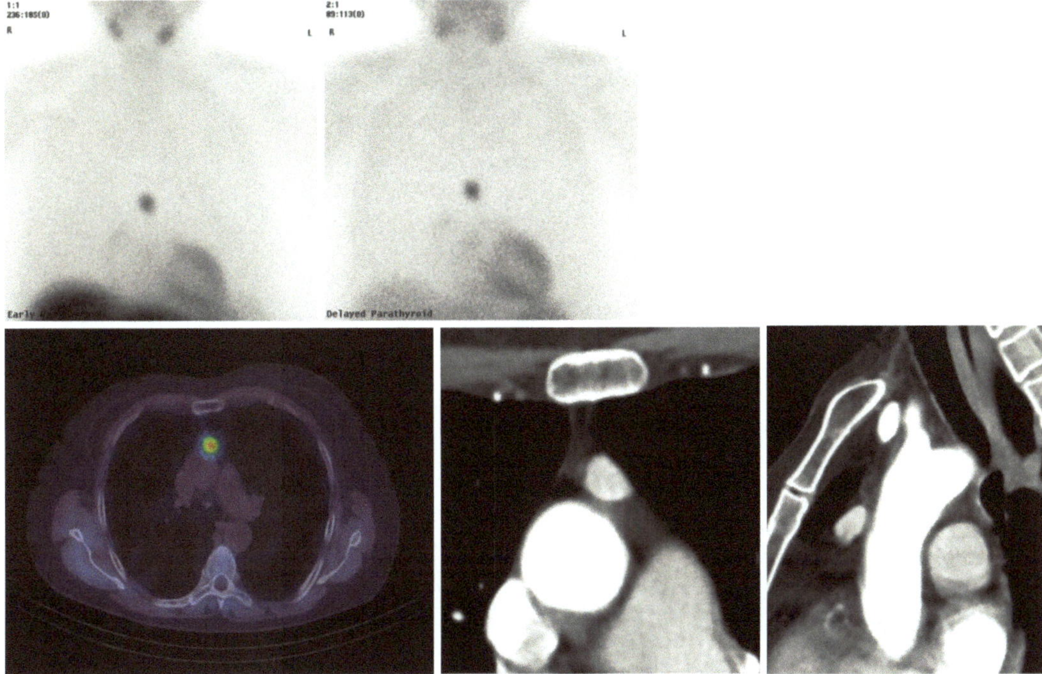

Fig. 19.2 Washout ^{99m}Tc-MIBI images demonstrating a mediastinal ectopic gland accurately localised with SPECT-CT. 4D CT images contemporaneously demonstrate the parathyroid adenoma with intense enhancement

increases with fused images and it has been shown that for smaller adenomas the increased sensitivity and specificity seen with SPECT-CT are more apparent [52]. As with all parathyroid imaging modalities the accuracy of SPECT-CT is adversely affected by multi-gland disease [53]. SPECT-CT can be performed at an early time point (10–30 min post-injection), a delayed time point (90–150 min post-injection) or both time points [54]. The need for dual-time-point SPECT-CT is debated with a study suggesting that an early-time-point SPECT-CT may suffice in the majority of cases [55] (Figs. 19.2 and 19.3).

Positron Emission Tomography (PET)

Three different radiopharmaceuticals have been shown to demonstrate uptake in parathyroid adenomas, namely FDG, choline and methionine. In general PET has not found widespread use in first-time imaging for PHPT but the high reported sensitivity of ^{11}C-methionine and ^{18}F-fluorocholine suggests a potential role in persistent and/or recurrent disease, as an alternative to 4D CT, particularly if conventional imaging with US and ^{99m}Tc-MIBI-SPECT is negative or inconclusive.

(a) ^{18}F-FDG-PET

Parathyroid adenomas demonstrate increased uptake as demonstrated by Newmann et al. [56] but due to lower specificity compared to ^{99m}Tc-MIBI-SPECT this type of investigation is not commonly undertaken.

(b) ^{11}C-methionine

^{11}C-methionine accumulates in parathyroid adenomas due to increased transmembrane transport and protein synthesis—the amino acid methionine is a component of parathyroid hormone. Sensitivities of ^{11}C-methionine for the localisation of parathyroid adenomas have been reported to be 69–94%, with a pooled sensitivity from a recent meta-analysis of 81 [57]. The disadvantage of the isotope ^{11}C is that its half-life is short (20 min), which makes its routine use logistically difficult and expensive.

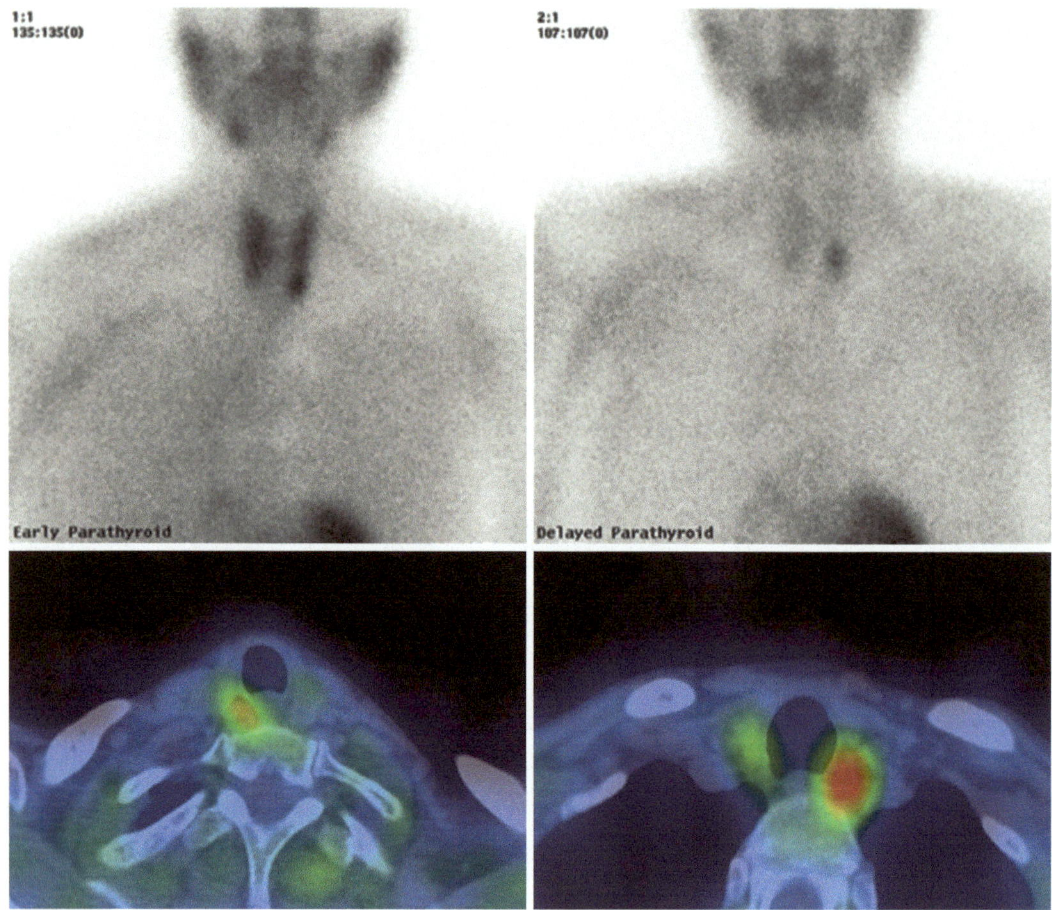

Fig. 19.3 ^{99m}Tc-MIBI images of the same patient demonstrating the greater sensitivity of SPECT-CT compared to planar imaging. Planar images demonstrate a left lower parathyroid adenoma. SPECT-CT demonstrates a right upper parathyroid adenoma in addition

(c) ^{11}C-choline/^{18}F-fluorocholine

Choline-based radiopharmaceuticals, which reflect lipid or cell membrane metabolism, can be utilised in parathyroid imaging. The same limitations of ^{11}C-methionine apply to ^{11}C-choline, due to the short half-life of ^{11}C, but ^{18}F-fluorocholine, with a half-life of 110 min, has been used as an alternative and found to be highly sensitive for parathyroid localisation (Table 19.3).

Computed Tomography (CT)

Conventional contrast-enhanced computed tomography is not generally used for parathyroid imaging due to its low sensitivity [32].

Four-dimensional CT is a technique that relies on the perfusion characteristics of parathyroid adenomas, i.e. rapid uptake and washout of contrast with time (the fourth dimension) for localisation. 4D CT has been shown to be particularly useful in re-operative parathyroid surgery [58] and when conventional imaging with US/^{99m}Tc-MIBI-SPECT is negative or inconclusive [20, 22, 59]. It is also an accurate technique for localisation in first-time surgery for PHPT with a reported sensitivity of 85.7% [59], though the thyroid-specific radiation exposure, which is higher than that in conventional parathyroid scintigraphy, would be a concern if it were to be used routinely in first-time surgery, particularly in young people (Table 19.4).

Table 19.3 Sensitivity and specificity of PET in preoperative parathyroid gland(s) localisation

	Number of patients	Sensitivity (%)	Specificity (%)	Radiopharmaceutical	Patient group
Melon 1995	7	28.5		^{18}F-FDG PET	PHPT
Neumann 1996	21	86	78	^{18}F-FDG PET	PHPT
Michaud 2014	12	89		^{18}F-fluorocholine PET-CT	PHPT/SHPT
Kluijfhout 2015	5	80		^{18}F-fluorocholine PET-CT	PHPT negative or discordant US/MIBI SPECT
Sundin 1996	34	85		^{11}C-methionine PET	Primary/recurrent PHPT/SHPT
Cook 1998	8	75		^{11}C-methionine PET	Recurrent PHPT/THPT
Otto 2004	18	94		^{11}C-methionine PET	PHPT negative or equivocal US/MIBI
	12	69		^{11}C-methionine PET	SHPT/THPT negative or equivocal US/MIBI

Table 19.4 Outcome of 4D CT localisation for first-time surgery for PHPT

	Imaging outcome	Number	Sensitivity (%)	Specificity (%)	PPV
Rodgers 2006	Lateralise	75	88	88	
	Localise	75	70	88	
Starker 2011	Lateralise	33	93.9		83.8
	Localise	33	85.7		93.5
Hunter 2012	Lateralise	143	93.7		
	Localise	143	86.6		
Kelly 2014	Lateralise	152	87.5		
Brown 2015	Lateralise	89	88	88	
Day 2015	Localise	37	89		74
	Lateralise	37	93		80
Hinson 2015	Localise	19	76.5	91.5	
	Lateralise	19	84.2	81.8	

Magnetic Resonance Imaging (MRI)

This study has possible advantage over other modalities as it outlines the anatomical landmark and different structures of the neck more accurately. It is usually more popular in redo neck surgery either for recurrent or persistent disease and those with previous neck surgery. Adenomas are generally hyperintense on T2-weighted images and hypointense in T1 intermediate images and light up after administration of contrast material.

The fundamental property of magnetic imaging lies in its ability to measure the difference in density of adjacent organs to increase confidence in detecting the abnormal gland [60]. Sensitivity has been reported to be between 69 and 88% with false-positive rate of 1.6–10%. When compared to USG and ^{99m}Tc-MIBI, MRI gives slightly higher sensitivity and accuracy (88% vs. 58%, 80% and 84% vs. 44% and 80%) [61]. Dynamic magnetic resonance angiography (MRA) improves sensitivity and specificity especially for lateralisation [62]. As with all other imaging modalities, MRI is more sensitive in detecting an adenoma compared to hyperplastic gland. Disadvantages include higher cost and unsuitability for patients with claustrophobia or ferrous implants.

Parathyroid Imaging in Multi-Gland Disease

The incidence of multi-gland disease is significantly increased in patients with negative localisation scans though interestingly a significant proportion of patients with negative localisation scans will still have a single adenoma [63–65].

The lower accuracy of parathyroid localisation in multi-gland disease is not restricted to any particular modality, but affects all types of parathyroid localisation [66] (see Table 19.5 which illustrates the most recent data on sensitivity, specificity and accuracy of imaging modalities comparing single-gland disease (SGD) and multi-gland disease (MGD)).

Strategy in Negative Localisation or Discordant Localisation

The absence of a target for surgery on preoperative parathyroid imaging should not influence the indication for parathyroidectomy, which is a decision, taking into account the patients' fitness for surgery, made on the basis of the biochemical diagnosis and the presence of symptoms and/or complications from PHPT. However, image-negative patients with PHPT are a more challenging group to manage with increased risks of failed surgery/persistent disease [64, 67]. The key question in this group is whether to proceed to bilateral neck exploration or undertake further imaging to try and identify a target for focussed approach. Both approaches are reasonable.

Despite an increase in the incidence of MGD in image-negative patients a significant proportion still have SGD—76% (79/104) of patients with PHPT and non-localising ^{99m}Tc-MIBI scans in a study by Chiu et al. [64]. Thus, with the advent of more sensitive imaging modalities such as 4D CT and PET-CT there is an argument to investigate these patients further, to identify a surgical target to enable focussed approach [1–4].

Day et al. [68] reported successful parathyroid localisation (sensitivity 89%, PPV 74%) with 4D CT in 37 patients with non-localised disease, after US and ^{99m}Tc-MIBI, which permitted a focussed approach in 38%. Similarly, Hinson et al. [69] found 4D CT to be clinically useful in parathyroid localisation (sensitivity 76.5%, specificity 91.5% and accuracy 88.2%) in 19 patients with non-localising US and ^{99m}Tc-MIBI-SPECT. Brown et al. [70] reported an 80% sensitivity of 4D CT in 21 patients with negative ^{99m}Tc-MIBI enabling focussed-approach surgery in 17 cases. However, numbers of PHPT patients from studies using PET in the context of non-localised or discordant conventional imaging are too small to make any general conclusions regarding the role of PET, though there are reports that this imaging modality may be useful for this purpose [71, 72].

Similar arguments for negative localisation apply to patients with discordant or contradictory imaging—i.e. imaging investigations that identify parathyroid adenomas in different locations or when parathyroid adenomas seen on one scan are not confirmed on another. Although the incidence of MGD is increased in patients with discordant imaging, the incidence of SGD is still high in this group, and did not differ from that seen in patients with negative preoperative imaging in a study by Philippon et al. [63]—69.5% (69/99) with discordant imaging versus 72% (20/28) with negative imaging. So there is a rationale for trying to identify SGD in patients with discordant results on US and ^{99m}Tc-MIBI SPECT-CT, with more sensitive imaging such as 4D CT, to potentially enable them to benefit from the focussed approach.

The strategy adopted in endocrine units will depend on local expertise and availability of imaging as well as surgeon and patient preference. The potential benefits of focussed-approach surgery need to be weighed up against the disadvantages and costs of multiple imaging investigations, particularly those using ionising radiation. It should not be forgotten that the cure rates of bilateral neck exploration in patients with negative localisation from traditional parathyroid imaging, though lower than patients with preoperatively localised disease, are still very good (89/92 or 97% at 6 months, Chiu et al. [64]). Surgical adjuncts such as ioPTH may also improve the outcome in those patients that undergo surgery without further imaging [67].

When concordant results are obtained from preoperative parathyroid localisation with US and ^{99m}Tc-MIBI then the European Society of Endocrine Surgeons recommends focussed approach without the need for ioPTH, and advises BNE without further investigation in image-negative patients [73] and BNE or MIP with ioPTH in patients with discordant imaging investigations.

Table 19.5 Most recent data (past 10 years) comparing sensitivity (SN), specificity (SP) and accuracy of preoperative parathyroid localisation studies

			SGD				MGD			
Author	Year	Modality	No. of patients	SN (%)	SP (%)	Accuracy (%)	No. of patients	SN (%)	SP (%)	Accuracy (%)
Soon et al.	2008		195	89.9	76.5		9	37.5	15.7	
Weber et al.	2010	^{11}C Met- PET-CT	30	83			3	67		
Saengsuda et al.	2012	^{99m}Tc-MIBI	18	90	100	97.2	48	67.1	92.3	71.7
Chazen et al.	2012	4D-CT	32	85.7	100	92.0	7	42.9	100.0	88.6
Nichols et al.	2012	^{99m}Tc MIBI	520	97.0	93.0		331	61.0	84.0	
Wakamatsu et al.	2015	US	35	55.2			35	46.7		
Galvin et al.	2016	^{99m}Tc MIBI		50.0			6	24.0		
		4D-CT		88.0				53.0		
Nocholas et al.[a]	2016	^{99m}Tc MIBI SPECT-CT	207	98.0	95.0		39	66.0	90.0	
	2016	4D-CT	34	76			6	53		
		^{99m}Tc MIBI		43				24		

SN sensitivity, *SP* specificity

[a]Note the high sensitivity and specificity of ^{99m}Tc-MIBI SPECT/CT

Single or Combined Imaging

Given the benefits and limitations of individual imaging modalities it is not surprising that the sensitivity of parathyroid localisation increases when the results of different studies are combined. Particularly US has limited accuracy in ectopic and posteriorly situated adenomas that may be identified on ^{99m}Tc-MIBI. But the accuracy of both scintigraphy and US is reduced in multi-gland disease which is therefore more likely to be present if both these imaging modalities are negative [65]. There is a strong argument therefore for routinely performing both US and ^{99m}Tc-MIBI in first-time surgery for PHPT (Table 19.6).

Parathyroid Localisation for Persistent/Recurrent Parathyroidectomy

Re-operative parathyroid surgery for persistent or recurrent PHPT is technically more challenging than first-time surgery due to the obliteration of tissue planes due to previous surgery, higher incidence of ectopic parathyroid glands, and familial/multi-gland disease. The importance of operative planning, with review of previous operation notes and pathology reports as well as surgical experience and knowledge of parathyroid anatomy and embryology, cannot be overemphasised to improve outcomes in reoperative surgery, which remain lower than first-time parathyroidectomy [74].

Accurate preoperative localisation with a view to focussed parathyroidectomy is the key to successful re-operative parathyroidectomy. Conventional imaging with US and ^{99m}Tc-MIBI SPECT/CT is usually repeated in this group of patients and if the results remain negative discordant or equivocal, then further localisation is undertaken. Traditionally these have included MRI or conventional CT, though the sensitivity of these cross-sectional modalities is limited, often with invasive localisation such as selective venous sampling (SVS) or USG FNAC.

SVS is an invasive procedure in which the cervical veins are accessed under fluoroscopic control via a cannula introduced percutaneously into the femoral vein. It regionalises an area in which the parathyroid adenoma is located, based on a 1.5–2.0-fold increase in the PTH compared to baseline levels, from a sample taken from a peripheral forearm vein [75]. Complications related to cannulation and adverse allergic reactions to contrast agents may occur but are rare. It is often reserved in re-operative neck cases secondary to persistent or recurrent disease when all other imaging modalities failed to localise an abnormal gland or are inconclusive [3]. Sensitivities for SVS in this scenario have been reported to range from 63 to 95% (Table 19.7).

Although reports of parathyroid localisation in re-operative PHPT with 4D CT do not include large patient numbers as yet, early indications suggest that this modality has a role, and may increase concordance of image and surgical findings over US and ^{99m}Tc-MIBI, enabling focussed re-operative parathyroid surgery and reduced operative time [76, 77]. Furthermore the sensitivity of parathyroid imaging with 4D CT does not seem to be reduced in high BMI or re-operative (50–91%) compared to first-time surgery

Table 19.6 Sensitivity of US and ^{99m}Tc-MIBI alone or combination in parathyroid localisation

	US (%)	^{99m}Tc MIBI (%)	Combined US + ^{99m}Tc MIBI (%)	Number of patients
Lumachi 2000	80.4	86.8	94.5	91
De Feo 2000	27	57	96	49
Haber 2002	80	92	Improved	74
Kebapci 2004	84	73	92	52
Freudenberg 2006	Ns	74	91	84
Whitson 2008	67	67	82	226

Table 19.7 Accuracy of parathyroid imaging in recurrent disease

	Number	Modality	Sensitivity	PPV
Nilsson 1994	29	SVS	93	
Marriette 1998		^{99m}Tc MIBI	69	
		US	50	
		SVS	63	
		MRI	29	
		Conventional CT	16	
Akerstrom 2008	44	^{99m}Tc MIBI	90	88
	41	US	72	93
	38	^{11}C-methionine PET	79	87
	11	SVS	91	100
Mortenson 2008	44	^{99m}Tc MIBI	54	
	42	US	21	
	45	4D CT	88	
Gotway 2001	98	^{99m}Tc MIBI	85	89
	98	MRI	82	89
Witteveen 2010		SVS	75–95	
Lubitz 2010	18	4D CT	50	
Brown 2015	11	^{99m}Tc MIBI	46	100
	11	US	30	
	11	4D CT	91	

(70–87%). Although the sensitivity of 4D CT is reduced in MGD, this was still significantly higher than ^{99m}Tc-MIBI or US in re-operative cases reported by Mortenson 2008 (80% vs. 27% and 17%, respectively) [58].

Another approach in re-operative patients with equivocal localisation on imaging is to perform USG FNAC with rapid PTH assay of suspected parathyroid adenomas, and this strategy has been shown to be effective in a study of 12 patients from 2006 by Maser et al. [78].

Is 99mTc-MIBI SPECT-CT Alone Adequate in Preoperative Imaging of PHPT?

There is a significant body of evidence supporting the benefits of ^{99m}Tc-MIBI SPECT-CT over US and planar ^{99m}Tc-MIBI for preoperative localisation of PHPT [50, 51, 79, 80]. Apart from improved parathyroid localisation, it has also been shown to be relatively more sensitive for hyperplastic lesions [53, 81], in re-operative surgery [82] and in cases with excessive thyroid gland retention of ^{99m}Tc-MIBI [83]. The high radiation exposure of 4D CT also makes ^{99m}Tc-MIBI SPECT-CT potentially a safer localising investigation, albeit with similar sensitivity and specificity to 4D CT [80]. One major drawback of ^{99m}Tc-MIBI SPECT-CT is its possibly higher cost when compared to planar ^{99m}Tc-MIBI, which becomes more evident in cases with an easily localised gland [84]; however a detailed cost-effectiveness analysis, and study of the sensitivity and PPV of US with ^{99m}Tc-MIBI -SPECT versus US with ^{99m}Tc-MIBI SPECT-CT, found no significant difference between these two imaging strategies in parathyroid localisation [85].

Some surgeons are reluctant to rely on single-modality imaging for preoperative parathyroid localisation due to misleading false-positive results and there have been very few publications comparing US and ^{99m}Tc-MIBI SPECT-CT with ^{99m}Tc-MIBI SPECT-CT alone. Tee MC et al. [86] did however report no incremental value on the extent of parathyroid surgery when US was added to ^{99m}Tc-MIBI SPECT-CT, but the high accuracy rate of parathyroid localisation with combined US and ^{99m}Tc-MIBI SPECT-CT, reported by

Satoru et al. [87] of 100%, versus 88.5% with single-modality imaging alone, demonstrates why multimodal imaging is still a popular strategy.

^{99m}Tc-MIBI SPECT-CT can be considered a multimodality imaging investigation, combining the functional information from ^{99m}Tc-MIBI SPECT with the anatomical cross-sectional information from CT, and is now not uncommonly used as the sole imaging technique in parathyroid localisation. The CT component can be optimised to help demonstrate nodules by adjusting imaging parameters and patients can be secured in position to ensure that there is minimal movement between the SPECT and CT components, to aid localisation. If ^{99m}Tc-MIBI SPECT demonstrates a hot spot, consistent with a hyper-functioning parathyroid adenoma that is not confirmed on the CT component or ^{99m}Tc-MIBI SPECT fails to demonstrate an adenoma, there is then a strong argument for using US, in addition to ^{99m}Tc-MIBI SPECT-CT.

US does however provide additional information about the thyroid gland which can be useful. It is a quick and relatively easy office-based procedure that is increasingly being used by trained clinicians without the need for a separate visit to the radiology department. In rare cases, US can identify further parathyroid adenomas that were not ^{99m}Tc-MIBI avid. US can also be performed perioperatively to determine the optimal skin incision and plane of dissection for parathyroidectomy, helping to plan surgery.

In conclusion, given the high sensitivity and specificity of ^{99m}Tc-MIBI SPECT-CT as a dual-modality contemporaneous technique, ^{99m}Tc-MIBI SPECT-CT can be used as the sole imaging modality for parathyroid localisation. But given the low cost, lack of radiation exposure and likely small increase in accuracy that US offers when combined with SPECT-CT, US should still be considered, in addition, prior to surgery, and especially when a hyper-functioning parathyroid adenoma is either not identified with ^{99m}Tc-MIBI SPECT-CT or identified with ^{99m}Tc-MIBI SPECT and not co-localised on CT. Each institution should consider the local expertise available when defining its preferred pathway.

Guideline for Imaging in Primary Hyperparathyroidism (Fig. 19.4)

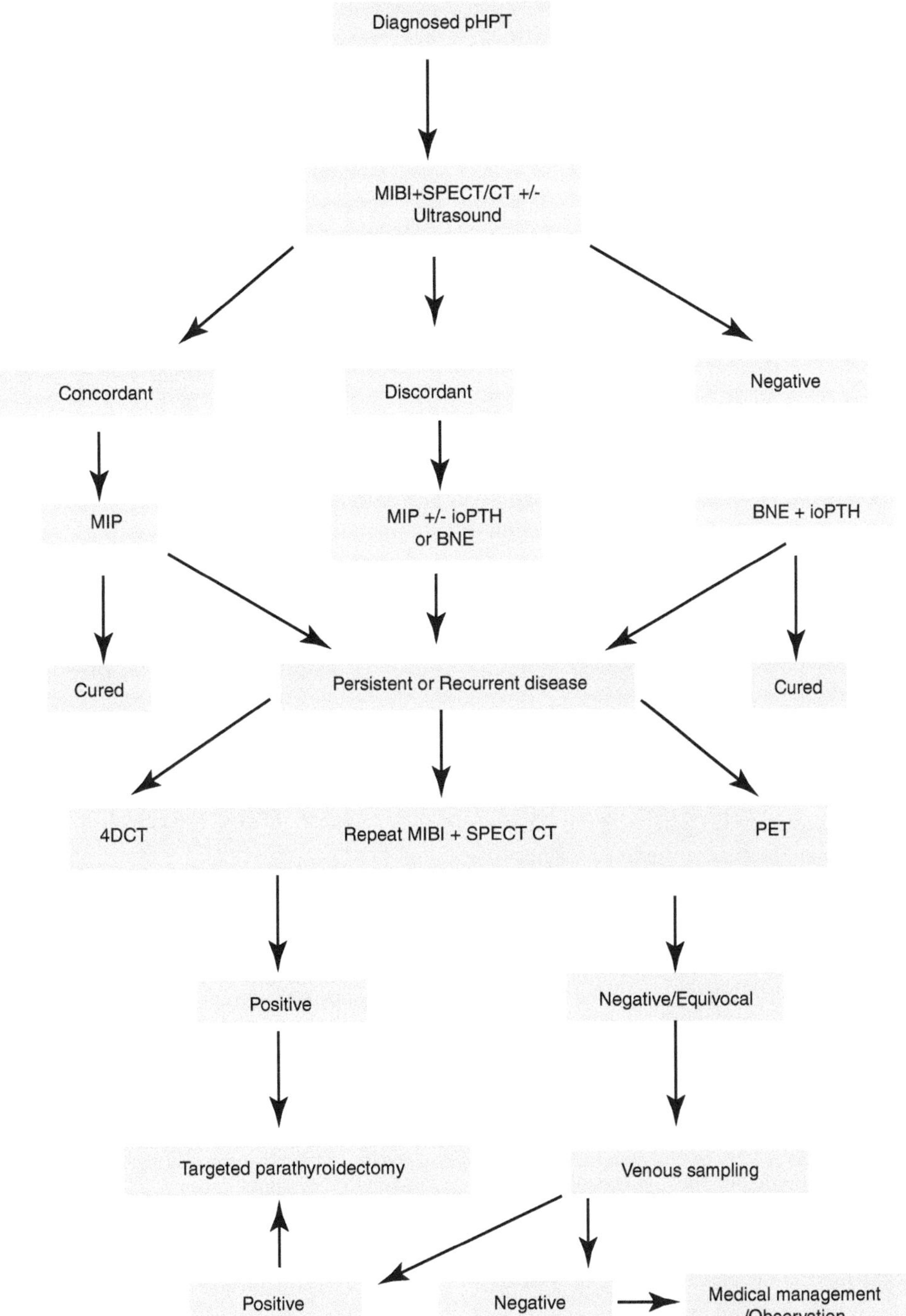

Fig. 19.4 Algorithm of a suggested approach to preoperative localisation strategy in sporadic primary hyperparathyroidism. ^{99m}Tc-MIBI SPECT-CT +/− US is proposed as the most accurate initial preoperative imaging modality that is able to identify mediastinal ectopic gland(s) as well as double adenomas. BNE is the suggested approach after a negative preoperative localisation or discordant results. The addition of ioPTH measurement is useful in discordant and negative localisation cases. In recurrent or persistent diseases, either one or a combination of 4D CT, ^{99m}Tc-MIBI SPECT-CT or PET is useful. Failing which, an invasive selective venous sampling can be performed

Conclusions

Preoperative localisation studies in patients with primary hyperparathyroidism are becoming a necessity nowadays to allow minimally invasive surgery and exclude the presence of an ectopic gland. The choice of imaging modalities is mainly based on the availability, cost and expertise of each method. This field is expected to further expand with the emergence of more sensitive methods of detection and advancement of technology.

Clinical Pearls

1. In low-resource countries BNE for PHPT without prior parathyroid imaging is a very reasonable approach in experienced hands.
2. Parathyroid imaging is undertaken to facilitate focussed-approach surgery and also identify those ectopically located glands not amenable to excision via a standard cervicotomy incision.
3. Though choice of parathyroid imaging depends on the availability and expertise in each centre ^{99m}Tc MIBI SPECT CT is the imaging modality of choice for first-time parathyroidectomy in PHPT. Fusion of functional information from scintigraphy with anatomical information from conventional CT improves the accuracy of this imaging modality.
4. Parathyroid surgeons should use US for parathyroid localisation in the outpatient department and operating theatre. It is quick, inexpensive and non-invasive, and enables assessment of concurrent thyroid pathology as well as helping to determine the optimal incision placement and direction of tissue dissection during parathyroidectomy.
5. Prior to re-operative surgery for persistent or recurrent disease a surgical target needs to be identified by imaging. Repeat initial imaging and/or, if available, perform 4D CT to identify the source of persistent or recurrent disease, particularly if initial imaging is negative or equivocal (alternatively MRI or ^{11}C-methionine/^{18}F-fluorocholine PET can be considered). If the results of non-invasive parathyroid imaging remain equivocal then SVS should be undertaken prior to re-operative surgery to confirm that the suspected target seen on imaging is the source of autonomous PTH secretion. Referral to tertiary centres with access to more specialist imaging and expertise is often undertaken in these cases.

References

1. Bergenfelz A, Lindblom P, Tibblin S, Westerdahl J. Unilateral versus bilateral neck exploration for primary hyperparathyroidism: a prospective randomized controlled trial. Ann Surg. 2002;236(5):543–51.
2. Russell CF, Dolan SJ, Laird JD. Randomized clinical trial comparing scan-directed unilateral versus bilateral cervical exploration for primary hyperparathyroidism due to solitary adenoma. Br J Surg. 2006;93(4):418–21.
3. Udelsman R. Approach to the patient with persistent or recurrent primary hyperparathyroidism. J Clin Endocrinol Metab. 2011;96(10):2950–8.
4. Singh Ospina NM, Rodriguez-Gutierrez R, Maraka S, Espinosa de Ycaza AE, Jasim S, Castaneda-Guarderas A, et al. Outcomes of parathyroidectomy in patients with primary hyperparathyroidism: a systematic review and meta-analysis. World J Surg. 2016;40(10):2359–77.
5. Pasieka JL. What should we tell our patients? Lifetime guarantee or is it 5- to 10-year warranty on a parathyroidectomy for primary hyperparathyroidism? World J Surg. 2015;39(8):1928–9.
6. Schneider DF, Mazeh H, Sippel RS, Chen H. Is minimally invasive parathyroidectomy associated with greater recurrence compared to bilateral exploration? Analysis of more than 1,000 cases. Surgery. 2012;152(6):1008–15.
7. Norman J, Lopez J, Politz D. Abandoning unilateral parathyroidectomy: why we reversed our position after 15,000 parathyroid operations. J Am Coll Surg. 2012;214(3):260–9.
8. McGill J, Sturgeon C, Kaplan SP, Chiu B, Kaplan EL, Angelos P. How does the operative strategy for primary hyperparathyroidism impact the findings and cure rate? A comparison of 800 parathyroidectomies. J Am Coll Surg. 2008;207(2):246–9.
9. Wang C. The anatomic basis of parathyroid surgery. Ann Surg. 1976;183(3):271–5.
10. Lappas D, Noussios G, Anagnostis P, Adamidou F, Chatzigeorgiou A, Skandalakis P. Location, number and morphology of parathyroid glands:

results from a large anatomical series. Anat Sci Int. 2012;87(3):160–4.
11. Hojaij F, Vanderlei F, Plopper C, Rodrigues CJ, Jacomo A, Cernea C, et al. Parathyroid gland anatomical distribution and relation to anthropometric and demographic parameters: a cadaveric study. Anat Sci Int. 2011;86(4):204–12.
12. Noussios G, Anagnostis P, Natsis K. Ectopic parathyroid glands and their anatomical, clinical and surgical implications. Exp Clin Endocrinol Diabetes. 2012;120(10):604–10.
13. Iacconi P, Puccini M, Bianchi A, Miccoli P. Ectopic parathyroid glands in primary hyperparathyroidism. Ann Ital Chir. 1992;63(5):599–603.
14. Moreno MA, Callender GG, Woodburn K, Edeiken-Monroe BS, Grubbs EG, Evans DB, et al. Common locations of parathyroid adenomas. Ann Surg Oncol. 2011;18(4):1047–51.
15. Jaskowiak N, Norton JA, Alexander HR, Doppman JL, Shawker T, Skarulis M, et al. A prospective trial evaluating a standard approach to reoperation for missed parathyroid adenoma. Ann Surg. 1996;224(3):308–20; discussion 20–1
16. Feliciano DV. Parathyroid pathology in an intrathyroidal position. Am J Surg. 1992;164(5):496–500.
17. Arnault V, Beaulieu A, Lifante JC, Sitges Serra A, Sebag F, Mathonnet M, et al. Multicenter study of 19 aortopulmonary window parathyroid tumors: the challenge of embryologic origin. World J Surg. 2010;34(9):2211–6.
18. Akerstrom G, Malmaeus J, Bergstrom R. Surgical anatomy of human parathyroid glands. Surgery. 1984;95(1):14–21.
19. Lindqvist V, Jacobsson H, Chandanos E, Bäckdahl M, Kjellman M, Wallin G. Preoperative 99Tcm-sestamibi scintigraphy with SPECT localizes most pathologic parathyroid glands. Langenbeck's Arch Surg. 2009;394(5):811–5.
20. Rodgers SE, Hunter GJ, Hamberg LM, Schellingerhout D, Doherty DB, Ayers GD, et al. Improved preoperative planning for directed parathyroidectomy with 4-dimensional computed tomography. Surgery. 2006;140(6):932–40; discussion 40–1
21. Starker LF, Mahajan A, Bjorklund P, Sze G, Udelsman R, Carling T. 4D parathyroid CT as the initial localization study for patients with de novo primary hyperparathyroidism. Ann Surg Oncol. 2011;18(6):1723–8.
22. Cheung K, Wang TS, Farrokhyar F, Roman SA, Sosa JA. A meta-analysis of preoperative localization techniques for patients with primary hyperparathyroidism. Ann Surg Oncol. 2012;19(2):577–83.
23. Yeh MW, Barraclough BM, Sidhu SB, Sywak MS, Barraclough BH, Delbridge LW. Two hundred consecutive parathyroid ultrasound studies by a single clinician: the impact of experience. Endocr Pract. 2006;12(3):257–63.
24. Aspinall SR, Nicholson S, Bliss RD, Lennard TW. The impact of surgeon-based ultrasonography for parathyroid disease on a British endocrine surgical practice. Ann R Coll Surg Engl. 2012;94(1):17–22.
25. Arora S, Balash PR, Yoo J, Smith GS, Prinz RA. Benefits of surgeon-performed ultrasound for primary hyperparathyroidism. Langenbeck's Arch Surg. 2009;394(5):861–7.
26. Solorzano CC, Carneiro-Pla DM, Irvin GL 3rd. Surgeon-performed ultrasonography as the initial and only localizing study in sporadic primary hyperparathyroidism. J Am Coll Surg. 2006;202(1):18–24.
27. Soon PS, Delbridge LW, Sywak MS, Barraclough BM, Edhouse P, Sidhu SB. Surgeon performed ultrasound facilitates minimally invasive parathyroidectomy by the focused lateral mini-incision approach. World J Surg. 2008;32(5):766–71.
28. Gotthardt M, Lohmann B, Behr TM, Bauhofer A, Franzius C, Schipper ML, et al. Clinical value of parathyroid scintigraphy with technetium-99m methoxyisobutylisonitrile: discrepancies in clinical data and a systematic metaanalysis of the literature. World J Surg. 2004;28(1):100–7.
29. Mihai R, Simon D, Hellman P. Imaging for primary hyperparathyroidism—an evidence-based analysis. Langenbeck's Arch Surg. 2009;394(5):765–84.
30. Erbil Y, Barbaros U, Yanik BT, Salmaslioglu A, Tunaci M, Adalet I, et al. Impact of gland morphology and concomitant thyroid nodules on preoperative localization of parathyroid adenomas. Laryngoscope. 2006;116(4):580–5.
31. Bandeira FAF, Oliveira RIRB, Griz LHM, Caldas G, Bandeira C. Differences in accuracy of 99mTc-sestamibi scanning between severe and mild forms of primary hyperparathyroidism. J Nucl Med Technol. 2008;36(1):30–5.
32. Kunstman JW, Kirsch JD, Mahajan A, Udelsman R. Clinical review: Parathyroid localization and implications for clinical management. J Clin Endocrinol Metab. 2013;98(3):902–12.
33. Goetze S, Lavely WC, Ziessman HA, Wahl RL. Visualization of brown adipose tissue with 99mTc-methoxyisobutylisonitrile on SPECT/CT. J Nucl Med. 2008;49(5):752–6.
34. Sandqvist P, Nilsson IL, Gryback P, Sanchez-Crespo A, Sundin A. SPECT/CT's advantage for preoperative localization of small parathyroid adenomas in primary hyperparathyroidism. Clin Nucl Med. 2017;42(2):e109–e14.
35. Tomas MB, Pugliese PV, Tronco GG, Love C, Palestro CJ, Nichols KJ. Pinhole versus parallel-hole collimators for parathyroid imaging: an intraindividual comparison. J Nucl Med Technol. 2008;36(4):189–94.
36. Klingensmith WC 3rd, Koo PJ, Summerlin A, Fehrenbach BW, Karki R, Shulman BC, et al. Parathyroid imaging: the importance of pinhole collimation with both single- and dual-tracer acquisition. J Nucl Med Technol. 2013;41(2):99–104.
37. Caveny SA, Klingensmith WC 3rd, Martin WE, Sage-El A, RC MI Jr, Raeburn C, et al. Parathyroid imaging: the importance of dual-radiopharmaceutical simultaneous acquisition with 99mTc-sestamibi and 123I. J Nucl Med Technol. 2012;40(2):104–10.
38. Casara D, Rubello D, Pelizzo M, Shapiro B. Clinical role of 99mTcO4/MIBI scan, ultrasound and intra-operative gamma probe in the performance of unilateral and minimally invasive surgery in

primary hyperparathyroidism. Eur J Nucl Med. 2001;28(9):1351–9.

39. Powell DK, Nwoke F, Goldfarb RC, Ongseng F. Tc-99m sestamibi parathyroid gland scintigraphy: added value of Tc-99m pertechnetate thyroid imaging for increasing interpretation confidence and avoiding additional testing. Clin Imaging. 2013;37(3):475–9.
40. Hindie E, Melliere D, Jeanguillaume C, Perlemuter L, Chehade F, Galle P. Parathyroid imaging using simultaneous double-window recording of technetium-99m-sestamibi and iodine-123. J Nucl Med. 1998;39(6):1100–5.
41. Tunninen V, Varjo P, Schildt J, Ahonen A, Kauppinen T, Lisinen I, et al. Comparison of five parathyroid scintigraphic protocols. Int J Mol Imaging. 2013;2013:1–12.
42. Guerin C, Lowery A, Gabriel S, Castinetti F, Philippon M, Vaillant-Lombard J, et al. Preoperative imaging for focused parathyroidectomy: making a good strategy even better. Eur J Endocrinol. 2015;172(5):519–26.
43. Sharma J, Mazzaglia P, Milas M, Berber E, Schuster DM, Halkar R, et al. Radionuclide imaging for hyperparathyroidism (HPT): which is the best technetium-99m sestamibi modality? Surgery. 2006;140(6):856–65.
44. Lorberboym M, Minski I, Macadziob S, Nikolov G, Schachter P. Incremental diagnostic value of preoperative 99mTc-MIBI SPECT in patients with a parathyroid adenoma. J Nucl Med. 2003;44(6):904–8.
45. Moka D, Voth E, Dietlein M, Larena-Avellaneda A, Schicha H. Technetium 99m-MIBI-SPECT: a highly sensitive diagnostic tool for localization of parathyroid adenomas. Surgery. 2000;128(1):29–35.
46. Slater A, Gleeson FV. Increased sensitivity and confidence of SPECT over planar imaging in dual-phase sestamibi for parathyroid adenoma detection. Clin Nucl Med. 2005;30(1):1–3.
47. Lavely WC, Goetze S, Friedman KP, Leal JP, Zhang Z, Garret-Mayer E, et al. Comparison of SPECT/CT, SPECT, and planar imaging with single- and dual-phase 99mTc-sestamibi parathyroid scintigraphy. J Nucl Med. 2007;48(7):1084–9.
48. Thomas DL, Bartel T, Menda Y, Howe J, Graham MM, Juweid ME. Single photon emission computed tomography (SPECT) should be routinely performed for the detection of parathyroid abnormalities utilizing technetium-99m sestamibi parathyroid scintigraphy. Clin Nucl Med. 2009;34(10):651–5.
49. Nichols KJ, Tomas MB, Tronco GG, Rini JN, Kunjummen BD, Heller KS, et al. Preoperative parathyroid scintigraphic lesion localization: accuracy of various types of readings. Radiology. 2008;248(1):221–32.
50. Wei WJ, Shen CT, Song HJ, Qiu ZL, Luo QY. Comparison of SPET/CT, SPET and planar imaging using 99mTc-MIBI as independent techniques to support minimally invasive parathyroidectomy in primary hyperparathyroidism: a meta-analysis. Hell J Nucl Med. 2015;18(2):127–35.
51. Treglia G, Sadeghi R, Schalin-Jantti C, Caldarella C, Ceriani L, Giovanella L, et al. Detection rate of (99m) Tc-MIBI single photon emission computed tomography (SPECT)/CT in preoperative planning for patients with primary hyperparathyroidism: a meta-analysis. Head Neck. 2016;38(Suppl 1):E2159–72.
52. Sandqvist P, Nilsson IL, Gryback P, Sanchez-Crespo A, Sundin A. SPECT/CT's advantage for preoperative localization of small parathyroid adenomas in primary hyperparathyroidism. Clin Nucl Med. 2017;42(2):e109–14.
53. Nichols KJ, Tronco GG, Palestro CJ. Influence of multigland parathyroid disease on 99mTc-sestamibi SPECT/CT. Clin Nucl Med. 2016;41(4):282–8.
54. Greenspan BS, Dillehay G, Intenzo C, Lavely WC, O'Doherty M, Palestro CJ, et al. SNM practice guideline for parathyroid scintigraphy 4.0. J Nucl Med Technol. 2012;40(2):111–8.
55. Mandal R, Muthukrishnan A, Ferris RL, de Almeida JR, Duvvuri U. Accuracy of early-phase versus dual-phase single-photon emission computed tomography/computed tomography in the localization of parathyroid disease. Laryngoscope. 2015;125(6):1496–501.
56. Neumann DR, Esselstyn CB, MacIntyre WJ, Chen EQ, Go RT, Kohse LM. Parathyroid adenoma localization by PET FDG. J Comput Assist Tomogr. 1993;17(6):976–7.
57. Braeuning U, Pfannenberg C, Gallwitz B, Teichmann R, Mueller M, Dittmann H, et al. 11C-methionine PET/CT after inconclusive 99mTc-MIBI-SPECT/CT for localisation of parathyroid adenomas in primary hyperparathyroidism. Nuklearmedizin. 2015;54(1):26–30.
58. Mortenson MM, Evans DB, Lee JE, Hunter GJ, Shellingerhout D, Vu T, et al. Parathyroid exploration in the reoperative neck: improved preoperative localization with 4D-computed tomography. J Am Coll Surg. 2008;206(5):888–95; discussion 95–6
59. Starker LF, Mahajan A, Björklund P, Sze G, Udelsman R, Carling T. 4D parathyroid CT as the initial localization study for patients with de novo primary hyperparathyroidism. Ann Surg Oncol. 2010;18(6):1723–8.
60. Ernst O. Hyperparathyroidism: CT and MR findings. J Radiol. 2009;90(3 Pt 2):409–12.
61. Numerow LM, Morita ET, Clark OH, Higgins CB. Persistent/recurrent hyperparathyroidism: a comparison of sestamibi scintigraphy, MRI, and ultrasonography. J Magn Reson Imaging. 1995;5(6): 702–8.
62. Aschenbach R, Tuda S, Lamster E, Meyer A, Roediger H, Stier A, et al. Dynamic magnetic resonance angiography for localization of hyperfunctioning parathyroid glands in the reoperative neck. Eur J Radiol. 2012;81(11):3371–7.
63. Philippon M, Guerin C, Taieb D, Vaillant J, Morange I, Brue T, et al. Bilateral neck exploration in patients with primary hyperparathyroidism and discordant imaging results: a single-centre study. Eur J Endocrinol. 2014;170(5):719–25.

64. Chiu B, Sturgeon C, Angelos P. What is the link between nonlocalizing sestamibi scans, multigland disease, and persistent hypercalcemia? A study of 401 consecutive patients undergoing parathyroidectomy. Surgery. 2006;140(3):418–22.
65. Sebag F, Hubbard JG, Maweja S, Misso C, Tardivet L, Henry JF. Negative preoperative localization studies are highly predictive of multiglandular disease in sporadic primary hyperparathyroidism. Surgery. 2003;134(6):1038–41; discussion 41–2
66. Levin KE, Clark OH. The reasons for failure in parathyroid operations. Arch Surg (Chicago, Ill : 1960). 1989;124(8):911–4; discussion 4–5
67. Bergenfelz AO, Wallin G, Jansson S, Eriksson H, Martensson H, Christiansen P, et al. Results of surgery for sporadic primary hyperparathyroidism in patients with preoperatively negative sestamibi scintigraphy and ultrasound. Langenbeck's Arch Surg. 2011;396(1):83–90.
68. Day KM, Elsayed M, Beland MD, Monchik JM. The utility of 4-dimensional computed tomography for preoperative localization of primary hyperparathyroidism in patients not localized by sestamibi or ultrasonography. Surgery. 2015;157(3):534–9.
69. Hinson AM, Lee DR, Hobbs BA, Fitzgerald RT, Bodenner DL, Stack BC Jr. Preoperative 4D CT localization of nonlocalizing parathyroid adenomas by ultrasound and SPECT-CT. Otolaryngol Head Neck Surg. 2015;153(5):775–8.
70. Brown SJ, Lee JC, Christie J, Maher R, Sidhu SB, Sywak MS, et al. Four-dimensional computed tomography for parathyroid localization: a new imaging modality. ANZ J Surg. 2015;85(6):483–7.
71. Otto D, Boerner AR, Hofmann M, Brunkhorst T, Meyer GJ, Petrich T, et al. Pre-operative localisation of hyperfunctional parathyroid tissue with 11C-methionine PET. Eur J Nucl Med Mol Imaging. 2004;31(10):1405.
72. Kluijfhout WP, Vorselaars WMCM, Vriens MR, Borel Rinkes IHM, Valk GD, de Keizer B. Enabling minimal invasive parathyroidectomy for patients with primary hyperparathyroidism using Tc-99m-sestamibi SPECT–CT, ultrasound and first results of 18F-fluorocholine PET–CT. Eur J Radiol. 2015;84(9):1745–51.
73. Bergenfelz AOJ, Hellman P, Harrison B, Sitges-Serra A, Dralle H. Positional statement of the European Society of Endocrine Surgeons (ESES) on modern techniques in pHPT surgery. Langenbeck's Arch Surg. 2009;394(5):761–4.
74. Carty SE, Norton JA. Management of patients with persistent or recurrent primary hyperparathyroidism. World J Surg. 1991;15(6):716–23.
75. Taslakian B, Trerotola SO, Sacks B, Oklu R, Deipolyi A. The essentials of parathyroid hormone venous sampling. Cardiovasc Intervent Radiol. 2017;40(1):9–21.
76. Cham S, Sepahdari AR, Hall KE, Yeh MW, Harari A. Dynamic parathyroid computed tomography (4DCT) facilitates reoperative parathyroidectomy and enables cure of missed hyperplasia. Ann Surg Oncol. 2015;22(11):3537–42.
77. Lubitz CC, Hunter GJ, Hamberg LM, Parangi S, Ruan D, Gawande A, et al. Accuracy of 4-dimensional computed tomography in poorly localized patients with primary hyperparathyroidism. Surgery. 2010;148(6):1129–37; discussion 37–8
78. Maser C, Donovan P, Santos F, Donabedian R, Rinder C, Scoutt L, et al. Sonographically guided fine needle aspiration with rapid parathyroid hormone assay. Ann Surg Oncol. 2006;13(12):1690–5.
79. Patel CN, Salahudeen HM, Lansdown M, Scarsbrook AF. Clinical utility of ultrasound and 99mTc sestamibi SPECT/CT for preoperative localization of parathyroid adenoma in patients with primary hyperparathyroidism. Clin Radiol. 2010;65(4):278–87.
80. Treglia G, Trimboli P, Huellner M, Giovanella L. Imaging in primary hyperparathyroidism: focus on the evidence-based diagnostic performance of different methods. Minerva Endocrinol. 2018;43(2):133–43.
81. Zhao M, Li X, Huang J, Yin X. [Value of single photon emission computed tomography/computerized tomography in the diagnosis of hyperparathyroidism and the comparative study with multiple imaging modality]. Zhong Nan Da Xue Xue Bao Yi Xue Ban. 2015;40(9):1016–22.
82. Yin L, Guo D, Liu J, Yan J. The role of 99mTc-MIBI SPECT-CT in reoperation therapy of persistent hyperparathyroidism patients. Open medicine (Warsaw). Open Med (Warsaw, Poland). 2015;10(1):462–7.
83. Hwang SH, Rhee Y, Yun M, Yoon JH, Lee JW, Cho A. Usefulness of SPECT/CT in parathyroid lesion detection in patients with thyroid parenchymal 99mTc-sestamibi retention. Nucl Med Mol Imaging. 2017;51(1):32–9.
84. Setabutr D, Vakharia K, Nogan SJ, Kamel GN, Allen T, Saunders BD, et al. Comparison of SPECT/CT and planar MIBI in terms of operating time and cost in the surgical management of primary hyperparathyroidism. Ear Nose Throat J. 2015;94(10–11):448–52.
85. Barber B, Moher C, Cote D, Fung E, O'Connell D, Dziegielewski P, et al. Comparison of single photon emission CT (SPECT) with SPECT/CT imaging in preoperative localization of parathyroid adenomas: a cost-effectiveness analysis. Head Neck. 2016;38(Suppl 1):E2062–5.
86. Tee MC, Chan SK, Nguyen V, Strugnell SS, Yang J, Jones S, et al. Incremental value and clinical impact of neck sonography for primary hyperparathyroidism: a risk-adjusted analysis. Can J Surg. 2013;56(5):325–31.
87. Noda S, Onoda N, Kashiwagi S, Kawajiri H, Takashima T, Ishikawa T, et al. Strategy of operative treatment of hyperparathyroidism using US scan and (99m)Tc-MIBI SPECT/CT. Endocr J. 2014;61(3):225–30.

Surgical Techniques and Adjuncts in Hyperparathyroidism

20

Heather C. Stuart and Janice L. Pasieka

Introduction

Parathyroid surgery has evolved significantly since its inception and is associated with many pivotal discoveries that have advanced the field. From the discovery of parathyroid glands to the intraoperative measurement of parathyroid hormone this endocrinopathy continues to produce new and innovative techniques to optimize patient outcomes. This chapter describes the historical highlights that have facilitated our current practices in parathyroid surgery, the surgical approaches that have been developed including the role of intraoperative parathyroid hormone (ioPTH) measurements, and additional intraoperative adjuncts that have been developed to maximize surgical cure and minimize patient morbidity.

Historical Aspects of Parathyroid Surgery

The first description of parathyroid glands is credited to Sir Richard Owen in 1862 [1]. His excitement over the "rare opportunity" to dissect an Indian rhinoceros following her death was justified when he later described "a small compact yellow glandular body attached to the thyroid" that would later be found to have profound physiologic impact [2]. The first human parathyroid was reported in 1887 by Ivan Sandstrom, a medical student from Uppsala, Sweden [3]. He noted these small glands in a number of animals, and then went on to describe the glands in variable anatomic locations in over 50 human cadaveric dissections. Sandstrom was the first to coin the term "glandulae parathyroideae" because of their proximity to the thyroid gland [4]. Eugene Gley, a French pathologist, was one of the first to have insight into the function of parathyroid glands. In 1891, he published his observations on the development of tetany in animals following parathyroidectomy. Functional studies continued throughout the early twentieth century with McCallum and Voegtlin describing the relationship between hypocalcaemia and tetany, inferring a relationship to parathyroid function [5]. These two, along with Halstead, were among the first to use calcium and PTH extract as a treatment for tetany [6]. This was confirmed by Collip in 1925 when he was able to show that purified PTH extract was able to reverse tetany in patients with hypocalcemia following parathyroidectomy [7]. Jakob Erdheim, in 1907, explored the role of parathyroid glands when he noted them to be enlarged in patients with severe bone

H. C. Stuart · J. L. Pasieka (✉)
Sections of General Surgery and Surgical Oncology, Department of Surgery, Faculty of Medicine, Cumming School of Medicine, University of Calgary, Calgary, AB, Canada
e-mail: janice.pasieka@ahs.ca

R. Parameswaran, A. Agarwal (eds.), *Evidence-Based Endocrine Surgery*,
https://doi.org/10.1007/978-981-10-1124-5_20

disease (osteitis fibrosa cystica); however he inferred incorrectly that the increased size was a consequence rather than a cause of bony destruction [8]. In 1915 Friedrich Schlagenhaufer proposed what would ultimately be accurate that enlarged hyperfunctional parathyroid glands were the cause of the bone destruction and that resection of the offending gland could offer surgical cure [4].

The first recorded parathyroidectomy was in 1925, performed by Felix Mandl, on a tram car driver named Albert Gahne. Unfortunately, the patient was a victim to the initial theories on the cause of enlarged parathyroid glands and was treated with parathyroid replacement prior to changing paths and undergoing a parathyroidectomy. Mandl removed a 2 cm gland that, in hindsight, was likely a parathyroid carcinoma. The patient developed recurrent hypercalcemia 6 years later and passed away after attempting a second surgery [9]. Probably the most famous hyperparathyroid patient was Captain Charles Martell, who was originally diagnosed in 1926 with von Recklinghausen bone disease and hypercalcemia felt to be secondary to hyperparathyroidism. He underwent seven surgeries attempting to locate the offending gland, but the first six were unsuccessful and unfortunately removed the several normal parathyroid glands. His seventh surgery in 1932 was performed by Edward Churchill and Oliver Cope where they removed a 2.5 cm mediastinal parathyroid gland. Sadly, Martell continued to struggle with nephrolithiasis and passed away 6 weeks after surgery from laryngospasm following kidney stone removal [10, 11]. The irony is that the struggle to isolate and remove the hyperfunctional gland(s) is an obstacle in treatment that we still face today. Despite many advances, recurrent or persistent parathyroid disease is often attributed to undiagnosed double adenomas or hyperplasia.

The importance of identifying and removing hyperfunctioning glands is demonstrated in patients like Captain Martell. The challenge becomes localizing and removing the gland or glands and ensuring that there is no residual hyperfunctioning tissue. The morphological determination of an abnormal gland was left to the discretion of the surgeon with the interpretation of "abnormal" being based on the size of the gland and its appearance in comparison to other glands (Fig. 20.1). Intraoperatively an enlarged gland may be interpreted as abnormal based on size criteria; however this does not always correlate with hyperfunctioning tissue [12]. Pathologically there is also variability in distinguishing an adenoma from parathyroid hyperplasia which decreases the accuracy of frozen section as an intraoperative adjunct. This difficulty in intraoperative diagnosis likely led to the wide variability in the incidence of multigland disease described in the twentieth century (3–65%) [13].

James Walton, in 1931, was one of the first to advocate for wide exploration for all parathyroid glands, arguing that if glands were not identified in the common locations less common locations should also be explored (retroesophageal, thymic, carotid sheath, etc.) [14]. The trend over the next 60 years was to perform a bilateral neck exploration (BNE) in order to assess each parathyroid gland and resect all abnormal glands. Over time it became clear that the majority of patients with primary HPT had a single-gland disease, so is the late 1970s Tibblin proposed the concept of a unilateral exploration if one normal and one abnormal gland were found on the first side of the neck explored [15]. Although this approach laid the groundwork for a limited exploration, it was not universally excepted until decades later with the introduction of ioPTH measurements and improved preoperative localization.

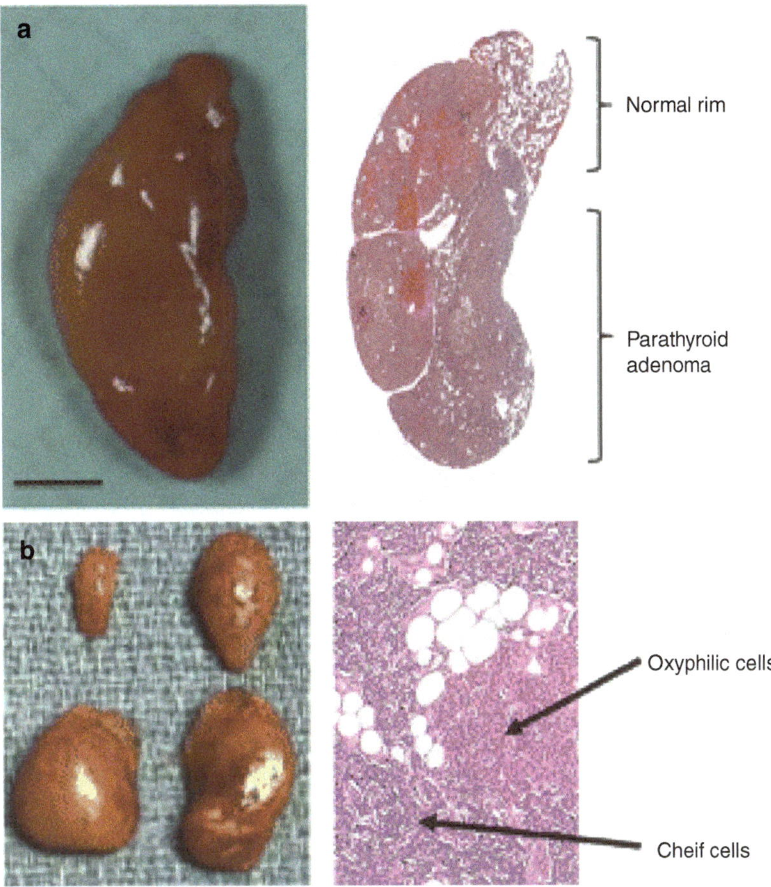

Fig. 20.1 Gross macroscopic photo of a parathyroid adenoma (**a**) and four-gland hyperplasia (**b**). (**a**, right) Microscopic section of parathyroid adenoma and a normal rim. In many cases, but not all, histopathological sections in parathyroid hyperplasia show nodules containing chief and oxyphilic cells (right in (**b**)). Photos are shown owing to courtesy of pathologist Dr. Christofer Juhlin, Karolinska Institutet, Sweden [78]

Evolution of Preoperative Imaging and ioPTH

The functional use of radionucleotide imaging with technetium-99m-sestamibi in the early 1990s revolutionized parathyroid surgery by providing a method of localizing hyperfunctioning glands preoperatively [16]. Patients were injected with Tc-sestamibi and then had cervicothoracic imaging at 15 min and 3 h. A parathyroid adenoma was identified by persistent focal uptake on late imaging that was separate from the thyroid gland (Fig. 20.2). This is thought to be secondary to the radionucleotide being retained in the mitochondria-rich adenoma. Initial studies showed up to 90% accuracy in localizing hyperfunctioning glands, but follow-up studies show more variable accuracy ranging from 70 to 90% [17]. However, it was established as a valuable imaging modality that would come to facilitate minimally invasive parathyroidectomies despite the recognition that patients with hyperplasia or double adenomas may be at higher risk for non- or inaccurate localization [18].

In the 1960s Rosalyn Yalow and Solomon Berson developed a radioimmunoassay that could be used to measure substances within the body, including parathyroid hormone. This technique was refined over time, but was a cornerstone in the development of PTH assays and set the stage for intraoperative PTH measurements

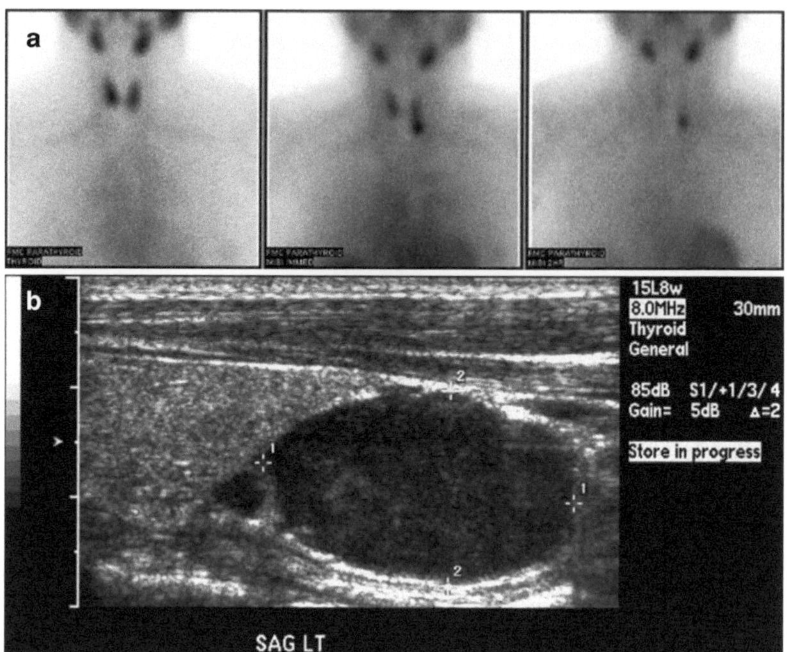

Fig. 20.2 Preoperative imaging in primary hyperparathyroidism. (**a**) Sestamibi with SPECT displaying focal retention in the left lower position seen on delayed 2 hour images. (**b**) Corresponding cervical ultrasound from the same patient showing a large hypoechoic parathyroid adenoma

which would help to restructure parathyroid surgery. Berson passed away suddenly in 1972, but Yalow went on to accept the Nobel Prize in Medicine in 1977 for their combined work on radioimmunoassays [19]. As serum PTH measurements became more readily accessible in the 1980s the assay evolved to be able to rapidly yield a result. This facilitated the intraoperative use of PTH testing. George Irvin was one of the first to publish on this in the early 1990s and showed that an intraoperative drop in PTH reflected the appropriate removal of hyperfunctioning parathyroid tissue [20]. Intraoperative PTH measurements developed quickly as an adjunct to parathyroid surgery and were found to be most useful in patients with preoperative imaging that suggested single-gland disease.

Preoperative localization studies in conjunction with ioPTH facilitated an increasingly less invasive approach to parathyroidectomy by providing additional confidence that all hyperfunctioning gland(s) were resected, thus allowing the era of minimally invasive parathyroidectomy (MIP) to evolve. A MIP is defined by either (1) a unilateral neck exploration (UNE) that identifies both parathyroid glands on one side of the neck or (2) a focused image-directed parathyroidectomy that locates a single gland on preoperative imaging and removes it without identifying any additional glands. There are multiple studies suggesting that the cure rate for primary hyperparathyroidism is similar between BNEs and MIPs when intraoperative PTH monitoring (ioPTH) is used [12, 21]. In addition there are potential benefits to MIP with some evidence to support shorter operative time [22], shorter hospital stays [23], and decreased risk of temporary hypocalcemia [24]. However, the caveat is that during a unilateral exploration if no abnormal glands are identified on the ipsilateral side or the ioPTH fails to drop appropriately the procedure is converted to a BNE which occurs in up to 40% of attempted unilateral explorations [21].

Surgical Approaches

Bilateral Neck Exploration

After the recognition that one or more parathyroid glands could be hyperfunctioning and that they could be in variable positions in the neck, BNE was adopted as the surgical approach of choice in the twentieth century. Performed through an approximately 3 cm cervical neck incision, all four glands are assessed prior to resecting the abnormal gland(s). The determination of an "abnormal gland" is made by the surgeon by means of increased size (greater than 50 mg) or atypical gland characteristics. Frozen section has limited value in differentiating hyperplastic from normal parathyroid tissue [25]. As such the BNE relies on the surgeon's experience and expertise to accurately diagnosis single- versus multi-gland disease.

The goal of a BNE was to excise 1–3.5 glands depending on whether an adenoma, double-adenoma, or four-gland hyperplasia was present. Now that a number of adjuncts including preoperative imaging and ioPTH are commonly utilized, the indications for BNE as the initial planned procedure have narrowed to focus on patients that are at higher risk for multi-gland disease. This includes patients that fail to localize on preoperative imaging and patients with preexisting conditions such as multiple endocrine neoplasia (MEN) 1, MEN 2a, familial primary hyperparathyroidism, and lithium-associated parathyroid disease. The risk of multi-gland disease ranges from 24% in patients that do not localize on imaging to 100% in patients with MEN 1 [26, 27]. For sporadic HPT, BNE in experienced hands has a durable cure rate of 98% without the utilization of preoperative localization or ioPTH measurements. In centers where these modalities are not readily available, BNE remains the most cost-effective operation.

In North America, many BNEs are performed following intraoperative failure to unilaterally localize an abnormal gland or if the ioPTH fails to drop appropriately. In this setting, ioPTH is often used in conjunction with bilateral exploration. However, if BNE is the initial planned procedure there is little reported benefit for using ioPTH intraoperatively as the cure rates are similar without it [28]. Early criticism of BNE involved the potential increased risk of complications with extended dissection, such as hypocalcemia or recurrent laryngeal nerve injury [29]. However, several studies have shown complication rates between BNE and MIP to be similar, especially when performed by an experienced endocrine surgeon [30, 31].

Minimally Invasive Parathyroidectomy (Unilateral and Image Directed)

A UNE involves the identification of one abnormal and one normal parathyroid gland on the ipsilateral side of the neck. Failure to meet these criteria necessitates the need for conversion to a BNE. Initially these operations were performed without the advantages of preoperative imaging or ioPTH measurements, and can still be done utilizing only the morphological assessment of the glands in experienced hands with excellent results. Initially conversion to a BNE occurred 50% of the time, yet despite this the success rate for a UNE was 97% [32]. Modern-day series still require conversion to a BNE up to 40% of the time because of either failure for the ioPTH to drop appropriately or failure to meet unilateral criteria [21, 33].

An image-directed MIP, as the name implies, is the removal of a single abnormal parathyroid gland seen preoperatively of imaging. Since there is no assessment of any of the other parathyroid glands to aid in the discovery of multi-gland disease, ioPTH is recommended for this approach [34]. Either of these techniques is typically performed through a slightly smaller incision and can be done with regional anesthetic. Traditionally this has been done using an open approach; however, video assisted or robotic are being popularized in some high-volume centers [35]. The basis for success of the MIP is that it is performed on patients with sporadic primary hyperparathyroidism that have preoperative imaging to suggest single-gland disease. If the sensitivity of preoperative imaging modalities was higher, there could be an argument made for performing MIP without ioPTH. However, despite significant advances in the accuracy of sestamibi, ultrasound, single-photon emission CT (SPECT), or 4-D CT, there is still a 10–15% margin of error for detecting multi-gland disease [36, 37]. In patients with concordant localization on sestamibi and US, operative success with ioPTH reaches up to 98% with the use of ioPTH changing management in only 2% of cases [34].

There have been many studies comparing the efficacy of BNE with that of MIP in treating HPT, including at least four randomized trials (Table 20.1). When ioPTH is used with MIP, the cure rate is greater than 95% up to 5 years postoperatively. There have been arguments for each approach for decreasing operative times, cost, and associated complications; however there is no conclusive evidence suggesting a significant difference [38]. Currently the majority of endocrine surgeons favor MIP as an initial approach for sporadic HPT in appropriately selected patients, but several groups have developed techniques using BNE or additional adjuncts that have similar outcomes.

Table 20.1 Randomized and retrospective series comparing focused neck exploration and bilateral neck exploration

Series	Study type	Outcome
Westerdahl and Bergenfelz (2007) [21]	Randomized	=Cure rate at 5 years
Bergenfelz et al. (2002) [80]	Randomized	=Cure rate; increased cost and operative time in FNE; increased postoperative hypocalcemia with BNE
Slepavicius et al. (2008) [81]	Randomized	=OR time and cure rate; increased cost with FNE; increased postoperative hypocalcemia with BNE
Aarum et al. (2007) [82]	Randomized	=Cure rate; =complication rate; increased cost with FNE
Grant et al. (2005) [83]	Retrospective	=Cure rate; =complication rate
Udelsman et al. (2011) [84]	Retrospective	Increased cure rate and lower complication rate with FNE

Note that studies do not compare all similar outcome measures
Abbreviations: = equivalent, *OR* operating room, *FNE* Focused neck exploration, *BNE* Bilateral neck exploration [38]

Adjuncts

Intraoperative PTH

Yalow was credited with the development of the first serum PTH assay; however the technique continued to be refined and in 1987 Nussbaum published on a rapid immune-radiometric assay that would eventually be used to measure PTH intraoperatively [39]. The attractive feature of circulating PTH is a half-life of only 3–5 min, whereas the hypercalcemia does not normalize for several hours. This allows almost real-time detection of a drop in systemic PTH levels following the resection of all autonomously hyperfunctioning parathyroid gland(s), while the normal gland remains suppressed. An appropriate hormone decrease indicates that additional exploration to look for additional abnormal glands is not necessary, which can lead to a shorter operation and less disruption to normal parathyroid glands [40]. The group at the University of Miami developed criteria for determining when all hyperfunctional tissue had been removed based on serial measurements of PTH prior to and following excision of the affected gland. PTH levels are measured prior to incision, prior to gland excision, and at 5 and 10 min post-gland excision. An intraoperative drop in PTH of greater than 50% from highest value of either the pre-incision or pre-excision value to the 10-min value provides the most accurate estimation of postoperative normocalcemia [41]. Although this is the most widely accepted criteria several other groups have proposed that, in addition to a greater than 50% drop, the PTH returns to within normal limits in order to more accurately discriminate against multi-gland disease [42].

Intraoperative PTH does require interpretation by the surgeon and thoughtfulness about unexpected trends. Additionally, it requires a facility prepared to process rapid PTH assays and an operative team available and educated in collecting samples. Its popularity grew rapidly in the United States, but given the variability of resources throughout the world it is not universally considered the standard of care.

Parathyroid Localization

There are other adjuncts that are used to confirm parathyroid tissue, visualize parathyroid glands, and assist in gland localization and functional status. Confirmation of parathyroid tissue is important when determining which tissue to resect, which to leave in vivo, and which to autotransplant. Although used more frequently prior to the advent of ioPTH, two described techniques that are still used in specific circumstances are frozen section and tissue aspirate. Frozen section has had two roles: (1) to confirm that tissue is parathyroid gland and (2) to attempt to differentiate adenomas from hyperplastic parathyroid tissue. The first of these is still used to differentiate parathyroid tissue from lymph nodes, cervical fat, thymus, or thyroid nodules. This has been validated and has shown accuracy up to 99.2% in determining parathyroid tissues [34, 43]. Frozen section to differentiate adenoma from hyperplasia has shown a high degree of inaccuracy in a number of studies [44, 45]. The general consensus is that if there is question about the diagnosis of single- versus multi-gland disease a BNE should be performed and subjectively abnormal glands should be removed regardless of histology [34]. Gland aspiration on the other hand has proven to be an accurate and cost-effective method to identify parathyroid tissue in institution with the infrastructure to perform ioPTH. A small-gage needle is inserted into the tissue and the aspirate is suspended in 1 mL of normal saline. The sample is sent for rapid PTH testing and if the value is greater than 1500 pg/mL there is a 100% sensitivity and specificity for parathyroid tissue [46].

Methylene Blue and Indocyanine Green

There are a number of other techniques that have been proposed with varying success to aid in the identification of parathyroid glands intraoperatively. These include but are not limited to the use of methylene blue and indocyanine green fluorescence with near-infrared fluorescence. Methylene blue was introduced in 1971 as an agent that collected in the parathyroid glands following intravenous administration. It localized to both normal and abnormal parathyroid glands, so it was originally proposed as a method of identifying and preserving tissue rather than identifying hyperfunctional tissue [47]. Over time, as the technique was refined, it showed some efficacy in staining only abnormal glands and had some potential to reduce operative duration [48]. However, use of the dye was associated with the risk of significant toxicities including cardiovascular instability and severe neurologic complications. As well, it is contraindicated during pregnancy and in patients taking serotonin reuptake inhibitors [49]. Recently, there have been some studies using lower dose methylene blue, 0.5 mg/kg rather than the traditional 7.5 mg/kg, that have a lower toxicity profile and showed potential when combined with the use of near-infrared fluorescent light in identifying parathyroid adenoma [50]. Despite some advances, the use of methylene blue for parathyroid identification is not used widely.

Indocyanine green (ICG) fluorescence imaging is an emerging technique. It has a potential dual purpose of assisting in parathyroid gland identification, but also assessing gland perfusion and as such viability. After adequate neck exposure, 5 mg of the dye is injected intravenously and near-infrared fluorescence imaging is used to visualize the glands. Many of the studies have used ICG fluorescence in conjunction with thyroidectomy rather than during parathyroid surgery, but the accuracy of detecting glands was up to 84% [51]. The ability to visualize at least one well-perfused gland with ICG fluorescence correlated with normal postoperative PTH levels [52]. This technique may not be relevant for patients with single-gland disease undergoing MIP, but has potential relevance in patients with multi-gland disease undergoing a subtotal parathyroidectomy.

The quality of parathyroid glands to take up various intravenous dyes can assist with localization after adequate exposure; however, techniques to localize hyperfunctional parathyroid tissue prior to exposure increase the potential for MIP. Several adjuncts have gained popularity including intraoperative ultrasound, jugular venous sampling, and radio-guided adenoma localization. Ultrasound is known to be an effective tool for localizing parathyroid adenomas especially when combined with sestamibi preoperatively [53, 54]. It has the advantage of being inexpensive, having no risk of radiation, or being noninvasive to the patient. However, it is user dependent and its accuracy and ability to detect parathyroid glands are reliant on the user's experience and technique. As well, patient size, gland size, and additional thyroid or neck pathology can limit the ability to locate glands. On ultrasound, parathyroid glands appear as solid, well-circumscribed, hypoechoic masses (Fig. 20.2). When in classic positions abnormal glands are usually easily detectable, but barriers to locating them include ectopic positions (retrotracheal, retro-esophageal, mediastinal), multi-gland disease, and previous surgery [55, 56]. The majority of ultrasound for parathyroid disease is performed preoperatively; however intraoperative ultrasound plays a role in real-time localization and has been shown to be beneficial especially in the reoperative setting and when other preoperative imaging has been discordant [57, 58].

Internal Jugular Venous Sampling

Differential internal jugular venous sampling (JVS) is another effective technique to lateralize the side of the neck that a hyperfunctioning parathyroid gland is located. It can be used preoperatively or intraoperatively and is indicative of gland localization when the PTH level on one side is greater than 10% of the contralateral side. The accuracy of localization is reported as up to 81% overall and in patients with negative preoperative sestamibi accuracy can be up to 65% [59–61]. Risk factors for non-lateralization include multi-gland disease, and ectopic location of parathyroid glands outside of the neck and in the reoperative setting. Overall, JVS is a simple and effective method of lateralizing parathyroid pathology and can increase the ability of the surgeon to perform an MIP.

Radio-Guided Parathyroid Localization

Radio-guided parathyroid localization uses the same principle as sestamibi scanning, in that technetium 99-m is injected into the patient and collected in mitochondria of hyperfunctioning parathyroid glands. When used for localization intraoperatively the patients are injected 1–2 h preoperatively and a handheld gamma probe is used to narrow the location of the adenoma, similar to localization in a sentinel lymph node biopsy. There are several applications for this technique: (1) to guide the location of incision, (2) to localize glands in classic and ectopic position, (3) to confirm activity in resected glands, and (4) to assess residual activity in the surgical bed. In 1999, the "20% rule" was proposed, stating that any resected tissue measuring greater than 20% of the background count, in the setting of a positive sestamibi scan, was the result of a parathyroid adenoma [62]. This provided a guideline for practitioners to use radio-guided localization to perform MIP with confidence that the hyperfunctioning gland had been removed. Other advantages to using radio guidance included verification that the correct glands have been removed and assistance in localization in difficult cases such as reoperative surgery or ectopic glands [63, 64]. As well, there is evidence that it is effective in multi-gland disease, in secondary and tertiary hyperparathyroidism, and in patients with negative preoperative sestamibi imaging [63, 65]. However, thyroid pathology, especially goiters, has been shown to decrease its accuracy [66, 67]. Contraindications to the use of radio guidance include pregnancy and allergy to the radioactive tracer. In one study by Chen et al. (2005) radio-guided localization had an accuracy of 83% for localizing a single hyperfunctioning gland, which alone was inferior to ioPTH (accuracy 98%) [17]. However, their combined use allows for the enhanced gland localization with radio guidance and greater accuracy with the use of ioPTH.

Additional techniques are evolving that use the principles of radio-guided localization such as a portable mini-gamma camera to take intraoperative images [68] or low-dose radio-guided localization using 37 MBq of technetium 99-m rather than the standard 600 MBq [66]. Radio-guided parathyroidectomy has been shown to be effective when used as part of an MIP combined with ioPTH or with BNE; however, there is no convincing evidence that its accuracy is adequate when used on its own. Although the use of radio guidance techniques has been growing over the last 20 years, it is still not universally utilized. Critics of the method report difficultly with the timing of administering the radio tracer, malfunctioning of the equipment, and unnecessary additional cost when most endocrine surgeons can find the glands without its use [69].

Recurrent Laryngeal Nerve Monitoring

Recurrent laryngeal nerve (RLN) monitoring has been described extensively in the thyroid surgery literature but has a much smaller role in parathyroid surgery. It is a technique that uses nerve stimulation to evaluate vocal cord function in an effort to prevent intraoperative nerve injury. However, despite extensive observation, there is no definitive evidence that intraoperative nerve monitoring decreases the risk of postoperative temporary or permanent vocal cord paralysis during thyroidectomy [70]. A proportion of surgeons do not routinely identify the RLN during parathyroidectomy and, only rarely, would be dissecting along its insertion into the larynx. So, although there is little literature evaluating nerve monitoring in parathyroid surgery given the low rate of nerve injury (<1%) there is little predicted benefit [71].

Clinical Pearls and Conclusion

Parathyroid surgery has had an exciting and, at times, controversial evolution over the last century. The development and ongoing refinement of surgical adjuncts continue to push parathyroid surgeons to achieve success rates far superior to other functional tumors. The significant population of people that suffer from HPT facilitate the creation of a large body of literature to evaluate and refine our approach to the surgical treatment. BNE remains the cornerstone for surgical management, and all endocrine surgeons must be familiar and facile in performing this operation safely and effectively. The development of MIP with ioPTH has been one of the largest contributions to treatment in the last 20 years. It has provided a consistent method of evaluating in vivo parathyroid function and can be applied to primary, secondary, tertiary, and reoperative disease.

Less invasive surgical exploration with similar success of normocalcemia postoperatively has helped to enhance recovery and improve patient care. Whether MIP has the same robust long-term cure as a BNE is currently debated among experts [72–77]. Appropriate patient selection is more than ever required in the era of MIP, as persistent disease is a surgical failure and should remain less than 3%. Efficiency, expense, and resources, in addition to optimizing patient outcome, need to be considered when selecting adjuncts for parathyroid surgery and understandably these factors will vary between institutions, countries, and surgeons. Ultimately if there is any question intraoperatively about residual disease or failure of adjuncts to determine pathology, the approach is converted to a BNE. An experienced endocrine surgeon understands the pathophysiology for parathyroid disease and should be able to develop an approach using the adjuncts available to them in their healthcare environment that will maximize surgical cure. This may not be the same worldwide, but each surgeon and institution will balance their resources and experience to provide the best care for patients.

References

1. Duke, W.S. and D.J. Terris, Sir Richard Owen, in J.L. Pasieka, J.A. Lee Surgical endocrinopathies: clinical management and the founding figures, Springer International Publishing: Cham. 2015 p. 131–134.

2. Owen R. On the anatomy of the Indian Rhinoceros (Rh. Unicornis L.). Trans Zool Soc Lond. 1862;4:31–58.
3. Sandstrom I. On new gland in man and several animals. Bull Inst Hist Med. 1938;6:192–222.
4. Organ CH Jr. The history of parathyroid surgery, 1850–1996: the Excelsior Surgical Society 1998 Edward D Churchill Lecture. J Am Coll Surg. 2000;191(3):284–99.
5. MacCallum WG, Voegtlin C. On the relation of tetany to the parathyroid glands and to calcium metabolism. J Exp Med. 1909;11(1):118–51.
6. Halsted WS. Hypoparathyreosis, status parathyreoprivus, and transplantation of the parathyroid glands. Am J Med Sci. 1907;134(1):12.
7. Collip JP. Extraction of a parathyroid hormone which will prevent or control parathyroid tetany and which regulates the levels of blood calcium. J Biol Chem. 1925;63:395–438.
8. Erdheim J. Tetania parathyreopriva. Mitt Grenzgeb Med Chir. 1906;16:632–744.
9. Mandl F. Attempt to treat generalized fibrous osteitis by extirpation of parathyroid tumor. Zentralbl Chir. 1926;53:260–4.
10. Richardson EPMD, Aub JCMD, Bauer WMD. Parathyroidectomy in Osteomalacia. Ann Surg. 1929;90(4):730–41.
11. Bauer W, Albright F, Aub JC. A case of osteitis fibrosa cystica (osteomalacia?) With evidence of hyperactivity of the para-thyroid bodies. Metabolic study II 1. J Clin Invest. 1930;8(2):229–48.
12. Irvin GL 3rd, Carneiro DM, Solorzano CC. Progress in the operative management of sporadic primary hyperparathyroidism over 34 years. Ann Surg. 2004;239(5):704–8; discussion 708–11
13. Kaplan EL, Yashiro T, Salti G. Primary hyperparathyroidism in the 1990s. Choice of surgical procedures for this disease. Ann Surg. 1992;215(4):300–17.
14. Schulte K-M, Röher H-D. History of thyroid and parathyroid surgery. In: Oertli D, Udelsman R, editors. Surgery of the thyroid and parathyroid glands. Berlin: Springer; 2012. p. 1–14.
15. Tibblin S, Bondeson AG, Ljungberg O. Unilateral parathyroidectomy in hyperparathyroidism due to single adenoma. Ann Surg. 1982;195(3):245–52.
16. Taillefer R, et al. Detection and localization of parathyroid adenomas in patients with hyperparathyroidism using a single radionuclide imaging procedure with technetium-99m-sestamibi (double-phase study). J Nucl Med. 1992;33(10):1801–7.
17. Chen H, Mack E, Starling JR. A comprehensive evaluation of perioperative adjuncts during minimally invasive parathyroidectomy: which is most reliable? Ann Surg. 2005;242(3):375–80; discussion 380–3
18. Shen W, et al. Sestamibi scanning is inadequate for directing unilateral neck exploration for first-time parathyroidectomy. Arch Surg. 1997;132(9):969–74; discussion 974–6
19. Media N. 2016. https://www.nobelprize.org/nobel_prizes/medicine/laureates.
20. Irvin GL 3rd, Dembrow VD, Prudhomme DL. Clinical usefulness of an intraoperative "quick parathyroid hormone" assay. Surgery. 1993;114(6):1019–22; discussion 1022–3
21. Westerdahl J, Bergenfelz A. Unilateral versus bilateral neck exploration for primary hyperparathyroidism: five-year follow-up of a randomized controlled trial. Ann Surg. 2007;246(6):976–80; discussion 980–1
22. Ryan JA Jr, et al. Efficacy of selective unilateral exploration in hyperparathyroidism based on localization tests. Arch Surg. 1997;132(8):886–90; discussion 890–1
23. Chen H, Sokoll LJ, Udelsman R. Outpatient minimally invasive parathyroidectomy: a combination of sestamibi-SPECT localization, cervical block anesthesia, and intraoperative parathyroid hormone assay. Surgery. 1999;126(6):1016–21; discussion 1021–2
24. Martin RC 2nd, Greenwell D, Flynn MB. Initial neck exploration for untreated hyperparathyroidism. Am Surg. 2000;66(3):269–72.
25. Elliott DD, Monroe DP, Perrier ND. Parathyroid histopathology: is it of any value today? J Am Coll Surg. 2006;203(5):758–65.
26. Chiu B, Sturgeon C, Angelos P. What is the link between nonlocalizing sestamibi scans, multigland disease, and persistent hypercalcemia? A study of 401 consecutive patients undergoing parathyroidectomy. Surgery. 2006;140(3):418–22.
27. Thakker RV, et al. Clinical practice guidelines for multiple endocrine neoplasia type 1 (MEN1). J Clin Endocrinol Metabol. 2012;97(9):2990–3011.
28. Starr FL, DeCresce R, Prinz RA. USe of intraoperative parathyroid hormone measurement does not improve success of bilateral neck exploration for hyperparathyroidism. Arch Surg. 2001;136(5):536–42.
29. Robertson GSM, et al. Long-term results of unilateral neck exploration for preoperatively localized nonfamilial parathyroid adenomas. Am J Surg. 1996;172(4):311–4.
30. Udelsman R. Six hundred fifty-six consecutive explorations for primary hyperparathyroidism. Ann Surg. 2002;235(5):665–72.
31. Abdulla AG, et al. Trends in the frequency and quality of parathyroid surgery: analysis of 17,082 cases over 10 years. Ann Surg. 2015;261(4):746–50.
32. Wang C-A. Surgical management of primary hyperparathyroidism. Curr Probl Surg. 1985;22(11):4–50.
33. Hughes DT, et al. Factors in conversion from minimally invasive parathyroidectomy to bilateral parathyroid exploration for primary hyperparathyroidism. Surgery. 2013;154(6):1428–34; discussion 1434–5
34. Wilhelm SM, et al. The American Association of Endocrine Surgeons guidelines for definitive management of primary hyperparathyroidism. JAMA Surg. 2016;151(10):959–68.
35. Greene AB, et al. National trends in parathyroid surgery from 1998 to 2008: a decade of change. J Am Coll Surg. 2009;209(3):332–43.

36. Hunter GJ, et al. Accuracy of four-dimensional CT for the localization of abnormal parathyroid glands in patients with primary hyperparathyroidism. Radiology. 2012;264(3):789–95.
37. Perez-Monte JE, et al. Parathyroid adenomas: accurate detection and localization with Tc-99m sestamibi SPECT. Radiology. 1996;201(1):85–91.
38. Laird AM, Libutti SK. Minimally invasive parathyroidectomy versus bilateral neck exploration for primary hyperparathyroidism. Surg Oncol Clin N Am. 2016;25(1):103–18.
39. Nussbaum SR, et al. Highly sensitive two-site immunoradiometric assay of parathyrin, and its clinical utility in evaluating patients with hypercalcemia. Clin Chem. 1987;33(8):1364–7.
40. Irvin GL 3rd, et al. Ambulatory parathyroidectomy for primary hyperparathyroidism. Arch Surg. 1996;131(10):1074–8.
41. Callender GG, Udelsman R. Surgery for primary hyperparathyroidism. Cancer. 2014;120(23):3602–16.
42. Richards ML, et al. An optimal algorithm for intraoperative parathyroid hormone monitoring. Arch Surg. 2011;146(3):280–5.
43. Westra WH, Pritchett DD, Udelsman R. Intraoperative confirmation of parathyroid tissue during parathyroid exploration: a retrospective evaluation of the frozen section. Am J Surg Pathol. 1998;22(5):538–44.
44. Bornstein-Quevedo L, et al. Histologic diagnosis of primary hyperparathyroidism: a concordance analysis between three pathologists. Endocr Pathol. 2001;12(1):49–54.
45. Saxe AW, et al. The role of the pathologist in the surgical treatment of hyperparathyroidism. Surg Gynecol Obstet. 1985;161(2):101–5.
46. Perrier ND, et al. Intraoperative parathyroid aspiration and parathyroid hormone assay as an alternative to frozen section for tissue identification. World J Surg. 2000;24(11):1319–22.
47. Dudley NE. Methylene blue for rapid identification of the parathyroids. Br Med J. 1971;3(5776):680–1.
48. Han N, et al. Intra-operative parathyroid identification using methylene blue in parathyroid surgery. Am Surg. 2007;73(8):820–3.
49. Pollack G, et al. Parathyroid surgery and methylene blue: a review with guidelines for safe intraoperative use. Laryngoscope. 2009;119(10):1941–6.
50. Tummers QRJG, et al. Intraoperative guidance in parathyroid surgery using near-infrared fluorescence imaging and low-dose methylene blue. Surgery. 2015;158(5):1323–30.
51. Zaidi N, et al. The feasibility of indocyanine green fluorescence imaging for identifying and assessing the perfusion of parathyroid glands during total thyroidectomy. J Surg Oncol. 2016;113(7):775–8.
52. Vidal Fortuny J, et al. Indocyanine green angiography in subtotal parathyroidectomy: technique for the function of the parathyroid remnant. J Am Coll Surg. 2016;223(5):e43–9.
53. Hajioff D, et al. Preoperative localization of parathyroid adenomas: ultrasonography, sestamibi scintigraphy, or both? Clin Otolaryngol Allied Sci. 2004;29(5):549–52.
54. Purcell GP, et al. Parathyroid localization with high-resolution ultrasound and technetium Tc 99m sestamibi. Arch Surg. 1999;134(8):824–8; discussion 828–30
55. Sugg SL, et al. Detection of multiple gland primary hyperparathyroidism in the era of minimally invasive parathyroidectomy. Surgery. 2004;136(6):1303–9.
56. Mazeh H, Chen H. Intraoperative adjuncts for parathyroid surgery. Expert Rev Endocrinol Metab. 2011;6(2):245–53.
57. Norton JA, et al. Intraoperative ultrasound and reoperative parathyroid surgery: an initial evaluation. World J Surg. 1986;10(4):631–9.
58. Al-Lami A, et al. Utility of an intraoperative ultrasound in lateral approach mini-parathyroidectomy with discordant pre-operative imaging. Eur Arch Otorhinolaryngol. 2013;270(6):1903–8.
59. Ito F, et al. The utility of intraoperative bilateral internal jugular venous sampling with rapid parathyroid hormone testing. Ann Surg. 2007;245(6):959–63.
60. Carneiro-Pla D. Effectiveness of "office"-based, ultrasound-guided differential jugular venous sampling (DJVS) of parathormone in patients with primary hyperparathyroidism. Surgery. 2009;146(6):1014–20.
61. Barczynski M, et al. Utility of intraoperative bilateral internal jugular venous sampling with rapid parathyroid hormone testing in guiding patients with a negative sestamibi scan for minimally invasive parathyroidectomy—a randomized controlled trial. Langenbeck's Arch Surg. 2009;394(5):827–35.
62. Murphy C, Norman J. The 20% rule: a simple, instantaneous radioactivity measurement defines cure and allows elimination of frozen sections and hormone assays during parathyroidectomy. Surgery. 1999;126(6):1023–8; discussion 1028–9
63. Chen H, Mack E, Starling JR. Radioguided parathyroidectomy is equally effective for both adenomatous and hyperplastic glands. Ann Surg. 2003;238(3):332–7; discussion 337–8
64. Nichol PF, et al. Radioguided parathyroidectomy in patients with secondary and tertiary hyperparathyroidism. Surgery. 2003;134(4):713–7; discussion 717–9
65. Somnay YR, et al. Radioguided parathyroidectomy for tertiary hyperparathyroidism. J Surg Res. 2015;195(2):406–11.
66. Rubello D, et al. Importance of radio-guided minimally invasive parathyroidectomy using hand-held gamma probe and low (99m)Tc-MIBI dose. Technical considerations and long-term clinical results. Q J Nucl Med. 2003;47(2):129–38.
67. Chen H, Sippel RS, Schaefer S. The effectiveness of radioguided parathyroidectomy in patients with negative technetium tc 99m-sestamibi scans. Arch Surg. 2009;144(7):643–8.
68. Casella C, et al. Radioguided parathyroidectomy with portable mini gamma-camera for the treatment of primary hyperparathyroidism. Int J Endocrinol. 2015;2015:134731.

69. Jaskowiak NT, et al. Pitfalls of intraoperative quick parathyroid hormone monitoring and gamma probe localization in surgery for primary hyperparathyroidism. Arch Surg. 2002;137(6):659–68; discussion 668–9
70. Pisanu A, et al. Systematic review with meta-analysis of studies comparing intraoperative neuromonitoring of recurrent laryngeal nerves versus visualization alone during thyroidectomy. J Surg Res. 2014;188(1):152–61.
71. Allendorf J, et al. 1112 consecutive bilateral neck explorations for primary hyperparathyroidism. World J Surg. 2007;31(11):2075–80.
72. Norman J, Lopez J, Politz D. Abandoning unilateral parathyroidectomy: why we reversed our position after 15,000 parathyroid operations. J Am Coll Surg. 2012;214(3):260–9.
73. Norman J, Politz D, Lopez J. Reply: Unilateral parathyroidectomy: delayed treatment with higher failures. J Am Coll Surg. 2012;215(2):297–300.
74. Hodin R, et al. No need to abandon unilateral parathyroid surgery. J Am Coll Surg. 2012;215(2):297; author reply 297–300
75. Stojadinovic A, et al. Unilateral vs. bilateral parathyroidectomy: a healthy debate. J Am Coll Surg. 2012;215(2):300–2.
76. Schneider DF, et al. Is minimally invasive parathyroidectomy associated with greater recurrence compared to bilateral exploration? Analysis of more than 1,000 cases. Surgery. 2012;152(6):1008–15.
77. Pasieka JL. What should we tell our patients? Lifetime guarantee or is it 5- to 10-year warranty on a parathyroidectomy for primary hyperparathyroidism? World J Surg. 2015;39(8):1928–9.
78. Barczyński M, et al. Sporadic multiple parathyroid gland disease—a consensus report of the European Society of Endocrine Surgeons (ESES). Langenbeck's Arch Surg. 2015;400(8):887–905.
79. Starker LF, et al. Minimally invasive parathyroidectomy. Int J Endocrinol. 2011;2011, Article ID 206502, 8 p.
80. Bergenfelz A, et al. Unilateral versus bilateral neck exploration for primary hyperparathyroidism: a prospective randomized controlled trial. Ann Surg. 2002;236(5):543–51.
81. Slepavicius A, et al. Focused versus conventional parathyroidectomy for primary hyperparathyroidism: a prospective, randomized, blinded trial. Langenbeck's Arch Surg. 2008;393(5):659–66.
82. Aarum S, et al. Operation for primary hyperparathyroidism: the new versus the old order. A randomised controlled trial of preoperative localisation. Scand J Surg. 2007;96(1):26–30.
83. Grant CS, et al. Primary hyperparathyroidism surgical management since the introduction of minimally invasive parathyroidectomy: Mayo Clinic experience. Arch Surg. 2005;140(5):472–8; discussion 478–9
84. Udelsman R, Lin Z, Donovan P. The superiority of minimally invasive parathyroidectomy based on 1650 consecutive patients with primary hyperparathyroidism. Ann Surg. 2011;253(3):585–91.

21 Hereditary Hyperparathyroidism

Christopher J. Yates and Julie A. Miller

Example Case

Mrs. JD is a 35-year-old woman with a past history of Cushing's disease successfully treated by transsphenoidal surgery at the age of 25 years. She presented 1 month earlier with renal colic and biochemical tests identified hypercalcaemia of 3.1 mmol/L with an elevated parathyroid hormone level of 15 pmol/L, normal renal function and a replete 25-hydroxy vitamin D level. The past history of a pituitary adenoma raised the possibility of multiple endocrine neoplasia type 1. A parathyroid sestamibi failed to localise a single adenoma, and surgical neck exploration revealed enlargement of all four parathyroid glands. A subtotal parathyroidectomy was performed and histopathology revealed hyperplasia of all four glands. The patient was referred to a clinical genetic service that confirmed the diagnosis of multiple endocrine neoplasia type 1. The patient was screened for associated tumours, including a recurrent pituitary tumour, thymic or bronchial carcinoid, and pancreatic neuroendocrine and adrenocortical tumours. These investigations identified a 1.5 cm cystic lesion in the pancreatic head and a raised neuroendocrine tumour marker, pancreatic polypeptide that is being monitored. Her family were offered genetic counselling and diagnostic testing and those who tested positive were referred for endocrine evaluation.

Clinical Pearls

1. Germline mutations are evident in approximately 10% of patients with primary hyperparathyroidism.
2. Inherited syndromes that cause hyperparathyroidism include multiple endocrine neoplasia types 1, 2 and 4 and hyperparathyroidism-jaw tumour syndrome.
3. Inherited causes of isolated hyperparathyroidism include familial isolated hyperparathyroidism, familial hypocalciuric hypercalcaemia, neonatal severe hyperparathyroidism and autosomal dominant moderate hyperparathyroidism.
4. Indications for mutational analysis in patients with primary HPT include:
   (a) Onset before the age of 40 years
   (b) Multi-gland disease
   (c) Parathyroid carcinoma or atypical parathyroid adenomas
   (d) First-degree relatives of known mutation carriers

C. J. Yates
Department of Endocrinology, The Royal Melbourne Hospital, Parkville, VIC, Australia

Department of Medicine, The University of Melbourne, Melbourne, VIC, Australia
e-mail: Christopher.Yates@mh.org.au

J. A. Miller (✉)
Endocrine Surgery Unit, The Royal Melbourne Hospital, Parkville, VIC, Australia

Department of Surgery, The University of Melbourne, Melbourne, VIC, Australia
e-mail: Julie.Miller@mh.org.au

R. Parameswaran, A. Agarwal (eds.), *Evidence-Based Endocrine Surgery*,
https://doi.org/10.1007/978-981-10-1124-5_21

   (e) Index cases with two or more MEN1-associated tumours
5. Early identification of hereditary hyperparathyroidism facilitates
   (a) Confirming the clinical diagnosis
   (b) Planning the optimal surgical approach
   (c) Recommending surveillance for associated conditions
   (d) Screening family members in order to enter affected relatives into a surveillance programme
6. For MEN1-associated hyperparathyroidism subtotal parathyroidectomy with transcervical thymectomy is currently the most common surgical technique used, and appears to offer the advantages of a single incision, a reduced risk of permanent hypoparathyroidism and an acceptable recurrence and reoperation rate.

Introduction

Primary hyperparathyroidism (PHPT) is the most common cause of hypercalcaemia and it is characterised by hyperactivity of one or more parathyroid glands with an increase in serum calcium and elevated or inappropriately normal parathyroid hormone levels (PTH). PHPT is a common endocrine disorder with an incidence of approximately 50 per 100,000 person-years that peaks in the sixth decade [1]. The majority of cases arise sporadically, with 80% due to a solitary benign adenoma. In approximately 15% of patients all four glands are hyperplastic, while multiple adenomas have been reported in 2–4% of cases [2–4]. Parathyroid carcinomas occur in <1% of cases [5]. Multi-gland disease and parathyroid carcinomas are more common with hereditary (familial) causes of PHPT.

More than 10% of patients with PHPT have a pathogenic germline gene mutation [6]. These gene mutations are identified in familial forms of PHPT; however they may also be seen in sporadic cases. This distinction between familial and sporadic PHPT may be complicated by a lack of family history because the affected parent may not have been investigated or may have died before symptoms developed, or alternatively the patient may have developed a de novo germline mutation [7].

Familial parathyroid diseases causing hyperparathyroidism may occur in isolation or as a component of a genetic syndrome involving other diseases. Syndromic causes of hyperparathyroidism include multiple endocrine neoplasia (MEN) types 1, 2 and 4 and hyperparathyroidism-jaw tumour syndrome (HPT-JT), while isolated hereditary hyperparathyroidism may occur due to familial isolated hyperparathyroidism, familial hypocalciuric hypercalcaemia (FHH), neonatal severe hyperparathyroidism (NSHPT) and autosomal dominant moderate hyperparathyroidism (ADMH) (Table 21.1).

Mutations in 11 genes have been identified to cause familial PHPT and these mutations are typically inherited in an autosomal dominant manner with variable penetrance (Table 21.1) [6]. These mutations involve inactivation of tumour-suppressor genes in the cases of MEN1, MEN4, FIPHT and HPT-JT; activation of an oncogene in the case of MEN2; or dysregulation of the calcium set point in FHH, NSHPT and ADMH [8–10].

Early identification of familial causes of PHPT is critical for (1) confirming the clinical diagnosis; (2) planning the optimal surgical approach; (3) recommending surveillance for associated conditions (e.g. MEN1 and HPT-JT); and (4) screening family members in order to enter affected relatives into a surveillance programme, and avoid unnecessary costly, time-consuming and potentially invasive investigations in unaffected members of the kindred.

Genetic counselling and testing for familial PHPT should therefore be considered in patients with early disease onset below the age of 40 years, presence of associated endocrine tumours in the patient or their relatives, presence of parathyroid carcinoma/atypical adenoma or presence of multi-gland parathyroid disease, especially in males or younger patients [6]. If a mutation is identified, then genetic counselling and analysis should also be offered to first-degree relatives.

In the context of hereditary PHPT, all parathyroid glands carry the genetic mutation and parathyroid gland involvement can be gradual

Table 21.1 Inherited causes of hyperparathyroidism

Disease	Gene	Gene product	Inheritance	Associated tumours
Multiple endocrine neoplasia 1 (MEN1)	*MEN1*	Menin	Autosomal dominant	Multiple
Multiple endocrine neoplasia 2 (MEN2)	*RET*	Ret	Autosomal dominant	Multiple
Multiple endocrine neoplasia 4 (MEN4)	*CDKN1B*	Cyclin dependent kinase inhibitor 1B	Autosomal dominant	Multiple
Hyperparathyroidism-jaw tumour syndrome (HPT-JT)	*CDC73*	Parafibromin	Autosomal dominant	Multiple
Familial isolated hyperparathyroidism (FIHPT)	*MEN1* *CDC73* *CaSR*	Menin Parafibromin Calcium-sensing receptor	Autosomal dominant	None
Familial hypocalciuric hypercalcaemia 2 (FHH2)	*GNA11*	Guanine nucleotide-binding protein subunit alpha-11	Autosomal dominant	None
Familial hypocalciuric hypercalcaemia 3 (FHH3)	*AP2S1*	AP-2 complex subunit sigma	Autosomal dominant	None
Neonatal severe hyperparathyroidism (NSHPT)	*CaSR*	Calcium-sensing receptor	Autosomal dominant or autosomal recessive	None
Autosomal dominant moderate hyperparathyroidism (ADMH)	*CaSR*	Calcium-sensing receptor	Autosomal dominant	None
Familial hypocalciuric hypercalcaemia 1 (FHH1)	*CaSR*	Calcium-sensing receptor	Autosomal dominant	None

and progressive. Thus the primary objective is to achieve normocalcaemia and avoid permanent hypoparathyroidism, rather than cure. Imaging using ultrasound, 99mTc-sestamibi scanning, four-dimensional CT or MRI is endorsed by some authors, and can be helpful in select cases. Recommended treatment varies according to the cause of hereditary HPTH and is discussed below.

Syndromic Causes of Hyperparathyroidism

Multiple Endocrine Neoplasia 1 (MEN1)

Diagnosis and Genetics

MEN1 is a highly penetrant autosomal dominant disorder characterised by tumours of the parathyroid glands, the pancreatic islets and the anterior pituitary gland (Table 21.2). Adrenocortical tumours, lipomas, carcinoid tumours, facial angiofibromas and collagenomas may also occur in affected patients [8]. A diagnosis of MEN1 can be established in an individual with two of more of the three characteristic MEN1-associated tumours, in an individual who has one MEN1-associated tumour and a first-degree relative with a clinical diagnosis of MEN1 or in an asymptomatic individual identified to have a germline *MEN1* gene mutation [11].

MEN1 is caused by mutations of the *MEN1* tumour-suppressor gene located on chromosome 11q13 that encodes a 610 amino-acid protein called menin [12]. Menin is ubiquitously expressed and is involved in the regulation of transcription, genome stability and cell division. More than 1300 different germline mutations have been identified throughout the *MEN1* gene and most result in a truncated inactive form of menin consistent with its role as a tumour-suppressor gene. There is no evident genotype-phenotype correlation [8, 13]. It is important to note that over 10% of germline *MEN1* mutations arise de novo and may be transmitted to subsequent generations and between 5 and 10% of patients with clinical MEN1 don't have an

Table 21.2 Clinical features of hereditary parathyroid disease

Disease	Age at presentation (years)	Clinical features	Parathyroid pathology	Associated diseases	Management
MEN1	20–25 (100% penetrance by 50 years)	Hypercalcaemia, hypercalciuria, nephrolithiasis, osteoporosis	Multi-gland disease (adenomas/ hyperplasia)	Pituitary, pancreatic neuroendocrine, adrenocortical and carcinoid tumours	Subtotal or total parathyroidectomy with transcervical thymectomy (with or without parathyroid autograft)
MEN2	>30	Mild hypercalcaemia	Single- or multi-gland disease (adenoma/ hyperplasia)	Medullary thyroid carcinoma, and phaeochromocytoma	Targeted parathyroidectomy
MEN4	>35	Hypercalcaemia, hypercalciuria, nephrolithiasis, osteoporosis	Multi-gland disease (adenomas/ hyperplasia)	Pituitary, pancreatic neuroendocrine, adrenal, kidney and reproductive organ tumours	Subtotal or Total parathyroidectomy with transcervical thymectomy (with or without parathyroid autograft)
HPT-JT	>30	Severe hypercalcaemia with hypercalcaemic crisis (up to 22% have parathyroid carcinoma)	Single- or multi-gland disease	Ossifying fibromas of the jaw, uterine tumours, Wilms' tumour, papillary renal carcinoma, polycystic kidney disease	Single-gland disease—targeted parathyroidectomy, multi-gland disease—subtotal or total parathyroidectomy (avoid autografting), carcinoma—en bloc resection
FHH	At birth	Asymptomatic	Multi-gland hyperplasia	Nil	No surgery
NSHPT	At birth	Severe hypercalcaemia, skeletal manifestations of hyperparathyroidism	Marked multi-gland hyperplasia	Nil	Urgent total parathyroidectomy
ADMH	45	Hypercalcaemia, hypercalciuria, hypomagnesaemia, nephrolithiasis	Single- or multi-gland disease (adenomas/ hyperplasia)	Nil	Subtotal or total parathyroidectomy
FIHPT	20–25	Hypercalcaemia, osteoporosis, nephrolithiasis or asymptomatic	Single- or multi-gland disease	Nil	Single-gland disease—targeted parathyroidectomy Multi-gland disease—Subtotal parathyroidectomy If MEN1 o3 CDC73 mutations treat as per MEN1 or HPT-JT syndrome

identified mutation within the coding region of the MEN1 gene [7, 8].

MEN1 is the most common familial cause of PHPT and accounts for between 2 and 4% of all PHPT cases [14]. The incidence of MEN1 has been estimated to be 0.25%; however this rises to between 1 and 18% among patients with PHPT [15]. Parathyroid tumours are the first manifestation of MEN1 in 85% of patients, and the penetrance of PHPT is approximately 90–95% by 50 years of age [11, 14, 16, 17]. The age of onset of MEN1-associated PHPT is typically 20–25 years, which is approximately 30 years earlier than sporadic cases of PHPT. Parathyroid adenomas have occurred as young as 8 years of age in MEN1 patients [11, 14, 17]. Pancreatic neuroendocrine tumours, which include gastrinomas, insulinomas and non-functioning tumours, occur in more than 80% of MEN1 patients and account for 50% of MEN1-related deaths, while pituitary tumours, most commonly prolactinomas, occur in 30% of MEN1 patients [18, 19]. Annual biochemical screening for PHPT is recommended from 5 years of age in *MEN1* gene mutation carriers using a serum calcium and PTH assessment, alongside biochemical tests for pancreatic neuroendocrine and pituitary tumours (prolactin, IGF-1, gastrin, fasting glucose, insulin, glucagon, vasoactive intestinal polypeptide, pancreatic polypeptide and chromogranin A) (Table 21.3) [11].

Timing and Extent of Parathyroid Surgery

Similar to sporadic PHPT, MEN1-associated PHPT may present with asymptomatic hypercalcaemia, symptomatic hypercalcaemia (e.g. polydipsia, polyuria, constipation or malaise), nephrolithiasis, nephrocalcinosis or osteitis fibrosa cystica. Hypercalcaemia may increase the secretion of gastrin from a gastrinoma. Clinical distinguishing factors between MEN1-associated and sporadic PHPT include younger age of onset, multi-gland disease, a milder biochemical presentation (lower calcium and PTH), a greater reduction in bone mineral density and an equal male/female ratio [11, 20]. All parathyroid glands are affected by MEN1; however variable parathyroid gland enlargement may be noted at the time of diagnosis. The parathyroid glands in MEN1 may have a lobulated rather than ovoid morphology compared with sporadic adenomas, and up to 30% of affected patients have supernumerary parathyroid glands [21]. Ectopic parathyroid glands within the thymus, anterior mediastinum or thyroid or carotid sheath may also be observed. The most frequent site is the thymus, which has been reported in 4.9–30% of MEN1 patients [21]. Small nests of parathyroid cells can also be located in the fat surrounding the trachea, oesophagus and carotid arteries [21]. Parathyroid carcinoma is rare in MEN1 with a prevalence of 0.28% [22].

Table 21.3 Recommended endocrine tumour surveillance for MEN1 gene mutation carriers (adapted from Thakker et al., JCEM 2012)

Tumour	Screening commencement age (years)	Biochemistry	Imaging
Hyperparathyroidism	8	Calcium and PTH	Nil
Pancreatic neuroendocrine tumours			
Gastrinoma	20	Gastrin	Nil
Insulinoma	5	Fasting insulin and glucose	Nil
Other	<10	Chromogranin-A, pancreatic polypeptide, glucagon, vasoactive intestinal peptide	MRI, CT or EUS annually
Pituitary	5	Prolactin, IGF-1	MRI every 3 years
Adrenal	<10	Nil	MRI or CT annually
Thymic and bronchial carcinoid	15	Nil	CT or MRI every 1–2 years

Although there is consensus that surgical excision of parathyroid glands is the most effective treatment for PHPT in MEN1 patients, the timing and nature of surgery remain contentious [23]. Typically the severity of symptoms, presence of kidney stones, magnitude of biochemical derangements and presence of reduced bone density dictate the timing of surgery. The goals of surgery are restoring calcium levels to normal, avoiding hypoparathyroidism and minimising the need for reoperations. Options include parathyroidectomy limited to enlarged glands, unilateral, subtotal parathyroidectomy (3 or 3½ glands), or total parathyroidectomy with autograft of parathyroid gland fragments into sites such as the brachiocephalic muscle in the forearm, sternomastoid or pectoralis major. The thymus should also be removed as it may harbour an ectopic parathyroid gland in 15% of patients or a thymic carcinoid tumour [24]. Part of the thymus deep in the mediastinum may not be successfully removed by cervical thymectomy and removal of the entire thymus, if required, is best done via a mediastinal approach.

Because of multi-gland parathyroid involvement, the use of preoperative imaging such as cervical US, nuclear scintigraphy, four-dimensional CT, MRI or PET is controversial prior to initial surgery, and depends upon whether the patient and treating team prefer a staged approach based on the principle of asymmetric and metachronous enlargement of the parathyroid glands in MEN I. However imaging is mandatory before reoperation to identify residual disease.

A French and Belgian series of 256 MEN1 patients revealed that the majority (51%) underwent subtotal parathyroidectomy and post-operatively 19% had persistent disease while 15% had hypocalcaemia [24]. A meta-analysis of 52 patients has shown that surgical strategies involving less than subtotal parathyroidectomy have the highest rates of persistent and recurrent PHPT, at 31% and 59%, respectively [25]. In the same study, subtotal parathyroidectomy was associated with a recurrence rate of 65% and although no recurrences were observed among patients who underwent total parathyroidectomy, 67% of the latter patients developed permanent hypoparathyroidism. A Dutch study including 73 patients showed that removal of less than three parathyroid glands was associated with a 53% risk of persistent or recurrent disease compared to just 17% for subtotal parathyroidectomy and 19% for total parathyroidectomy. Long-term hypoparathyroidism occurred in 24%, 39% and 66% of patients who underwent less than subtotal, subtotal and total parathyroidectomy, respectively [26]. Among those who underwent subtotal or total parathyroidectomy, risk of persistent or recurrent disease was more frequent in those who didn't undergo bilateral transcervical thymectomy [26]. In a recent randomised trial of 32 patients followed for 7.5 years, the rate of recurrent hyperparathyroidism was 24% for patients treated with subtotal parathyroidectomy and 13% in patients treated with total parathyroidectomy, while the rates of permanent hypoparathyroidism were 12% and 7% in each group, respectively [27]. These differences were not statistically significant. Thus, subtotal parathyroidectomy with transcervical thymectomy is currently the most common surgical technique selected for the management of PHPT in MEN1 patients, and appears to offer the advantages of a single incision, a reduced risk of permanent hypoparathyroidism and an acceptable recurrence and reoperation rate [23]. If total parathyroidectomy is selected, the rapid intraoperative PTH assay, if available, can be used to determine if removal of all functioning parathyroid tissue has been achieved, and if not this allows further evaluation for supernumerary or ectopic glands. Having a PTH level near the detectable limit 20 min after excision of the parathyroid glands indicates successful parathyroidectomy [28]. However, intraoperative PTH is not widely available in many countries.

Recurrence rates after parathyroidectomy are variable, and the time for recurrence varies from months to 10 years [29]. Risk of recurrence is increased by a lack of MEN1 diagnosis at the time of surgery and therefore inadequate treatment, limited surgeon experience, a short duration of HPT, young patient age, absence of thymectomy, less than subtotal parathyroidectomy, lack of use of intraoperative parathyroid assays and a long follow-up time [21, 24, 29–32]. In the future,

MEN1 genotyping may prove helpful. A single study has shown that among patients undergoing less than subtotal parathyroidectomy, patients with nonsense or frameshift mutations of exons 2, 9 and 10 have a lower risk of persistent or recurrent PHPT compared to patients with other [26]. Previously very little genotype:phenotype correlations have been noticed with MEN1.

Reoperations for recurrent PHPT in MEN1 usually involve focused exploration in a scarred neck. Review of previous operation and histopathology reports, and accurate localisation studies, including parathyroid sestamibi, US 4DCT, and selective venous sampling may be helpful in some cases. There are increased risks with reoperation including permanent vocal cord palsy, haemorrhage and hypoparathyroidism. Therefore reoperation is reserved for patients with high urinary calcium excretion, significant osteoporosis or symptomatic hypercalcaemia. Intraoperative PTH is useful in the case of cervical reoperation for recurrent HPT as surgical dissection can be stopped when circulating PTH falls to normal or decreases 50% from basal levels [33, 34]. As an alternative to re-operative surgery, percutaneous injection of ethanol via ultrasound guidance has been described; however more than one infusion of 0.3 mL is required in approximately half of patients to destroy the parathyroid gland. This approach has been studied in 37 patients with recurrent HPT and 73% became normocalcaemic, 6 became hypocalcaemic and 14 remained hypercalcaemic. The mean duration of normocalcaemia was 24 months and 7 required surgical intervention post-ethanol infusion [35]. Cinacalcet which increases the sensitivity of the calcium-sensing receptor to extracellular calcium has also been shown to reduce serum calcium and PTH levels and increase bone mineral density during 1 year of treatment in patients with MEN1 and recurrent or persistent HPTH [36–39]. However, the medication is expensive and the results are not durable (Table 21.4).

Table 21.4 Comparison of surgical techniques for the management of MEN1-associated hyperparathyroidism

Surgical technique	Advantages	Disadvantages	Conclusion
• Unilateral or less than subtotal parathyroidectomy	• Lowest risk of hypoparathyroidism • Some patients have asymmetric enlargement	• Highest rate of both recurrent and persistent hyperparathyroidism	• SP with a bilateral cervical thymectomy is most commonly recommended • Alternatively TP/AT to forearm with bilateral cervical thymectomy is also a good option • Procedures should ideally be performed in high-volume centres • Discuss pros and cons of each approach with patient • Recommendation level: B (supported by small randomised trials and moderate to high risk for error)[b] • Strength of recommendation: strong • Quality of evidence: moderate (further research is likely to have an important impact on confidence in the estimate of effect and may change the estimate)[b]
• Subtotal parathyroidectomy[a] (SP)	• Avoids a forearm incision for parathyroid autograft • Reduces the risk of permanent hypoparathyroidism	• Increased risk of recurrent hyperparathyroidism compared with TP/AT	
• Total parathyroidectomy with autotransplantation[a] • (TP/AT)	• Lowest risk of persistent and recurrent hyperparathyroidism • Enables a low-risk procedure for the management of most recurrent hyperparathyroidism	• Obligate period of transient hypoparathyroidism • Highest risk of permanent hypoparathyroidism • Very high rates of parathyroid graft function must be achieved • Potential risk of parathyromatosis	

[a]Concurrent cervical thymectomy is recommended due to a 15% change of finding parathyroid tissue and the risk of thymic carcinoid tumours [26]

[b]Recommendations according to the modified Sackett's classification and the Grading of Recommendations, Assessment, Development and Evaluation (GRADE) system

Multiple Endocrine Neoplasia 4 (MEN4)

Five to ten percent of patients with MEN1 do not have mutations of the MEN1 gene and these patients may have mutations of other genes [8]. MEN4 is a phenocopy syndrome of MEN1 characterised by the occurrence of tumours of the parathyroid glands, anterior pituitary and pancreatic islets, in association with tumours of the adrenals, kidneys and reproductive organs (Table 21.2). It occurs due to an autosomal dominant inactivating mutation in the *CDKN1B* gene on chromosome 12p13 that encodes the cell cycle regulator cyclin-dependent kinase inhibitor p27^{kip1} [8, 40]. Only 15 cases of MEN4 have been reported in the literature, with all clinically affected patients being female. PHPT has been present in 81% and is multiglandular in most cases. Resection similar to that performed in MEN1 has been proposed [23, 41].

Multiple Endocrine Neoplasia 2 (MEN2)

Diagnosis and Genetics

MEN2 (previously known as MEN2A) is characterised by the presence of medullary thyroid cancer, phaeochromocytomas and parathyroid adenomas (Table 21.2). Primary hyperparathyroidism does not occur in MEN3 (previously known as MEN2B), which is characterised by familial medullary thyroid carcinoma and phaeochromocytomas, mucosal neuromas and often a Marfanoid habitus. MEN2 occurs in <2.5/100,000, and hyperparathyroidism occurs in only 20–40% of patients compared to medullary thyroid carcinoma, which occurs in virtually all patients, and phaeochromocytomas, which occur in ~50% of patients [14, 31, 42–45].

MEN2 occurs due to an autosomal dominant activating mutation of the *RET* proto-oncogene on 10q11.21. In contrast to MEN1, there is a good genotype-phenotype correlation in MEN2, and primary hyperparathyroidism occurs more frequently with mutations at codon 634, and just in a minority of patients with mutations of codons 609, 611, 618, 620, 790, 791 and 804. It is rare in patients with mutations of codons 630, 649, 768, 790, 804 and 891 and it does not occur with mutations of codons 883, 913 and 922 that are responsible for MEN3 [14, 44, 46]. The specific RET codon mutation also predicts the age of onset of medullary thyroid carcinoma and likelihood of nodal involvement, allowing tailoring of timing and extent of prophylactic thyroidectomy to the individual.

PHPT is usually mild or asymptomatic and is rarely the first manifestation of MEN2, typically occurring in the fourth decade; however it has occurred in a patient as young as 5 years [21, 23]. It is often detected at the time of thyroidectomy for medullary thyroid carcinoma in normocalcaemic patients. There is a female predominance for MEN2-associated HPTH of 1.5–2.6. Single adenomas are found in 27–54% of cases and approximately half of patients develop enlargement of all four parathyroid glands. A single case of parathyroid carcinoma has been reported, and ectopic and supernumerary glands are found in up to 43% and 8.6% of cases, respectively [23, 44].

RET gene mutation testing should be performed in all patients with a personal or familial history of medullary thyroid carcinoma or phaeochromocytoma and considered in young patients with multi-gland or familial PHPT. Screening for PHPT is recommended from age 11 in patients with codon 634 mutations and by age 16 years in carriers of other *RET* gene mutations [14, 46].

Timing and Extent of Parathyroid Surgery

Surgery is the mainstay of treatment for MEN2-associated PHPT, but should always be preceded by screening for phaeochromocytoma first, and resection should it be present. Resection of enlarged parathyroid glands at the time of total thyroidectomy for medullary thyroid carcinoma is justifiable since it may avoid reoperation. Therefore parathyroid function testing and pre-operative localisation studies as required are performed prior to thyroidectomy in patients with suspected MEN2.

Although selective parathyroidectomy, subtotal parathyroidectomy and total parathyroidectomy are all performed, most favour a conservative approach of selective resection of only grossly enlarged parathyroid glands, reserving total parathyroidectomy and autografting for those cases where all four glands are abnormal [23, 31, 43, 44]. Prophylactic parathyroidectomy is not undertaken as the sequelae of mild asymptomatic PHPT are less than those of permanent hypoparathyroidism.

Approximately 77–100% of patients with MEN2-related PHPT are cured after surgery and about 20% develop permanent hypoparathyroidism, a risk increased by bilateral level VI neck node dissection for medullary thyroid carcinoma [43]. Recurrence of PHPT occurs in 0–12% over a 5-year follow-up and imaging studies should be performed before reoperation [31, 43–45].

Hyperparathyroidism-Jaw Tumour Syndrome (HPT-JT)

Diagnosis and Genetics

HPT-JT is a rare autosomal dominant syndrome characterised by highly penetrant parathyroid tumours (single or multiple), uterine tumours in 57%, ossifying fibromas of the mandible or maxilla in 30% and renal abnormalities in 13% (Wilms' tumour, papillary renal carcinoma, polycystic kidney disease) (Table 21.2) [23, 47, 48]. The ossifying fibromas of the mandible or maxilla must be differentiated from brown tumours that occur with PHPT. It occurs due to inactivating mutations of the tumour-suppressor gene CDC73 on chromosome 1q31.2 that encodes parafibromin [49]. Parafibromin is a component of the polymerase-associated factor 1 complex that mediates key transcriptional events in histone modification, chromatic remodelling, initiation and elongation and activates the wnt/β-catenin and hedgehog signalling pathways [50–52]. HPT-JT-associated PHPT exhibits a more aggressive course than other hereditary causes of PHPT and has occurred as young as 7 years old; however it typically occurs in early adulthood. It is usually caused by a single benign parathyroid adenoma that often displays cystic or atypical histology; however parathyroid carcinomas have been observed in up to 22% of cases [23, 53]. CDC73 germline analysis should be performed in cases of hereditary PHPT with negative MEN1 gene testing; a personal or family history of HPT-JT syndrome; atypical, cystic or malignant parathyroid histology; absent nuclear parafibromin staining on parathyroid tumour tissue; early onset <40 years; and multi-glandular or recurrent HPTH [53–55].

Timing and Extent of Surgery

The optimal surgical treatment of PHPT in HPT-JT syndrome is unclear. Historically, due to the increased risk of malignancy and multiple-gland involvement, bilateral neck exploration and subtotal/total parathyroidectomy have been proposed [56]. However, autografting of parathyroid tissue has been discouraged due to the risk of seeding parathyroid cancer cells. More recently when the probability of a parathyroid malignancy is low, selective parathyroidectomy based on preoperative localisation studies has been proposed with benefits including a lower risk of hypoparathyroidism and minimal tissue trauma, facilitating reoperations if required [57]. An en bloc resection including the ipsilateral thyroid lobe, adjacent soft tissue and ipsilateral parathyroid is recommended for suspected parathyroid carcinomas to avoid fracture of the tumour and local seeding of malignant cells [55, 58]. Central compartment node dissection may be required if node involvement is suspected. The overall survival for patients with parathyroid carcinoma who undergo surgery is 8.9 years [59]. From age 5 years, 6-monthly biochemical testing for PHPT is recommended for all patients, with annual renal ultrasonography and gynaecology assessment, and 5-yearly dental X-ray [23]. Prompt surgery is necessary as soon as calcium and parathyroid hormone increase in order to prevent parathyroid carcinoma metastases.

Non-syndromic Causes of Hyperparathyroidism

Familial Hypocalciuric Hypercalcaemia (FHH)

FHH is a benign autosomal dominant condition associated with hypocalciuria (urinary calcium clearance/creatinine clearance ratio (CCR)

<0.01) with a mild hypercalcaemia and normal circulating PTH concentrations in 80% (Table 21.2) [6, 11, 60]. Mild hypermagnesaemia is typical. Twenty per cent have raised PTH concentrations and 20% may have a CCR >0.01 and therefore be indistinguishable from HPT. Additionally, a CCR <0.01 may be seen in patients with HPT in the presence of vitamin D deficiency, renal insufficiency or African ethnicity [6, 11, 60, 61]. Therefore genetic mutational analysis may help to identify FHH patients.

There are three known variants responsible for FHH. FHH1 accounts for two-thirds of cases and is due to an inactivating mutation of the extracellular domain of the *CaSR* gene [60]. The calcium-sensing receptor (CaSR) is a G protein-coupled receptor that senses changes in the circulating calcium concentration and when activated inhibits PTH secretion and increases renal calcium excretion. Therefore there is an increase in the calcium ion-dependent set point for PTH release [60]. FHH2 accounts for less than 5% of cases and occurs due to loss-of-function mutations of *GNA11* that encodes for the G protein subunit α11 [62]. FHH3 accounts for >5% of cases and occurs due to a loss-of-function mutation of the *AP2S1* gene that encodes the adaptor-protein 2 σ subunit and plays a central role in the endocytosis of plasma membrane constituents such as the CaSR [62].

Hypercalcaemia in FHH is present at all ages and patients are usually asymptomatic; however chondrocalcinosis, premature vascular calcification, pancreatitis and gallstones have been observed [63–65]. The parathyroid glands are often moderately enlarged. Distinguishing FHH from PHPT is important, as parathyroidectomy is not indicated for FHH because it does not correct the inactivation of the calcium receptor and therefore patients remain hypercalcaemic. FHH should be screened for prior to parathyroid surgery especially in patients <40 years old, those who have had prior unsuccessful parathyroid surgery or patients with a family history of hypercalcaemia or unsuccessful parathyroid surgery. Because clinical and biochemistry parameters may not differentiate between PHPT and FHH, gene testing may be helpful for diagnostic and therapeutic reasons.

Neonatal Severe Hyperparathyroidism (NSHPT)

NSHPT is characterised by the development of severe hypercalcaemia with skeletal manifestation of HPT within the first 6 months of life (Table 21.2) [60]. The parathyroid glands are markedly hyperplastic in this condition and untreated NSHPT can be a severe neurodevelopmental disorder. Therefore urgent parathyroidectomy is recommended in the first month of life. NSHPT is often associated with inactivating homozygous *CaSR* mutations in the children of consanguineous parents; however many other cases appear sporadic or only one parent had clinically apparent FHH [60].

Autosomal Dominant Moderate Hyperparathyroidism (ADMH)

ADMH is a rare syndrome associated with hypercalcaemia and hypercalciuria, plus hypomagnesaemia, elevated serum PTH and nephrolithiasis in some patients (Table 21.2) [66]. Single- or multi-gland parathyroid hyperplasia or adenomas have been observed. This condition was found to be due to a mutation in the intracytoplasmic tail domain of the CaSR. Regression of hypercalcaemia has been observed after subtotal or radical parathyroidectomy.

Familial Isolated Hyperparathyroidism (FIHPT)

FIHPT is a rare familial cause of HPT that appears to be inherited in an autosomal dominant manner and is characterised by single- or multi-glandular parathyroid lesions occurring at a young age (20–25 years) in the absence of other endocrine tumours (Table 21.2). It can be asymptomatic or present with symptomatic hypercalcaemia, osteoporosis and nephrolithiasis. The responsible genes remain largely unknown; however studies of ten kindred have identified a locus on chromosome 2p12.3-p14 [67]. In affected families mutations of *MEN1* have been detected in 20–23%, *CaSR* in 14–18% and *CDC73* less frequently and these genes should be tested [11, 68–72]. It is important to exclude clinical features of MEN1 and HPT-JT before making a diagnosis of FIHPT. Surgery is the principal treatment and intraoperative visualisation of all four parathyroid glands is recommended as FIHPT may be either caused by a single-adenoma or multiple-gland disease that is often asymmetrical [23]. In the presence of *MEN1* and *CDC73* gene mutations, patients should be treated as in MEN1 and HPT-JT syndromes, respectively.

Nonfamilial PHPT Due to De Novo Germline Mutations

Approximately 10% of patients presenting with PHPT below the age of 45 and >5% of patients presenting after 50 years may have de novo germline mutations of *MEN1*, *CDC73*, *CaSR*, *CDKIs (CDKN1A* (p21)*, CDKN2B* (p15) *or CDKN2C* (p18)) or *PTH* genes [6, 11, 73–77]. Just one *PTH* gene mutation has been reported in a patient who had hypercalcaemia and an undetectable serum concentration of intact PTH; however following removal of the parathyroid adenoma, normocalcaemia was achieved [76]. The occurrence of germline mutations in nonfamilial PHPT has implications for the management of HPT in these patients, screening for tumours associated with the specific syndrome and screening of children who may have inherited the mutation.

Recommendations for Genetic Testing in PHPT

As germline mutations are evident in approximately 10% of PHPT patients, indications for mutational analysis include:

(a) Onset before the age of 40 years
(b) Multi-gland disease
(c) Parathyroid carcinoma or atypical parathyroid adenomas
(d) First-degree relatives of known mutation carriers
(e) Index cases with two or more MEN1-associated tumours [6, 11]

Genetic testing should involve a genetic counsellor and informed consent and testing should be performed at accredited centres. Mutational analysis should use DNA obtained from non-tumour cells (e.g. leucocyte DNA) to look for germline mutations of *MEN1*, *CaSR*, AP2S1, *GNA11*, *CDC73*, *CDKN1A*, *CDKN1B*, *CDKN2B*, *CDKN2C*, *RET* and *PTH* genes (Fig. 21.1) [78]. The identification of a germline mutation should prompt entry into surveillance programmes for clinical manifestations of the relevant syndromes and screening of first-degree relatives for the mutation. Asymptomatic first-degree relatives that have the mutation should be offered period surveillance for clinical manifestations of the relevant syndromes, while those without the mutation can be reassured. A careful clinical history should be taken for patients over the age of 40 years and, if there is a clinical suspicion of a syndromic form of PHPT, targeted genetic testing is indicated with appropriate genetic counselling.

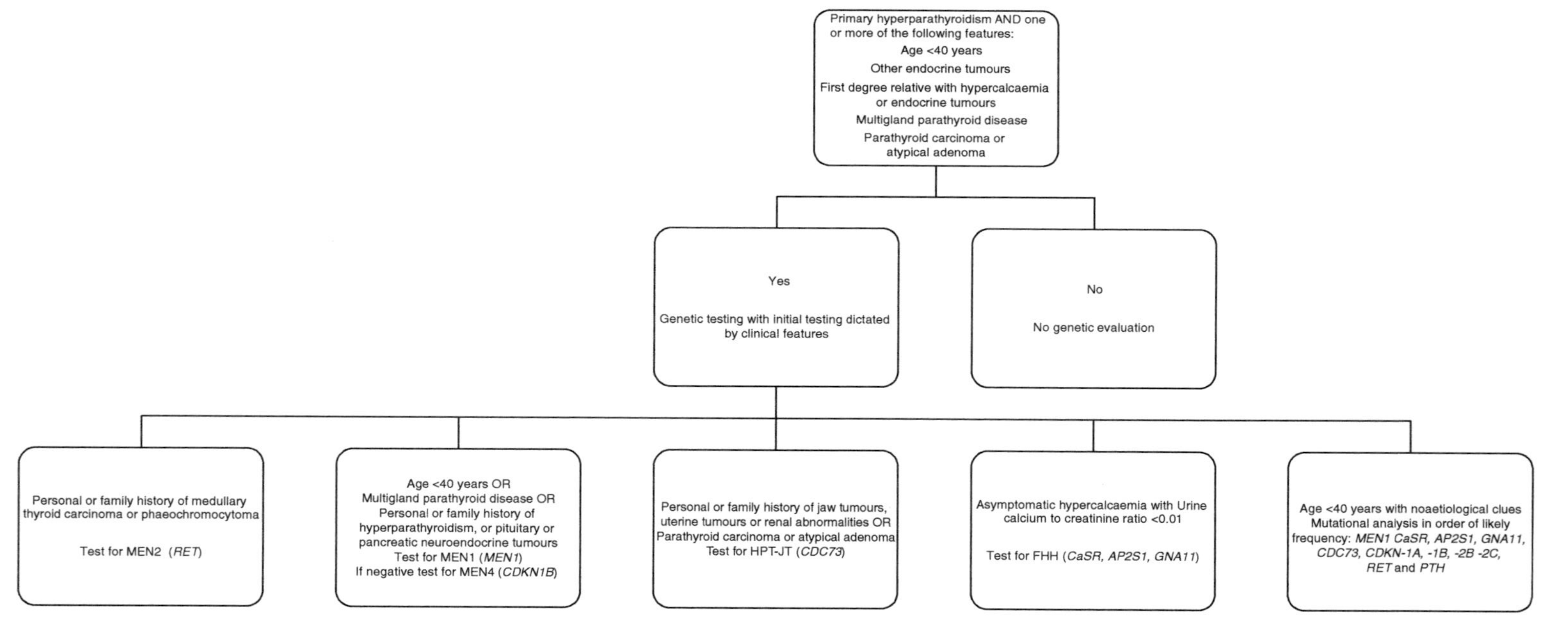

Fig. 21.1 A clinical approach to genetic screening of PHPT

References

1. Griebeler ML, Kearns AE, Ryu E, Hathcock MA, Melton LJ, Wermers RA. Secular trends in the incidence of primary hyperparathyroidism over five decades (1965–2010). Bone. 2015;73:1–7.
2. Verdonk CA, Edis AJ. Parathyroid double adenomas—fact or fiction. Surgery. 1981;90(3):523–6.
3. Harness JK, Ramsburg SR, Nishiyama RH, Thompson NW. Multiple adenomas of the parathyroids—do they exist. Arch Surg. 1979;114(4):468–74.
4. Attie JN, Bock G, Auguste LJ. Multiple parathyroid adenomas—report of 33 cases. Surgery. 1990;108(6):1014–20.
5. Ruda JM, Hollenbeak CS, Stack BC. A systematic review of the diagnosis and treatment of primary hyperparathyroidism from 1995 to 2003. Otolaryngol Head Neck Surg. 2005;132(3):359–72.
6. Eastell R, Brandi ML, Costa AG, D'Amour P, Shoback DM, Thakker RV. Diagnosis of asymptomatic primary hyperparathyroidism: Proceedings of the Fourth International Workshop. J Clin Endocrinol Metab. 2014;99(10):3570–9.
7. Bassett JHD, Forbes SA, Pannett AAJ, Lloyd SE, Christie PT, Wooding C, et al. Characterization of mutations in patients with multiple endocrine neoplasia type 1. Am J Hum Genet. 1998;62(2):232–44.
8. Thakker RV. Multiple endocrine neoplasia type 1 (MEN1) and type 4 (MEN4). Mol Cell Endocrinol. 2014;386:2–15.
9. Hannan FM, Thakker RV. Calcium-sensing receptor (CaSR) mutations and disorders of calcium, electrolyte and water metabolism. Best Pract Res Clin Endocrinol Metab. 2013;27(3):359–71.
10. Thakker RV. Multiple endocrine neoplasia. Harrison's principles of internal medicine. 19th ed. New York: McGraw-Hill; 2013.
11. Thakker RV, Newey PJ, Walls GV, Bilezikian J, Dralle H, Ebeling PR, et al. Clinical practice guidelines for multiple endocrine neoplasia type 1 (MEN1). J Clin Endocrinol Metab. 2012;97(9):2990–3011.
12. Lemmens I, VandeVen WJM, Kas K, Zhang CX, Giraud S, Wautot V, et al. Identification of the multiple endocrine neoplasia type 1 (MEN1) gene. Hum Mol Genet. 1997;6(7):1177–83.
13. Lemos MC, Thakker RV. Multiple endocrine neoplaslia type 1 (MEN 1): analysis of 1336 mutations reported in the first decade following identification of the gene. Hum Mutat. 2008;29(1):22–32.
14. Brandi ML, Gagel RF, Angeli A, Bilezikian JP, Beck-Peccoz P, Bordi C, et al. Guidelines for diagnosis and therapy of MEN type 1 and type 2. J Clin Endocrinol Metab. 2001;86(12):5658–71.
15. Thakker RV. Multiple endocrine neoplasia 1. In: Jameson JL, DeGroot LJ, editors. Endocrinology. Philadelphia: Elsevier; 2010. p. 2719–41.
16. Thakker RV, Bouloux P, Wooding C, Chotai K, Broad PM, Spurr NK, et al. Association of parathyroid tumors in multiple endocrine neoplasia type-1 with loss of alleles on chromosome-11. N Engl J Med. 1989;321(4):218–24.
17. Machens A, Schaaf L, Karges W, Frank-Raue K, Bartsch DK, Rothmund M, et al. Age-related penetrance of endocrine tumours in multiple endocrine neoplasia type 1 (MEN1): a multicentre study of 258 gene carriers. Clin Endocrinol (Oxf). 2007;67(4):613–22.
18. Yates CJ, Newey PJ, Thakker RV. Challenges and controversies in management of pancreatic neuroendocrine tumours in patients with MEN1. Lancet Diabetes Endocrinol. 2015;3(11):895–905.
19. Thakker RV. Genetics of parathyroid tumours. J Intern Med. 2016;280:574.
20. Eller-Vainicher C, Chiodini I, Battista C, Viti R, Mascia ML, Massironi S, et al. Sporadic and MEN1-related primary hyperparathyroidism: differences in clinical expression and severity. J Bone Miner Res. 2009;24(8):1404–10.
21. Brandi ML, Tonelli F. Genetic syndromes associated with primary hyperparathyroidism. In: Gasparri G, Camandona M, Palestini N, editors. Primary, secondary and tertiary hyperparathyroidism: diagnostic and therapeutic updates, Updates in surgery. Italy: Springer; 2016. p. 153–81.
22. Ospina NS, Sebo TJ, Thompson GB, Clarke BL, Young WF. Prevalence of parathyroid carcinoma in 348 patients with multiple endocrine neoplasia type 1-case report and review of the literature. Clin Endocrinol (Oxf). 2016;84(2):244–9.
23. Iacobone M, Carnaille B, Palazzo FF, Vriens M. Hereditary hyperparathyroidism—a consensus report of the European Society of Endocrine Surgeons (ESES). Langenbeck's Arch Surg. 2015;400(8):867–86.
24. Goudet P, Cougard P, Verges B, Murat A, Carnaille B, Calender A, et al. Hyperparathyroidism in multiple endocrine neoplasia type I: surgical trends and results of a 256-patient series from Groupe d'Etude des Neoplasies Endocriniennes Multiples study group. World J Surg. 2001;25(7):886–90.
25. Schreinemakers JMJ, Pieterman CRC, Scholten A, Vriens MR, Valk GD, Rinkes I. The optimal surgical treatment for primary hyperparathyroidism in MEN1 patients: a systematic review. World J Surg. 2011;35(9):1993–2005.
26. Pieterman CRC, van Hulsteijn LT, den Heijer M, van der Luijt RB, Bonenkamp JJ, Hermus A, et al. Primary hyperparathyroidism in MEN1 patients. A cohort study with longterm follow-up on preferred surgical procedure and the relation with genotype. Ann Surg. 2012;255(6):1171–8.
27. Lairmore TC, Govednik CM, Quinn CE, Sigmond BR, Lee CY, Jupiter DC. A randomized, prospective trial of operative treatments for hyperparathyroidism in patients with multiple endocrine neoplasia type 1. Surgery. 2014;156(6):1326–35.
28. Montenegro FLD, Lourenco DM, Tavares MR, Arap SS, Nascimento CP, Neto LMM, et al. Total parathyroidectomy in a large cohort of cases with hyperparathyroidism associated with multiple endocrine

neoplasia type 1: experience from a single academic center. Clinics. 2012;67:131–9.
29. Kraimps JL, Duh QY, Demeure M, Clark OH, Liechty D, Shaha AR, et al. Hyperparathyroidism in multiple endocrine neoplasia syndrome. Surgery. 1992;112(6):1080–8.
30. Hellman P, Skogseid B, Oberg K, Juhlin C, Akerstrom G, Rastad J. Primary and reoperative parathyroid operations in hyperparathyroidism of multiple endocrine neoplasia type 1. Surgery. 1998;124(6):993–9.
31. Oriordain DS, Obrien T, Grant CS, Weaver A, Gharib H, Vanheerden JA, et al. Surgical-management of primary hyperparathyroidism in multiple endocrine neoplasia type-1 and type-2. Surgery. 1993;114(6):1031–9.
32. Salmeron MDB, Gonzalez JMR, Insenser JS, Goday A, Perez NMT, Zambudio AR, et al. Causes and treatment of recurrent hyperparathyroidism after subtotal parathyroidectomy in the presence of multiple endocrine neoplasia 1. World J Surg. 2010;34(6):1325–31.
33. Nilubol N, Weisbrod AB, Weinstein LS, Simonds WF, Jensen RT, Phan GQ, et al. Utility of intraoperative parathyroid hormone monitoring in patients with multiple endocrine neoplasia type 1-associated primary hyperparathyroidism undergoing initial parathyroidectomy. World J Surg. 2013;37(8):1966–72.
34. Kivlen MH, Bartlett DL, Libutti SF, Skarulis MC, Marx SJ, Simonds WF, et al. Reoperation for hyperparathyroidism in multiple endocrine neoplasia type 1. Surgery. 2001;130(6):991–8.
35. Ospina NS, Thompson GB, Lee RA, Reading CC, Young WF. Safety and efficacy of percutaneous parathyroid ethanol ablation in patients with recurrent primary hyperparathyroidism and multiple endocrine neoplasia type 1. J Clin Endocrinol Metab. 2015;100(1):E87–90.
36. Moyes VJ, Monson JP, Chew SL, Akker SA. Clinical use of cinacalcet in MEN1 hyperparathyroidism. Int J Endocrinol. 2010;2010:1.
37. Filopanti M, Verga U, Ermetici F, Olgiati L, Eller-Vainicher C, Corbetta S, et al. MEN1-related hyperparathyroidism: response to cinacalcet and its relationship with the calcium-sensing receptor gene variant Arg990Gly. Eur J Endocrinol. 2012;167(2):157–64.
38. Falchetti A, Cilotti A, Vagelli L, Masi L, Amedei A, Cioppi F, et al. A patient with MEN1-associated hyperparathyroidism, responsive to cinacalcet (vol 4, pg 351, 2008). Nat Clin Pract Endocrinol Metab. 2008;4(7):420.
39. Giusti F, Cianferotti L, Gronchi G, Cioppi F, Masi L, Faggiano A, et al. Cinacalcet therapy in patients affected by primary hyperparathyroidism associated to Multiple Endocrine Neoplasia Syndrome type 1 (MEN1). Endocrine. 2016;52(3):495–506.
40. Molatore S, Pellegata NS. The MENX syndrome and p27: relationships with multiple endocrine neoplasia. In: Martini L, Chrousos GP, Labrie F, Pacak K, Pfaff DW, editors. Neuroendocrinology: pathological situations and diseases. Prog Brain Res. 2010;182:295–320.
41. Tonelli F, Marcucci T, Giudici F, Falchetti A, Brandi ML. Surgical approach in hereditary hyperparathyroidism. Endocr J. 2009;56(7):827–41.
42. Giusti F, Cavalli L, Cavalli T, Brandi ML. Hereditary hyperparathyroidism syndromes. J Clin Densitom. 2013;16(1):69–74.
43. Kraimps JL, Denizot A, Carnaille B, Henry JF, Proye C, Bacourt F, et al. Primary hyperparathyroidism in multiple endocrine neoplasia type IIa: Retrospective French multicentric study. World J Surg. 1996;20(7):808–13.
44. Herfarth KKF, Bartsch D, Doherty GM, Wells SA, Lairmore TC. Surgical management of hyperparathyroidism in patients with multiple endocrine neoplasia type 2A. Surgery. 1996;120(6):966–73.
45. Raue F, Kraimps JL, Dralle H, Cougard P, Proye C, Frilling A, et al. Primary hyperparathyroidism in multiple endocrine neoplasia type 2a. J Intern Med. 1995;238(4):369–73.
46. Wells SA, Asa SL, Dralle H, Elisei R, Evans DB, Gagel RF, et al. Revised American Thyroid Association guidelines for the management of medullary thyroid carcinoma. Thyroid. 2015;25(6):567–610.
47. Bradley KJ, Hobbs MR, Buley ID, Carpten JD, Cavaco BM, Fares JE, et al. Uterine tumours are a phenotypic manifestation of the hyperparathyroidism-jaw tumour syndrome. J Intern Med. 2005;257(1):18–26.
48. Carpten JD, Robbins CM, Villablanca A, Forsberg L, Presciuttini S, Bailey-Wilson J, et al. HRPT2, encoding parafibromin, is mutated in hyperparathyroidism-jaw tumor syndrome. Nat Genet. 2002;32(4):676–80.
49. Bradley KJ, Cavaco BM, Bowl MR, Harding B, Cranston T, Fratter C, et al. Parafibromin mutations in hereditary hyperparathyroidism syndromes and parathyroid tumours. Clin Endocrinol. 2006;64(3):299–306.
50. Yart A, Gstaiger M, Wirbelauer C, Pecnik M, Anastasiou D, Hess D, et al. The HRPT2 tumor suppressor gene product parafibromin associates with human PAF1 and RNA polymerase II. Mol Cell Biol. 2005;25(12):5052–60.
51. Rozenblatt-Rosen O, Hughes CM, Nannepaga SJ, Shanmugam KS, Copeland TD, Guszczynski T, et al. The parafibromin tumor suppressor protein is part of a human Paf1 complex. Mol Cell Biol. 2005;25(2):612–20.
52. Mosimann C, Hausmann G, Basler K. Parafibromin/hyrax activates Wnt/Wg target gene transcription by direct association with beta-catenin/armadillo. Cell. 2006;125(2):327–41.
53. Kelly TG, Shattuck TM, Reyes-Mugica M, Stewart AF, Simonds WF, Udelsman R, et al. Surveillance for early detection of aggressive parathyroid disease: carcinoma and atypical adenoma in familial isolated hyperparathyroidism associated with a germline HRPT2 mutation. J Bone Miner Res. 2006;21(10):1666–71.
54. Cetani F, Pardi E, Borsari S, Viacava P, Dipollina G, Cianferotti L, et al. Genetic analyses of the HRPT2 gene in primary hyperparathyroidism: germline and somatic mutations in familial and spo-

radic parathyroid tumors. J Clin Endocrinol Metab. 2004;89(11):5583–91.
55. Iacobone M, Masi G, Barzon L, Porzionato A, Macchi V, Ciarleglio F, et al. Hyperparathyroidism—jaw tumor syndrome: a report of three large kindred. Langenbeck's Arch Surg. 2009;394(5):817–25.
56. Sarquis MMS, Dias EP, Eng C, De Marco LA. Familial hyperparathyroidism: surgical outcome after 30 years of follow-up in 3 families with germline HRPT2 mutations. Surgery. 2009;145(2):249–50.
57. Iacobone M, Barzon L, Porzionato A, Masi G, Macchi V, Viel G, et al. The extent of parathyroidectomy for HRPT2-related hyperparathyroidism. Surgery. 2009;145(2):250–1.
58. Iacobone M, Lumachi F, Favia G. Up-to-date on parathyroid carcinoma: analysis of an experience of 19 cases. J Surg Oncol. 2004;88(4):223–8.
59. Mehta A, Patel D, Rosenberg A, Boufraqech M, Ellis RJ, Nilubol N, et al. Hyperparathyroidism-jaw tumor syndrome: results of operative management. Surgery. 2014;156(6):1315–25.
60. Hannan FM, Nesbit MA, Zhang C, Cranston T, Curley AJ, Harding B, et al. Identification of 70 calcium-sensing receptor mutations in hyper- and hypo-calcaemic patients: evidence for clustering of extracellular domain mutations at calcium-binding sites. Hum Mol Genet. 2012;21(12):2768–78.
61. Eldeiry LS, Ruan DT, Brown EM, Gaglia JL, Garber JR. Primary hyperparathyroidism and familial hypocalciuric hypercalcemia: relationships and clinical implications. Endocr Pract. 2012;18(3):412–7.
62. Nesbit MA, Hannan FM, Howles SA, Babinsky VN, Head RA, Cranston T, et al. Mutations affecting G-protein subunit alpha(11) in hypercalcemia and hypocalcemia. N Engl J Med. 2013;368(26):2476–86.
63. Marx SJ. Familial hypocalciuric hypercalcemia. N Engl J Med. 1980;303(14):810–1.
64. Volpe A, Guerriero A, Marchetta A, Caramaschi P, Furlani L. Familial hypocalciuric hypercalcemia revealed by chondrocalcinosis. Joint Bone Spine. 2009;76(6):708–10.
65. Heath H. Familial benign (hypocalciuric) hypercalcemia—a troublesome mimic of mild primary hyperparathyroidism. Endocrinol Metab Clin North Am. 1989;18(3):723–40.
66. Carling T, Szabo E, Bai M, Ridefelt P, Westin G, Gustavsson P, et al. Familial hypercalcemia and hypercalciuria caused by a novel mutation in the cytoplasmic tail of the calcium receptor. J Clin Endocrinol Metab. 2000;85(5):2042–7.
67. Warner J, Nyholt DR, Busfield F, Epstein M, Burgess J, Stranks S, et al. Familial isolated hyperparathyroidism is linked to a 1.7 Mb region on chromosome 2p13.3-14. J Med Genet. 2006;43(3):e12.
68. Simonds WF, James-Newton LA, Agarwal SK, Yang B, Skarulis MC, Hendy GN, et al. Familial isolated hyperparathyroidism—clinical and genetic characteristics of 36 kindreds. Medicine. 2002;81(1):1–26.
69. Simonds WF, Robbins CM, Agarwal SK, Hendy GN, Carpten JD, Marx SJ. Familial isolated hyperparathyroidism is rarely caused by germline mutation in HRPT2, the gene for the hyperparathyroidism-jaw tumor syndrome. J Clin Endocrinol Metab. 2004;89(1):96–102.
70. Warner J, Epstein M, Sweet A, Singh D, Burgess J, Stranks S, et al. Genetic testing in familial isolated hyperparathyroidism: unexpected results and their implications. J Med Genet. 2004;41(3):155–60.
71. Hannan FM, Nesbit MA, Christie PT, Fratter C, Dudley NE, Sadler GP, et al. Familial isolated primary hyperparathyroidism caused by mutations of the MEN1 gene. Nat Clin Pract Endocrinol Metab. 2008;4(1):53–8.
72. Villablanca A, Wassif WS, Smith T, Hoog A, Vierimaa O, Kassem M, et al. Involvement of the MEN1 gene locus in familial isolated hyperparathyroidism. Eur J Endocrinol. 2002;147(3):313–22.
73. Newey PJ, Bowl MR, Cranston T, Thakker RV. Cell division cycle protein 73 homolog (CDC73) mutations in the hyperparathyroidism-jaw tumor syndrome (HPT-JT) and parathyroid tumors. Hum Mutat. 2010;31(3):295–307.
74. Starker LF, Akerstrom T, Long WD, Delgado-Verdugo A, Donovan P, Udelsman R, et al. Frequent germline mutations of the MEN1, CASR, and HRPT2/CDC73 genes in young patients with clinically nonfamilial primary hyperparathyroidism. Horm Cancer. 2012;3(1–2):44–51.
75. Hannan FM, Nesbit MA, Christie PT, Lissens W, Van der Schueren B, Bex M, et al. A homozygous inactivating calcium-sensing receptor mutation, Pro339Thr, is associated with isolated primary hyperparathyroidism: correlation between location of mutations and severity of hypercalcaemia. Clin Endocrinol. 2010;73(6):715–22.
76. Au AYM, McDonald K, Gill A, Sywak M, Diamond T, Conigrave AD, et al. PTH mutation with primary hyperparathyroidism and undetectable intact PTH. N Engl J Med. 2008;359(11):1184–6.
77. Costa-Guda J, Soong CP, Parekh VI, Agarwal SK, Arnold A. Germline and somatic mutations in cyclin-dependent kinase inhibitor genes CDKN1A, CDKN2B, and CDKN2C in sporadic parathyroid adenomas. Horm Cancer. 2013;4(5):301–7.
78. Thakker RV. Familial and hereditary forms of primary hyperparathyroidism. In: Bilezikian JP, editor. The parathyroids. 3rd ed. London: Academic; 2015. p. 341–63.

22 Renal Hyperparathyroidism

Kee Yuan Ngiam

"A 56 year-old female with a background of diabetic end-stage renal failure on haemodialysis for the last 12 years is referred to the endocrine surgical clinic for 6-month history of severe back pain, skin itch and poor sleep. She has multiple co-morbid conditions such as non-ST elevation myocardial infarction treated conservatively with aspirin and clopidogrel; left ischaemic stroke with good functional recovery and poorly controlled diabetes mellitus. Her intact PTH levels are 930 pg/mL and alkaline phosphatase levels are 823 IU/L. She is on multiple medications to regulate her calcium and phosphate levels including phosphate binders, cinacalcet and vitamin D analogues. Despite being on these increasing does of these medications, her serum phosphate and PTH levels are progressively increasing. With no possibility of receiving a renal transplant she is undergoes total parathyroidectomy with deltoid autoimplantation. Post surgery, she develops severe hungry bone syndrome, a result of long-term hyperparathyroidism, but is effectively supported with calcium infusion and oral replacements by protocol. In one month, she makes a full recovery with resolution of physical symptoms and improvement in mood. Her calcium and phosphate levels are normalized and she is able to stop phosphate binders".

K. Y. Ngiam
Division of Thyroid and Endocrine Surgery, Department of Surgery, National University Hospital, Singapore, Singapore
e-mail: kee_yuan_ngiam@nuhs.edu.sg

Introduction

End-stage renal failure (ESRF) is a global epidemic driven by increasing incidence of type 2 diabetes mellitus and hypertension [1]. In Singapore, 2.3% of the residents aged between 18 and 69 years had renal impairment as defined by eGFR less than 60 mL/min/1.73m^2. The age-standardised incidence rate has increased by 43% from 1999 to 2014. In the USA, ESRF affects 14% of the population [2], including approximately 660,000 patients who are dialysis dependent [3]. Singapore has the second highest incidence of kidney failure due to diabetes mellitus and one of the lowest kidney transplant rates in the world. Renal transplantation rates have decreased in between 2010 and 2012 from 225 to 179 despite laws in 2009 to permit paired donations of unrelated donors to recipients and the use of cadaveric donors about 60 years of age.

Due to the low rate of transplantation relative to the increased incidence of ESRF, renal hyperparathyroidism (rHPT) develops as a complication marked by derangements in calcium, phosphorus and vitamin D metabolism [4]. rHPT is associated with increased cardiovascular morbidity and mortality [5–9], and in patients with no access to transplantation; patients are often offered parathyroid surgery late into their dialysis vintages with its attendant challenges and complications.

Renal hyperparathyroidism encompasses both secondary and tertiary hyperparathyroidism.

R. Parameswaran, A. Agarwal (eds.), *Evidence-Based Endocrine Surgery*,
https://doi.org/10.1007/978-981-10-1124-5_22

Secondary hyperparathyroidism (sHPT) is the condition when renal failure results in hypocalcaemia, hyperphosphataemia and reduced hydroxylation of 25-OH vitamin D into its active form causing four-gland parathyroid hyperplasia and increase in PTH levels. Tertiary hyperparathyroidism (tHPT) occurs in the setting of long-standing sHPT and the parathyroid gland develops autonomous PTH secretion that is not reversible with renal transplantation. This results in hypercalcaemia, and in up to 20% of cases it is caused by adenomas.

Aetiology

Normal Homeostasis of Calcium and Phosphorus

Two major hormones tightly regulate serum calcium and phosphate levels: parathyroid hormone (PTH) and calcitonin. Parathyroid glands are chiefly responsible for maintaining extracellular calcium concentrations through the secretion of an 84-amino-acid polypeptide hormone. PTH regulates serum calcium concentrations through regulating absorption in the intestines and kidneys and resorption of bone. PTH secretion is in turn regulated directly though plasma concentration of ionised calcium mediated by the calcium-sensing receptor (CaSR) on the surface of the parathyroid gland.

There are three mechanisms through which PTH regulates serum calcium. PTH increases the concentration of serum calcium through resorption of calcium and phosphate from bone matrix. It acts directly on PTH receptors on osteoblasts in bone fluid which secrete RANKL, resulting in a chronic increase in osteoclastic activity and net bone resorption. Another way PTH increases serum calcium is via increasing calcium reabsorption by the kidney through activating 1-α-hydroxylase in the proximal tubules in the kidney, thus increasing hydroxylation of 25-dihydroxyvitamin D (calcidiol) to the active 1,25-dihydroxyvitamin D-3 (calcitriol). This mediates intestinal absorption of calcium and phosphorus. PTH also increases reabsorption of calcium in the kidney but decreases reabsorption of phosphorus causing phosphaturia. However, in the setting of end-stage renal failure (ESRF) there is a lack of 25-hydroxy (25-OH) vitamin D hydroxylation and a lack of reabsorption of calcium from the kidney resulting in an initial state or low or normal serum calcium. Phosphorus tends to accumulate in ESRF patients due to the loss of renal elimination, together with obligatory absorption of dietary phosphate and high PTH levels causing bone resorption and release of phosphate into serum.

Whilst PTH is the main regulator of intra- and extracellular calcium, other hormones are important in phosphate regulation. Fibroblast growth factor 23 (FGF-23) is a phosphaturic hormone secreted by bone in response to hyperphosphataemia. FGF-23 acts on Klotho and FGF receptor complex on the parathyroid cell membrane to reduce parathyroid cell proliferation and secretion of PTH. Its action in the kidney is mediated through suppressing sodium-phosphate co-transporter in the proximal tubule, thus causing phosphorus excretion. It also decreases 1-α-hydroxylase activity, leading to reduced 1,25-OH vitamin D levels [10]. Decreased active vitamin D causes hypocalcaemia and hyperphosphataemia and increases parathyroid cell proliferation and hence excessive secretion of PTH. In chronic ESRF, FGF-23 levels will rise in concert with hyperphosphataemia as parathyroid cell becomes resistant to FGF23 through downregulation of CaSR, vitamin D receptor (VDR) and Klotho [11–14]. This results in increased cardiovascular mortality in patients with ESRF [15].

The point at which parathyroid cell proliferation becomes deregulated is complex and poorly understood. What is clear is that a combination of hyperphosphataemia, hypocalcaemia, vitamin D deficiency and increased FGF23 stimulates proliferation of parathyroid cells [11]. This typically occurs when glomerular filtration rate (GFR) drops below 60 mL/min/1.73 m^2, which is CKD stage 3 and above, and forms the cut-off for screening for hyperparathyroidism in CKD patients. Abnormal serum phosphate and calcium level occur much later in the course of CKD (when the GFR drops below 40 mL/min/1.73 m^2) [4].

With further GFR reduction, serum phosphorus levels start to rise and induce hypocalcaemia by binding bioavailable calcium as $CaHPO_4$, which indirectly leads to a further rise in PTH production and causes systemic calcium deposition when the calcium × phosphate product exceeds 72 mg^2/dL^2. This is the postulated mechanism for increasing cardiovascular morbidity and mortality in ESRF patients [9].

The apocryphal notion that sHPT leads to diffuse parathyroid cell hyperplasia can be debunked immediately by the macroscopic examination of excised parathyroid glands in these patients. They are almost always asymmetric and can have a variety of appearances indicating an underlying polyclonal, hyperplastic phenomenon. Although the mechanism has not been elucidated, the appearance of hyperplastic parathyroid glands can be divided into four types as proposed by Tominaga [16]: diffuse hyperplasia, early nodularity in diffuse hyperplasia, nodular hyperplasia and single-nodular hyperplasia. It is postulated that the cells progressively develop monoclonal nodules due to the loss of genetic regulation triggered by downregulation of the vitamin D receptor and CaSR. Single-nodular gland grows progressively to suppress surrounding diffuse hyperplasia and can function like an adenoma. However, there is no evidence that rHPT patients that have predominant nodular hyperplasia or single-nodular hyperplasia share the same underlying genetic mechanisms of a primary parathyroid adenoma. Although incidental adenomatous parathyroid glands have been found in early CKD patients, it arises from a different genetic mechanism involving cyclin D1 located in the long arm of chromosome 11 [17]. The downregulation of the VDR and hence resistance to calcimimetic and vitamin D analogues may the mechanism for development of tHPT due to loss of negative feedback [16, 18].

Presentation

The presentation of rHPT is highly variable depending on the severity of disease. In countries where renal transplantation is limited, patients may present with florid renal osteodystrophy. This is described by the National Kidney Foundation as "CKD-mineral and bone disorder" (CKD-MBD) to connote the systemic effects of CKD. Bone pain, back pain and arthralgia of major joints are the commonest modes of presentation in this group of patients. Chronic dialysis-related amyloid arthropathy is a severe complication of rHPT caused by β^2-microglobulin deposition in joints featuring destructive osteoarthropathies, destructive spondyloarthropathy and carpal tunnel syndrome. These symptoms may be effectively reversed with parathyroidectomy (PTx) except for amyloid arthropathy.

Other presentations include neuromuscular psychiatric symptoms (such as low mood, poor sleep, lethargy, asthenia), which may be related to hypercalcaemia and/or hyperparathyroidism. Itching and coughing are other symptoms but may be related to uraemia. Paradoxically, these symptoms are relieved with PTx which suggests that hyperparathyroidism may be the underlying mechanism rather than hypercalcaemia or uraemia.

According to NKF/KDOQI guidelines [2], renal osteodystrophy can be divided into adynamic bone disease (at low PTH levels <120 pg/mL), osteomalacia, mixed (high turnover with mineralisation defect; PTH >450 pg/mL) bone disease, amyloid and aluminium bone disease.

Adynamic bone disease is caused by excessive use of calcimimetics, phosphate binders and, in cases of total parathyroidectomy with autoimplantation, failure of the autoimplant to function. This results in brittle bones and resultant fractures.

High-turnover disease is manifested as osteitis fibrosa cystica including subperiosteal resorption, salt and pepper skull, rugger jersey spine, deformity of skeleton and shrinking man syndrome. Chronic high-turnover disease may result in brown tumours which resemble osteolytic bone metastases.

Complications related to rHPT are related to widespread calcium deposition due to high Ca $\times PO_4$ quotients. Ectopic calcification may be deposited in arteries, in particular intimal and medial calcification. Other manifestations include calciphylaxis, tumoural calcinosis and calcification of lung, stomach, conjunctiva and heart valves.

A combination of arteriolar calcification and uraemia, termed "calcific uraemic arteriopathy" increases cardiovascular risk by more than eight times [19]. Moreover, high PTH levels (≥600 pg/mL) can result in anaemia resistant to erythropoietin and can cause in diastolic cardiomyopathy. It has been suggested that FGF-23 may induce arterial smooth muscle myocytes differentiated into osteoblast-like cells which may lead to vascular calcification [4].

Investigations

The workup for rHPT includes blood tests such as iPTH, alkaline phosphatase (ALP), corrected calcium, phosphate, magnesium, 25-hydroxyvitamin D and any preoperative blood tests that are required for safe general anaesthesia. Bone isoforms of ALP may be sent if there is any concern that elevated ALP may be related to liver diseases.

It is routine to perform a preoperative ultrasound of the thyroid to localise the parathyroid glands before surgery. Any discordance between the PTH levels and parathyroid gland sizes (e.g. high PTH levels but no parathyroids seen on ultrasound) should alert the surgeon to perform additional imaging to exclude mediastinal or ectopic parathyroid glands [20]. Ultrasound of the thyroid is also important to exclude thyroid nodules which require fine-needle aspiration cytology to exclude a thyroid malignancy as well as to map the location of any intra-thyroid parathyroids which would aid the surgeon during surgery to locate such lesions.

Tc99m-sestamibi scans are not routinely done for rHPT unless ectopic, mediastinal or recurrent parathyroid glands are suspected. Large hypertrophic parathyroid glands will take up Tc99m-sestamibi avidly and produce a dense scintigram that may falsely mask smaller parathyroid glands adjacent to it. Furthermore, thyroid nodules might also take up Tc99m-sestamibi and lead to a false-positive result. If functional and anatomical localisation is desired, a SPECT-CT is the modality of choice, especially in the setting of recurrent neck or mediastinal parathyroids. Other modalities include a 4D CT scan which is ideal for anatomic localisation of early recurrences where PTH is mildly elevated and the recurrence is small. It must be noted that 4D CT scan incurs a high radiation load and is relatively contraindicated in children and young adults. Lastly, if cases where recurrences are equivocal on axial imaging, suspected parathyroid glands may be sampled with FNA and PTH washings.

Treatment

Medical Treatment Options

Medical management of rHPT is a combination of optimal treatment of CKD and risk factors (e.g. control of blood pressure, diabetes mellitus) followed by appropriate initiation of dialysis. KDIGO guidelines recommend screening for CKD stage 3 (GFR <60 mL/min) with serum PTH, calcium and phosphate. Patients should be offered renal transplantation where possible and early referral for PTx where indications for surgery are met. Meanwhile, the medical goals are optimisation of serum phosphate and calcium levels through a combination of a low-phosphate diet, phosphate binders, vitamin D analogues and lastly calcimimetic medications. All medical treatments lead to the inexorable rise of PTH resulting in CKD-MBD and its associated complications. The size of enlarged parathyroid glands is an important factor in determining the effectiveness of medical treatment. Gland sizes exceeding 500mm^3 should consider PTx instead of medical therapy.

Phosphate Binders

Despite low-phosphate diets, ESRF patients still find it difficult to reduce phosphate levels due to obligatory intestinal uptake of phosphate. Loss of clearance by the kidney and continuous resorption of bone releasing phosphate into the serum result in chronic hyperphosphataemia. Phosphate binders are effective in decreasing serum phosphorus and PTH levels, and decreasing mortality compared with no treatment [21].

Phosphate binders can be divided into calcium- and non-calcium-based binders. Older phosphate binders such as aluminium hydroxide should not be used given the availability of newer agents due to the risk of aluminium toxicity and adynamic bone disease. Calcium salts are cheap and effective phosphate binders that form insoluble calcium phosphate complexes in the gut when taken with meals. However, some calcium is absorbed and can cause hypercalcaemia. Newer agents such as lanthanum and sevelamer hydrochloride are highly effective and are not absorbed. They have gastrointestinal side effects and are costly.

The Kidney Disease Outcomes Quality Initiative (KDOQI) guidelines recommend the use of phosphate binders in CKD 3 and 4 in patients who have hyperphosphataemia despite dietary restriction [22]. Combinational therapy may be initiated if phosphate levels cannot be controlled.

Vitamin D Analogues

1,25-Hydroxy vitamin D deficiency is one of the causes of rHPT due to reduced 1-α-hydroxylation. Replacement with active forms of vitamin D such as calcitriol, paricalcitol and doxercalciferol has been shown in observational studies to improve survival although one meta-analysis showed no difference in symptom reduction and mortality [23]. Despite this, the KDIGO guidelines still suggest treatment with vitamin D analogues or calcitriol in CKD 3 to 5. For patients on dialysis, active forms must be used to control rHPT.

Calcimimetics

The only calcimimetic agent available is cinacalcet and it works by allosteric modulation of the CaSR on the parathyroid gland resulting in increased sensitivity to extracellular calcium, thus suppressing PTH secretion [24]. Although the cinacalcet has been shown to be effective in lowering PTH and reducing symptoms [25], the EVOLVE randomised controlled trial in 2012 did not show a decrease in cardiovascular and overall mortality [26]. Further reviews confirmed these findings and showed that cinacalcet has increased rates of vomiting and hypocalcaemia. However, cinacalcet is still used despite its high cost and lack of long-term effectiveness due to its ability to control PTH levels. Nevertheless, many patients on cinacalcet and maximal medical management still require parathyroidectomy to control their symptoms in the long term. There is some anecdotal evidence that cinacalcet induces haemorrhagic infarction resulting in adherence to surrounding tissues and recurrent laryngeal nerves, thus increasing the risk of nerve damage during surgery [27].

Ethanol Ablation of Parathyroids

Parathyroid ablation using ultrasound-guided ethanol injection has been used since 1985 to control sHPT in patients who are unable to undergo parathyroidectomy [28]. The technique for injecting dehydrated absolute alcohol was initially intended for single parathyroid adenoma but has evolved to treat sHPT due to the poor operative risk in this group of patients. However, multiple treatments are required and there is significant risk of recurrent laryngeal nerve palsy due to the close proximity of the nerve to the parathyroid. Treatments should be adequately spaced and performed unilaterally at any one sitting to avoid bilateral nerve palsy. It is imperative to protect the nerve through injecting a saline buffer around the nerve and accurate needle positioning within the parathyroid. Despite these precautions, there might be some transient nerve palsy and pain due to extravasation of ethanol to the surrounding tissues and patients must be warned for these side effects [29].

Indications for Surgical Treatment

The KDOQI guidelines recommend parathyroidectomy for patients with severe hyperparathyroidism (persistent serum levels of intact PTH >800 pg/mL [88.0 pmol/L]), associated with hypercalcaemia and/or hyperphosphataemia that are refractory to medical therapy for more than 6 months [30]. Other indictors include calciphylaxis, osteoporosis (T-score >2.5 SD below mean), pathological bone fracture and symptomatic hyperparathyroidism (such as pruritus, bone pain, severe vascular calcifications and myopathy).

Surgical Technique

There are three surgical procedures used to treat rHPT: total parathyroidectomy (TPX) alone, TPX with autotransplantation and subtotal parathyroidectomy. They are typically accompanied with bilateral cervical thymectomy to reduce the risk of recurrence [31]. These operations are accepted surgical treatment options for rHPT, each with specific advantages and disadvantages, but none has been shown to be superior to another [32]. The most important factor that determines the success of PTx is the experience of the surgeon.

Total parathyroidectomy alone involves removal of all parathyroid glands with bilateral thymectomy. This operation has the lowest rate of recurrent hyperparathyroidism but has the disadvantage of permanent hypoparathyroidism. Patients undergoing TPX alone would require lifelong calcium and vitamin D replacement. It should not be performed in patients with the potential for renal transplantation, as PTH is required for normal graft function. Fluctuations in calcium in these patients may cause urinary calculus formation and further threaten the kidney transplant.

In TPX with autotransplantation, all four glands are excised and half a gland is transplanted into the brachioradialis muscle or deltoid muscle. Approximately 50 mg of normal-appearing parathyroid tissue is cut into small 1 mm pieces and implanted into a muscular pocket and marked with metal clips and non-absorbable sutures. This method provides a predictable location and landmarks to identify recurrences, if any. Alternative methods include injection of finely minced parathyroid tissue into the muscle or subcutaneous tissue using a specialised large-bore plastic needle with the advantage being a simple procedure performed through a small incision. However, in the event of a recurrence, it may be difficult to locate all the hypertrophic lesions, which may spread deep to and laterally in the muscle. In addition, wide or repeated resection of parathyroid recurrences can result in significant loss of muscle strength in the affected muscle. Another advantage of reimplantation of parathyroid tissue at ectopic sites is ease of access, usually under local anaesthetic, if there is a recurrence and reoperation is required. This avoids the risks associated with re-exploration of the neck. This autoimplant typically takes 3–4 weeks to revascularise and resume its function.

It is imperative that normal parathyroid tissue be autoimplanted instead of nodular parathyroid tissue. This can be confirmed on direct visual inspection of the parathyroid or with a stereomicroscope to look for fat-rich stroma and lobular features. This is because graft-dependent recurrent hyperparathyroidism is associated with autotransplantation of nodular hyperplastic tissue compared to autotransplantation of diffusely hyperplasic gland.

Subtotal parathyroidectomy is the removal of 3½ parathyroid glands, leaving the remaining partial gland intact in its original anatomic location with its blood supply. Typically, the most normal-appearing gland in the superior position is selected. Its advantages are minimising the period of post-operative hypoparathyroidism and risk of permanent hypoparathyroidism. This is therefore suitable for patients who might be kidney-transplant candidates, as they need to reduce the risk of permanent hypoparathyroidism and graft failure. However, if there is a recurrence, there might be an increased risk of injury to the recurrent laryngeal nerve during reoperation.

The risks of PTx include recurrent laryngeal nerve injury (2%), haematoma requiring re-exploration (<1%) and post-operative symptomatic hungry bone syndrome (~90%). Recurrence is dependant on the identification and removal of all four parathyroids, presence of ectopic or mediastinal parathyroids, parathyromatosis (caused by capsular rupture of the parathyroid gland during surgery) and removal of bilateral thymi.

The most important post-operative complication of PTx especially in patients with high dialysis vintages is the risk of hungry bone syndrome resulting in severe hypocalcaemia. This is typically treated with a combination of intravenous calcium infusions, oral calcium replacement, vitamin D replacement with calcitriol and high-calcium bath dialysis.

A protocol-driven approach is shown to reduce the morbidity associated with post-operative hypocalcaemia. This is achieved through preoperative calcium and vitamin D loading, cessation of calcimimetics and phosphate binders and establishing central line access for high-dose calcium infusions. Intraoperatively, standardised calcium infusions are initiated once parathyroid glands are removed and infusion rates are then titrated post-operatively according to protocol. Oral calcium and calcitriol are adjusted post-operatively to reduce the need for intravenous calcium infusions, potentially reducing length of stay and complication related to calcium infusions.

Post-parathyroidectomy, patients experience significant improvement in symptoms within weeks. There are significant improvements in bone pain, arthralgia, myalgia, mood and other psychological manifestations [33]. Most of the improvements of bone-related symptoms are attributed to an increase in trabecular bone mineral content and accelerated bone formation within 1 week after surgery [34]. In the USA, the 30-day post-operative mortality of parathyroidectomy is approximately 3.1% [35]. However, the long-term survival benefits of PTx, including reductions in cardiovascular events and all-cause mortality, are reduced by up to 15%, outweighing the risk of surgery [36, 37]. Other benefits include improving anaemia, immune function and nutrition in these patients [38, 39]. Compared to cinacalcet, parathyroidectomy is more cost effective in ESRF patients who are eligible for surgery. Early screening of CKD patients who meet the criteria for surgery would thus reduce their risk of surgery and improve overall outcomes for these patients.

Conclusion

In conclusion, rHPT is a complex disease characterised by derangements in calcium, phosphorus and vitamin D metabolism. There is a significant risk of skeletal and cardiovascular complications as a result of CKD-MBD, which increases the risk of fractures and death. These complications can be screened and treated expediently especially in CKD 3 patients. Medical treatment forms the mainstay of treatment in the initial stages but almost all patients progress to symptomatic hyperparathyroidism without kidney transplantation. For patients who are fit for surgery, parathyroidectomy provides the best long-term outcome in terms of improvement in symptoms and overall mortality. Hence, early screening of CKD patients who meet the criteria for surgery would reduce their risk of surgery and improve overall outcomes for these patients.

References

1. Mallamaci F. Highlights of the 2015 ERA-EDTA congress: chronic kidney disease, hypertension. Nephrol Dial Transplant. 2016;31(7):1044–6. https://doi.org/10.1093/ndt/gfw006.
2. K/DOQI clinical practice guidelines for chronic kidney disease: evaluation, classification, and stratification. Am J Kidney Dis. 2002;39(2 Suppl 1):S1–266.
3. Collins AJ, Foley RN, Gilbertson DT, et al. United States Renal Data System public health surveillance of chronic kidney disease and end-stage renal disease. Kidney Int Suppl. 2015;5(1):2–7. https://doi.org/10.1038/kisup.2015.2.
4. Levin A, Bakris GL, Molitch M, et al. Prevalence of abnormal serum vitamin D, PTH, calcium, and phosphorus in patients with chronic kidney disease: results of the study to evaluate early kidney disease. Kidney Int. 2007;71(1):31–8. https://doi.org/10.1038/sj.ki.5002009.
5. De Boer IH, Gorodetskaya I, Young B, et al. The severity of secondary hyperparathyroidism in chronic

renal insufficiency is GFR-dependent, race-dependent, and associated with cardiovascular disease. J Am Soc Nephrol. 2002;13(11):2762–9.
6. Fellner SK, Lang RM, Neumann A, et al. Parathyroid hormone and myocardial performance in dialysis patients. Am J Kidney Dis. 1991;18(3):320–5. https://doi.org/10.1016/S0272-6386(12)80090-4.
7. Block GA, Klassen PS, Lazarus JM, et al. Mineral metabolism, mortality, and morbidity in maintenance hemodialysis. J Am Soc Nephrol. 2004;15(8):2208–18.
8. Kalantar-Zadeh K, Kuwae N, Regidor DL, et al. Survival predictability of time-varying indicators of bone disease in maintenance hemodialysis patients. Kidney Int. 2006;70(4):771–80. https://doi.org/10.1038/sj.ki.5001514.
9. Ganesh SK, Stack AG, Levin NW, et al. Association of elevated serum PO(4), Ca x PO(4) product, and parathyroid hormone with cardiac mortality risk in chronic hemodialysis patients. J Am Soc Nephrol. 2001;12(10):2131–8.
10. Farrow EG, White KE. Recent advances in renal phosphate handling. Nat Rev Nephrol. 2010;6(4):207–17. https://doi.org/10.1038/nrneph.2010.17.
11. Galitzer H, Ben-Dov IZ, Silver J, et al. Parathyroid cell resistance to fibroblast growth factor 23 in secondary hyperparathyroidism of chronic kidney disease. Kidney Int. 2010;77(3):211–8. https://doi.org/10.1038/ki.2009.464.
12. Komaba H, Goto S, Fujii H, et al. Depressed expression of Klotho and FGF receptor 1 in hyperplastic parathyroid glands from uremic patients. Kidney Int. 2010;77(3):232–8. https://doi.org/10.1038/ki.2009.414.
13. Fukuda N, Tanaka H, Tominaga Y, et al. Decreased 1,25-dihydroxyvitamin D3 receptor density is associated with a more severe form of parathyroid hyperplasia in chronic uremic patients. J Clin Invest. 1993;92(3):1436–43. https://doi.org/10.1172/JCI116720.
14. Gogusev J, Duchambon P, Hory B, et al. Depressed expression of calcium receptor in parathyroid gland tissue of patients with hyperparathyroidism. Kidney Int. 1997;51(1):328–36. https://doi.org/10.1038/ki.1997.41.
15. Quarles LD. Role of FGF23 in vitamin D and phosphate metabolism: implications in chronic kidney disease. Exp Cell Res. 2012;318(9):1040–8. https://doi.org/10.1016/j.yexcr.2012.02.027.
16. Tominaga Y, Tanaka Y, Sato K, et al. Histopathology, pathophysiology, and indications for surgical treatment of renal hyperparathyroidism. Semin Surg Oncol. 1997;13(2):78–86. https://doi.org/10.1002/(SICI)1098-2388(199703/04)13:2<78::AID-SSU3>3.0.CO;2-Z.
17. Imanishi Y, Hosokawa Y, Yoshimoto K, et al. Primary hyperparathyroidism caused by parathyroid-targeted overexpression of cyclin D1 in transgenic mice. J Clin Invest. 2001;107(9):1093–102. https://doi.org/10.1172/JCI10523.
18. Madorin C, Owen RP, Fraser WD, et al. The surgical management of renal hyperparathyroidism. Eur Arch Otorhinolaryngol. 2012;269(6):1565–76. https://doi.org/10.1007/s00405-011-1833-2.
19. Mazhar AR, Johnson RJ, Gillen D, et al. Risk factors and mortality associated with calciphylaxis in end-stage renal disease. Kidney Int. 2001;60(1):324–32. https://doi.org/10.1046/j.1523-1755.2001.00803.x.
20. Hu J, Ngiam KY, Parameswaran R. Mediastinal parathyroid adenomas and their surgical implications. Ann R Coll Surg Engl. 2015;97(4):259–61. https://doi.org/10.1308/003588415X14181254789088.
21. Isakova T, Gutierrez OM, Chang Y, et al. Phosphorus binders and survival on hemodialysis. J Am Soc Nephrol. 2009;20(2):388–96.
22. Goodman WG. The consequences of uncontrolled secondary hyperparathyroidism and its treatment in chronic kidney disease. Semin Dial. 2004;17(3):209–16. https://doi.org/10.1111/j.0894-0959.2004.17308.x.
23. Palmer SC, McGregor DO, Macaskill P, et al. Meta-analysis: vitamin D compounds in chronic kidney disease. Ann Intern Med. 2007;147(12):840–53. https://doi.org/10.7326/0003-4819-147-12-200712180-00004.
24. Cunningham J, Danese M, Olson K, et al. Effects of the calcimimetic cinacalcet HCl on cardiovascular disease, fracture, and health-related quality of life in secondary hyperparathyroidism. Kidney Int. 2005;68(4):1793–800. https://doi.org/10.1111/j.1523-1755.2005.00596.x.
25. Block GA, Martin KJ, de Francisco AL, et al. Cinacalcet for secondary hyperparathyroidism in patients receiving hemodialysis. N Engl J Med. 2004;350(15):1516–25. https://doi.org/10.1056/NEJMoa031633.
26. Chertow GM, Block GA, Correa-Rotter R, et al. Effect of cinacalcet on cardiovascular disease in patients undergoing dialysis. N Engl J Med. 2012;367(26):2482–94. https://doi.org/10.1056/NEJMoa1205624.
27. Sumida K, Nakamura M, Ubara Y, et al. Histopathological alterations of the parathyroid glands in haemodialysis patients with secondary hyperparathyroidism refractory to cinacalcet hydrochloride. J Clin Pathol. 2011;64(9):756–60. https://doi.org/10.1136/jclinpath-2011-200100.
28. Solbiati L, Giangrande A, De Pra L, et al. Percutaneous ethanol injection of parathyroid tumors under US guidance: treatment for secondary hyperparathyroidism. Radiology. 1985;155(3):607–10. https://doi.org/10.1148/radiology.155.3.3889999.
29. Takeda S, Michigishi T, Takazakura E. Successful ultrasonically guided percutaneous ethanol injection for secondary hyperparathyroidism. Nephron. 1992;62(1):100–3.
30. K/DOQI clinical practice guidelines for bone metabolism and disease in chronic kidney disease. Am J Kidney Dis. 2003;42(4 Suppl 3):S1–201.
31. Schneider R, Bartsch DK, Schlosser K. Relevance of bilateral cervical thymectomy in patients with renal hyperparathyroidism: analysis of 161 patients undergoing reoperative parathyroidectomy. World J Surg. 2013;37(9):2155–61. https://doi.org/10.1007/s00268-013-2091-9.

32. Higgins RM, Richardson AJ, Ratcliffe PJ, et al. Total parathyroidectomy alone or with autograft for renal hyperparathyroidism? Q J Med. 1991;79(288):323–32. https://doi.org/10.1093/oxfordjournals.qjmed.a068553.
33. Dumasius V, Angelos P. Parathyroid surgery in renal failure patients. Otolaryngol Clin N Am. 2010;43(2):433–40., , x–xi. https://doi.org/10.1016/j.otc.2010.01.010.
34. Yajima A, Ogawa Y, Takahashi HE, et al. Changes of bone remodeling immediately after parathyroidectomy for secondary hyperparathyroidism. Am J Kidney Dis. 2003;42(4):729–38. https://doi.org/10.1016/S0272-6386(03)00909-0.
35. Kestenbaum B, Andress DL, Schwartz SM, et al. Survival following parathyroidectomy among United States dialysis patients. Kidney Int. 2004;66(5):2010–6. https://doi.org/10.1111/j.1523-1755.2004.00972.x.
36. Costa-Hong V, Jorgetti V, Gowdak LH, et al. Parathyroidectomy reduces cardiovascular events and mortality in renal hyperparathyroidism. Surgery. 2007;142(5):699–703. https://doi.org/10.1016/j.surg.2007.06.015.
37. Sharma J, Raggi P, Kutner N, et al. Improved long-term survival of dialysis patients after near-total parathyroidectomy. J Am Coll Surg. 2012;214(4):400–7; discussion 407–8
38. Chow TL, Chan TT, Ho YW, et al. Improvement of anemia after parathyroidectomy in Chinese patients with renal failure undergoing long-term dialysis. Arch Surg. 2007;142(7):644–8. https://doi.org/10.1001/archsurg.142.7.644.
39. Yasunaga C, Nakamoto M, Matsuo K, et al. Effects of a parathyroidectomy on the immune system and nutritional condition in chronic dialysis patients with secondary hyperparathyroidism. Am J Surg. 1999;178(4):332–6. https://doi.org/10.1016/S0002-9610(99)00194-4.

Revision Parathyroidectomy 23

Anatoliy V. Rudin and Geoffrey Thompson

Goals

The objective of this chapter is to discuss the evaluation of recurrent and persistent hyperparathyroidism, including definition, etiology, diagnosis, indications for reoperation, preoperative planning, localization studies, and operative strategies.

Introduction

Primary hyperparathyroidism (PHPT) is the most common cause of hypercalcemia in the outpatient setting. As a result of excessive and autonomous parathyroid hormone production, the majority of cases are sporadic, with approximately 80–85% of patients presenting with a single-adenoma, multiglandular hyperplasia in 10–15%, double adenoma in 2–5%, and parathyroid cancer in <1%.

PHPT is biochemically diagnosed, and a surgical cure rate can be achieved in up to 95–97% of cases in nonfamilial, nonmalignant cases. Postoperatively, patients are considered cured if they maintain normal calcium levels 6 months after parathyroidectomy. However, 1–10% of patients may develop persistent or recurrent disease after initial operation, having been reported as high as 30% in some series [1–6]. If hyperparathyroidism does not resolve postoperatively or recurs within a 6-month period the patient is considered to have persistent disease. If a patient has a presumed postoperative cure and hyperparathyroidism recurs after 6 months, the patient is considered to have recurrent disease. Persistent PHPT is more common than recurrent, and is usually the result of a missed adenoma by a less than experienced surgeon.

G. Thompson (✉) · A. V. Rudin
Endocrine Surgery, Mayo Clinic,
Rochester, MN, USA
e-mail: thompson.geoffrey@mayo.edu;
rudin.anatoliy@mayo.edu

Etiology

The reasons for recurrent or persistent disease can be associated with multiple factors, including failure to find abnormal adenoma, inadequate surgical resection, and inaccurate diagnosis (failure to find, failure to treat, failure to diagnose). In addition, studies have demonstrated that a surgeon's experience can have a major impact on operative success rate [2, 7–9]. Moreover, the risk of recurrent or persistent disease is increased in patients with multigland disease, familiar syndromes, and parathyroid carcinoma [7].

Missed Adenoma

The majority of patients reviewed in literature for reoperative hyperparathyroidism were discovered to have a missed adenoma as the most com-

R. Parameswaran, A. Agarwal (eds.), *Evidence-Based Endocrine Surgery*,
https://doi.org/10.1007/978-981-10-1124-5_23

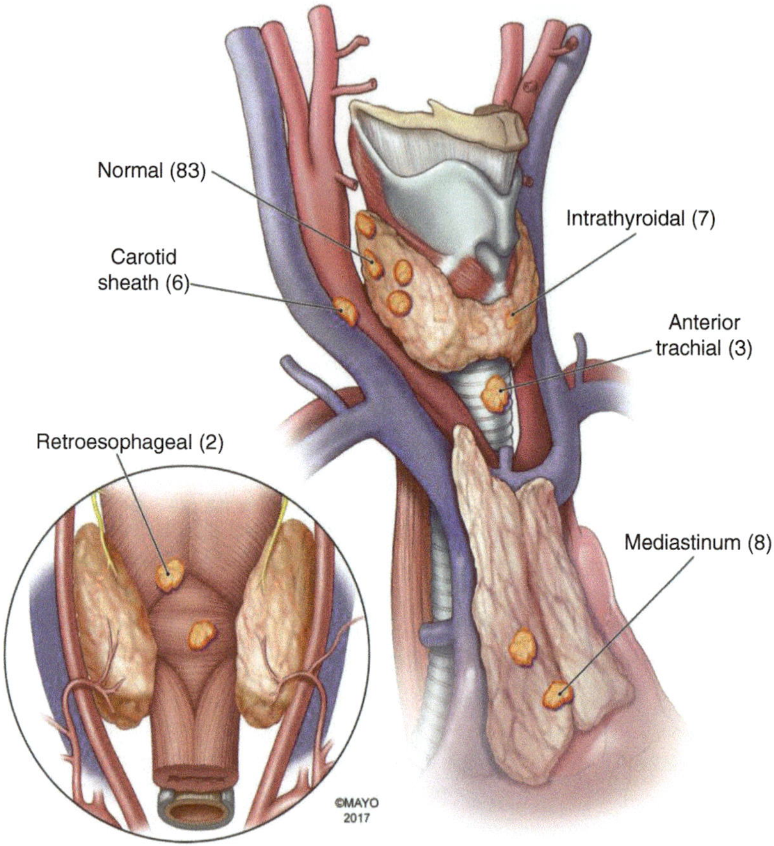

Fig. 23.1 Preoperative parathyroid surgeries at Mayo. Number and anatomic location of abnormal glands removed at preoperative parathyroid surgery (Thompson [1], image modified)

mon reason for both persistent and recurrent diseases [9, 10]. During reoperation, the majority of adenomas have been found in their expected anatomic location, with the inferior parathyroid gland contributing to more variability [1, 9, 11]. If a parathyroid is not in the expected location, it is considered ectopic. Ectopic adenomas vary by location and contribute to persistent or recurrent PHPT in reoperative cases [1, 2, 7, 8] (Fig. 23.1). Most common ectopic locations are the thymus (17–26%) and paraesophageal regions (28%), followed by mediastinum (27%), intrathyroidal (4–10%), pterygopalatine fossa (2–9%), and within the carotid sheath (3.6–9%) [1, 7, 9, 12, 13]. Uncommon locations include the aortopulmonary window (5%), and anterior to the trachea [7].

Multiple Adenomas

The incidence of multiple adenomas ranges from 2 to 12% in various studies [14]. Failure to identify multiple adenomas on preoperative imaging may lead to focused unilateral exploration instead of the warranted bilateral exploration, which can lead to inadequate tissue resection and postoperative hyperparathyroidism (HPT). In addition, the recurrence rate of HPT is higher among patients with double adenoma compared to single adenoma [6], suggesting the possibility of early asymmetric hyperplasia. The use of intraoperative PTH with preoperative ultrasound and sestamibi may assist in detecting double adenomas and ensuring that adequate resection is performed [14].

Moreover, supernumerary glands have been detected in up to 13% of random autopsies, and can occur in a small subset of cases, especially in patients with MEN syndromes and up to 30% of patients with renal hyperparathyroidism [15, 16]. If not detected on preoperative imaging this can lead to operative failure especially in the presence of hyperplasia or cancer.

Parathyroid Hyperplasia

Parathyroid hyperplasia occurs in approximately 15% of patients with PHPT; however, it is responsible for approximately 38% of reoperations [7, 12]. This suggests incomplete resection at the initial operation with continued growth of the remaining hyperplasic tissue. Failure is therefore attributed to inadequate tissue resection of tissue and failure to diagnose multigland hyperplasia preoperatively or intraoperatively. The usual treatment involves bilateral exploration with subtotal or total parathyroidectomy with autotransplantation.

Parathyroid Carcinoma

Rare causes of recurrent or persistent disease include parathyroid carcinoma, which accounts for 0.4–4% of PHPT cases [17, 18]. The majority of recurrent disease is within the neck; however, metastases to lungs and bones do occur [19]. Suspicion of parathyroid carcinoma should be considered preoperatively by a thorough history and physical examination, including excessively high preoperative calcium and PTH levels, a palpable mass, and positive family history of parathyroid carcinoma. However, the majority of patients with parathyroid cancer are not diagnosed preoperatively [18]. When parathyroid carcinoma is recognized, most authors recommend en bloc resection (parathyroid, thyroid, RLN, and lymph nodes), although up to 78% of patients were treated with simple parathyroidectomy in one study [18]. Overall, given the high local recurrence rate, recognition of parathyroid carcinoma is imperative. Parathyroid carcinoma requires en bloc resection of the tumor along with other involved structures as indicated.

Local Recurrence

Local recurrence of disease can be seen in the context of malignant disease or benign parathyromatosis. The most common is recurrence due to hypertrophy or hyperplasia of small benign nodules of parathyroid tissue at previous resection sites due to tumor spillage. It is imperative to ensure delicate handling of the parathyroid gland and avoid capsular rupture [20].

Incorrect Diagnosis

Operating for the incorrect diagnosis is another cause for failure [2]. One commonly reported reason is benign familial hypocalciuric hypercalcemia (FHH) [21]. This hereditary disease should be suspected in patients with inappropriately normal PTH concentration in the presence of mild hypercalcemia, and a positive family history. These patients have had lifelong hypercalcemia. It is important to distinguish FHH from PHPT because FHH does not require parathyroidectomy. Testing for the calcium-sensing receptor mutation is diagnostic. Other causes for incorrect diagnosis include the use of lithium or thiazide diuretics.

Preoperative Diagnosis and Planning

When patients present for evaluation of persistent or recurrent hyperparathyroidism, it is imperative to review the patient's old records and reestablish the initial diagnosis. Patients should have a thorough history, physical examination, and repeat biochemical confirmation, including serum calcium, PTH, creatinine, and 24-h urine to rule out FHH. Once the diagnosis has been established, the indications for reoperation should be guided by the current NIH guidelines [22]. Reoperative success is reduced as compared to first-time operation with both increased morbidity and cost. Therefore, the risks associated with reoperation have to be weighed. These risks include higher incidence of recurrent laryngeal nerve injury, permanent hypoparathyroidism, and increased rates of failure to cure [7, 13, 23, 24].

Once the diagnosis and indication for reoperation have been established, it is important to review prior operative notes to determine the extent of surgery, how many parathyroid glands were identified and removed, if the recurrent laryngeal nerve (RLN) was visualized, and the intraoperative PTH values if available. If the operative report is unclear, attempts should be made to contact the operative surgeon. Also, the pathology report and slides need to be reviewed to verify the histopathology. Evaluation of concordance with previous localization studies is very helpful.

Given the increased risk of injury to the recurrent laryngeal nerve with reoperation, preoperative vocal cord check should be performed in all cases considered for reoperation. Studies have shown that patients with recurrent laryngeal nerve palsy have reconstitution of function in the majority of cases at 6 months, and up to 2 years [25]. Therefore, in a patient with a known vocal cord palsy from prior surgery, up to 6 months should be allowed for recovery before considering reoperation. Additional injury to the contralateral recurrent laryngeal nerve can result in greater morbidity, including the need for tracheostomy. The status of RLN may, therefore, impact the decision-making process and should be weighed heavily.

Localization Studies

Multiple studies have shown that preoperative localization improves outcomes, reduces morbidity, decreases operative time, and is essential when treating recurrent or persistent hyperparathyroidism [12, 26]. Increased failure rates can be seen in patients with non-localizing studies [27]. In general, localization studies can be divided into two categories: noninvasive and invasive. Noninvasive studies should be done before considering invasive studies. Typically, at least two or more concordant imaging studies should be obtained prior to proceeding with a reoperation [5]. Currently, the optimal imaging modality or combinations thereof have not been established [28].

Noninvasive Localization

Sestamibi Scintigraphy

Sestamibi parathyroid scintigraphy has been established as cost effective, reliable, and the first choice for localization of abnormal parathyroid tissue [29, 30]. It utilizes technetium-99m-methoxyisobutylisonitrile (99mTc sestamibi), which is absorbed and retained longer by the parathyroid tissue than thyroid [31]. Studies have demonstrated 64–88% sensitivity for detecting a single adenoma and 98.9% specificity [31–33]. However, 99mTc sestamibi has been associated with false-negative rates up to 25%, which is more common in patients with multigland disease, small adenomas, nodular thyroid disease, and normocalcemia [31]. At our institution, we utilize I123 in addition to sestamibi, performing a subtraction scan along with SPECT and planar imaging, providing better accuracy (Figs. 23.2 and 23.3).

Ultrasound

Ultrasonography is a relatively inexpensive, noninvasive, readily available localization tool with good sensitivity when done by experienced operators, and can be used in reoperative cases to localize a parathyroid adenoma (Fig. 23.4) [1]. The sensitivity of ultrasound for detecting a single adenoma ranges from 61 to 92% of patients [32]. The sensitivity can be increased with concurrent fine-needle aspiration for cytology and washout PTH levels. Studies have shown that a combination of neck ultrasound and 99mTC sestamibi increases sensitivity to greater than 90% for localizing an adenoma [32]. However, ultrasound is limited because it is operator dependent, with a sensitivity range of 33–92%, and has reduced success in detecting ectopic adenomas,

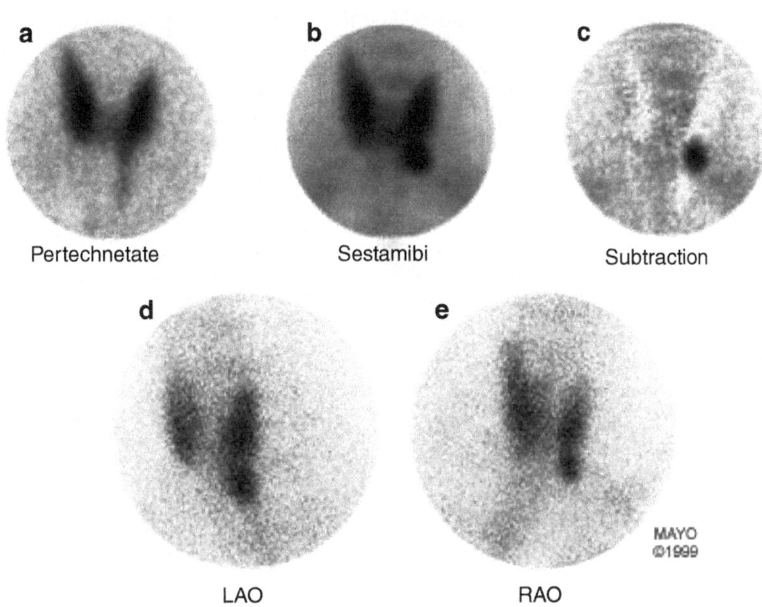

Fig. 23.2 Sestamibi scan demonstrating left inferior parathyroid gland adenoma on subtraction view (**c**). The left and right oblique images are concordant with a left inferior adenoma

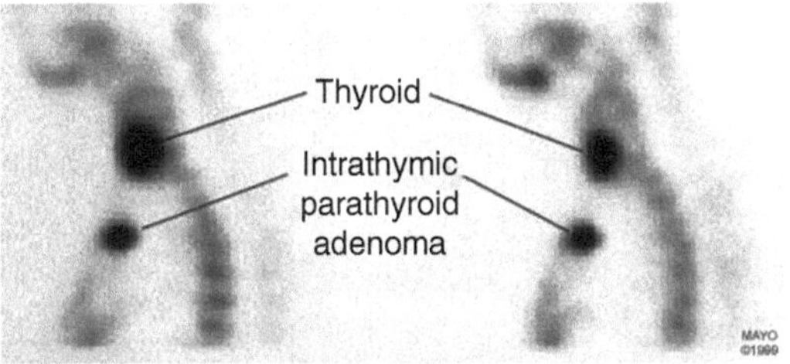

Fig. 23.3 Sestamibi with sagittal SEPCT shows an intrathymic left inferior parathyroid adenoma in the anterior mediastinum

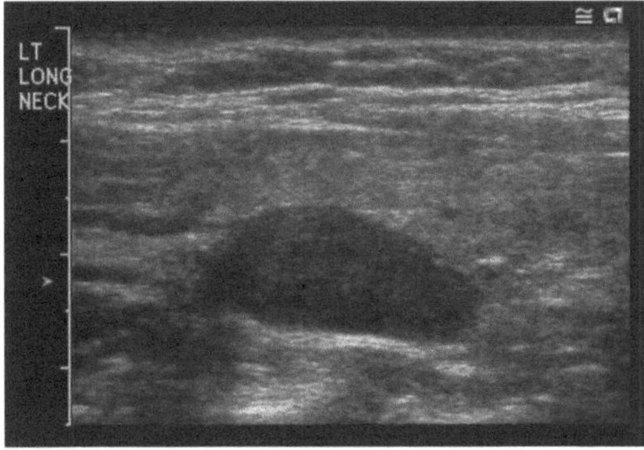

Fig. 23.4 Neck ultrasound demonstrating single parathyroid adenoma

especially in the presence of thyroid nodules and those within the mediastinum [32, 34].

Single-Photon Emission Computed Tomography

Single-photon emission computed tomography (SPECT) can be a useful adjunct to sestamibi, especially in detecting ectopic adenomas. Both modalities can be combined for increased sensitivity [31, 35]. In patients undergoing reoperation, sensitivity can be improved from 79.5 to 87% for adenoma detection [31]. In addition, SPECT provides higher resolution images and additional tomography aids in mapping the relationship of the abnormal parathyroid to the surrounding structures, including trachea, esophagus, thyroid, thymus, and carotid artery. However, SPECT imaging can still fall short with multiglandular disease [31].

Four-Dimensional Computed Tomography

4D CT can be helpful when there are equivocal or negative conventional imaging findings [36]. One study looked at 45 patients undergoing reoperative parathyroidectomy and found that 4D CT had an 88% sensitivity compared to 54% with sestamibi [37]. The main disadvantage of this test is the increased radiation exposure and contrast load.

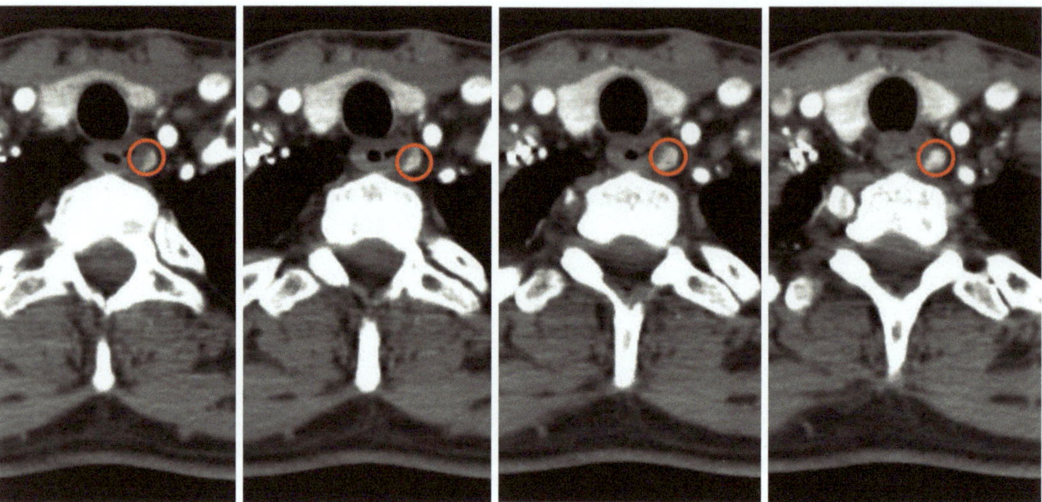

Fig. 23.5 CT scan demonstrating a left parathyroid adenoma along the left posterolateral border of the cervical esophagus (arterial phase, 2 mm slices, adenoma measured 8 × 4 × 14 mm)

Computed Tomography

Computed tomography has been shown to be helpful in identifying ectopic adenomas (Fig. 23.5), particularly in the mediastinum, with an overall sensitivity from 46 to 87%.

Magnetic Resonance Imaging

The role of magnetic resonance imaging (MRI) is very similar to that of a CT scan. Magnetic resonance has a reported sensitivity and positive predictive value of 79.9% and 84.7%, respectively. Moreover, addition of MRI to sestamibi and ultrasound has been shown to increase sensitivity to 91.5% [38]. The drawbacks of MRI include higher cost, patient tolerance, and availability.

Invasive Localization

Invasive localization studies are indicated when noninvasive studies have failed to reveal the pathology. Since there is increased risk associated with an invasive procedure, these should be reserved for select patients who have biochemically confirmed hyperparathyroidism with equivocal or negative imaging studies that clearly need reoperation. Selective venous sampling is the most commonly utilized invasive study. However, with advent of new imaging modalities and improvement in radiology techniques, this is indicated far less frequently. Selective venous sampling of cervical and mediastinal veins can help focus the extent of dissection when a gradient is identified in relation to the value in a peripheral vein.

Selective Venous Sampling

This modality is the most common invasive technique utilized for localizing parathyroid glands; however, it is time consuming and expensive [39]. It requires catheterization of perithyroidal and mediastinal veins under fluoroscopic guidance with subsequent measurement of PTH hormone levels. These levels are then analyzed and compared to the contralateral neck and mediastinal samples as well as a peripheral sample to determine the region involved. More recently, interventionalist can obtain samples from smaller venous branches to increase sensitivity, with the sampling method referred to as “super selective” venous sampling (sSVS) [39]. The adenoma will typically be localized in an area with twice the

PTH values compared to peripheral levels. In a single-institutional study, sensitivity and positive predictive values of 86% and 93%, respectively, were achieved using sSVS [39]. Prior surgery and subsequent venous remodeling, however, can negatively impact the results [39].

Nonoperative Ablation Therapies

Angiographic Embolization

Angiographic catheter ablation has been reported for some mediastinal glands with reasonable outcomes and cure rates of up to 60% [40]. It is especially useful in patients with previously failed neck surgery and the risk of increased operative morbidity. The technique involves insertion of catheter in the feeding artery branch and chemically ablating the adenoma. Contrast media and ethanol have been reported [40]. Peripheral nerve symptoms, bradycardia, and renal failure have been seen. In addition, there is a risk of possible embolic complications [40].

Percutaneous Ethanol Injection

Percutaneous ethanol injection (PEI) has been reported as a treatment modality in patients with both primary and secondary hyperparathyroidism, either with remnant or graft-dependent tissue or in those at high surgical risk [41]. Following washout confirmation, the therapy involves insertion of an ultrasound-guided needle and injection of 95% ethanol into the target parathyroid tissue. Additional treatment sessions can be performed as needed [41, 42]. Complications of REI include pain, hematoma, transient laryngeal nerve palsy, as well as permanent palsy [42, 43]. The overall success has been reported anywhere from 35 to 80% [42]. Ethanol injection has been associated with fibrosis and can negatively impact subsequent reoperations if ever indicated [43]. This approach should only be used in select cases.

Operative Management

Reoperation for persistent or recurrent hyperparathyroidism can be successful in 89–95% of cases with proper preoperative localization studies and a focused approach [12, 44]. It is important to plan the reoperation based on localization studies, previous surgical dissection, and knowledge of parathyroid embryology. The operative approach is tailored according to the location of disease, neck versus mediastinum, and the pathology, solitary versus multigland. Intraoperative laryngeal nerve monitoring is recommended in hopes of reducing the risk of RLN injury. Patients should only be considered for reoperation when NIH guidelines are met or the patient has symptomatic disease (kidney stones, fragility fractures, pancreatitis, hypercalcemic crisis).

Focused Neck Exploration

The most common reason for revision parathyroidectomy is a missed adenoma. If confirmed on preoperative evaluation, the previous neck incision can be used in most cases [9, 10, 12]. Often, the parathyroid glands can be approached through either a central or a lateral neck approach. Utilizing the central approach, the dissection is carried out through the previously operated field with the disadvantage of having to deal with a scarred field. The central approach usually provides the easiest route to the inferior parathyroid glands, especially if intrathymic. The lateral approach is best suited to access the superior parathyroid glands. The lateral approach can be done using the previous cervical incision. Dissection is carried out lateral to the median raphe, between the strap muscles and the anterior border of sternocleidomastoid muscle. The strap muscles are retracted medially and the sternocleidomastoid laterally. The omohyoid muscle can be divided to gain exposure to the carotid sheath, which is retracted laterally to expose to the tracheoesophageal groove (Fig. 23.6a, b). The recurrent laryngeal nerve should be identified prior to gland removal. In case of an undescended parathyroid adenoma, a direct approach can be

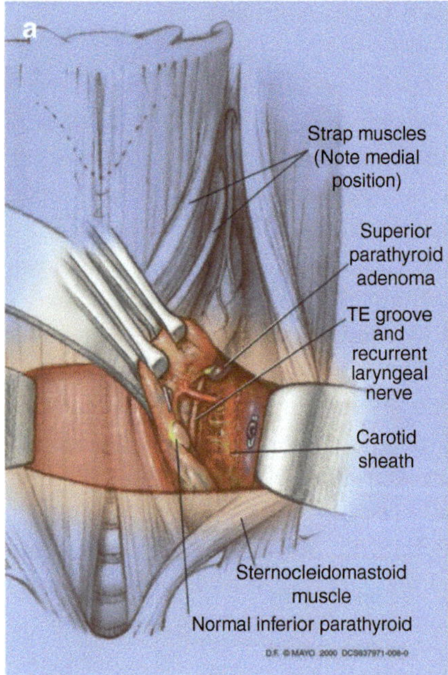

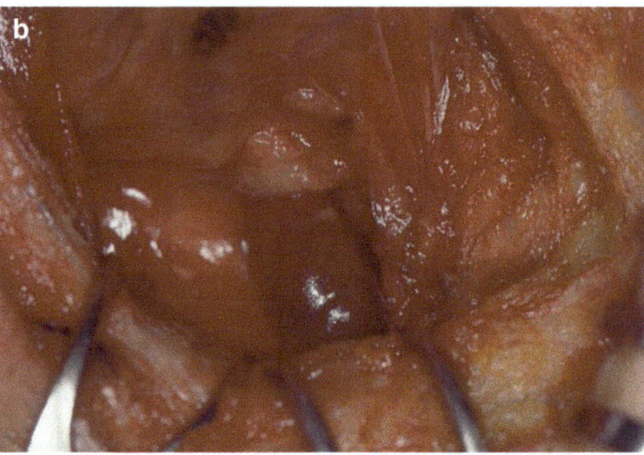

Fig. 23.6 (**a**) Reoperation for a superior parathyroid adenoma. Lateral approach is used using the previous collar incision, developing a plane between the anterior border or sternocleidomastoid and lateral border of strap muscles. (**b**) Lateral approach for a reoperative case showing a superior adenoma located in the tracheoesophageal groove

used (Fig. 23.7). This can be achieved using a transverse incision either over the carotid bifurcation or along the anterior border of sternocleidomastoid. The hypoglossal nerve courses deep to the adenoma and should be carefully avoided during dissection.

Bilateral Neck Exploration

Multigland parathyroid hyperplasia is responsible for hyperparathyroidism in approximately 15% of cases [7, 12]. If preoperative evaluation and workup suggest multiglandular disease, the goal with reoperation is to remove most of the residual disease. The surgical options include bilateral exploration or directed approach with either subtotal or total parathyroidectomy with autotransplantation or cryopreservation. Autotransplantation can be performed subcutaneously in the anterior chest wall or intramuscularly in the forearm brachioradialis muscle. The advantage of the subcutaneous route is that the parathyroid tissue can be removed at bedside the day after surgery if PTH levels indicate normal functioning tissue in the neck.

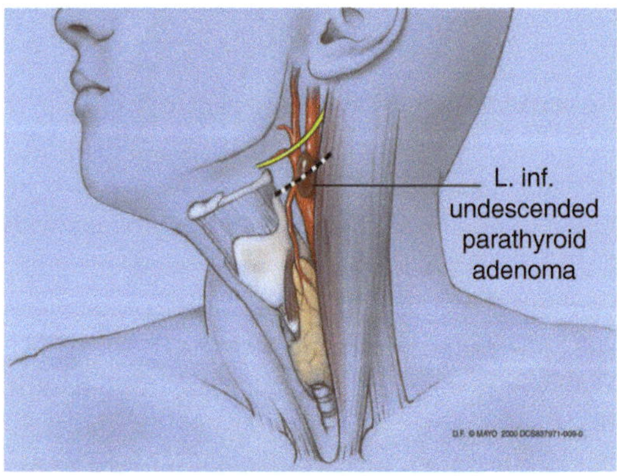

Fig. 23.7 Shows an undescended parathyroid adenoma anterior to the carotid bifurcation

Mediastinal Disease

The rate of mediastinal adenomas accounts for up to 27% of reoperative cases [7, 9, 12, 13]. In most instances, these represent inferior parathyroid glands that have descended into the chest during the embryologic development. In one series, they evaluated 38 patients that underwent revision parathyroidectomy via median sternotomy for parathyroid adenomas [45]. In those patients 47% of the adenomas were located in the thymus, in 21% it was found in the anterior mediastinum, 24% para-aortic, and 5% pericardial [45]. The approach to mediastinal disease can be based on the relationship to the aortic arch. When the adenoma is located above the aortic arch, it can generally be approach through the previous collar incision. If it is located below the aortic arch and deep in the mediastinum, a median sternotomy either total or partial may be required [1, 3, 9, 12]. More recently, minimally invasive techniques for ectopic mediastinal parathyroidectomy have been reported. The techniques utilized include video and robotic assisted thoracoscopy, the transcervical approach with a Cooper retractor, and mediastinoscopy [46]. A retrospective review showed comparable outcomes between minimally invasive and open techniques, but with significantly shorter hospital stays for minimally invasive approaches [46].

Intraoperative Adjuncts

There are multiple intraoperative adjuncts that can be utilized to help locate the adenoma. These adjuncts include methylene blue injection, intraoperative ultrasound, IOPTH, radioguided sestamibi scanning, bilateral jugular venous sampling, and frozen section. However, the majority of patients should have preoperative localization with two or more concordant studies before proceeding with reoperation, thus avoiding the need for some of these techniques. Intravenous methylene blue injection has been reported as an adjunct to localize parathyroid glands intraoperatively [47]. However, it has untoward side effects, including neurotoxic sequelae, pseudocyanosis, pseudohypoxia, and temporary urine discoloration [47]. The efficacy of this adjunct in the context of other techniques has not been proven [47]. However, we do find that the most useful adjuncts are intraoperative PTH and frozen section. Frozen section is useful when there is uncertainty regarding tissue removal. If intraoperative frozen section is not available, intraoperative specimen FNA with washout IOPTH has been reported as a possible alternative.

Autotransplantation and Cryopreservation

One of the most common complications after a parathyroidectomy is hypocalcemia, and in most instances this is a transient phenomenon; however a small subset of patients develop permanent hypocalcemia and require long-term calcium and vitamin D supplementation [48]. The decision has to be made intraoperatively if autotransplantation should be carried out. If a patient had a total parathyroidectomy or if there is a question of remaining parathyroid tissue, autotransplantation should be performed. Autotransplanted parathyroid tissue is successful in reestablishing meaningful function in approximately 80% of cases when performed at the time of re-exploration.

Cryopreservation should be considered in reoperative cases with the goal of providing a treatment option for patients experiencing permanent hypocalcemia after reoperation [49, 50]. However, the practice of cryopreservation has been decreasing as compared to the past, and is selectively practiced. In general it is considered costly and time consuming, with limited success [49, 51]. Cryopreserved parathyroid grafts can regain functionality in anywhere from 8 to 83% of reported cases [51, 52]. The success of function is dependent on multiple factors, including cryopreservation, thawing, and autotransplantation techniques [49, 51]. In one study, of all the patients who had cryopreserved tissue, only 1% required delayed autotransplantation. Thus, given the low utility of cryopreserved tissue and the variable success of delayed autotransplant, cryopreservation should be considered on a case-by-case basis as well as institutional availability. Subcutaneous autotransplantation is our preferred option (Fig. 23.8).

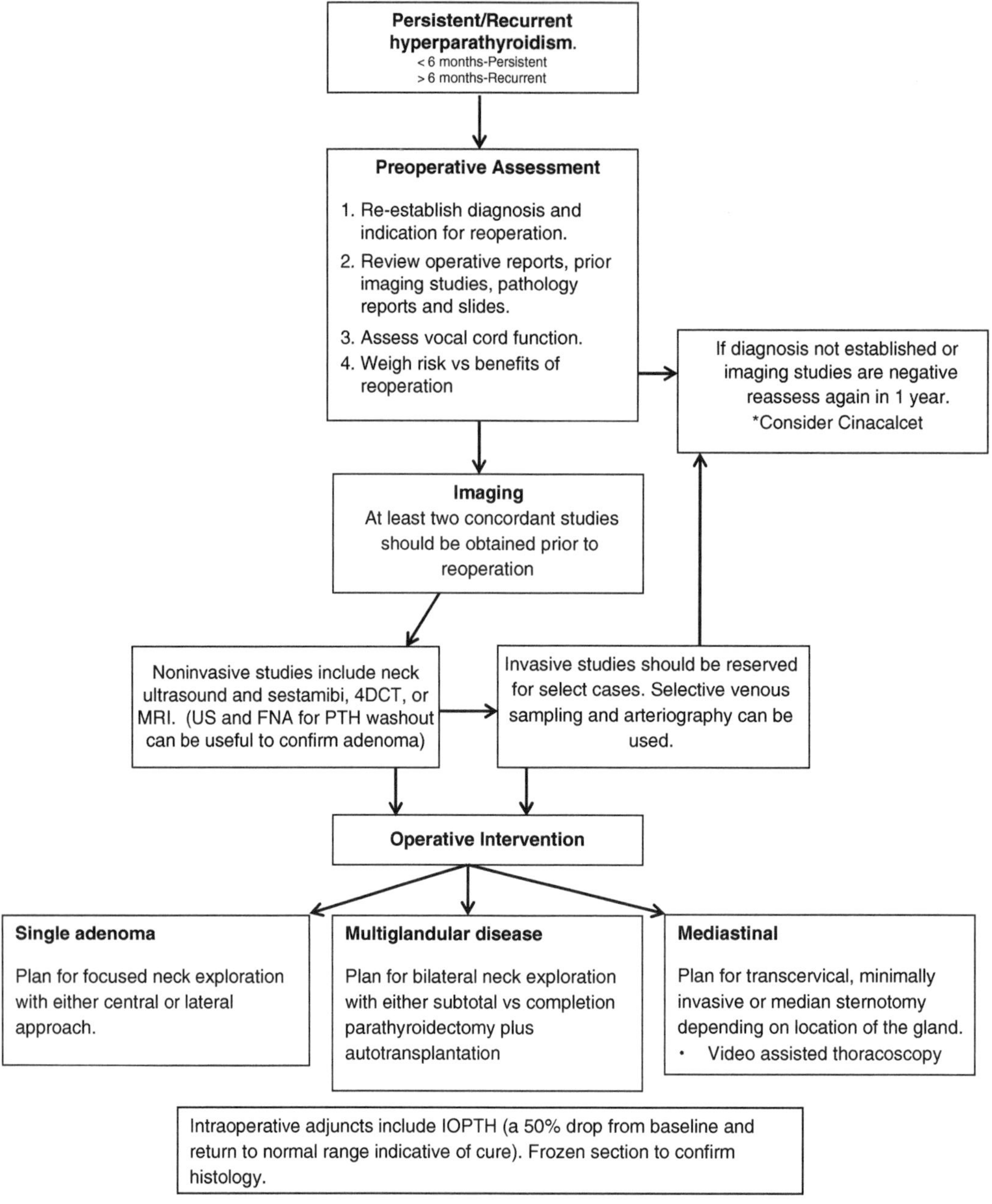

Fig. 23.8 Approach to patients with recurrent or persistent hyperparathyroidism

Conclusion

Persistent and recurrent hyperparathyroidism can occur after initial parathyroidectomy. The best practise is to avoid reoperation by optimizing the success of the initial operation. Reoperation is associated with increased morbidity and cost, and the decision to reoperate should be made by analyzing the patient's risk/benefit ratio. The patient record should be thoroughly reviewed and at least two concordant localizing studies should be obtained prior to proceeding with reoperation. There are multiple approaches available for reintervention and should be tailored for each patient.

Pearls

1. Most missed glands are in eutopic locations.
2. Avoid first-time failures. Experience is key.
3. Reoperations for PHPT are associated with a lower success rate and greater morbidity than with first-time operations.
4. Reestablish the diagnosis. Rule out FHH, thiazides, and lithium.
5. Weigh benefits of surgery versus risks.
6. Obtain at least two concordant localizing studies.

References

1. Thompson GB, Grant CS, Perrier ND, Harman R, Hodgson SF, Ilstrup D, et al. Reoperative parathyroid surgery in the era of sestamibi scanning and intraoperative parathyroid hormone monitoring. Arch Surg. 1999;134(7):699–704; discussion 704–5
2. Mundschenk J, Klose S, Lorenz K, Dralle H, Lehnert H. Diagnostic strategies and surgical procedures in persistent or recurrent primary hyperparathyroidism. Exp Clin Endocrinol Diabetes. 1999;107(6):331–6.
3. Wadstrom C, Zedenius J, Guinea A, Reeve TS, Delbridge L. Re-operative surgery for recurrent or persistent primary hyperparathyroidism. Aust N Z J Surg. 1998;68(2):103–7.
4. McIntyre CJ, Allen JL, Constantinides VA, Jackson JE, Tolley NS, Palazzo FF. Patterns of disease in patients at a tertiary referral Centre requiring reoperative parathyroidectomy. Ann R Coll Surg Engl. 2015;97(8):598–602.
5. Henry JF. Reoperation for primary hyperparathyroidism: tips and tricks. Langenbeck's Arch Surg. 2010;395(2):103–9.
6. Alhefdhi A, Schneider DF, Sippel R, Chen H. Recurrent and persistence primary hyperparathyroidism occurs more frequently in patients with double adenomas. J Surg Res. 2014;190(1):198–202.
7. Mariette C, Pellissier L, Combemale F, Quievreux JL, Carnaille B, Proye C. Reoperation for persistent or recurrent primary hyperparathyroidism. Langenbeck's Arch Surg. 1998;383(2):174–9.
8. Tezelman S, Shen W, Siperstein AE, Duh QY, Clark OH. Persistent or recurrent hyperparathyroidism in patients with double adenomas. Surgery. 1995;118(6):1115–22; discussion 22–4
9. Jaskowiak N, Norton JA, Alexander HR, Doppman JL, Shawker T, Skarulis M, et al. A prospective trial evaluating a standard approach to reoperation for missed parathyroid adenoma. Ann Surg. 1996;224(3):308–20; discussion 20–1
10. Dotzenrath C, Goretzki PE, Roher HD. [Surgical strategy in persistence and recurrence in surgery of primary hyperparathyroidism]. Langenbecks Arch Chir. 1994;379(4):218–23.
11. Nawrot I, Chudzinski W, Ciacka T, Barczynski M, Szmidt J. Reoperations for persistent or recurrent primary hyperparathyroidism: results of a retrospective cohort study at a tertiary referral center. Med Sci Monit. 2014;20:1604–12.
12. Shen W, Duren M, Morita E, Higgins C, Duh QY, Siperstein AE, et al. Reoperation for persistent or recurrent primary hyperparathyroidism. Arch Surg. 1996;131(8):861–7. discussion 7-9
13. Silberfein EJ, Bao R, Lopez A, Grubbs EG, Lee JE, Evans DB, et al. Reoperative parathyroidectomy: location of missed glands based on a contemporary nomenclature system. Arch Surg. 2010;145(11):1065–8.
14. Haciyanli M, Lal G, Morita E, Duh QY, Kebebew E, Clark OH. Accuracy of preoperative localization studies and intraoperative parathyroid hormone assay in patients with primary hyperparathyroidism and double adenoma. J Am Coll Surg. 2003;197(5):739–46.
15. d'Alessandro AF, Montenegro FL, Brandao LG, Lourenco DM Jr, Toledo Sde A, Cordeiro AC. Supernumerary parathyroid glands in hyperparathyroidism associated with multiple endocrine neoplasia type 1. Rev Assoc Med Bras (1992). 2012;58(3):323–7.
16. Pattou FN, Pellissier LC, Noel C, Wambergue F, Huglo DG, Proye CA. Supernumerary parathyroid glands: frequency and surgical significance in treatment of renal hyperparathyroidism. World J Surg. 2000;24(11):1330–4.
17. Hakaim AG, Esselstyn CB Jr. Parathyroid carcinoma: 50-year experience at The Cleveland Clinic Foundation. Cleve Clin J Med. 1993;60(4):331–5.
18. Lee PK, Jarosek SL, Virnig BA, Evasovich M, Tuttle TM. Trends in the incidence and treatment of parathyroid cancer in the United States. Cancer. 2007;109(9):1736–41.
19. Morita SY, Brownlee NA, Dackiw AP, Westra WH, Clark DP, Zeiger MA. An unusual case of recurrent hyperparathyroidism and papillary thyroid cancer. Endocr Pract. 2009;15(4):349–52.
20. Twigt BA, van Dalen T, Vroonhoven TJ, Consten EC. Recurrent hyperparathyroidism caused by benign neoplastic seeding: two cases of parathyromatosis and a review of the literature. Acta Chir Belg. 2013;113(3):228–32.
21. Marx SJ, Stock JL, Attie MF, Downs RW Jr, Gardner DG, Brown EM, et al. Familial hypocalciuric hypercalcemia: recognition among patients referred after unsuccessful parathyroid exploration. Ann Intern Med. 1980;92(3):351–6.
22. Bilezikian JP, Brandi ML, Eastell R, Silverberg SJ, Udelsman R, Marcocci C, et al. Guidelines for the management of asymptomatic primary hyperparathyroidism: summary statement from the Fourth International Workshop. J Clin Endocrinol Metab. 2014;99(10):3561–9.
23. Palmer JA, Rosen IB. Reoperative surgery for hyperparathyroidism. Am J Surg. 1982;144(4):406–10.

24. Patow CA, Norton JA, Brennan MF. Vocal cord paralysis and reoperative parathyroidectomy. A prospective study. Ann Surg. 1986;203(3):282–5.
25. Steurer M, Passler C, Denk DM, Schneider B, Niederle B, Bigenzahn W. Advantages of recurrent laryngeal nerve identification in thyroidectomy and parathyroidectomy and the importance of preoperative and postoperative laryngoscopic examination in more than 1000 nerves at risk. Laryngoscope. 2002;112(1):124–33.
26. Doherty GM, Weber B, Norton JA. Cost of unsuccessful surgery for primary hyperparathyroidism. Surgery. 1994;116(6):954–7; discussion 957–8
27. Shin JJ, Milas M, Mitchell J, Berber E, Ross L, Siperstein A. Impact of localization studies and clinical scenario in patients with hyperparathyroidism being evaluated for reoperative neck surgery. Arch Surg. 2011;146(12):1397–403.
28. Alexander HR Jr, Chen CC, Shawker T, Choyke P, Chan TJ, Chang R, et al. Role of preoperative localization and intraoperative localization maneuvers including intraoperative PTH assay determination for patients with persistent or recurrent hyperparathyroidism. J Bone Miner Res. 2002;17(Suppl 2):N133–40.
29. Wei JP, Burke GJ, Mansberger AR Jr. Prospective evaluation of the efficacy of technetium 99m sestamibi and iodine 123 radionuclide imaging of abnormal parathyroid glands. Surgery. 1992;112(6):1111–6; discussion 1116–7
30. Peeler BB, Martin WH, Sandler MP, Goldstein RE. Sestamibi parathyroid scanning and preoperative localization studies for patients with recurrent/persistent hyperparathyroidism or significant comorbid conditions: development of an optimal localization strategy. Am Surg. 1997;63(1):37–46.
31. Palestro CJ, Tomas MB, Tronco GG. Radionuclide imaging of the parathyroid glands. Semin Nucl Med. 2005;35(4):266–76.
32. Adkisson CD, Koonce SL, Heckman MG, Thomas CS, Harris AS, Casler JD. Predictors of accuracy in preoperative parathyroid adenoma localization using ultrasound and Tc-99m-Sestamibi: a 4-quadrant analysis. Am J Otolaryngol. 2013;34(5):508–16.
33. Fayet P, Hoeffel C, Fulla Y, Legmann P, Hazebroucq V, Luton JP, et al. Technetium-99m sestamibi scintigraphy, magnetic resonance imaging and venous blood sampling in persistent and recurrent hyperparathyroidism. Br J Radiol. 1997;70(833):459–64.
34. Haber RS, Kim CK, Inabnet WB. Ultrasonography for preoperative localization of enlarged parathyroid glands in primary hyperparathyroidism: comparison with (99m)technetium sestamibi scintigraphy. Clin Endocrinol. 2002;57(2):241–9.
35. Neumann DR, Esselstyn CB Jr, Kim EY, Go RT, Obuchowski NA, Rice TW. Preliminary experience with double-phase SPECT using Tc-99m sestamibi in patients with hyperparathyroidism. Clin Nucl Med. 1997;22(4):217–21.
36. Cham S, Sepahdari AR, Hall KE, Yeh MW, Harari A. Dynamic parathyroid computed tomography (4DCT) facilitates Reoperative parathyroidectomy and enables cure of missed hyperplasia. Ann Surg Oncol. 2015;22(11):3537–42.
37. Mortenson MM, Evans DB, Lee JE, Hunter GJ, Shellingerhout D, Vu T, et al. Parathyroid exploration in the reoperative neck: improved preoperative localization with 4D-computed tomography. J Am Coll Surg. 2008;206(5):888–95; discussion 95–6
38. Kluijfhout WP, Venkatesh S, Beninato T, Vriens MR, Duh QY, Wilson DM, et al. Performance of magnetic resonance imaging in the evaluation of first-time and reoperative primary hyperparathyroidism. Surgery. 2016;160(3):747–54.
39. Lebastchi AH, Aruny JE, Donovan PI, Quinn CE, Callender GG, Carling T, et al. Real-time super selective venous sampling in remedial parathyroid surgery. J Am Coll Surg. 2015;220(6):994–1000.
40. Howell P, Kariampuzha S, Kipgen W, Baker MZ, Tytle TL, Williams GR, et al. Non-surgical therapy of primary hyperparathyroidism. J Okla State Med Assoc. 2001;94(12):561–5.
41. Douthat WG, Cardozo G, Garay G, Orozco S, Chiurchiu C, de la Fuente J, et al. Use of percutaneous ethanol injection therapy for recurrent secondary hyperparathyroidism after subtotal parathyroidectomy. Int J Nephrol. 2011;2011:246734.
42. Caron NR, Sturgeon C, Clark OH. Persistent and recurrent hyperparathyroidism. Curr Treat Options in Oncol. 2004;5(4):335–45.
43. Bennedbaek FN, Karstrup S, Hegedus L. Percutaneous ethanol injection therapy in the treatment of thyroid and parathyroid diseases. Eur J Endocrinol. 1997;136(3):240–50.
44. Richards ML, Thompson GB, Farley DR, Grant CS. Reoperative parathyroidectomy in 228 patients during the era of minimal-access surgery and intraoperative parathyroid hormone monitoring. Am J Surg. 2008;196(6):937–42; discussion 42–3
45. Russell CF, Edis AJ, Scholz DA, Sheedy PF, van Heerden JA. Mediastinal parathyroid tumors: experience with 38 tumors requiring mediastinotomy for removal. Ann Surg. 1981;193(6):805–9.
46. Said SM, Cassivi SD, Allen MS, Deschamps C, Nichols FC 3rd, Shen KR, et al. Minimally invasive resection for mediastinal ectopic parathyroid glands. Ann Thorac Surg. 2013;96(4):1229–33.
47. Patel HP, Chadwick DR, Harrison BJ, Balasubramanian SP. Systematic review of intravenous methylene blue in parathyroid surgery. Br J Surg. 2012;99(10):1345–51.
48. Liu HG, Chen ZC, Zhang XH, Yang K. Replantation with cryopreserved parathyroid for permanent hypoparathyroidism: a case report and review of literatures. Int J Clin Exp Med. 2015;8(3):4611–9.
49. Shepet K, Alhefdhi A, Usedom R, Sippel R, Chen H. Parathyroid cryopreservation after parathyroidectomy: a worthwhile practice? Ann Surg Oncol. 2013;20(7):2256–60.
50. Caccitolo JA, Farley DR, van Heerden JA, Grant CS, Thompson GB, Sterioff S. The current role of para-

thyroid cryopreservation and autotransplantation in parathyroid surgery: an institutional experience. Surgery. 1997;122(6):1062–7.

51. Schneider R, Ramaswamy A, Slater EP, Bartsch DK, Schlosser K. Cryopreservation of parathyroid tissue after parathyroid surgery for renal hyperparathyroidism: does it really make sense? World J Surg. 2012;36(11):2598–604.

52. Cohen MS, Dilley WG, Wells SA Jr, Moley JF, Doherty GM, Sicard GA, et al. Long-term functionality of cryopreserved parathyroid autografts: a 13-year prospective analysis. Surgery. 2005;138(6):1033–40; discussion 40–1

Parathyroid Carcinoma: Current Concepts

24

Roma Pradhan, Sabaretnam Mayilvaganan, and Amit Agarwal

Parathyroid cancer is a rare tumor accounting for less than 1% of primary hyperparathyroidism [1]. De Quervain in 1904 described the first case of parathyroid carcinoma which was nonfunctioning.

Etiology and Pathogenesis

Largely unknown though few reports of parathyroid hyperplasia transforming to PC in long-standing secondary HPT are there. Other risk factors may be prior neck irradiation and genetic predisposition as seen in HPT-JT syndrome, MEN1, 2A, and isolated familial HPT. It must be remembered that HRPT2 gene mutation is an early event in the development of parathyroid carcinoma. The origins of parathyroid cancer have been a subject of debate but recent evidence suggests that these cancers originate de novo [2] rather than progression from a benign adenoma or hyperplastic glands, which is extremely rare. Parathyroid tumors can be both monoclonal and polyclonal in origin [3]. A significant monoclonal component has been shown in MEN1-related familial parathyroid tumors, nonfamilial parathyroid hyperplasia, renal parathyroid disease, and also parathyroid carcinoma. Oncogenes play a role in the development of parathyroid tumors that include the CCND1/PRAD1 oncogene [4–8] and MEN1 tumor-suppressor gene. While these mutations have been shown in a third of parathyroid adenomas, rarely have they been seen in parathyroid cancer.

Germline Predisposition

It is important for clinicians to consider underlying genetic cause.

Patients with germline HRPT2 mutations develop parathyroid carcinomas especially in about 15% of patients with hyperparathyroidism jaw-tumor syndrome (HPT-JT) and a small subset of families with familial isolated hyperparathyroidism [9]. The *HRPT2* gene encodes the protein parafibromin. *HPRT2* mutations are commonly seen in parathyroid carcinoma but uncommon in adenomas [10]. Another gene that has been postulated to play a role in malignant transformation of the parathyroid gland includes loss of function of retinoblastoma (RB1) tumor-suppressor gene [11] in a secondary fashion.

Preoperative Diagnosis of PC

There are no absolute clinical or biochemical features diagnostic of parathyroid carcinoma. However, there is evidence in literature about

R. Pradhan
Dr Ram Manohar Lohia Institute of Medical Sciences, Lucknow, Uttar Pradesh, India

S. Mayilvaganan · A. Agarwal (✉)
Department of Endocrine Surgery, SGPGIMS, Lucknow, UP, India

R. Parameswaran, A. Agarwal (eds.), *Evidence-Based Endocrine Surgery*,
https://doi.org/10.1007/978-981-10-1124-5_24

some features which may suggest a high index of suspicion of parathyroid carcinoma, prompting the surgeon to consider it in differential diagnosis.

1. *Serum Calcium*: Though the review by Talat and Schulte [12] suggested that calcium cannot be taken as a surrogate parameter for PC, there is evidence in literature to suggest that unlike mild hypercalcemia of benign PHPT, serum calcium levels are generally much higher(3–4 mg/dL) above the upper unit of normal [13–15].
2. *PTH* is elevated 4.5-fold above the upper normal limit as compared to benign PHPT [12] where PTH is usually less than twice normal, except in these cases of benign PHPT presenting as OFC, especially seen in developing countries.
3. *ALP* levels are also much higher in parathyroid carcinoma except in these cases of benign PHPT presenting as OFC, especially seen in developing countries [12, 16].
4. Newer makes like urinary α-β subunit of HCG may be elevated in parathyroid carcinoma [17, 18].
5. There is evidence in literature [9] that renal involvement (nephrocalcinosis and/or decreased GFR) is seen in one-third of patients whereas osteitis fibrosa cystica is seen in another one-third patients. More importantly, concomitant bone and renal disease is seen in at least 50% of patients of parathyroid carcinoma unlike benign PHPT where simultaneous involvement is distinctly unusual.
6. Similarly the incidence of recurrent pancreatitis, peptic ulcer, and anemia is higher in PC as compared to benign PHPT.
7. More patients of PC are likely to present with hypercalcemic crisis (10%) [19, 20] than benign PHPT.
8. A palpable neck mass has been observed in 70% of patients with PC [15, 21, 22].
9. *Clinical features* like RLN palsy, lymph node metastasis, and distant metastasis in a patient with PHPT are sine qua non of parathyroid carcinoma [23, 24].
10. *Imaging:* On USG or CT PC may have ill-defined margins and signs of invasion of surrounding structures as well as LN metastasis [25]. Typically PC are lobulated, hypoechoic, and relatively large and with ill-defined borders [26–29]. In a retrospective study 69 patients with parathyroid lesions larger than 15 mm were evaluated by ultrasound. A high positive predictive value (PPV) for cancer was identified for infiltration (PPV 100%) and calcification (PPV 100%) and a high negative predictive value (NPV) was found for the absence of suspicious vascularity (NPVV 97.6%), a thick capsule (NPV 96.7%), and inhomogeneity (NPV 100%). The investigators concluded that in parathyroid lesions larger than 15 mm, USG for specific features provides a valuable tool to identify parathyroid cancers before surgery [26]. M1B1 cannot distinguish between benign and malignant PHPT.
11. FNA of primary lesions should be avoided as it has been associated with tumor seeding of needle tract [30]. FNA cytology will not be able to distinguish benign from malignant PHPT [31].

There is no evidence to show that age and gender can be of help in distinguishing between benign and malignant PHPT. It should be noted that in patients who present with severe/advanced PHPT as is commonly seen in developing countries [32] distinction between benign and malignant parathyroid disease is even more difficult on the basis of profound hypercalcemia/hyperparathyroidism, concomitant renal and bone disease, or a palpable neck mass.

Intraoperative Pathology

In the absence of local invasion or regional metastasis, intraoperative diagnosis of PC can be difficult. Frozen section analysis is of little value and is unreliable [11]. In the analysis by Koea and Shaw [19] of the 358 patients intraoperative diagnosis of parathyroid carcinoma was made only in 178 patients based on local invasion (ipsilateral thyroid gland in 89%, strap muscles in 71%, RLN in 26%, esophagus in 18%, and trachea in 17%) and in 46 patients on the basis of dense fibrous capsule.

Histopathology

1. Intraoperative findings: The following findings help to make an intraoperative diagnosis of parathyroid carcinoma:
   (a) Lobulated, firm/stony-hard parathyroid mass [33]
   (b) Presence of a dense, grayish-white fibrous capsule that tenaciously adheres to surrounding structures [33]
   (c) Gross infiltration of adjacent thyroid, RLN, strap muscles, and esophagus [34]
   (d) Enlarged central compartment (level VI) or lateral neck nodes
   (e) Size of the PC has been reported to range from 0.75 to >6 cm [35, 36]

Histological Features

In the absence of gross intraoperative finding suggestive of parathyroid carcinoma, histopathological distinction between benign and malignant parathyroid tumors is difficult. Schantz and Cattlemen [37] proposed the set of criteria which are (1) uniform sheets of chief cells arranged in a lobular pattern separated by dense fibrous trabeculae, (2) capsular or vascular invasion, and (3) mitotic figures with tumor parenchymal cells that must be distinguished from endothelial cell mitoses. However these have been challenged by many authors. Mckeown et al. [38] pointed out that cellular pleomorphism and atypia are not reliable indicators of malignancy in endocrine tumors. Similarly, invasion has to be assessed carefully as nests of parathyroid tumor within the capsule of the gland may represent benign entrapment.

Similarly a multicenter study of 56 carcinomas by Bondenon [39] found that mitotic activity was variable and fibrous band pattern was not present in 20%. Thus different authors consider different criteria:

Okamoto et al. [40] consider capsular invasion as the most important feature.

Obara et al. [41]: Mitotic rate is a good predictor.

Chang et al. [42]: Fibrous trabeculae, capsular and vascular invasion.

Mckeown et al. [38] and Bondeson [39]: Don't rely on above features but rely on cellular atypia and macronuclear pleomorphism.

The best predictors of malignant histology were presence of invasion, a fibrotic capsule, and nuclear atypia [43]. In another study [42] presence of vascular or capsular invasion and fibrosis trabeculae was the most common indicator of malignancy. Thus there is overall consensus that the overall histological pattern is much more useful than relying on a single histological feature.

In the review by Talat and Schulte [12], results of all five commonly used HPE criteria were:

Fibrous lesions 100/206 (49%)
Capsular invasion 149/177 (84%)
Vascular invasion 113/167 (68%)
Infiltration into adjacent tissue 96/186 (52%)
Lymph nodes 27/43 (63%)

The authors concluded that in these 330 patients there was no significant homogeneity of distribution of pathology findings.

Impact of HPE Features on Outcome

Only Talat and Schulte [12] studied the factual outcome relevance of individual criteria. Presence of fibrous bands and local invasion is associated with lower recurrence and mortality rate at 5 years overall. In stark contrast, vascular invasion carries a fourfold higher risk to experience death or recurrence at 5 years and 2.8/2.6-fold higher risk over all recurrence and death.

Ultrastructural Features

Electron microscopy is not much useful in diagnosing PC [44].

Flow cytometric analysis can be of some value in diagnosing PC based on higher nuclear DNA content and an aneuploidy pattern [45]. However aneuploidy occurs frequently in parathyroid adenomas as well; hence this technique is not of much use in differentiating benign and malignant disease [46].

Immunohistochemical Staining

A number of immunohistochemical markers for malignant potential in parathyroid tumors have been studied to complement the histopathological examination; however, only few have displayed the sensitivity and specificity that are needed. Initial studies focused on immunohistochemical analyses of well-established proteins controlling the cell cycle process as well as apoptosis such as p53, RB gene, and Ki67 [47–49]. However, these markers showed low sensitivity and specificity. Subsequently promising markers like parafibromin, APC, galectin-3, and PGP 9.5 expression were studied [50–54]. The use of parafibromin immunostaining in the differential diagnosis of parathyroid tumors was first introduced by Tan et al. [55] who reported a diagnostic value of 96% for sensitivity and 99% for specificity. However, subsequent studies could not replicate the high sensitivity and specificity that are needed [56, 57].

Detection of gelatinase A mRNA in PC looks promising [58].

Management

There are still some unresolved issues in surgical management of parathyroid carcinoma because this disease presents the clinician with three essential difficulties.

- The first problem is recognizing the presence and extent of malignant parathyroid disease prior to surgery, i.e., a correct surgical staging.
- The second problem relates to the choice of the surgical approach. Even when cancer is diagnosed pre- or intraoperatively, there is no agreement on the extent of surgery.
- The third problem relates to the high rate of locoregional recurrence and death in parathyroid cancer patients, even when an en bloc resection had been performed.

Staging

Shaha and Shah proposed a staging system based on tumor size, extent of local invasion, presence of LN, and distant metastasis [23]. When the authors of a multicentric study [12] applied Shaha's system to 185 patients, they found that the increased stages in Shaha's system did not indicate a progressive worsening of the prognosis and thus cast doubt on the usefulness of this staging system. The authors attempted to construct a staging system based on increased local and locoregional aggressiveness and excluded size as a criterion. When Villar-del-Moral et al. [59] applied the above staging system proposed by Talat and Schulte [12] they found that RFS and DSS were best predicted by this staging system as compared to Shaha's classification system.

The clinical management of a common clinical scenario where the diagnosis of PC is made postoperatively for a patient who had undergone a simple parathyroidectomy for a benign pathology is controversial. Some authors consider a re-exploration while others do not recommend re-exploration. The indicators of re-exploration suggested by various authors [13, 35, 60] are:

- Gross characteristic of the lesion typical of a carcinoma
- HP features with aggressive features like capsular and vascular invasion
- Patient remains hypercalcemia
- In an article by Christine et al. [61], O'Neill diagnosis of PC was made postoperatively in seven patients who had undergone a simple parathyroidectomy. Despite re-exploration with further radical surgery (unilateral thyroid lobectomy and lymphadenectomy) in six patients, no further malignancy was identified in any specimen. Also it has not been proven that the thyroid lobectomy gives an advantage in preventing local recurrence and increasing OS when thyroid lobe is clearly not involved [62].

- One approach may be to reserve radical reoperation to patients with evidence of HRPT2 mutation (parafibromin-negative, PGP9.5-positive pattern of staining). For patients without evidence of HRPT2 mutation, further radical surgery may not be mandated if there is no macroscopic impression of residual disease [63].

Surgical Management: There Are Following Unresolved Issues:

- What should be the extent of resection: en bloc or simple parathyroidectomy?
- What should be the extent of lymph node resection?
- What are the predictive factors of recurrence and cause specific mortality?
- What are the indications of re-exploration following histopathological diagnosis of parathyroid carcinoma in an unsuspected case?
- What are the immunohistochemical markers that can complement or replace the histopathological diagnosis of parathyroid carcinoma?
- What is the role of adjuvant radiotherapy in preventing recurrences?

The Extent of Resection: En Bloc or Simple Parathyroidectomy (Table 24.1)

Most authors agree that bilateral neck exploration with examination of all PTG should be routinely performed, to exclude the presence of parathyroid hyperplasia even though carcinoma of multiple glands is exceedingly rare [64]. One important precaution to observe is to avoid rupture of gland capsule. In HPT-JT syndrome all parathyroid glands should be explored but prophylactic parathyroidectomy is not recommended. Now there are reports that suggest that MIP can be safely performed in parathyroid carcinoma and that if parathyroid carcinoma diagnosis is made after performing MIP then routine reoperation may be avoided but for certain situations.

Second controversial issue is whether to perform an en bloc resection or limited resection. Surgical resection is the only curative treatment for patients with parathyroid cancer and the two most commonly performed resections are simple tumor excision (parathyroidectomy) and en bloc resection. En bloc excision involves en bloc removal of tumor with ipsilateral thyroid lobe and isthmus, and surrounding soft tissue especially which is adherent to tumor, along with removal of contiguous LN (paratracheal, tracheo-

Table 24.1 Impact of the type of resection performed on the long-term outcomes in terms of local recurrence and mortality

Study	Level of evidence	Study type	No. of patients	Surgical procedure	Results
Koea and Shaw [19]	III	Review (1933–1999)	301	Simple PTx (192): En bloc (104):	92 (48%) 8 (7.6%)
Talat and Schulte [12]	IV	Review	330	Simple PTx:158 En bloc excision:172	103 (65%) 54 (31.3%)
Busaidy et al. [65]	III	Retrospective (1980–2004)	27	Simple PTx: 18 En bloc: 9	7 (38.8%) 3 (33.3)
Villar-del-Moral [59]	III	Cohort study (2014)	62	Simple PTx: 18 En bloc: 44	14 (22.6%) Recurrences were not separately mentioned for the two surgical procedures
Wang and Gaz [74]	III	Retrospective (1966–2005)	28	Simple PTx: 8 En bloc: 14	8 (100%) 0 (0%)
Ihihara et al. [17]	III	Retrospective	38	Simple PTx: 16 En bloc: 22	8 (50%) 4 (18%)

There is only level III or IV evidence in favor of en bloc excision for parathyroid carcinoma

esophageal, and upper mediastinal), and skeletonization of trachea while RLN is not typically sacrificed.

Different studies have highlighted the impact of the type of resection performed on the long-term outcomes in terms of local recurrence and mortality.

Evidence in support of this comes from the following studies.

- Koea and Shaw [19]: The authors showed that en bloc resection of the carcinoma and the adjacent structures in the neck is the surgical treatment and is associated with an 8% local recurrence rate and a long-term overall survival rate of 89% (mean follow-up 69 months). In contrast simple parathyroidectomy results in a 51% local recurrence rate and 53% long-term survival rate (mean follow-up 62 months). Adverse prognostic factors for survival were initial management with simple parathyroidectomy alone, presence of nodal or distant metastatic disease at presentation, and non-functioning PTC.
- The second study is a meta-analysis of 330 patients with mean follow-up duration—6.1 years [12]: Authors reported mortality of 35 with 63% cases developing locoregional recurrence. The authors reported that local excision alone carried a 2-fold higher risk of needing at least one redo surgery and 2.9-fold higher risk of needing three or more redo surgeries. The authors concluded that failure to perform oncological surgery carries a high risk for recurrence and death (local vs. en bloc resection RR 2.0, CI 1.2–3.2, $P < 0.01$) and recommended en bloc resection.
- The third study is the paper by Busaidy et al. [65]: Out of 27 patients, 9 underwent en bloc excision out of which only 3 relapsed while 18 underwent local excision out of which 7 had local recurrences.
- In another multicenter review of patients by the Spanish Parathyroid Carcinoma Group (SPCSG) [59] authors reported 62 parathyroid carcinoma, 44 (71%) underwent en bloc resection and the rest underwent simple parathyroidectomy alone. In their cohort the rate of recurrence was low (20.1%) and the authors commented that the high rates of radical surgery in their cohort of patients could explain differences in terms of recurrence and mortality between their data and some of the previously reported outcomes.
- In the study by Kebebew et al. [66] out of the 14 patients who had recurrence and underwent reoperation, 8 had en bloc excision at first operation, but all were referred from outside so the extent of en bloc excision carries a question mark.
- Thus the conclusion of most studies is that surgery was an important outcome predictor with more radical surgery protecting against early and late recurrences and death.

Extent of Lymph Node Resection

The incidence of regional LN metastasis has been reported in 15–30% [12, 35, 65, 67]. Nodal involvement has been shown as an independent risk factor for local recurrence but its impact on cancer-related death is controversial [68].

Reviews give varying advice and fall into five categories:

- Advice for en bloc tumor resection but no explicit advice for lymphadenectomy
- Advice for en bloc resection with systematic central lymphadenectomy
- Advice for systematic central and lateral lymphadenectomy
- Advice for an indication for lateral lymphadenectomy based on specific findings only
- Explicit caution against prophylactic lateral lymph node dissection

- The remarkable variation of opinion and review of the underlying evidence for such advice indicates a relative paucity of data. One must remember that soft-tissue infiltration is more common (56.7%) than LN involvement (32.1%). Similarly soft-tissue recurrence is more common (58.7%) while recurrence in LN accounts for only 41.3%. Also, recurrence is a strong predictor of death in parathyroid cancer. So there is a possibility that performance of a distinct form of LND indicates a higher quality of surgery and is thus linked with performance of a true en bloc resection with free margins.

- In the present literature, majority of authors recommend ipsilateral central compartment lymph node clearance as part of initial en bloc resection though the rate of lymph node dissection is lacking.
- Only one study suggests routine central neck dissection [12]. Of the 1027 cases collected from literature, only 193 (18.8%) provided a description of some sort of lymph node clearance.
- In the American National Cancer Data Base report by Hundahl et al. [35], nodal status was only evaluated in 37% of cases.
- Similarly in the multicenter study by the Spanish parathyroid carcinoma group [59], only 19 cases (30.6%) had undergone some kind of nodal dissection.

Risk factors for decreased DSS: positive correlation with intraoperative tumor rupture, positive margin resection, nodal invasion, and locoregional and distant relapse [59].

However, in a large NCB data of 1000 patients [69], only age and positive LNs were associated with higher death rates.

Predictive Factors of Recurrence and Cause-Specific Mortality

The third problem relates to the high rate of locoregional recurrence and death in parathyroid cancer patients, even when an en bloc resection had been performed. RR to die of parathyroid cancer is 2.3-fold higher in patients without sufficient staging system compared with those assigned stage I–IV. This points towards an important observation: patients who undergo limited or ill-described resections are at least in part understaged and undertreated.

- The Spanish multicenter [59] study identified variables after a multivariate analysis that predicted tumor relapse and death due to disease. These included intraoperative tumor rupture, presence of mitotic figures in tumor cells, and stage III in the Schulte risk classification.
- In the TNM staging system proposed by Shaha and Shah [23], a stepwise worsening of prognosis was not associated with a greater stage. In fact when Talat and Schulte [12] applied this system to their185 patients, they found that stage IIIa has a lesser mortality and recurrence than stage I. The same authors attempted to reconstruct a staging system based on an increased local and locoregional aggressiveness and excluded size as a criterion. Separation of patients into low risk and high risk identified a 3.5–7.0-fold higher risk of recurrence and death (<0.01) for the high-risk group. The Spanish study assessed the proposed PC staging systems to predict outcomes with the log-rank test. The authors showed that RFS was best predicted using the stages of Schulte risk staging compared with the Shaha classification.

Role of Adjuvant Radiotherapy in Preventing Recurrences

It is not radiosensitive; however it may help in local control and therefore may be of some benefit in patients who are at high risk of local recurrence. There are few retrospective studies which have shown some benefit with postoperative radiotherapy but the results should be interpreted with caution because of small number of patients [65, 70, 71]. The data for chemotherapy is inadequate for definite opinion due to rarity of disease [72, 73]. Recently biological therapy in the form of anti-parathyroid immunotherapy (tumor-suppressor gene product) MOA inducing cell cycle arrest by repressing cyclin D1, octreotide therapy, and azidothymidine (AZT) that inhibits telomerase activity has been tried with varying success.

Management of hypercalcemia

- Goal of treatment:
  - Lowering of hypercalcemia
- Modalities:
  - Forced saline diuresis
  - Bisphosphonates
  - Plicamycin
  - Calcitonin/gallium nitrate
  - Immunotherapy

Management of Recurrent and Metastatic PC

In contrast to many other tumors including many endocrine cancers, management of recurrent or metastatic PC is primarily surgical because significant palliation of hypercalcemia results from the resection of local and regional recurrences in the neck and mediastinum as well as resection of solitary distant metastasis in the lungs or liver [35]. In a retrospective review of 12 reoperations for locoregional recurrences and 2 pulmonary metastases, symptomatic relief was achieved in 86% of patients [17]. Similarly in a series of pulmonary metastasis in six patients, three of those patients had complete biochemical resolution of hypercalcemia [74].

Adverse Prognostic Factors

1. Clinical: Male gender, younger age, and higher calcium levels [12]
2. Cytological: Mitosis [59]
3. Histopathology-vascular invasion [12]
4. Anatomical cancer-progressing features: Lymph node and periglandular invasion, distant metastasis
5. Oncological features: Simple parathyroidectomy
6. Nonfunctioning tumors are likely to be lethal with high number of recurrences and requirement of high number of calcium-lowering medications [66]
7. Increased staging: High risk

Natural History/Survival

PC has a high recurrence rate of 60% and death rate of 35% [12].

Average time between surgery and first occurrence is 3 years.

5-year OS: 40–80% [21, 23, 35, 66]

10-year OS: 35–79% [21, 35, 65]

Median OS: 14.3 years [21, 35, 65]

Concluding Remarks

Parathyroid carcinoma is a rare malignancy whose recognition requires a high index of suspicion. Best opportunity to cure parathyroid carcinoma is to diagnose it before or at the time of surgery for the tumor to be completely removed at the time of initial operation. Histological diagnosis can be difficult and nonspecific but immunohistochemical markers (PF, galectin-3, PGP 9.5) can be used as a complement to histological diagnosis. En bloc excision reduces soft-tissue recurrence and, even though evidence base for LN involvement by parathyroid cancer is sparse, a systematic central LN resection may improve outcomes. Thus failure to perform oncological surgery (en bloc resection) predicts higher recurrence and death rates. Staging into a low- and high-risk groups allows significant outcome predictions and could help to stratify therapy decisions. New TNM staging system helps in predicting cancer progression. Finally a moderate enhancement of the surgical approach to meet oncological criteria is likely to greatly improve outcome. Cinacalcet and bisphosphonates are the most effective treatments for hypercalcemia.

References

1. Fraker DL. Parathyroid tumors. In: DeVita Jr VT, Hellman S, Rosenberg SA, editors. Cancer: principles and practice of oncology. 6th ed. Philadelphia: Lippincott Williams and Wilkins; 2001. p. 1763–9.
2. Sharretts JM, Simonds WF. Clinical and molecular genetics of parathyroid neoplasms. Best Pract Res Clin Endocrinol Metab. 2010;24(3):491–502.
3. Gill AJ. Understanding the genetic basis of parathyroid carcinoma. Endocr Pathol. 2014;25(1):30–4.
4. Goswamy J, Lei M, Simo R. Parathyroid carcinoma. Curr Opin Otolaryngol Head Neck Surg. 2016;24(2):155–62.
5. Shi Y, Hogue J, Dixit D, Koh J, Olson JA Jr. Functional and genetic studies of isolated cells from parathyroid tumors reveal the complex pathogenesis of parathyroid neoplasia. Proc Natl Acad Sci U S A. 2014;111(8):3092–7.
6. Friedman E, Sakaguchi K, Bale AE, Falchetti A, Streeten E, Zimering MB, et al. Clonality of parathyroid tumors in familial multiple endocrine neoplasia type 1. N Engl J Med. 1989;321(4):213–8.
7. Shattuck TM, Kim TS, Costa J, Yandell DW, Imanishi Y, Palanisamy N, et al. Mutational analyses of RB and BRCA2 as candidate tumour suppressor genes in parathyroid carcinoma. Clin Endocrinol. 2003;59(2):180–9.
8. Arnold A. The cyclin D1/PRAD1 oncogene in human neoplasia. J Investig Med. 1995;43(6):543–9.

9. Simonds WF, Robbins CM, Agarwal SK, Hendy GN, Carpten JD, Marx SJ. Familial isolated hyperparathyroidism is rarely caused by germline mutation in HRPT2, the gene for the hyperparathyroidism-jaw tumor syndrome. J Clin Endocrinol Metab. 2004;89(1):96–102.
10. Cetani F, Pardi E, Borsari S, Viacava P, Dipollina G, Cianferotti L, et al. Genetic analyses of the HRPT2 gene in primary hyperparathyroidism: germline and somatic mutations in familial and sporadic parathyroid tumors. J Clin Endocrinol Metab. 2004;89(11):5583–91.
11. Cryns VL, Thor A, Xu HJ, Hu SX, Wierman ME, Vickery AL Jr, et al. Loss of the retinoblastoma tumor-suppressor gene in parathyroid carcinoma. N Engl J Med. 1994;330(11):757–61.
12. Talat N, Schulte KM. Clinical presentation, staging andlong-term evolution of parathyroid cancer. Ann Surg Oncol. 2010;17:2156–74.
13. Holmes EC, Morton DL, Ketcham AS. Parathyroid carcinoma: a collective review. Ann Surg. 1969;169(4):631–40.
14. Schaapveld M, Jorna FH, Aben KK, et al. Incidence and prognosis of parathyroid gland carcinoma: a population-based study in The Netherlands estimating the preoperative diagnosis. Am J Surg. 2011;202(5):590–7.
15. Harari A, Waring A, Fernandez-Ranvier G, et al. Parathyroid carcinoma: a 43-year outcome and survival analysis. J Clin Endocrinol Metab. 2011;96(12):3679–86.
16. Robert JH, Trombetti A, Garcia A, et al. Primary hyperparathyroidism: can parathyroid carcinoma be anticipated on clinical and biochemical grounds? Report of nine cases and review of the literature. Ann Surg Oncol. 2005;12(7):526–32.
17. Iihara M, Okamoto T, Suzuki R, et al. Functional parathyroid carcinoma: longterm treatment outcome and risk factor analysis. Surgery. 2007;142(6):936–43; discussion 943.e1
18. Rubin MR, Bilezikian JP, Birken S, et al. Human chorionic gonadotropin measurements in parathyroid carcinoma. Eur J Endocrinol. 2008;159(4):469–74.
19. Koea JB, Shaw JH. Parathyroid cancer: biology and management. Surg Oncol. 1999;8:155–65l.
20. Singh DN, Gupta SK, Kumari N, Krishnani N, Chand G, Mishra A, Agarwal G, Verma AK, Mishra SK, Agarwal A. Primary hyperparathyroidism presenting as hypercalcemic crisis: twenty-year experience. Indian J Endocrinol Metab. 2015;19(1):100–5.
21. Shane E. Clinical review 122: parathyroid carcinoma. J Clin Endocrinol Metab. 2001;86(2):485–93.
22. Levin KE, Galante M, Clark OH. Parathyroid carcinoma versus parathyroid adenoma in patients with profound hypercalcemia. Surgery. 1987;101(6):649–60.
23. Shaha AR, Shah JP. Parathyroid carcinoma: a diagnostic and therapeutic challenge. Cancer. 1999;86(3):378–80.
24. Shaha AR, Ferlito A, Rinaldo A. Distant metastases from thyroid and parathyroid cancer. ORL J Otorhinolaryngol Relat Spec. 2001;63(4):243–9.
25. Fang SH, Lal G. Parathyroid cancer. Endocr Pract. 2011;17(Suppl 1):36–43.
26. Sidhu PS, Talat N, Patel P, et al. Ultrasound features of malignancy in the preoperative diagnosis of parathyroid cancer: a retrospective analysis of parathyroid tumours larger than 15 mm. Eur Radiol. 2011;21(9):1865–73.
27. Hara H, Igarashi A, Yano Y, et al. Ultrasonographic features of parathyroid carcinoma. Endocr J. 2001;48(2):213–7.
28. Edmonson GR, Charboneau JW, James EM, et al. Parathyroid carcinoma: highfrequency sonographic features. Radiology. 1986;161(1):65–7.
29. Tamler R, Lewis MS, LiVolsi VA, et al. Parathyroid carcinoma: ultrasonographic and histologic features. Thyroid. 2005;15(7):744–5.
30. Spinelli C, Bonadio AG, Berti P, et al. Cutaneous spreading of parathyroid carcinoma after fine needle aspiration cytology. J Endocrinol Invest. 2000;23(4):255–7.
31. Kumari N, Mishra D, Pradhan R, Agarwal A, Krishnani N. Utility of fine-needle aspiration cytology in the identification of parathyroid lesions. J Cytol. 2016;33:17–21.
32. AgarwalA, GuptaSK, SukumarR. Hyperparathyroidism and malnutrition with severe Vitamin D deficiency. World J Surg. 2009;33(11):2303–13.
33. Smith JF, Coombs RR. Histological diagnosis of carcinoma of the parathyroid gland. J Clin Pathol. 1984;37(12):1370–8.
34. Delellis RA. Challenging lesions in the differential diagnosis of endocrine tumors: parathyroid carcinoma. Endocr Pathol. 2008;19(4):221–5.
35. Hundahl SA, Fleming ID, Fremgen AM, et al. Two hundred eighty-six cases of parathyroid carcinoma treated in the U.S. between 1985–1995: a National Cancer Data Base Report. The American College of Surgeons Commission on Cancer and the American Cancer Society. Cancer. 1999;86(3):538–44.
36. Cohn K, Silverman M, Corrado J, et al. Parathyroid carcinoma: the Lahey Clinic experience. Surgery. 1985;98(6):1095–100.
37. Schantz A, Castleman B. Parathyroid carcinoma. A study of 70 cases. Cancer. 1973;31(3):600–5.
38. McKeown PP, McGarity WC, Sewell CW. Carcinoma of the parathyroid gland: is it overdiagnosed? A report of three cases. Am J Surg. 1984;147:292–7.
39. Bondeson L, Sandelin K, Grimelius L. Histopathological variables and DNA cytometry in parathyroid carcinoma. Am J Surg Pathol. 1993;17:820–9.
40. Okamoto T, Iihara M, Obara T, Tsukada T. Parathyroid carcinoma: etiology, diagnosis, and treatment. World J Surg. 2009;33:2343–54.
41. Obara T, Okamoto T, Kanbe M, et al. Functioning parathyroid carcinoma: clinicopathologic features and rational treatment. Semin Surg Oncol. 1997;13(2):134–41.
42. Chang YJ, Mittal V, Remine S, et al. Correlation between clinical and histological findings in para-

thyroid tumors suspicious for carcinoma. Am Surg. 2006;72(5):419–26.
43. Fujimoto Y, Obara T. How to recognize and treat parathyroid carcinoma. Surg Clin North Am. 1987;67:343–57.
44. Holck S, Pedersen N. Carcinoma of the parathyroid gland. A light and electron microscopic study. Acta Pathol Microbiol Scand. 1981;89:297–302.
45. Levin K, Chew K, Ljung B, Mayall B, Siperstein A, Clark O. Deoxyribonucleic acid flow cytometry helps identify parathyroid carcinomas. J Clin Endocrinol Metab. 1988;67:779–84.
46. Mallette LE. DNA quantitation in the study of parathyroid lesions. A review. Am J Clin Pathol. 1992;98:305–11.
47. Cryns VL, Rubio MP, Thor AD, Louis DN, Arnold A. p53 abnormalities in human parathyroid carcinoma. J Clin Endocrinol Metab. 1994;78:1320–4.
48. Cetani F, Pardi E, ViacavaP Pollina GD, Fanelli G, Picone A, Borsari S, Gazzerro E, Miccoli P, Berti P, Pinchera A, Marcocci C. A reappraisal of the Rb1 gene abnormalities in the diagnosis of parathyroid cancer. Clin Endocrinol. 2004;60:99–10.
49. Lloyd RV, Carney JA, Ferreiro JA, Jin L, Thompson GB, Van Heerden JA, Grant CS, Wollan PC. Immunohistochemical analysis of the cell cycle-associated antigens Ki-67 and retinoblastoma protein in parathyroid carcinomas and adenomas. Endocr Pathol. 1995;6(4):279–87.
50. Juhlin CC, Nilsson IL, Johansson K, Haglund F, Villablanca A, Höög A, Larsson C. Parafibromin and APC as screening markers for malignant potential in atypical parathyroid adenomas. Endocr Pathol. 2010;21(3):166–77.
51. Bergero N, De Pompa R, Sacerdote C, Gasparri G, Volante M, Bussolati G, Papotti M. Galectin-3 expression in parathyroid carcinoma: immunohistochemical study of 26 cases. Hum Pathol. 2005;36(8):908–14.
52. Tezel E, Hibi K, Nagasaka T, Nakao A. PGP9.5 as a prognostic factor in pancreatic cancer. Clin Cancer Res. 2000;6(12):4764–7.
53. Takano T, Miyauchi A, Matsuzuka F, Yoshida H, Nakata Y, Kuma K, Amino N. PGP9.5 mRNA could contribute to the molecular-based diagnosis of medullary thyroid carcinoma. Eur J Cancer. 2004;40(4):614–618 27.
54. Yamazaki T, Hibi K, Takase T, Tezel E, Nakayama H, Kasai Y, Ito K, Akiyama S, Nagasaka T, Nakao A. PGP9.5 as a marker for invasive colorectal cancer. Clin Cancer Res. 2002;8(1):192–5.
55. Tan MH, Morrison C, Wang P, Yang X, Haven CJ, Zhang C, Zhao P, Tretiakova MS, Korpi-Hyovalti E, Burgess JR, Soo KC, Cheah WK, Cao B, Resau J, Morreau H, Teh BT. Loss of parafibromin immunoreactivity is a distinguishing feature of parathyroid carcinoma. Clin Cancer Res. 2004;10:6629–37.
56. Gill AJ, Clarkson A, Gimm O, Keil J, Dralle H, Howell VM, Marsh DJ. Loss of nuclear expression of parafibromin distinguishes parathyroid carcinomas and hyperparathyroidismjaw tumor (HPT-JT) syndrome related adenomas from sporadic parathyroid adenomas and hyperplasias. Am J Surg Pathol. 2006;30(9):1140–9.
57. Agarwal A, Pradhan R, Kumari N, Krishnani N, Shukla P, Gupta SK, Chand G, Mishra A, Agarwal G, Verma AK, Mishra SK. Molecular characteristics of large parathyroid adenomas. World J Surg. 2016;40(3):607–14.
58. Farnebo F, Svensson A, Thompson NW, et al. Expression of matrix metalloproteinase gelatinase A messenger ribonucleic acid in parathyroid carcinomas. Surgery. 1999;126:1183–7.
59. Villar-del-Moral J, Jimenez-Garcıa A, Salvador-Egea P, Martos-Martınez JM, Nuño-Vazquez-Garza JM, Serradilla-Martın M, Gómez-Palacios A, Moreno-Llorente P, Ortega-Serrano J, de la Quintana-Basarrate A. Prognostic factors and staging systems in parathyroid cancer: a multicenter cohort study. Surgery. 2014;156:1132–44.
60. Medas F, et al. Controversies in the management of parathyroid carcinoma: a case series and review of the literature. Int J Surg. 2015;28:S94. https://doi.org/10.1016/j.ijsu.2015.12.040
61. Christine J, Chan O'NC, Symons J, Learoyd DL, Sidhu SB, Delbridge LW, Gill A, Sywak MS. Parathyroid carcinoma encountered after minimally invasive focused parathyroidectomy may not require further radical surgery. World J Surg. 2011;35:147–53.
62. Lee PK, Jarosek SL, Virnig BA, Evasovich M, Tuttle TM. Trends in the incidence and treatment of parathyroid cancer in the United States. Cancer. 2007;109:1736–41.
63. Enomoto K, Uchino S, Ito A, et al. The surgical strategy and the molecular analysis of patients with parathyroid cancer. World J Surg. 2010;34:2604–10.
64. Kameyama K, Takami H. Double parathyroid carcinoma. Endocr J. 2003;50:477–9.
65. Busaidy NL, Jimenez C, Habra MA, Schultz PN, El-Naggar AK, Clayman GL, Asper JA, Diaz EM Jr, Evans DB, Gagel RF, Garden A, Hoff AO, Lee JE, Morrison WH, Rosenthal DI, Sherman SI, Sturgis EM, Waguespack SG, Weber RS, Wirfel K, Vassilopoulou-Sellin R. Parathyroid carcinoma: a 22-year experience. Head Neck. 2004;26(8):716–26.
66. Kebebew E, et al. Localization and reoperation results for persistent and recurrent parathyroid carcinoma. Arch Surg. 2001;136:878–85.
67. Mohebati A, Shaha A, Shah J. Parathyroid carcinoma: challenges in diagnosis and treatment. Hematol Oncol Clin North Am. 2012;26(6):1221–38.
68. Sandelin K, Auer G, Bondeson L, Grimelius L, Farnebo LO. Prognostic factors in parathyroid cancer: a review of 95 cases. World J Surg. 1992;16(4):724–31.
69. Sadler C, Gow KW, Beierle EA, Doski JJ, Langer M, Nuchtern JG, Vasudevan SA, Goldfarb M. Parathyroid

carcinoma in more than 1,000 patients: a population-level analysis. Surgery. 2014;156(6):1622–9.
70. Munson ND, Foote RL, Northcutt RC, et al. Parathyroid carcinoma: is there a role for adjuvant radiation therapy? Cancer. 2003;98(11):2378–84.
71. Chow E, Tsang RW, Brierley JD, et al. Parathyroid carcinoma—the Princess Margaret Hospital experience. Int J Radiat Oncol Biol Phys. 1998;41(3):569–72.
72. Bukowski RM, Sheeler L, Cunningham J, et al. Successful combination chemotherapy for metastatic parathyroid carcinoma. Arch Intern Med. 1984;144(2):399–400.
73. Chahinian AP. Chemotherapy for metastatic parathyroid carcinoma. Arch Intern Med. 1984;144(9):1889.
74. Wang CA, Gaz RD. Natural history of parathyroid carcinoma. Diagnosis, treatment, and results. Am J Surg. 1985;149:522–7.

Part III

Adrenal

The Adrenal Incidentaloma

25

Richard Egan and David Scott-Coombes

Introduction

An adrenal incidentaloma is an asymptomatic adrenal mass discovered by chance during investigation for non-adrenal disease. Most authorities would consider a mass ≥1 cm to be an incidentaloma [1–5]. The basic aims of subsequent investigation are to quantify the risk of malignancy, to determine the functional status of the tumour, to assess the need for surgical intervention and to develop a suitable, individualised follow-up protocol [3]. There have been several attempts to standardise the management of this increasingly common clinical entity, taking into account the natural history of the condition, the cost-effectiveness of treatment and follow-up regimens, and patient-specific factors [6, 7].

Epidemiology

The incidence of adrenal incidentaloma in autopsy studies is between 2.3 and 8.7%, and increases with age [3–5, 8–10]. With modern imaging methods incidentalomas are noted in up to 5% of abdominal scans [4, 11–13]. As technology improves yet further, this percentage will approach the value observed in the postmortem studies. Kim et al. reported an increased incidence of incidentaloma with age, with the majority discovered in the sixth and seventh decades of life [14], whilst radiological evidence of an incidental adrenal tumour is apparent in 7% of those aged over 70 years [15]. The increasing prevalence with age has also been reported by other groups, with incidental adrenal tumours noted on 3% of radiological studies at 50 years old, increasing to 10% in the elderly [3]. In centres where the case mix contains higher proportions of patients undergoing scanning for a history of extra-adrenal malignancy, the rate of incidentaloma may be as high as 12% [16].

R. Egan · D. Scott-Coombes (✉)
Endocrine Surgery, University Hospital of Wales, Cardiff, UK
e-mail: david.scott-coombes@wales.nhs.uk

Differential Diagnosis

Myriad conditions constitute the differential diagnosis of adrenal incidentaloma (Table 25.1), although the vast majority are benign, non-secreting adrenal tumours.

The reporting of the frequency distribution of the variety of diagnoses is likely subject to considerable selection bias [3]. This may be either due to the reporting of a purely surgical cohort or due to the selective referral patterns to specialist centres. In both situations, smaller benign lesions may be filtered out of any reported cohort. As a consequence, the frequency at which individual diagnoses are reported varies considerably.

Adenoma, for example, is reported to account for a median 80% of adrenal incidentalomas in

R. Parameswaran, A. Agarwal (eds.), *Evidence-Based Endocrine Surgery*,
https://doi.org/10.1007/978-981-10-1124-5_25

Table 25.1 Differential diagnosis of an adrenal incidentaloma

Adenoma	Nodular hyperplasia	Carcinoma
Ganglioneuroma	Phaeochromocytoma	Angiomyolipoma
Abscess	Amyloidosis	Cyst
Fibroma	Granulomatosis	Hamartoma
Haematoma	Lipoma	Liposarcoma
Myelolipoma	Teratoma	Pseudocyst
Metastasis	Schwannoma	Neuroblastoma

cohorts including all patients with an adrenal mass [3, 13]: this compares to a median 55% in purely surgical cohorts [3, 4]. There is a corresponding increase in the prevalence of adrenocortical cancer (ACC) (median 11% vs. 8% in general incidentaloma cohorts), phaeochromocytoma (10% vs. 7%) and metastasis (7% vs. 5%) in surgical cohorts [3, 4]. In some surgical cohorts, the proportion of patients with a diagnosis of phaeochromocytoma is as high as 25% [14]. Studies based on a radiological cohort identify functioning tumours in less than 1% of the total, although the vast majority of cases in this retrospective cohort were characterised radiologically and not clinically [13]. In almost all series, benign, non-functioning adenoma constitutes the majority of the diagnoses.

Thompson et al. performed a literature review of 2000 cases of adrenal incidentalomas and found that 82% of cases were benign, non-functioning tumours [17]. Benign secreting tumours accounted for a further 11%, with malignant adrenal tumours responsible for only 7% of the overall total [17]. Of those benign secreting tumours, phaeochromocytoma and cortisol-secreting (Cushing's) tumours made up 5% of the total each, respectively, with aldosterone-producing Conn's tumours responsible for only 1% [17]. In patients with incidental adrenal tumours and coexisting hypertension, the prevalence of Conn's tumours may be as high as 10% [18]. ACC constitutes 4.7% of incidentalomas, but with an incidence of 0.72 per million population per year remains a very rare malignancy. Adrenal metastasis constitutes the remaining 2.5% of adrenal incidentalomas, with metastases arising from a variety of solid organ tumours. The risk of primary malignancy in unselected incidentaloma is approximately 0.1% [17]. In a retrospective study of abdominal scanning in one US centre there were no cases of malignancy in 973 consecutive incidental adrenal tumours in patients without a history of malignancy [13].

Some diagnoses are found with such infrequency that their reporting is limited to case reports [19]. There are also cases reported in the literature of retroperitoneal pathology being misdiagnosed as an adrenal incidentaloma, and diagnoses such as leiomyosarcoma should be considered if imaging is not characteristic [20].

Investigation

Investigation of the adrenal incidentaloma aims to address several key questions:

- Is the tumour functioning or non-functioning?
- Is the tumour benign or malignant?
- Are there indications to resect the tumour?

The answer to the latter question will, to a large extent, be based upon the conclusions of the first two questions whilst also taking into consideration the size of the adrenal mass and the general medical condition of the patient. As a general rule, if bilateral adrenal incidentalomas are identified on imaging, both tumours should be assessed and managed independently, as outlined below. It is recommended that adrenal tumours be managed in the context of a multidisciplinary team (MDT) in the majority of cases. An MDT should generally consist of a minimum of a radiologist, an endocrinologist and a surgeon, each with an interest in adrenal disease, with additional members if local expertise allows. In addition, there is some evidence to suggest that management of patients in high-volume centres (≥10 adrenalectomies per annum) can lead to improved outcomes in surgical cases, particularly in cases of malignancy, for example [21]. Current UK guidelines suggest that surgeons performing adrenalectomy should perform a minimum of six such procedures per annum to maintain competence [22].

Assessing Functional Status

As a minimum, the vast majority of patients should be evaluated with a low-dose [1 mg] overnight dexamethasone suppression test (ODST) and a 24-h urinary metanephrine analysis or plasma-free catecholamine assay, to screen for a cortisol-secreting tumour or a phaeochromocytoma, respectively [3, 5, 23, 24]. For patients with hypertension, either treated or not, plasma potassium (sodium) and aldosterone:renin activity should be measured to exclude a Conn's tumour. Virilisation, as well as alerting the clinician to the high possibility of malignancy, should prompt assessment of the sex hormone precursors DHEA and DHEAS. Similarly, the presence of gynaecomastia warrants oestradiol assay [3]. Imaging features consistent with ACC are another indication to assay sex hormones [3]. Genetic testing associated with a diagnosis of phaeochromocytoma is discussed in detail in Chap. 28.

When performing an ODST, a cut-off value to exclude excess cortisol secretion of ≤50 nmol/L is recommended [3]. For patients without clinical manifestations of excess cortisol but a post-ODST cortisol level of >138 nmol/L, the term 'autonomous cortisol secretion' should be applied, and such patients screened for hypertension and type 2 diabetes mellitus, respectively, with the prefix 'possible' added if the value falls between the aforementioned levels [3]. The association between autonomous cortisol secretion and type 2 diabetes, hypertension and cardiovascular events has been demonstrated in several cohort studies [25, 26], although not all studies concur [27]. Although an increased risk of mortality in patients with impaired cortisol suppression has been reported in some studies, further work is required to assess this potential association [28].

For patients with bilateral incidentalomas measurement of serum 17-hydroxyprogesterone should be considered to exclude congenital adrenal hyperplasia [3]. In addition, testing for adrenal insufficiency should be considered in patients with radiological evidence of bilateral infiltrative lesions or evidence of haemorrhage. The preferred method to screen for adrenal insufficiency is the short synACTHen test.

Assessment of Malignant Potential: Imaging

Cross-sectional imaging provides a crucial component of the investigation of adrenal incidentaloma. The first-line imaging modality requested depends very much on the nature of the initial investigation that highlighted the adrenal incidentaloma. For example, a high-quality non-contrast CT scan performed to investigate renal calculi may provide comprehensive imaging for an adrenal tumour negating the need for further radiological evaluation. Several suggested imaging algorithms for the investigation of the adrenal incidentaloma have been devised [2, 29].

The European Society of Endocrinology (ESE) and European Network for the Study of Adrenal Tumours (ENSAT) in their collaborative guidelines for the management of adrenal incidentaloma recommend the use of non-contrast computed tomography (CT) scanning to assess such lesions for benignity [3]. Furthermore, they suggest that no further imaging is required if the lesion itself is <4 cm, homogenous and lipid rich and has a density of <10 Hounsfield units [3]. Magnetic resonance imaging (MRI) scanning is preferable to CT imaging in children, adolescents, pregnancy and adults under the age of 40 [3].

Clinical Pearl

- In incidentalomas less than 4 cm, which are lipid rich on scanning (<10 HU), malignancy can effectively be ruled out.

The main purpose of cross-sectional imaging is to aid in the distinction between benign and malignant tumours, although some functional tumours may also display characteristic radiological appearances. Whereas CT and MRI are generally utilised with the purpose of confirming benignity, positron emission tomography (PET)/CT is generally the imaging modality employed to detect malignancy. In any case of adrenal incidentaloma, where there is a lack of clear characteristics of benign disease, a referral to the regional MDT should be made [22].

Local invasion and distant metastases are diagnostic of malignancy, but are infrequent radiological findings. More subtle radiological features are typically called upon to stratify the risk of malignancy in adrenal tumours. Such features include a rapid increase in size on sequential scans, an irregular outline, necrosis, heterogeneous contrast uptake and relative contrast washout [2] (Fig. 25.1). Adenomas are classically lipid rich with a corresponding tissue density of <10 Hounsfield units (HU) on non-contrast CT [30]. A recently published systematic review and meta-analysis agrees that adrenal masses with ≤10 HU are unlikely to be malignant, although the authors stop short of making definitive statements regarding use of this parameter as a definitive diagnostic tool, largely due to insufficient evidence [12] (Fig. 25.2). If one considers patients with a history of extra-adrenal malignancy, the evidence is less convincing. In this setting 7% of adrenal metastases were reported as having a tumour density of <10 HU [12].

Clinical Pearl

- Keep in perspective the fact that the risk of malignancy in unselected incidentaloma cases is 0.1%.

However, 30–40% of adenomas are lipid poor, which may lead to elevated HU measurements on non-contrast CT imaging, and diagnostic uncertainty [20]. In addition to being low-attenuation lesions on non-enhanced scans, adenomas are also predicted by an absolute enhancement washout of ≥60% and/or relative contrast washout of ≥40% on contract-enhanced CT, or signal loss in opposed-phase MRI [2, 31, 32]. Malignant lesions will tend towards a slower contrast washout on [contrast] CT and, as with phaeochromocytomas, will remain unchanged in out-of-phase images [33]. A 15-min delayed image contrast 'adrenal protocol' CT is the preferred method for calculating adrenal washout [2, 3], and care should be taken in interpretation of contrast CT scans requested for an alternative

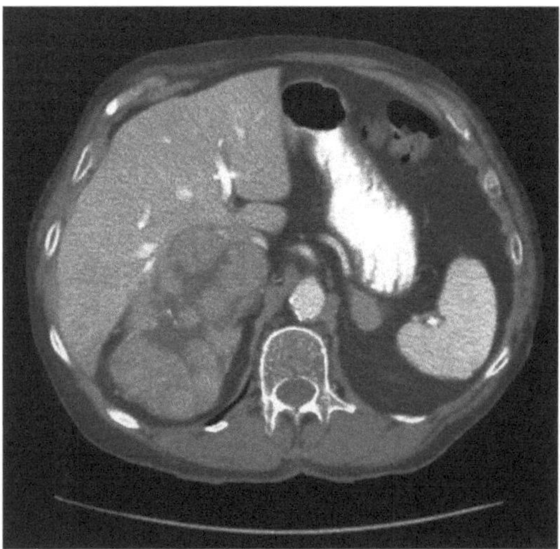

Fig. 25.1 A large right adrenal ACC with an irregular margin and heterogenous contrast enhancement

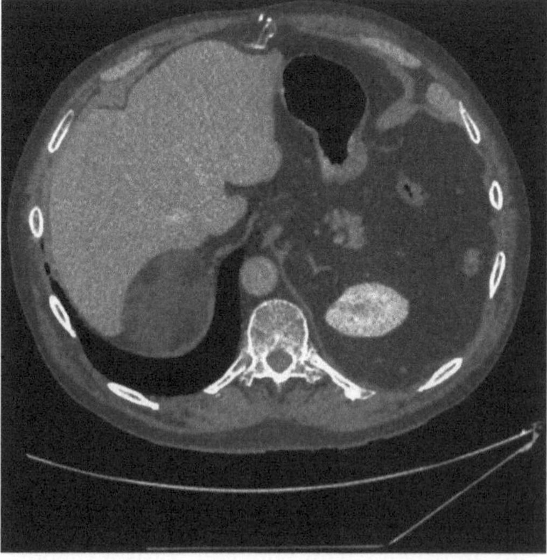

Fig. 25.2 A very-low-density fatty (negative HU) right-sided adrenal tumour which has a typical appearance of a myelolipoma

reason. In studies comparing MRI to CT in true adrenal incidentalomas, MRI was slightly inferior in terms of sensitivity and specificity, when predicting malignancy [12].

Novel risk stratification tools have been developed to aid with the diagnosis of malignancy and rationalise the use of surgical resection for potentially indeterminate lesions [34]. This tool, based on tumour size and HU on non-contrast CT, was developed with a retrospective analysis of historic patients. Despite initial promise, these results have not been replicated when applied to other retrospective cohorts [35].

Frilling et al. investigated the ability of a variety of imaging modalities to predict malignancy in adrenal tumours in oncology patients undergoing adrenalectomy [36]. In this small study comprising 31 adrenal metastases and 13 benign adenomas, both MRI and PET scanning had 100% sensitivity for predicting malignancy preoperatively [36]. Although MRI predicted benignity in each case, the specificity of PET scanning was inferior. CT scanning had 81% sensitivity and 39% specificity, whilst ultrasound scanning (USS) was generally inferior [36]. A large-scale meta-analysis of PET scanning in adrenal tumours demonstrated PET +/− CT to be both highly sensitive and specific in its ability to distinguish malignancy from benign pathology [37]. Combination scanning with non-contrast and delayed adrenal washout contrast-enhanced CT scanning has demonstrated sensitivity and specificity of 98% and 92%, respectively, for the identification of adenomas in 166 adrenal masses investigated [38].

^{18}F-2-deoxy-D-glucose (^{18}FDG)-PET scanning is growing in popularity as an imaging modality in some units. FDG-avid tumours include primary ACC, lymphoma, paraganglioma and adrenal metastasis [31] (Fig. 25.3). Recent UK guidelines recommend the use of preoperative ^{18}FDG-PET in addition to standard cross-sectional imaging in all patients with suspected ACC [22]. PET/CT is the most commonly used technique, combining the ability of PET to differentiate tissues with high metabolic requirements with the anatomical detail needed for localisation afforded by CT imaging. A tumour to liver standardised uptake value (T/L SUVmax ratio) of >1.53 is reported to be an independent prognostic factor for malignancy in FDG-PET/CT scans [39].

In certain cases of phaeochromocytoma, consideration to request ^{18}F-dihydroxyphenylalanine (DOPA) or ^{123}I-metaiodobenzylguanidine (MIBG) scanning can be given to provide more information and guide subsequent management [24, 31], especially when either paraganglioma or metastases are suspected. More recent advances, such as utilisation of ^{123}I-iodometomidate single-photon emission computed tomography (SPECT)/CT images to classify adrenal lesions, have not yet become mainstream imaging modalities but offer promise for the future [40].

Patient evaluation should include enquiries as to previous imaging, especially in patients referred from peripheral hospitals. Review of prior imaging may confirm not only the presence of an initially overlooked adrenal mass, but also a lack of interval change in the mass, conferring some degree of reassurance to patient and clinician alike. In certain circumstances stability for a period of ≥12 months may eliminate the need for follow-up [2].

Clinical Pearl

- A thorough review of a patient's previous imaging may reassure the clinician and negate the need for further radiological investigation and, in some cases, follow-up.

Assessment of Malignant Potential: Biopsy

The main indication to biopsy an adrenal incidentaloma is to diagnose a metastasis in patients with known or suspected extra-adrenal malignancy. A biopsy should only be undertaken when the information gained is predicted to alter or inform clinical management [3]. In practice the only other situation where an adrenal biopsy might be contemplated is when histological confirmation of malignancy in an otherwise irresectable tumour

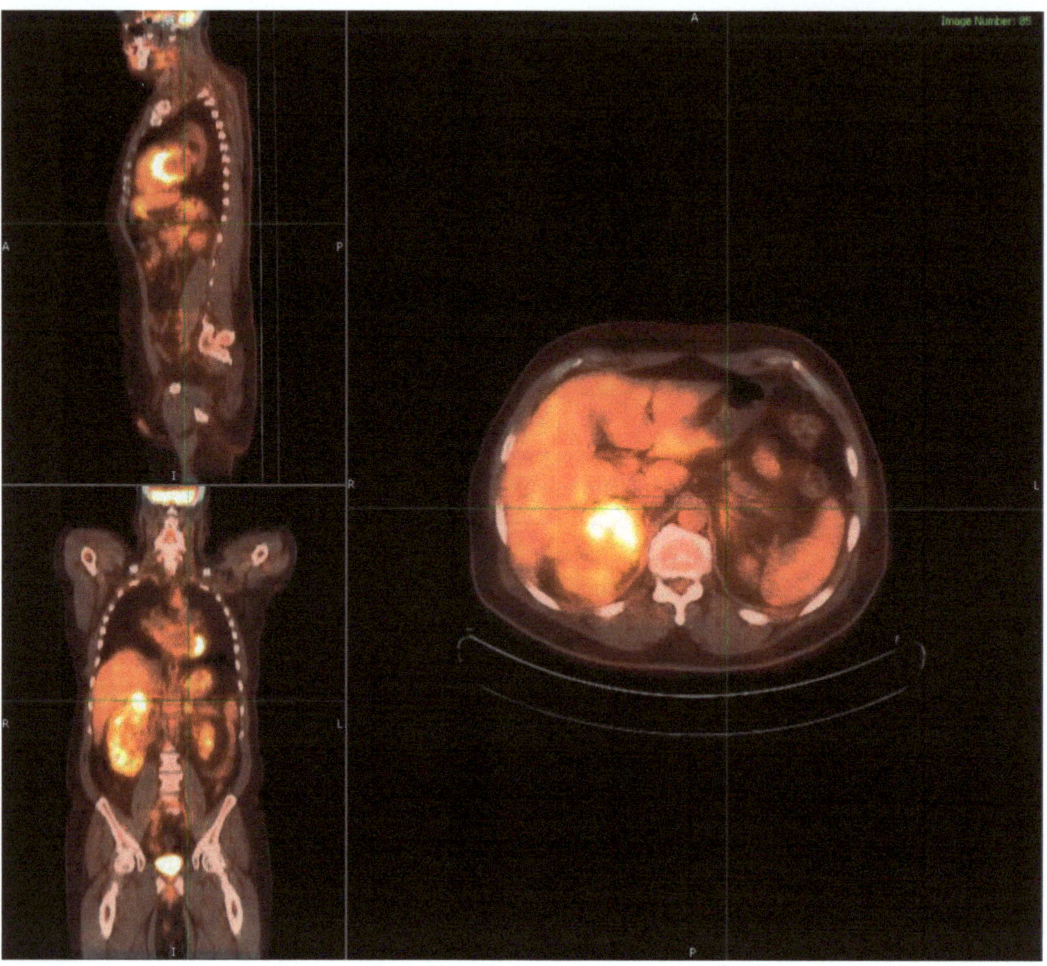

Fig. 25.3 A fused PET-CT image demonstrating avid FDG uptake in a right adrenal metastasis

might permit the use of adjuvant treatments, either as a palliative measure or as part of a clinical trial [3]. Fine-needle aspiration cytology cannot distinguish readily between adrenal adenoma and carcinoma, and is not suitable for the diagnosis of primary adrenal cancer [41]. Biopsy of phaeochromocytoma may precipitate a life-threatening hypertensive crisis, whilst histological evaluation of ACC is unreliable and the biopsy itself may lead to tumour seeding and compromise both the ability to achieve an R0 resection and disease prognosis [3]. Although one US study of patients with ACC found no negative impact on recurrence-free or overall survival in patients undergoing transcutaneous biopsy, when compared to those that had not undergone biopsy [42], the prevailing guidance is to avoid biopsy. Autopsy studies of patients with known malignancy report the prevalence of adrenal metastasis to be 8–38%. Conversely, in patients with no known primary malignancy the overall rate for discovering and adrenal metastasis is low [11]. Although the incidence of adrenal metastasis is rare in unselected incidentalomas, metastasis is the cause of the adrenal incidentaloma in approximately half of patients who have a history of malignant disease [43]. In some centres, rates of metastatic disease in apparent incidentaloma in oncology patients as high as 70–75% have been reported [36, 44]. As a general rule, patients with known extra-adrenal metastatic disease and an adrenal mass are more likely to have adrenal metastasis than benign pathology, whereas oncology patients with an isolated adrenal incidentaloma without overt radiological features of malignancy are still more likely to have a benign adrenal tumour [2].

In a recent systematic review and meta-analysis evaluating the diagnostic value of adrenal incidentaloma biopsy, the non-diagnostic rate was estimated at 8.7%, and the complication rate at 2.5% [3, 44], although rates up to 11% have been reported [42]. Potential complications include bleeding, pneumothorax, viscus injury, pain and tumour spread through the needle track. These figures may underestimate the true values, due to a variety of methodological factors. The sensitivity of adrenal biopsy to detect malignancy overall was 87% (95% CI; 78–93%), falling to 70% (42–88%) when analysing ACC as an individual entity [3, 42].

Assessment of Malignant Potential: Other

ACC is most often a sporadic occurrence but can occasionally be associated with a genetic syndrome. A known family history of Li-Fraumeni syndrome, Carney complex, familial adenomatous polyposis coli, Beckwith-Wiedemann syndrome or, rarely, multiple endocrine neoplasia type 1, should alert the clinician to an elevated risk of ACC once an adrenal mass has been identified [33]. Whether an adrenal tumour in this context is truly an incidentaloma is debateable.

Indications for Resection

As a general guide, the decision to offer surgical resection of an adrenal incidentaloma should be based on both the likelihood of malignancy and the degree of hormone excess, in conjunction with the patient's age, general health and personal wishes.

NIH guidelines from 2002 suggested a simple algorithm for the resection of adrenal incidentalomas. The recommendation for functioning tumours was to either offer surgical resection or manage them medically. For non-functioning tumours greater than 6 cm, surgical resection is recommended, whilst for those under 4 cm a conservative approach is suggested, although no formal follow-up regimen is proposed [23]. In addition, it concluded that for suspected metastases, surgical resection conferred no benefit [23].

These guidelines contained several clinical 'grey areas' where a lack of available evidence limited the development of firm recommendation. These included the management of non-functioning tumours whose size ranges between 4 and 6 cm, the size at which excision of a functioning tumour should be considered best practice, and the follow-up regimens that should be utilised for non-functioning tumours of 1–4 cm and those 4–6 cm tumours managed conservatively.

The reason for this lack of clarity lies in the fact that malignant potential of an adrenal tumour is not related to its size in a linear fashion. The malignant potential of incidentalomas <4 cm is low, but may rise to 10% once this size threshold has been surpassed. A large retrospective Chinese study reporting on 634 patients found only 1 malignancy (3 cm) in a total of 249 adrenalectomy procedures performed when the incidentaloma was ≤4 cm [45]. The risk of malignancy in patients undergoing adrenalectomy in this study increased to 9.4% (8/85) and 33.3% (48/144) in patients with tumours of >4–≤6 cm and >6 cm, respectively [45]. Of interest in this cohort, two-thirds of patients (249/376) with a tumour ≤4 cm underwent surgical intervention, of which only 40 patients had biochemical evidence of excess hormone secretion [45]. When compared against current European guidelines, this may be considered over treatment in the low-risk patient cohort.

Once a size of >6 cm has been reached the risk of malignancy rises markedly to 25–90% [23, 46, 47]. In a large retrospective review of a US cancer registry, Kebebew et al. found that only 4.2% of ACC were ≤6 cm in diameter [48].

Establishing a definitive size threshold for surgical excision has proven difficult. In all cases some degree of compromise needs to be sought. If the bar is set too high, it risks missing early cases of malignancy that would be treatable and potentially curable; too low, and many patients will undergo unnecessary surgery in order to identify the occasional small, malignant tumour. Whether such small tumours pose a realistic malignant potential is also controversial.

A more pragmatic approach might be to adopt a policy of observation and serial imaging. However such an approach may only heighten patient anxiety for those tumours that remain quiescent and harmless whilst allowing the rapid growth that may accompany malignant transformation to be missed for such a period so as to delay treatment, worsen prognosis or even render the tumour inoperable.

Population-based studies have suggested that the incidence of localised ACC diagnosed was essentially unchanged from 1973 until 2000. Although more operations for adrenal incidentaloma are being performed, patients with ACC are not being diagnosed earlier or treated at an earlier stage [48]. Any case that is suspicious for ACC should be managed in a specialist, high-volume unit, as better outcomes following surgery have been reported [21].

As a result of current best available evidence, many centres have adopted a policy to offer resection to patients with adrenal incidentalomas exceeding 4 cm in size, providing that the patient is a suitable surgical candidate [41, 49], and such parameters have been included in some guidelines [10]. More recent guidelines produced by ESE/ENSAT have recommended against performing surgery for asymptomatic tumours with no evidence of hormone excess and clear features of benignity on imaging [3]. The validity of this has been questioned, with some authors instead preferring to follow up patients for a minimum of 5 years irrespective of the evidence of benignity and lack of function at the initial assessment [50]. Another approach to patients with non-functioning tumours <40 mm and <10 HU may be to simply repeat a CT scan and screen for hypercortisolism at 5 years only [51]. In addition, some groups have adopted a policy where one indication for surgical resection is an adrenal tumour of >3 cm [52].

Surgical resection should be considered in patients with autonomous cortisol secretion, especially when associated with cortisol excess-related comorbidities [3]. There is weak evidence that comorbid conditions such as type 2 diabetes, hypertension and dyslipidaemia improve in some patients with autonomous cortisol secretion following resection; such improvements are not seen when patients are managed conservatively [53–55]. The increased hazard ratio for mortality in patients with autonomous cortisol secretion reported in a recent retrospective UK trial adds support to resection of responsible lesions [28]. In this context most deaths were attributable to cardiovascular disease or infective causes, whilst an association between abnormal cortisol secretion and cardiovascular disease and mortality has been replicated elsewhere [25]. Adrenalectomy is recommended for any unilateral tumour with clinically significant hormone excess, whereas bilateral adrenalectomy should be reserved only for those with evidence of overt Cushing's syndrome in the presence of bilaterally enlarged adrenals [3].

Choice of Procedure

Current guidelines have suggested that laparoscopic adrenalectomy is a feasible option, even for patients with radiological suspicion of malignancy, in unilateral tumours that are ≤6 cm and do not show frank local invasion [3]. One key benefit associated with laparoscopic surgery is a reduction in length of stay [56].

In contrast, evidence of local invasion mandates an open procedure [3]. Despite the recommendation for open surgery in suspected malignant disease, the evidence supporting this management is weak, with no conclusive evidence suggesting improvements in complete resection rates, or overall or disease-specific survival in open surgery compared to laparoscopic surgery [56–59].

It has been suggested that open resection improves the outcome for patients with ACC, both in terms of local recurrence and overall survival [60, 61]. One potential explanation for this is the locoregional lymph node dissection associated with an open procedure [60]. This is a controversial issue, however, and consensus on what constitutes the lymphatic basin for adrenal tumours has not been widely agreed. Alternatively it may be that increases in positive resection margins or tumour spillage [56] increase the risk of peritoneal recurrence rates [61]. Open resection for >6 cm phaeochromocytomas is also recommended in recent Endocrine Society guidelines, in order to prevent incomplete excision, local recurrence or tumour rupture [24].

Partial adrenalectomy for small tumours in patients that have previously undergone contralateral adrenalectomy can be considered in certain circumstances, such as phaeochromocytoma, to prevent adrenal insufficiency [24, 62]. Such a scenario is exceptionally rare, except in the context of hereditary disease such as MEN2 or von Hippel-Lindau, in which case any contralateral tumour is unlikely to represent a true incidentaloma.

Any patients undergoing surgery that may result in post-operative adrenal insufficiency require adequate counselling and have perioperative care pathways in place [22]. All patients with a preoperative cortisol that does not suppress to ≤50 nmol/L following low-dose ODST should be given high-dose glucocorticoid cover perioperatively [3].

Natural History and Follow-Up

The natural history of apparently benign, non-functioning adrenal incidentaloma is poorly understood. This has made the development of robust follow-up protocols problematic. In addition, follow-up of adrenal lesions has two facets, namely the size of the lesion, and its functional status. Current UK guidance suggests that any adrenal incidentaloma lacking clear characteristics of benignity should be referred to a specialist multidisciplinary team for ongoing investigation and management [22].

There is a significant body of evidence that patients with cortisol excess without overt clinical features rarely develop Cushing's syndrome [3, 63]. Despite this, a thorough clinical evaluation should seek to identify the presence of any additional cortisol-related comorbidities, which may include obesity, dyslipidaemia and osteoporosis, respectively, although their association with autonomous cortisol secretion is debatable [64]. Several studies have reported a reduction in bone density and an increased fracture rate in patients with adrenal incidentaloma and 'subclinical hypercortisolism' [65, 66]. Once cortisol excess has been established, all potential surgical candidates should be investigated to ensure ACTH independence [3]. For patients with incidentaloma and a normal initial hormone status evaluation, further hormonal screening has been advised against, unless new signs of endocrine dysfunction develop, or existing comorbidities worsen [3]. For patients with autonomous cortisol secretion without clinical signs of Cushing's syndrome, an annual assessment of cortisol-related comorbidities should be undertaken [3].

Bülow et al. reported a large prospective Swedish study that involved 229 patients with adrenal incidentalomas followed up with serial CT scans and hormonal assessment. At a median follow-up of 25 months, they noted either no change or a reduction in size in 92.6% of patients. Seventeen (7.4%) patients had adrenal tumours that grew by 5 mm or more, 12 of which grew by ≥1 cm [67]. Of the 17 patients with enlarging tumours, 11 had the mass excised; 7 due to an increase in size (to between 3.0 and 6.5 cm) and 4 owing to the development of hormone hypersecretion [67]. A similar prospective cohort study involving both serial cross-sectional imaging and hormonal assessment for 24 months demonstrated no cases of malignancy or hormonal hypersecretion in 226 patients [52]. A prospective Finnish cohort study of 69 non-functioning, lipid-laden incidentalomas found no case of significant growth, malignancy or new autonomous hormone secretion at 5 years [51]. A large systematic review that included 1410 apparently benign incidentalomas estimated a 0.2% pooled risk for developing malignancy in such patients [68]. The very low rate of progression to malignancy has also been reported in other cohort studies [52]. At the extreme end of this argument, some authors have concluded that the risk of developing a fatal malignancy from the ionisation radiation associated with certain follow-up protocols is equivalent to the risk of malignant transformation in an adrenal incidentaloma [68].

When considering the development of autonomous hormone secretion as the end point of follow-up it has been suggested that any tumour over 3 cm confers an increased risk of developing hyperfunction, although this may be confined to the first 2 years of follow-up [69]. The risk of an apparently benign incidental tumour developing 'autonomous cortisol secretion' is estimated at between 0 and 11.6% [3], with the highest figure corresponding to a study reporting greater than 5-year follow-up [26]; a systematic review, however, suggests a pooled risk of developing Cushing's syndrome at only 0.3% [68]. The risk of non-functioning tumours developing a Conn's adenoma or a phaeochromocytoma is lower still at 0–2%, respectively [3]. Taking both this and the associated risk of malignancy into account, Libè et al. suggest 6-monthly follow-up for the first 2 years followed by annual screening [69]. Other groups have reported that for small, benign lesions at baseline, follow-up regimens, both hormonal and radiological, do not increase the sensitivity for a diagnosis of hypersecretion or malignancy [52]. More recent consensus guidelines have recommended against follow-up imaging of clearly benign, non-functioning tumours of <4 cm [3]. These guidelines also suggest repeating a non-contrast CT or MRI scan at 6–12 months for indeterminate lesions, with surgical resection proposed in those exhibiting enlargement of >20% during this time interval [3]. Interval growth of ≤20% should undergo an additional scan within 6–12 months [3]. The exact interval between scans should be guided by the MDT and the perceived risk of malignancy. A period of 12 months would be adequate in indeterminate lesions with a low risk of malignancy, reducing to 6 or even 3 months in patients with an elevated risk, based on the initial radiological findings or clinical scenario. In such cases, a lack of interval growth is seen as an indicator of benignity.

Clinical Pearl

- Every MDT needs to write its own policy regarding follow-up. A policy of discharging patients in whom there is no interval growth for lesions <4 cm can be justified.

Follow-up protocols for adrenal incidentaloma have been well tolerated by patients. A patient-reported quality-of-life study bolted on to a prospective Swedish study that followed up non-progressive adrenal incidentalomas for 2 years, and reported reassuring patient satisfaction levels [70]. Although only 4% of 111 patients reported the follow-up programme as a negative experience, these patients were more likely to report anxiety [70]. However, a retrospective Chinese study stated that >80% of patients undergoing surveillance chose to undergo adrenalectomy due to anxiety relating to potential malignant change, including two-thirds of those with a tumour <4 cm [45].

Clinical Pearl

- Clinicians should be mindful that even when they have no concerns regarding malignancy/ hyperfunction, this episode of clinical evaluation can lead to significant anxiety for the patient.

Despite the fact that both diagnostic and follow-up protocols for adrenal tumours are becoming more widely available as the evidence base expands, the vast majority of adrenal incidentalomas are ignored. In one Dutch study, based on a cancer centre, the rate of adrenal incidentalomas in 356 scans was 7% [16]. Only 16% of these patients were referred for specialist endocrine investigations, and, following a focused re-evaluation of the scans, the rate of reported incidentaloma rose to 12%. A UK study that evaluated 4028 CT scans performed in district general hospitals reported an adrenal incidentaloma rate of 1.8% (75 patients) [71]. In common with the Dutch study, only 17% of the UK patients were referred for specialist review by an endocrine team, whilst 80% underwent absolutely no hormonal testing [71], with similar findings reported in US community hospitals [72].

References

1. Menegaux F, Chereau N, Peix J, Christou N, Lifante J, Paladino N, et al. Management of adrenal incidentaloma. J Visc Surg. 2014;151(5):355–64.
2. Berland L, Silverman S, Gore R, Mayo-Smith W, Megibow A, Yee J, et al. Managing incidental findings on abdominal CT: White Paper of the ACR Incidental Findings Committee. J Am Coll Radiol. 2010;7:754–73.
3. Fassnacht M, Arlt W, Bancos I, Dralle H, Newell-Price J, Sahdev A, et al. Management of adrenal incidentalomas: European Society of Endocrinology Clinical Practice Guideline in collaboration with the European Network for the Study of Adrenal Tumors. Eur J Endocrinol. 2016;175(2):G1–G34.
4. Barzon L, Sonino N, Fallo F, Palu G, Boscaro M. Prevalence and natural history of adrenal incidentalomas. Eur J Endocrinol. 2003;149:273–85.
5. Grumbach M, Biller B, Braunstein G, Campbell K, Carney J, et al. Management of the clinically inapparent adrenal mass ("incidentaloma"). Ann Intern Med. 2003;138(5):424–9.
6. Arnaldi G, Boscaro M. Adrenal incidentaloma. Best Pract Res Clin Endocrinol Metab. 2012;26(4):405–19.
7. Kaltsas G, Chrisoulidou A, Piaditis G, Kassi E, Chrousos G. Current status and controversies in adrenal incidentalomas. Trends Endocrinol Metab. 2012;23(12):602–9.
8. Kloos R, Gross M, Francis I, Korobkin M, Shapiro B. Incidentally discovered adrenal masses. Endocr Rev. 1995;16(4):460–84.
9. Herrera M, Grant C, van Heerden J, Sheedy P, Ilstrup D. Incidentally discovered adrenal tumours: an institutional perspective. Surgery. 1991;110:1014–21.
10. Zeiger M, Thompson B, Duh Q, Hamrahian A, Angelos P, Elaraj D, et al. American Association of Clinical Endocrinologists and American Association of Endocrine Surgeons medical guidelines for the management of adrenal incidentalomas. Endocr Pract. 2009;15(Suppl 1):S1–20.
11. Bertherat J, Mosnier-Pudar H, Bertagna X. Adrenal incidentalomas. Curr Opin Oncol. 2002;14(1):58–63.
12. Dinnes J, Bancos I, di Ruffano L, Chortis V, Davenport C, et al. Imaging for the diagnosis of malignancy in incidentally discovered adrenal masses: a systematic review and meta-analysis. Eur J Endocrinol. 2016;175:R51–64.
13. Song J, Chaudhry F, Mayo-Smith W. The incidental adrenal mass on CT: prevalence of adrenal disease in 1,049 consecutive adrenal masses in patients with no known malignancy. AJR Am J Roentgenol. 2008;190(5):1163–8.
14. Kim J, Bae K, Choi Y, Jeong J, Park K, Kim J, et al. Clinical characteristics for 348 patients with adrenal incidentaloma. Endocrinol Metab. 2013;28:20–5.
15. Ross N, Aron D. Hormonal evaluation of the patient with an incidentally discovered adrenal mass. N Engl J Med. 1990;323(20):1401–5.
16. Minnaar E, Human K, Henneman D, Nio C, Bisschop P, Nieveen J e a. An adrenal Incidentaloma: how often is it detected and what are the consequences? ISRN Radiol. 2013;2013:1.
17. Thompson G, Jn YW. Adrenal incidentaloma. Curr Opin Oncol. 2003;15(1):84–90.
18. Funder J, Carey R, Fardella C, Gomez-Sanchez C, Mantero F, Stowasser M, et al. Case detection, diagnosis, and treatment of patients with primary aldosteronism: an Endocrine Society Clinical Practice Guideline. J Clin Endocrinol Metab. 2008;93:3266–81.
19. Kumar S, Karthikeyan V, Manohar C, Sreelakshmi K, Shivalingaiah M. Adrenal schwannoma: a rare incidentaloma. J Clin Diag Res. 2016;10(8):PD01–2.
20. Khan I, Adlan M, Stechman M, Premawardhana L. A retroperitoneal leiomyosarcoma presenting as an adrenal incidentaloma in a subject on warfarin. Case Rep Endocrinol. 2015;2015:830814.
21. Lombardi C, Raffaelli M, Boniardi M, De Toma G, Marzano L, Miccoli P, et al. Adrenocortical carcinoma: effect of hospital volume on patient outcome. Langenbeck's Arch Surg. 2012;397(2):201–7.
22. F. Palazzo, A. Dickinson, B. Phillips, A. Sahdev, R. Bliss and A. Rasheed, et al. Adrenal surgery practice guidance for the UK 2016. 2016 [Online]. www.baets.org.uk/wp-content/uploads/Adrenal-Surgery-Practice-Guidance-for-the-UK-2016.pdf. Accessed 29 Jan 2017.
23. National Institutes of Health. NIH state-of-the-science statement on management of the clinically inapparent adrenal mass ("incidentaloma"). NIH Consens State Sci Statements. 2002;19(2):1–25.
24. Lenders J, Duh Q, Eisenhofer G, Gimenez-Roqueplo A, Grebe S, et al. Pheochromocytoma and paraganglioma: an Endocrine Society Clinical Practice Guideline. J Clin Endocrinol Metab. 2014;99(6):1915–42.
25. Di Dalmazi G, Vicennati V, Garelli S, Casadio E, Rinaldi E, Giampalma E, et al. Cardiovascular events and mortality in patients with adrenal incidentalomas that are either non-secreting or associated with intermediate phenotype or subclinical Cushing's syndrome: a 15-year retrospective study. Lancet Diabetes Endocrinol. 2014;2(5):396–405.
26. Morelli V, Reimondo G, Giordano R, Della Casa S, Policola C, Palmieri S, et al. Long-term follow-up in adrenal incidentalomas: an Italian multicentre study. J Clin Endocrinol Metab. 2014;99(3):827–34.
27. Giordano R, Marinazzo E, Berardelli R, Picu A, Maccario M, et al. Long-term morphological, hormonal, and clinical follow-up in a single unit on 118 patients with adrenal incidentalomas. Eur J Endocrinol. 2010;162:779–85.
28. Debono M, Bradburn M, Bull M, Harrison B, Ross R, Newell-Price J. Cortisol as a marker for increased mortality in patients with incidental adrenocortical adenomas. J Clin Endocrinol Metab. 2014;99(12):4462–70.
29. Boland G, Blake M, Hahn P, Mayo-Smith W. Incidental adrenal lesions: principles, techniques, and algorithms for imaging characterization. Radiology. 2008;249(3):756–75.

30. Boland G, Lee M, Gazelle G, Halpern E, McNicholas M, Mueller P. Characterization of adrenal masses using unenhanced CT: an analysis of the CT literature. Am J Roentgenol. 1998;171:201–4.
31. Wale D, Wong K, Viglianti B, Rubello D, Gross M. Contemporary imaging of incidentally discovered adrenal masses. Biomed Pharmacother. 2017;87:256–62.
32. Young W Jr. Conventional imaging in adrenocortical carcinoma: update and perspectives. Horm Cancer. 2011;2(6):341–7.
33. Bharwani N, Rockall A, Sahdev A, Gueorguiev M, Drake W, et al. Adrenocortical carcinoma: the range of appearances on CT and MRI. AJR Am J Roentgenol. 2011;196:W706–14.
34. Birsen O, Akyuz M, Dural C, Aksoy E, Aliyev S, Mitchell J, et al. A new risk stratification algorithm for the management of patients with adrenal incidentalomas. Surgery. 2014;156(4):959–65.
35. Foo E, Turner R, Wang K, Aniss A, Gill A, Sidhu S, et al. Predicting malignancy in adrenal incidentaloma and evaluation of a novel risk stratification algorithm. ANZ J Surg. 2018;88(3):E173–7.
36. Frilling A, Tecklenborg K, Weber F, Kuhl H, Muller S, Stamatis G, et al. Importance of adrenal incidentaloma in patients with a history of malignancy. Surgery. 2004;136(6):1289–96.
37. Boland G, Dwamena B, Jagtiani Sangwaiya M, Goehler A, Blake M, Hahn P, et al. Characterization of adrenal masses by using FDG PET: a systematic review and meta-analysis of diagnostic test performance. Radiology. 2011;259(1):117–26.
38. Caoili E, Korobkin M, Francis I, Cohan R, Platt J, Dunnick N, et al. Adrenal masses: characterization with combined unenhanced and delayed enhanced CT. Radiology. 2002;222(3):629–33.
39. Kunikowska J, Matyskiel R, Toutounchi S, Grabowska-Derlatka L, Koperski L, Krolicki L. What parameters from 18F-FDG PET/CT are useful in evaluation of adrenal lesions? Eur J Nucl Med Mol Imaging. 2014;41:2273–80.
40. Hahner S, Kreissl M, Fassnacht M, Haenscheid H, Bock S, et al. Functional characterization of adrenal lesions using [123I]IMTO-SPECT/CT. J Clin Endocrinol Metab. 2013;98(4):1508–18.
41. Nieman L. Approach to the patient with an adrenal Incidentaloma. J Clin Endocrinol Metab. 2010;95(9):4106–13.
42. Williams A, Hammer G, Else T. Transcutaneous biopsy of adrenocortical carcinoma is rarely helpful in diagnosis, potentially harmful, but does not affect patient outcome. Eur J Endocrinol. 2014;170(6):829–35.
43. Lenert J, Barnett C Jr, Kudelka A, Sellin R, Gagel R, Prieto V, et al. Evaluation and surgical resection of adrenal masses in patients with a history of extra-adrenal malignancy. Surgery. 2001;130(6):1060–7.
44. Bancos I, Tamhane S, Shah M, Delivanis D, Alahdab F, Arlt W, et al. The diagnostic performance of adrenal biopsy: a systematic review and meta-analysis. Eur J Endocrinol. 2016;175:R65–80.
45. Ye Y, Yuan X, Chen M, Dai Y, Qin Z, Zheng F. Management of adrenal incidentaloma: the role of adrenalectomy may be underestimated. BMC Surg. 2016;16:41.
46. Terzolo M, Ali A, Osella G, Mazza E. Prevalence of adrenal carcinoma among incidentally discovered adrenal masses. A retrospective study from 1989 to 1994. Gruppo Piemontese Incidentalomi Surrenalici. Arch Surg. 1997;132(8):914–9.
47. Bermini G, Miccoli P, Moretti A, Vivaldi M, Iacconi P, Salvetti A. Sixty adrenal masses of large dimentions: hormonal and morphologic evaluation. Urology. 1998;51(6):920–5.
48. Kebebew E, Reiff E, Duh Q, Clark O, McMillan A. Extent of disease at presentation and outcome for adrenocortical carcinoma: have we made progress? World J Surg. 2006;30(5):872–8.
49. Mantero F, Terzolo M, Arnaldi G, Osella G, Masini A, Ali A. A survey on adrenal incidentaloma in Italy. Study Group on Adrenal Tumors of the Italian Society of Endocrinology. J Clin Endocrinol Metab. 2000;85(2):637–44.
50. Morelli V, Scillitani A, Arosio M, Chiodini I. Follow-up of patients with adrenal incidentaloma, in accordance with the European society of endocrinology guidelines: could we be safe? J Endocrinol Investig. 2017;40(3):331–3.
51. Schalin-Jantti C, Raade M, Hamalainen E, Sane T. A 5-year prospective follow-up study of lipid-rich adrenal Incidentalomas: no tumor growth or development of hormonal hypersecretion. Endocrinol Metab. 2015;30:481–7.
52. Muth A, Hammarstedt L, Hellstrom M, Sigurjonsdottir H, Almqvist E, Wangberg B, et al. Cohort study of patients with adrenal lesions discovered incidentally. Br J Surg. 2011;98(10):1383–91.
53. Toniato A, Merante-Boschin I, Opocher G, Pelizzo M, Schiavi F, Ballotta E. Surgical versus conservative management for subclinical Cushing syndrome in adrenal incidentalomas: a prospective randomized study. Ann Surg. 2009;249(3):388–91.
54. Tsuiki M, Tanabe A, Takagi S, Naruse M, Takano K. Cardiovascular risks and their long-term clinical outcome in patients with subclinical Cushing's syndrome. Endocr J. 2008;55(4):737–45.
55. Iacobone M, Citton M, Viel G, Boetto R, Bonadio I, Mondi I. Adrenalectomy may improve cardiovascular and metabolic impairment and ameliorate quality of life in patients with adrenal incidentalomas and subclinical Cushing's syndrome. Surgery. 2012;152(6):991–7.
56. Donatini G, Caiazzo R, Do Cao C, Aubert S, Zerrweck C, El-Kathib Z, et al. Long-term survival after adrenalectomy for stage I/II adrenocortical carcinoma (ACC): a retrospective comparative cohort study of laparoscopic versus open approach. Ann Surg Oncol. 2014;21(1):284–91.

57. Mir M, Klink J, Guillotreau J, Long J, Miocinovic R, Kaouk J, et al. Comparative outcomes of laparoscopic and open adrenalectomy for adrenocortical carcinoma: single, high-volume Centre experience. Ann Surg Oncol. 2013;20(5):1456–61.
58. Miller B, Ammori J, Gauger P, Broome J, Hammer G, Doherty G. Laparoscopic resection is inappropriate in patients with known or suspected adrenocortical carcinoma. World J Surg. 2010;34(6):1380–5.
59. Miller B, Gauger P, Hammer G, Doherty G. Resection of adrenocortical carcinoma is less complete and local recurrence occurs sooner and more often after laparoscopic adrenalectomy than after open adrenalectomy. Surgery. 2012;152(6):1150–7.
60. Reibetanz J, Jurowich C, Erdodan I, Nies C, Rayes N, Dralle H, et al. Impact of lymphadenectomy on the oncological outcome of patients with adrenocortical carcinoma. Ann Surg. 2012;255(2):263–9.
61. Cooper A, Habra M, Grubbs E, Bednarski B, Ying A, Perrier N. Does laparoscopic adrenalectomy jeopardize oncologic outcomes for patients with adrenocortical carcinoma? Surg Endosc. 2013;27(11):4026–32.
62. Castinetti F, Taieb D, Henry J, Walz M, Guerin C, Brue T. Outcome of adrenal sparing surgery in heritable pheochromocytoma. Eur J Endocrinol. 2016;174(1):R9–18.
63. Nieman L. Update on subclinical Cushing's syndrome. Curr Opin Endocrinol Diabetes Obes. 2015;22(3):180–4.
64. Terzolo M, Bovio S, Pia A, Conton P, Reimondo G e a. Midnight serum cortisol as a marker of increased cardiovascular risk in patients with a clinically inapparent adrenal adenoma. Eur J Endocrinol. 2005;153:307–15.
65. Chiodini I, Viti R, Coletti F, Guglielmi G, Battista C e a. Eugonadal male patients with adrenal incidentalomas and subclinical hypercortisolism have increased rate of vertebral fractures. Clin Endocrinol. 2009;70(2):208–13.
66. Eller-Vainicher C, Morelli V, Ulivieri F, Palmieri S, Zhukouskaya V. Bone quality, as measured by trabecular bone score in patients with adrenal incidentalomas with or without subclinical hypercortisolism. J Bone Miner Res. 2012;27(10):2223–30.
67. Bulow B, Jansson SJC, Steen L, Thoren M, Wahrenberg H, et al. Adrenal incidentaloma- follow-up results from a Swedish prospective study. Eur J Endocrinol. 2006;154(3):419–23.
68. Cawood THP, O'Shea D, Cole D, Soule S. Recommended evaluation of adrenal incidentalomas is costly, has high false-positive rates and confers a risk of fatal cancer similar to the risk of the adrenal lesion becoming malignant; time for a rethink? Eur J Endocrinol. 2009;161:513–27.
69. Libe R, Dall'Asta C, Barbetta L, Baccarelli A, Beck-Peccoz P, Ambrosi B. Long-term follow-up study of patients with adrenal incidentalomas. Eur J Endocrinol. 2002;147(4):489–94.
70. Muth A, Taft C, Hammarstedt L, Bjorneld L, Hellstrom M, WAngberg B. Patient-reported impacts of a conservative management programme for the clinically inapparent adrenal mass. Endocrine. 2013;44(1):228–36.
71. Davenport E, Lang Ping Nam P, Wilson M, Reid A, Aspinall S. Adrenal incidentalomas: management in British district general hospitals. Postgrad Med J. 2014;90(1065):365–9.
72. Sahni P, Trivedi A, Omer A, Trivedi N. Adrenal incidentalomas: are they being worked up appropriately? J Community Hosp Intern Med Perspect. 2016;6:32913.

26 Cushing's Syndrome

Roy Lirov and Paul G. Gauger

Introduction

Cushing's syndrome is a rare clinical entity resulting from pathologic hypercortisolemia [1]. Patients may present along a spectrum of severity from classical signs and symptoms of cortisol excess to subclinical or entirely asymptomatic disease [1–3]. The most common endogenous causes are ACTH-producing pituitary adenomas, cortisol-secreting adrenal adenomas, and ectopic ACTH-secreting tumors [4, 5]. Arriving at an accurate diagnosis of the underlying etiology and initiating appropriate treatment in a timely manner are essential to preventing morbidity and mortality [6, 7]. Diagnostic evaluation requires a systematic approach and significant expertise [2, 4]. Although surgery is often the primary treatment modality, multispecialty care is often necessary for optimal outcomes [8].

Pathophysiology

Cortisol is produced in the adrenal cortex by iterative enzymatic modifications of its precursor cholesterol. The hypothalamic-pituitary-adrenal (HPA) axis upregulates cortisol production via pituitary secretion of adrenocorticotropic hormone (ACTH) and receives negative feedback by cortisol [9]. ACTH and cortisol are released in a circadian rhythm, with levels starting to rise at 3–4 a.m., peaking at approximately 8–9 a.m., and slowly tapering to a nadir near midnight [2, 4]. Loss of this diurnal pattern is a cardinal feature of Cushing's syndrome, and forms the basis for screening tests aimed at differentiating pathologic hypercortisolism from other conditions with overlapping clinical or biochemical findings [5]. Up to 95% of circulating cortisol is protein bound, mostly to cortisol-binding protein (CBG) [9, 10]. Non-pathologic increases in total cortisol can be observed in conditions affecting the level of CBG such as pregnancy and oral contraceptive use, an important consideration in laboratory testing [2, 5, 6]. Free, unbound cortisol is filtered by the kidneys and is in equilibrium with salivary cortisol [4, 11, 12]. At plasma levels exceeding 20 mcg/dL, free cortisol saturates CBG, resulting in precipitous increases in urinary levels [13].

Autonomous overproduction of cortisol due to intrinsic adrenal pathology such as a functional adrenocortical neoplasm or primary adrenal hyperplasia results in ACTH-independent hypercortisolism, with attendant suppression of pituitary corticotroph cells [1]. Alternatively, ACTH-producing lesions (most commonly pituitary adenomas) are responsible for secondary, ACTH-dependent hypercortisolism [4]. Effects of hypercortisolemia are

R. Lirov
Capital Surgeons Group, Austin, Texas, USA

P. G. Gauger (✉)
Division of Endocrine Surgery, Department of Surgery, Michigan Medicine, Ann Arbor, MI, USA
e-mail: pgauger@med.umich.edu

R. Parameswaran, A. Agarwal (eds.), *Evidence-Based Endocrine Surgery*,
https://doi.org/10.1007/978-981-10-1124-5_26

mediated by the affinity of cortisol for both glucocorticoid and mineralocorticoid receptors, which are widely expressed throughout the body [9, 14]. Hypercortisolemia causes profound derangements in metabolism and multimodal blockade of immune response [4, 9, 10]. Direct sequelae include insulin resistance, dyslipidemia, and hypertension, with attendant increases in atherosclerosis and cardiovascular risk profile as discussed below [2, 4, 15, 16]. Catabolism of skeletal muscle proteins to support increased gluconeogenesis by the liver results in severe proximal muscle weakness and physical deconditioning despite weight gain and truncal obesity [9]. Impaired immunity results from deficiencies in neutrophil and macrophage function, and downregulation of inflammatory cytokines [9, 17, 18]. An increase in procoagulant factors and decrease in fibrinolysis lead to a prothrombotic state [19, 20]. Hypercortisolemia also predisposes to bone mineral density loss by inhibiting osteoblast activity, and can have a profound effect on neuropsychiatric function [9, 10]. Hypercortisolism of any etiology may result in suppression of thyroid-stimulating hormone (TSH) and gonadotropins, and can lead to hypothyroidism and hypogonadotropic hypogonadism [4, 8, 21].

Etiologies

ACTH Dependent

Cushing's disease is the most common endogenous cause of Cushing's syndrome [4, 8]. This condition is usually caused by an ACTH-secreting adenoma of the pituitary gland, the vast majority of which are benign microadenomas, measuring <1 cm in diameter [2, 21]. These tumors are usually sporadic, but may be associated with familial isolated pituitary adenoma syndrome or multiple endocrine neoplasia type 1 [5]. A far less common cause of ACTH-dependent Cushing's syndrome, ectopic ACTH syndrome (EAS) is a rare paraneoplastic syndrome that has been observed with a variety of non-pituitary neuroendocrine tumors including small-cell lung cancer; neuroendocrine tumors of the bronchus, thymus, and pancreas; pheochromocytoma; and medullary thyroid cancer [22–25].

ACTH Independent

ACTH-independent hypercortisolism may be caused by a functional adrenocortical neoplasm or primary hyperplastic process of the adrenal cortex [2, 4]. Primary hyperplastic processes include ACTH-independent bilateral macronodular adrenal hyperplasia (AIMAH) and primary pigmented nodular adrenal disease (PPNAD) [26]. PPNAD is the pigmented form of micronodular adrenal hyperplasia [27, 28]. Familial in 50% of cases, PPNAD is the most common endocrine manifestation of Carney complex, an inherited multiple neoplasia syndrome featuring cutaneous lesions, cardiac myxomas, testicular tumors, and other manifestations [26, 29]. Characteristically, the adrenal glands of patients with PPNAD are normal in size or atrophic, but contain innumerable pigmented nodules measuring <1 cm [29, 30]. By contrast, AIMAH involves remarkable enlargement of both adrenal glands with many intraglandular nodules, each measuring up to 4 cm in diameter, although more diffuse enlargement may also be observed [26, 31]. Combined gland weight is commonly 5–10× that of normal adrenals, and weights up to 60-fold heavier (600 mg) have been reported [10]. Although most cases of AIMAH appear to be sporadic, several familial cases have been reported, and the disorder may also be rarely observed in patients with MEN1 and McCune–Albright syndrome [10, 11, 26, 32, 33].

In general, adrenal tumors are common and may result from a variety of etiologies, although the vast majority are benign and not hormonally active [34–36]. Adrenocortical neoplasms are usually monoclonal tumors that may be benign (adrenocortical adenoma) or malignant (adrenocortical carcinoma) [4, 37]. Over half of adrenocortical adenomas are nonfunctioning, although cortisol hypersecretion can be seen in up to 30% of cases [34]. Adrenocortical carcinoma is a rare but aggressive malignancy with a 5-year survival of only 40% for patients with resectable disease and median overall survival of only 2 years [38, 39]. Approximately half of adrenocortical carcinomas are hormonally functional, of which

50–80% produce glucocorticoid excess and 40–60% produce adrenal androgens [10, 40]. In approximately half of patients with hormonally active adrenocortical carcinoma concurrent production of both glucocorticoids and adrenal androgen may be observed [40].

In patients with ACTH-independent hypercortisolism of any cause, atrophy of uninvolved adrenal tissue as a result of ACTH suppression is observed. In patients with discrete adrenocortical tumors this phenomenon often manifests as contralateral gland atrophy, and in those with primary adrenal hyperplasia atrophic islands of adrenocortical cells between hyperplastic nodules may be observed [10, 26]. Chronic atrophy of residual adrenal tissue reflects that patients undergoing surgical management for Cushing's syndrome are at risk for postoperative adrenal insufficiency [10].

Epidemiology

It is generally accepted that most cases of Cushing's syndrome are iatrogenic, caused by administration of exogenous glucocorticoids [2, 4, 10, 28, 41]. The incidence of endogenous Cushing's syndrome was estimated at 2–3 cases per million person-years in two large European population-based studies, with a prevalence of 4 per 100,000 individuals [2, 42, 43]. The prevalence among patients with Cushing's-associated comorbidities may be substantially higher [2]. One study found that the rate of unsuspected Cushing's syndrome was 11% among elderly patients with osteoporosis and vertebral fractures. Among patients with obesity and poorly controlled diabetes in another study, prevalence of Cushing's syndrome was up to 2% [4]. In two large studies of patients with hypertension, a positive screening test for Cushing's syndrome was reported in 0.5–1% [2]. ACTH-dependent causes account for 80–85% of endogenous Cushing's syndrome, of which 75–80% are due to Cushing's disease and 15–25% are due to ectopic ACTH secretion [5]. Cushing's disease is more common in females, with a ratio of 3–4:1, whereas paraneoplastic ectopic ACTH syndrome does not seem to have a sex predisposition [24]. ACTH-independent etiologies cause Cushing's syndrome in 15–20% of cases, of which 90% are due to unilateral adrenal lesions [5]. It has been reported that one in five such lesions will prove malignant, although adrenocortical carcinoma is otherwise considered rare among cancers, with an estimated incidence of only 2.7 per 1,000,000 person-years, and is similarly uncommon among incidentally identified adrenal lesions [31].

Clinical Features and Presentation

Signs and symptoms of hypercortisolism are myriad and no individual feature is pathognomonic for Cushing's syndrome [4, 6, 18, 21, 41]. When a variety of manifestations are present in the setting of overt disease, the syndrome is unmistakable [2, 8]. However, cases involving more subtle or fewer features can present significant diagnostic challenges [6, 21]. The clinical features of Cushing's syndrome are presented in Table 26.1 [5]. The most common physical features are weight gain, which occurs in 70–95% of patients, and moon facies or facial plethora, which occur in 70–90% [5, 44]. Patients with a malignant cause of Cushing's syndrome may have a paraneoplastic wasting syndrome, which can mask weight gain [5, 10]. Characteristically, adiposity is centrally distributed (truncal obesity) with visceral fat that may be demonstrable as hepatosteatosis by CT in 20% of patients [45]. Patients may also display increased fat in the dorsocervical and supraclavicular regions, which is uncommon for normal individuals [4]. Hypertension is observed in 70–85% of patients, with a characteristic blunting of the nighttime decrease in blood pressure that is otherwise evident in normal individuals and even those with non-glucocorticoid-mediated hypertension [1, 16]. Hyperlipidemia is reported in 70% of patients [46], with measurable increases in very-low-density lipoprotein, low-density lipoprotein, and triglycerides, as well as decreases in high-density lipoprotein [47]. Insulin resistance is reported in 45–70% of patients [1, 5, 48],

Table 26.1 Manifestations of Cushing's syndrome in adults [6, 9, 10]

Symptoms
Easy bruising[a]
Proximal muscle weakness[a]
Weight gain
Irritability
Emotional lability
Impaired concentration/memory
Fatigue
Insomnia
Decreased libido
Menstrual dysfunction
Physical findings
Wide violaceous striae[a]
Facial plethora[a]
Moon facies
Truncal obesity/lipodystrophy
Dorsocervical fat pad
Supraclavicular fat pad
Thin skin
Acne
Hirsutism
Comorbidities
Hypertension
Glucose intolerance/diabetes mellitus
Osteoporosis/fractures
Hypokalemia
Fungal infectious

[a]Denotes more discriminatory for features for Cushing's syndrome

manifesting as glucose intolerance in 20–30% and overt diabetes in 30–40% [4, 5]. Neuropsychiatric disturbances are among the most common features in Cushing's syndrome, presenting in 70–85% of cases overall, with 80% of patients meeting the criteria for a major affective disorder including depression or bipolar [5, 49, 50]. These symptoms are often intermittent, distinguishing them from manifestations of non-glucocorticoid psychiatric illness, which are characteristically persistent [4]. Neuropsychiatric symptoms may correlate with the degree of hypercortisolemia and in severe cases suicidality and acute psychosis have been reported and may require emergent treatment [4, 8, 50–52]. Irritability may be one of the earliest findings, and other manifestations can include restlessness, insomnia, as well as impairments in memory and concentration [4, 21].

Although metabolic derangements and neuropsychiatric complaints are among the most common features of Cushing's syndrome, these manifestations are nonspecific by virtue of their high prevalence in the general population [5, 8]. Features that are more discriminatory for Cushing's syndrome are wide violaceous striae, easy bruising, proximal muscle weakness, and osteoporosis in younger populations [2, 53, 54]. Although striae are commonly seen in obesity or following pregnancy, when purple in color and exceeding 1 cm in width, these are highly suspicious for the presence of Cushing's syndrome [1, 2, 5, 6]. The presence of proximal muscle weakness may be assessed with directed questions about difficulty climbing stairs or squatting and reaching above shoulder level, performance of tasks such as rising from a chair without using the arms for assistance, and specific attention to testing the strength of proximal muscle groups on physical exam [4]. Decreases in bone mineral density or fractures are evident in 40–70% of patients with Cushing's syndrome and are particularly suspicious when occurring at a young age or in males [5]. Osteoporosis is reported in 50% of patients with Cushing's syndrome undergoing DEXA scan [55]. In males, a history of unexplained fractures may be the only evidence of Cushing's syndrome [4]. Males are also more likely to present with Cushing's syndrome at a younger age and in general tend to present with more overt manifestations of the syndrome [56]. Cushing's syndrome causes sexual dysfunction in up to 80% of patients, with menstrual irregularity seen in females and erectile dysfunction in males [5]. Infertility and decreased libido may be seen in both genders, although paradoxically libido may be increased in females due to mild virilization, which may also cause acne and hirsutism [4, 5, 21]. Severe virilization should always raise suspicion for adrenocortical carcinoma [4, 6, 40].

Although it is rarely a presenting sign of the disease, venous thromboembolism is prevalent in 2–3% of patients with Cushing's syndrome, occurring with an incidence approximately tenfold higher than that of the general population [19, 20, 57, 58]. Although routine prophylaxis against venous thromboembolism is not universally recommended in patients with Cushing's syndrome, hypercoagulability in this patient population is an important perioperative concern [19, 58, 59]. The powerful immunosuppressive effect of hypercortisolemia is another consideration in patients undergoing surgery for Cushing's syndrome due to its implications for impaired wound healing and predisposition to infection [4, 9, 60, 61]. A blunted inflammatory response due to hypercortisolemia may mask classic clinical signs such as fever or peritonitis in a patient presenting with severe infection or acute abdominal catastrophe [4, 9, 10, 60] (Figs. 26.1, 26.2, 26.3, 26.4, and 26.5).

The presentation of patients with Cushing's syndrome can vary significantly even among those with similar degrees of cortisol elevation [5, 62]. Most patients will present in middle adulthood with a selection of these clinical features that have gradually accumulated over years until the diagnosis is made [4, 42, 43]. Because of the diversity of features associated with Cushing's syndrome, patients may be seen for individual complaints by multiple subspecialists, among whom the suspicion for an endocrinopathy may be lower [6]. If the initial presentation lacks sufficiently compelling features to warrant further diagnostic evaluation for hypercortisolism, clinical follow-up is advised because the development of additional or progressive features over time increases the likelihood that Cushing's syndrome is present and should motivate laboratory evaluation at a subsequent visit [2]. Although Cushing's syndrome is often persistent and progressive, some patients may present with episodic symptoms (cyclical Cushing's syndrome) [2, 4]. In these cases, clinical and biochemical evidence of hypercortisolism is only present intermittently precluding a definitive diagnosis in the intervening periods of disease quiescence, underscoring the importance of scheduled follow-up. It is also important in the initial evaluation to differentiate the pathologic hypercortisolemia of Cushing's syndrome from states of physiologic hypercortisolemia secondary

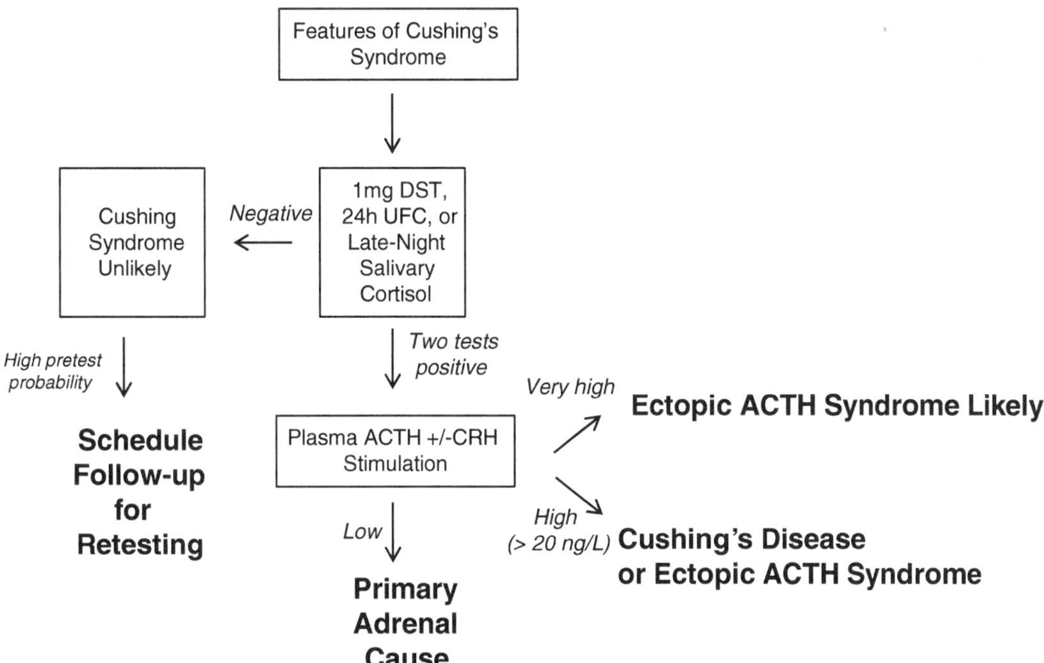

Fig. 26.1 Diagnostic algorithm for Cushing's syndrome [2, 6, 10, 111]

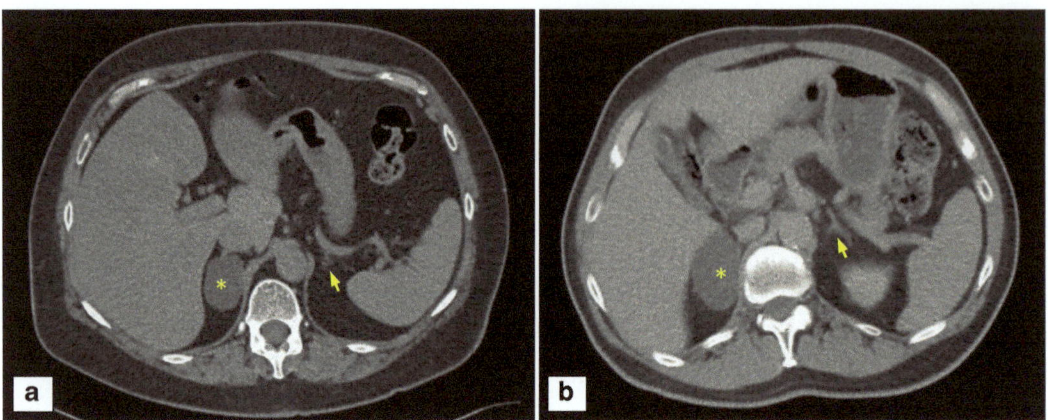

Fig. 26.2 Non-contrast axial CT scan of two different patients with right adrenocortical adenoma (asterisk). (**a**) Patient with Cushing's syndrome, notice atrophy of normal contralateral (left) adrenal gland (arrow). (**b**) Patient with nonfunctional adrenal adenoma, notice normal size of contralateral (left) adrenal gland (arrow)

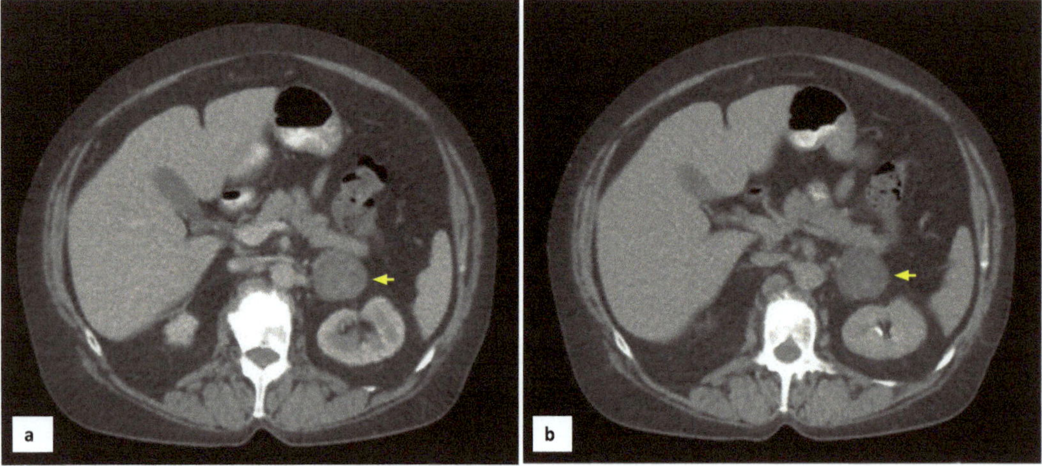

Fig. 26.3 Contrast-enhanced axial CT scan of a patient with left cortisol-producing adrenocortical adenoma (arrow) demonstrating rapid contrast washout (calculation below). (**a**) 60-second delay phase (attenuation 42 HU), (**b**) 15-min delay phase (attenuation 12 HU); notice atrophy of contralateral (right) adrenal gland. APW absolute percentage washout, RPW relative percentage washout

$$\text{APW} = \frac{\textit{CT Attenuation}\ (60\ \text{sec}) - \textit{CT Attenuation}\ (10-15\,\text{min})}{\textit{CT Attenuation}\ (60\ \text{sec}) - \textit{CT Attenuation}\ (\text{non-contrast})}$$

$$\left(\text{APW not calculated because non-contrastenhanced phase not available}\right)$$

$$\text{RPW} = \frac{\textit{CT Attenuation}\ (60\ \text{sec}) - \textit{CT Attenuation}\ (10-15\,\text{min})}{\textit{CT Attenuation}\ (60\ \text{sec})}$$

$$\text{RPW} = \frac{42-12}{42} = 71\%$$

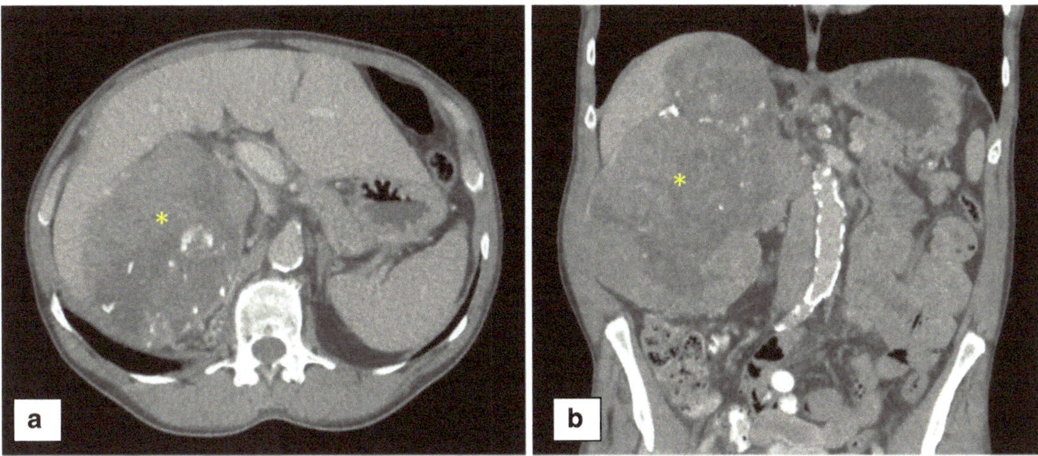

Fig. 26.4 CT scan of a patient with very large (18.1 cm) adrenocortical carcinoma of the right adrenal gland (asterisk). (**a**) Axial section, (**b**) coronal section; note border irregularity and local invasion, heterogeneous contrast enhancement, and internal calcifications

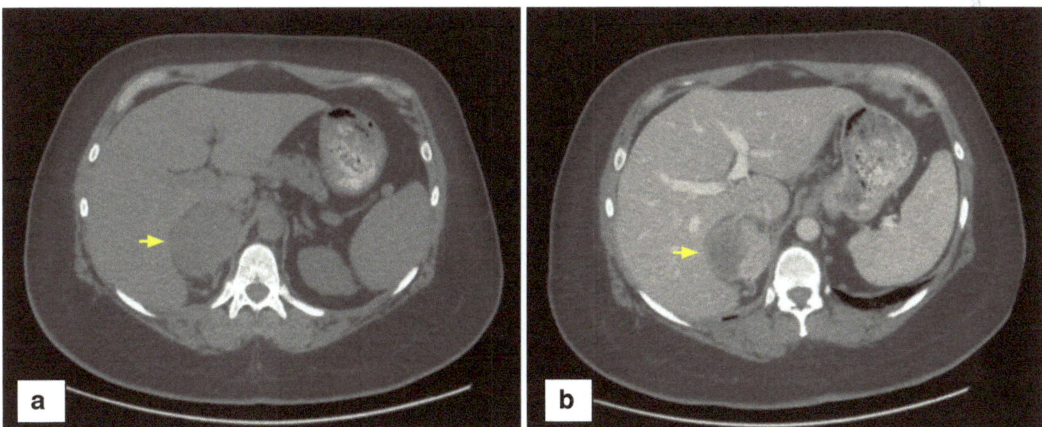

Fig. 26.5 CT scan of a patient with 5.8 cm adrenocortical carcinoma of the right adrenal gland (arrow). (**a**) Non-contrast enhanced. (**b**) Contrast enhanced (60-s delay) demonstrating heterogeneous contrast uptake and border irregularity

to another illness (so-called pseudo-Cushing's state) [2]. This is suggested by the concomitant presence of an acute illness or stressor, pregnancy, psychiatric disease, eating disorders, alcoholism, or morbid obesity [2, 5]. Overlapping clinical and biochemical features with true Cushing's syndrome may present a diagnostic challenge, but the hallmark of pseudo-Cushing's is resolution upon treatment of the underlying contributing illness [2, 4, 6].

To the extent that the clinical picture is dominated by features of hypercortisolism, Cushing's syndrome may present in an identical fashion regardless of underlying etiology, although specific manifestations of particular subtypes are noteworthy. Patients with enlarging pituitary macroadenomas may additionally complain of headaches and visual disturbances [4, 21]. Rare cases of invasive pituitary lesions may also cause cranial neuropathies or facial neuralgias [4]. Patients with ectopic ACTH syndrome may rapidly develop exceedingly high plasma ACTH levels (>500 pg/mL) and demonstrate urinary cortisol levels exceeding 10× the normal upper limit [4, 5, 10]. Acute onset of symptoms, hypokalemia, alkalosis, skin pigmentation, weight loss, and virilization are also classically described features of ectopic ACTH syndrome [4, 5, 10, 43, 60]. Weight loss and virilization may also be observed in patients with adrenocortical carcinoma [40]. Production of cortisol by adrenocortical cancers is often less efficient, and these lesions may be large enough to cause local symptoms such as palpable mass and abdominal pain by the time patients come to clinical attention for Cushing's syndrome [10, 39, 40]. Increasingly, patients are referred to surgeons for evaluation and management of incidentally identified adrenal lesions associated with biochemically evident hypercortisolism in the absence of compelling clinical features of Cushing's syndrome [3, 63, 64]. The quality of supporting evidence remains limited, but there is an evolving consensus that such patients are at elevated risk for cardiovascular consequences associated with hypercortisolism and appear to benefit from adrenalectomy [3, 63–68].

Initial Laboratory Evaluation

Appropriate diagnostic evaluation of patients for Cushing's syndrome requires a systematic approach and a thorough understanding of the utility and limitations of currently available laboratory tests [2, 69, 70]. Understanding when to initiate a diagnostic evaluation is an important first step [41]. Although some studies discussed previously show increased prevalence of Cushing's syndrome among groups with a subset of associated conditions, there are no conclusive data to justify screening for Cushing's syndrome in the general population [2, 5, 71]. Current guidelines recommend that initial screening for Cushing's syndrome be performed upon discovery of an adrenal incidentaloma or in patients presenting with clinical features of hypercortisolism [2, 35].

Prior to laboratory testing, a thorough history should be performed to rule out exogenous sources of glucocorticoids and to evaluate for conditions associated with pseudo-Cushing's syndrome [2, 4, 6]. Glucocorticoids are among the most commonly prescribed pharmaceuticals and a variety of preparations have been associated with development of exogenous Cushing's syndrome [2, 5, 59]. Endocrine Society Practice Guidelines recommend initial testing for Cushing's syndrome using any two of the following studies: 24-h urinary free cortisol, late-night salivary cortisol, or 1 mg dexamethasone suppression test (DST) [2]. Familiarity with the idiosyncrasies of each test is essential to increasing the likelihood of an accurate diagnostic result [2, 4, 6].

24-h urinary free cortisol is the only screening test for Cushing's syndrome that is independent of diurnal variation of cortisol secretion because it is an integrated assessment of tissue exposure to free cortisol over a 24-h period [4]. When performing this test, urine volume and creatinine must also be measured to ensure an appropriate collection. Fluid intake exceeding 5 l over the collection period can falsely elevate results [2, 6]. This test may be less sensitive in cases of mild hypercortisolism and may be less useful in the setting of an incidentaloma [2]. This test is also not recommended in patients with impaired renal function because cortisol clearance decreases linearly with GFR, potentially leading to false-negative results in patients with kidney disease [6]. In addition, choice of assay may influence results, as cross-reactivity between cortisol and its metabolites can be observed in immunoassays such as ELISA or RIA, but not structural based assays such as tandem mass spectrometry and high-performance liquid chromatography [2, 6].

The 1 mg DST detects the presence of an intact negative feedback loop in the HPA axis [4]. As described earlier, the diurnal pattern of cortisol secretion involves an ACTH-mediated rise in cortisol level beginning at 3–4 a.m. and peaking at 8–9 a.m. [2]. In the absence of Cushing's syndrome, a normally functioning HPA axis with an intact negative feedback loop will suppress this early morning secretion of ACTH in response to a supraphysiological dose of glucocorticoid administered late at night, whereas autonomous secretion of ACTH or cortisol will be exposed by detection of an unsuppressed morning cortisol level [4, 21]. The protocol involves administration of 1 mg of oral dexamethasone between 11 p.m. and midnight, followed by a serum cortisol level drawn between

8 and 9 a.m. the following morning [1, 2]. Morning serum cortisol level exceeding 1.8 mcg/dL is over 95% sensitive for Cushing's syndrome [8]. Although it is a reliable test with similar performance to the other screening studies, the 1 mg DST is the only study discussed that measures total cortisol rather than free cortisol, and is therefore more susceptible to variations in CBG that may occur in conditions such as liver disease, pregnancy, and oral contraceptive use [4, 9]. Another limitation is that dexamethasone is metabolized by the cytochrome enzyme CYP3A4 [6, 8]. Many common medications affect the activity of this enzyme complex and concurrent use of these drugs can lead to inaccurate results by affecting the availability of dexamethasone following administration of the standard dose [2].

Late-night salivary cortisol is an accurate and convenient study that assesses whether a nighttime nadir in cortisol is reached [4, 8]. Salivary cortisol is in equilibrium with free cortisol in the bloodstream and is unaffected by levels of CBG [8]. Saliva may be kept at room temperature following collection and is mailed by the patient to a laboratory [6]. The assay has a sensitivity of 92–100% and specificity of 93–100% [2]. False elevations may occur with smoking, chewing tobacco, or licorice use [2]. Stressful conditions such as depression or critical illness, and lifestyle affecting the timing of the sleep-wake cycle, can affect results as well [6].

A positive screening test warrants further evaluation by an endocrinologist at an institution with expertise in Cushing's syndrome [2]. Referral may also be beneficial in patients with compelling clinical features despite negative testing so that optimal second-line testing strategies may be selected, and repeated testing arranged when progression of disease is observed or if there is clinical suspicion for cyclical Cushing's syndrome [2, 8].

Subsequent Diagnostic Testing

Once the diagnosis of Cushing's syndrome is established, further testing begins with determination of a baseline plasma ACTH level, which may be followed by a corticotropin-releasing hormone (CRH)-stimulated level if initial results are in an indeterminate range between 10 and 20 ng/L [4, 21]. Baseline or CRH-stimulated plasma ACTH below 5–10 ng/L is consistent with suppression due to an ACTH-independent source of cortisol, whereas levels exceeding 20 ng/L suggest an ACTH-dependent process [4, 5, 10].

Cross-sectional abdominal imaging is obtained to assess for a primary adrenal lesion when ACTH-independent Cushing's syndrome is identified [4, 10]. Either CT or MRI may be used for initial imaging, and in such cases a unilateral adrenal lesion is most often identified. Bilateral adrenal enlargement with multiple nodules up to 5 cm in size is typical of AIMAH, whereas in PPNAD, normal or smaller-than-normal adrenal glands are observed [1, 10]. When initial imaging reveals a unilateral adrenal lesion, assessment of its malignant potential is essential for choosing appropriate surgical treatment [10]. Size is an important criterion, as the rate of adrenocortical cancer has been estimated at 2% in adrenal lesions smaller than 4 cm in diameter and 25% in lesions exceeding 6 cm [72, 73]. A CT performed under an adrenal protocol provides thin cuts at the level of the adrenal glands and contrast timing to assist further with determining malignant potential [74–76]. On the initial non-contrast phase, lipid-rich adrenal adenomas appear round and homogeneous, with distinct borders and enhancement of <10 Hounsfield units (HU) [75]. Otherwise similar lesions exceeding this attenuation threshold (>10 HU) may be further characterized by assessing the rate of contrast washout on delayed imaging: those demonstrating absolute percentage contrast washout >60% (or relative percentage washout >40%) may be classified as lipid-poor adenomas [40, 74, 76]. On T1-weighted chemical-shift MRI, benign lipid-rich adenomas characteristically demonstrate signal dropout from in- to out-of-phase images [40, 77, 78]. Adrenal tumors demonstrating heterogeneity, calcifications, or indistinct borders should be considered suspicious for adrenocortical cancer [79, 80]. Evidence of invasion, lymphadenopathy, or thrombosis in the adrenal vein is virtually diagnostic of malignancy [40]. Percutaneous biopsy of adrenal lesions in this setting is to be avoided as biopsy rarely provides beneficial clinical information and risks disseminating a contained malignancy [81].

When ACTH-dependent hypercortisolism is likely, studies directed at localizing the tumor to the pituitary or an ectopic source are necessary [5, 18]. In these cases, evaluation can be challenging and often requires both cross-sectional imaging and additional biochemical testing [2, 4, 21]. Gadolinium-enhanced pituitary MRI is preferred over CT for its higher sensitivity, and identifies a pituitary lesion in approximately 50% of such patients [2, 10]. However, most cases of Cushing's disease in adults are caused by microadenomas, which may be too small to identify on imaging. In addition, the incidence of pituitary incidentalomas in healthy individuals is approximately 10% [24, 82], and therefore the finding of a pituitary lesion in the setting of ACTH suppression may not be sufficient evidence of Cushing's disease. Where available, inferior petrosal sinus sampling (IPSS) with CRH stimulation is the recommended approach to assist with localization, but requires significant procedural expertise to execute reliably [8, 21]. Demonstration by IPSS of a central-to-peripheral ACTH ratio exceeding 2 (pre-CRH) and 3 (post-CRH) has a sensitivity of approximately 94% and specificity of nearly 100% for a pituitary source of ACTH [83, 84]. More widely accessible modalities include the high-dose dexamethasone suppression test and the CRH stimulation test, which rely on partial retention of native regulatory control among corticotroph adenomas [5, 8]. Pituitary tumors classically demonstrate suppression by glucocorticoids and stimulation by CRH to some extent, whereas ectopic ACTH-secreting tumors usually do not. These tests can be used to confirm the activity of a pituitary adenoma exceeding 6 mm on MRI, but reported diagnostic accuracies for these studies are significantly lower than for IPSS [5, 22, 85].

Identifying the source of an ectopic ACTH-secreting tumor can be challenging due to the many possible locations of such tumors [5, 18]. Both anatomic and functional imaging are typically used in this setting [86]. As described above, ectopic ACTH secretion can be caused by a variety of neuroendocrine tumors in various locations [22–25]. In a review of five retrospective studies, the most common causes of ectopic ACTH syndrome were bronchical carcinoid (23%), small-cell lung cancer, (22%), gastrointestinal/pancreatic neuroendocrine tumor (13%), thymic carcinoid (6.8%), medullary thyroid cancer (5.5%), pheochromocytoma/paraganglioma (3.4%), and disseminated neuroendocrine tumor with no known primary (6.5%) [22]. Imaging evaluation should be individualized and should include neck ultrasound to evaluate for medullary thyroid cancer and high-resolution contrast-enhanced CT of the chest to evaluate for small-cell lung cancer or bronchial carcinoid tumor [5]. Abdominal MRI or CT performed under a pancreas protocol can be used to identify neuroendocrine tumors of pancreas and include fine cuts at the level of the adrenal glands to evaluate for pheochromocytoma as well [86–88]. Endoscopic ultrasound can be a useful study for identification of occult pancreatic neuroendocrine tumors [88]. Although it is generally used as a biomarker for medullary thyroid cancer, calcitonin elevation has been reported in 44–75% of non-medullary thyroid tumors producing ACTH, and may be nonspecific in this setting [24]. Functional imaging including 111-In-pentetreotide scintigraphy (octreoscan) has been used to confirm activity in neuroendocrine tumors identified on anatomic imaging, and may occasionally identify tumors not detected on conventional studies [5, 86]. However, octreoscan has a reported sensitivity of only 49–60% in unselected patients [22–24]. Newer functional imaging techniques may have higher utility and are becoming more widely adopted in clinical practice, although sample sizes in studies reporting on their relative accuracies remain small. A recent systematic review of 107 case series and reports including 231 patients with ectopic ACTH syndrome demonstrated an overall sensitivity of 82% when utilizing 68-gallium-SSTR-PET/CT techniques including 18-F-fluorodopa, 68-Ga-DOTATATE, and 68-Ga-DOTATOC, with extremely high sensitivity reported for occult lesions in particular [86]. Despite an exhaustive imaging evaluation, ACTH-producing tumors may remain occult in 2–16% of cases [22–24].

Surgical Management of Cushing's Syndrome

General Considerations

Patients with Cushing's syndrome are at significantly elevated risk for morbidity and mortality [41]. In early series predating the widespread availability of effective treatment options, median survival for patients with Cushing's syndrome was only 4.6 years and 5-year survival was only 50%, with most deaths due to myocardial infarction, stroke, and infectious complications [2, 89]. Modern studies of patients with active Cushing's syndrome following attempted curative treatment demonstrate standardized mortality ratios of 1.7–5.0 times the general population [2, 8, 10, 42, 43]. Accumulation of additional features and progression of disease severity over time are characteristics of Cushing's syndrome [2, 4], and therefore early diagnosis and treatment are essential for minimizing morbidity and mortality [6, 7, 90].

Surgery is the primary treatment modality in the vast majority of cases of Cushing's syndrome. Successful treatment results in measurable improvements in standardized mortality, comorbidities, and healthcare-related quality of life [43, 91–96]. The degree of improvement following treatment is an area of ongoing investigation and depends on the underlying etiology, disease duration, and whether remission is achieved [10, 43, 57, 90]. In a study of 161 patients followed for an average of 8.7 years after successful treatment of Cushing's disease, survival was similar to age- and sex-matched controls [95]. Similarly, in another retrospective study of 289 patients, those with initial remission after transsphenoidal microsurgery for Cushing's disease had no statistically significant differences in long-term survival compared to the general population, whereas patients with persistent disease following surgery were shown to have increased mortality [94]. A retrospective study of 50 patients undergoing unilateral adrenalectomy for ACTH-independent Cushing's syndrome reported resolution of obesity in 60% and hypertension in 58%, as well as measurable improvements in bone mineral density. In that study, subjective recovery was reported in 96% of patients and long-term mortality was similar to the general population [97]. A recent meta-analysis including 688 patients with Cushing's disease and 109 patients with a benign adrenal adenoma causing Cushing's syndrome likewise reported no statistically significant difference in standardized mortality compared to the general population in patients undergoing successful surgical management for either condition, whereas those with persistent hypercortisolism following surgery for Cushing's disease had an increased standardized mortality ratio of 3.73 (95% CI 2.3–6.0) [98]. However, other studies demonstrate persistently elevated mortality following treatment of Cushing's syndrome regardless of remission status [57, 90–92], which may be explained in part by cardiovascular risk factors remaining elevated in long-term follow-up despite resolution of hypercortisolism [44, 99–101]. Regardless, it is clear that mortality and morbidity are significantly reduced following successful treatment of Cushing's syndrome, if not normalized [2, 43]. In addition, improvements in physical features, cardiovascular comorbidities [99, 102], bone mineral density [97, 103], cognitive status [93], and quality of life [96, 104] have all been demonstrated following successful treatment of Cushing's syndrome. The timeframe for resolution of individual features can be highly variable, from a few weeks to several years, and features such as psychiatric disturbances and quality-of-life impairments may persist in the long term [93, 97, 104–106].

The choice of operation depends on the underlying etiology and location of the offending lesion [8, 21]. In Cushing's disease, transsphenoidal endoscopic surgery (TSS) is the current modality of choice [10, 21], whereas unilateral adrenalectomy is used for cortisol-secreting primary adrenal tumors [4, 7]. In cases of ectopic ACTH syndrome, primary resection of the causative ACTH-producing lesion is recommended if oncologically appropriate [8, 22, 24]. Bilateral adrenalectomy may be used in selected patients with recurrent Cushing's disease, non-localized or unresectable tumors causing ectopic ACTH syndrome, or in primary adrenal hyperplasia due to either AIMAH or PPNAD [4, 21, 26]. Underlying etiology is the most important factor in determining outcome following surgery [90, 96, 97, 101, 107]. The highest rates of remission and lowest rates of recurrence are reported after surgical management of benign primary adrenal and pituitary lesions, whereas cure rates for adrenocortical carcinoma and ectopic ACTH-secreting tumors are often considerably lower and are dependent on tumor biology, stage at diagnosis, and completeness of resection [21, 23, 40, 96, 97, 101, 108].

Perioperative Considerations

The complexity of perioperative care of patients with hypercortisolism must not be underestimated [19, 21, 59, 109–112]. Patients undergoing operative management who have suffered from long-standing, severe hypercortisolism are highly susceptible to perioperative electrolyte and glucose instability, cardiac and infectious complications, venous thromboembolism, and impaired wound healing [8, 10, 59]. Severe physical deconditioning from a prolonged catabolic state impairs mobility and recovery, and may occasionally cause difficulties with postoperative ventilator weaning [5, 112]. In moderate-to-severe cases of hypercortisolism, initiating medical therapy and delaying surgery for several weeks may be necessary to partially reverse the catabolic effects of hypercortisolism, as increased perioperative mortality is observed in patients with poorly controlled cortisol levels preoperatively [10, 112–116].

Hypercoagulability is another important consideration in the perioperative period for patients with Cushing's syndrome [19]. In a systematic review, the rate of postoperative venous thromboembolism in patients undergoing surgery for Cushing's syndrome was up to 5.6% [57], with one study reporting a rate of 20% in patients undergoing surgery without perioperative prophylaxis [117]. Although an analysis of the Nationwide Inpatient Sample database reported that the rate of postoperative venous thromboembolism in a large cohort of patients undergoing surgery for Cushing's syndrome was only 0.7%, this risk was likely underestimated because patients with postoperative venous thromboembolism typically present after discharge, whereas this study reported only on in-hospital complications [57, 118]. In a review of four studies specifying the timeframe of postoperative venous thromboembolism in patients with Cushing's syndrome, 80% were reported within 4 weeks following surgery [19]. Postoperative prophylaxis against venous thromboembolism is routinely practiced by many institutions for patients with Cushing's syndrome and some have advocated for prolonged courses up to 4 weeks following surgery [19, 119]. Current treatment guidelines for Cushing's syndrome do not make specific recommendations in this regard, and therefore treatment should be individualized, weighing risk of venous thromboembolism against the potential for bleeding complications [8, 19, 21] (Tables 26.2 and 26.3).

After successful resection of the source of Cushing's syndrome, hypocortisolemia may ensue rapidly [10]. Adrenal insufficiency is an important cause of postoperative mortality and initiation of glucocorticoid replacement in the perioperative period is necessary, initially with hydrocortisone 50–100 mg delivered intravenously every 8 h [21, 59, 120]. After their immediate postoperative recovery, patients are transitioned to 10–25 mg of

Table 26.2 Etiologies of Cushing's syndrome [2, 6, 10, 111]

ACTH dependent
Cushing's disease (pituitary Cushing's syndrome)
Ectopic ACTH syndrome
ACTH independent
Adrenocortical adenoma
Adrenocortical carcinoma
Primary adrenal hyperplasias
Primary pigmented nodular adrenal disease (PPNAD)
ACTH-independent macronodular adrenal hyperplasia (AIMAH)

Table 26.3 Tumor types associated with ectopic ACTH syndrome [83, 84, 86]

Unfavorable prognosis
Small-cell lung cancer
Medullary thyroid cancer
Gastrinoma
Thymic carcinoid
Disseminated neuroendocrine tumor
Intermediate prognosis
Bronchial carcinoid
Pancreatic neuroendocrine tumor
Pheochromocytoma/paraganglioma
Occult primary

oral hydrocortisone (occasionally higher), divided over 2–3 doses daily (e.g., 10 mg in the morning, 10 mg at midday, and 5 mg in the evening) [1, 21]. In patients undergoing bilateral adrenalectomy lifelong replacement of both glucocorticoids and mineralocorticoids is necessary [10]. For those in whom functional adrenal tissue remains, it must be emphasized that chronic ACTH-independent hypercortisolemia leads to atrophy of uninvolved adrenal tissue [4, 21, 109, 110], and therefore recovery of the HPA axis following curative surgery for Cushing's syndrome may take up to 18 months or longer [8, 104, 110]. Glucocorticoid replacement is titrated in tandem with HPA axis recovery [8, 104, 110], and during this prolonged period of HPA axis recovery patients are at ongoing risk for life-threatening adrenal insufficiency during times of stress or illness [8]. All patients undergoing surgery for Cushing's syndrome should be educated regarding the signs of adrenal insufficiency such as fatigue, nausea, emesis, arthralgias, and headache [8]. Those at higher risk for this complication should be given a medic-alert bracelet and an emergency supply of injectable hydrocortisone in addition to their replacement dose with detailed instructions for use [21, 108, 121]. Patients undergoing bilateral adrenalectomy for the indications discussed below are at lifelong risk of adrenal insufficiency [10]. In a systematic review of patients undergoing bilateral adrenalectomy for Cushing's syndrome, adrenal insufficiency was reported in a median of 28% of cases, with a range of 9–64%, and was an important contributor to mortality in another series [112, 122].

Paradoxically, following establishment of eucortisolemia, patients often report initially feeling worse [8]. Patients that have acclimated to chronic supraphysiologic glucocorticoid levels experience a relative state of hypocortisolemia despite physiologic glucocorticoid replacement doses following surgery. In some cases, long-standing concurrent autoimmune disorders such as lupus, rheumatoid arthritis, psoriasis, and others that may have been quiescent due to the immunosuppressive effects of hypercortisolemia undergo reactivation following cure of Cushing's syndrome [8, 123–127]. Hypothyroidism and hypogonadism resulting from suppression of TSH and pituitary gonadotropins may resolve in tandem with HPA axis recovery and hormonal replacement may be necessary until recovery of these axes can be demonstrated [8].

Management of Cushing's Disease

Pituitary surgery is recommended as first-line treatment for patients confirmed to have Cushing's disease [8, 10, 21], and modern endoscopic TSS has supplanted older techniques for this procedure [21]. The operation should be performed by a neurosurgeon with significant experience to maximize the chance of remission and minimize morbidity. Among five modern studies published between 2007 and 2013, patients undergoing TSS for Cushing's disease experienced a median remission of 77%, with a range of 72–96%, and a median recurrence rate of 7.1% with a range of 0–15% [128–132]. Remission is associated with tumor size, surgeon experience, and younger patient age [8, 133, 134]. In a larger review of 74 studies including 6869 patients, those with macroadenomas were found to have lower median remission (64%), compared to patients with microadenomas (85%) [21]. Unsurprisingly, invasive pituitary tumors were found to have the lowest median rate of remission (43%), with a median recurrence of 25% [21]. Median time to recurrence overall was 41 months with a range of 1–345 months [21]. These data demonstrate that a significant proportion of patients undergoing curative treatment for Cushing's disease will require second-line treatment at some point in their course, and that postoperative surveillance for recurrence is necessary [5, 8, 135].

In general, TSS is considered a safe operation when performed by an experienced neurosurgeon, but complications following this procedure for patients with Cushing's syndrome are more frequent than for other indications [136–139]. In a review of 61 studies, median mortality following TSS for Cushing's syndrome was 0% with a range of 0–7.1%. The most common causes of postoperative death among these studies were myocardial infarction, pneumonia, and meningitis [21, 94, 140–145]. More common perioperative complications include diabetes insipidus (8%), cerebrospinal fluid leak (4.8%), visual disturbances (3.5%), meningitis (2.8%), sinusitis (2.3%), and syndrome of inappropriate antidiuretic hormone (2.2%) [21]. Other complications include adrenal insufficiency and venous thromboembolism. Recovery of the HPA axis may occur more rapidly (over a 6–12-month period) following surgery for Cushing's disease compared to other indications [8]. Finally, the rate of pituitary hormone deficiency following TSS increases with more extensive resection [21]. In patients undergoing hemi- or total hypophysectomy, the mean rates of hypopituitarism are 20% and 80%, respectively, whereas in seven studies in which selective adenomectomy was performed no cases of hypopituitarism were reported [146–151].

Management of recurrent Cushing's disease can be challenging, and the evidence available to guide treatment is limited [8, 135]. Treatment options for achieving eucortisolemia include reoperative pituitary surgery, radiation treatment, medical treatment, and bilateral adrenalectomy [8, 21]. Reoperative pituitary surgery has a higher rate of complications and lower remission rate compared to initial surgery but may be preferable in the setting of an obvious residual tumor on imaging [135, 152–155]. Pituitary radiotherapy may be considered as a second- or third-line option for refractory Cushing's disease in selected patients [8, 21, 135]. Disease control following pituitary radiotherapy is reported in 61% of patients with recurrence in 12%, and complications include hypopituitarism, optic neuropathy and other cranial nerve palsies, temporal lobe necrosis, cognitive impairment, cerebrovascular accident, and secondary brain tumors [21, 156]. Months to years may elapse before the treatment effect of radiotherapy is evident and therefore effective control of hypercortisolism should be established for such patients in the interim, typically with medical therapy [8].

In cases of severe or prolonged refractory disease, bilateral adrenalectomy has been used to effectively and rapidly control hypercortisolism [8, 21, 135, 156]. Bilateral adrenalectomy may also be an appropriate option for management of refractory Cushing's disease in reproductive-age females for whom avoiding the risk of infertility following repeat TSS or pituitary radiotherapy is the highest priority [21, 135]. In a recent systematic review of six studies involving patients undergoing bilateral adrenalectomy for recurrent Cushing's disease, surgical mortality was <1%, with a complication rate of 9% (range 0–44%) [21, 122]. A reported rate of hypercortisolism recurrence following bilateral adrenalectomy of <2% was attributed to residual adrenal tissue or adrenal rests [122]. Median long-term mortality in patients with refractory Cushing's disease undergoing bilateral adrenalectomy was 9% (range 0–45) at a median follow-up of 49 months (range 23–294) in a review of 20 studies involving 505 patients with this condition [122]. In light of these results, some authors have begun to advocate for earlier use of bilateral adrenalectomy in the setting of recurrent Cushing's disease [120, 122, 156–159]. The potential benefits of rapid control of hypercortisolemia must be weighed carefully against the potential for fatal long-term complications, including adrenal insufficiency and Nelson's syndrome [112, 116, 135]. Nelson's syndrome is a potentially fatal condition involving uncontrolled growth of pituitary corticotroph cells, presumably in response to removal of negative feedback inhibition following bilateral adrenalectomy, and is characterized by plasma ACTH levels exceeding 300 mg/dL and skin hyperpigmentation [21, 112, 160]. This condition was observed in a median of 22% (range 0–42%) of patients following bilateral adrenalectomy for Cushing's disease in studies specifically reporting this complication, and ongoing surveillance is therefore necessary for these patients [21, 112].

Management of Ectopic ACTH Syndrome

The underlying etiology of the ACTH-secreting lesion is the most important determinant of treatment and prognosis for patients with ectopic ACTH syndrome [23]. In two recent series involving 87 patients with ectopic ACTH syndrome, the proportion of patients with small-cell lung cancer was 18–21% [22, 23]. Largely influenced by the dismal prognosis of small-cell lung cancer, reported mortality rate in these series was 63%, whereas an earlier study containing only 3.3% of patients with small-cell lung cancer reported a much lower mortality rate of 21% [22–24]. Patients with ectopic ACTH syndrome caused by medullary thyroid cancer and gastrinoma also have a poor prognosis; however, survival for those with bronchial carcinoid, thymic carcinoid, neuroendocrine tumors of the appendix and pancreas, and occult ectopic ACTH-secreting tumors appears to be much better [24, 161, 162]. A determination of oncologic appropriateness and technical feasibility of surgery based on tumor type and stage at presentation should therefore heavily influence decision-making with regard to resection [8, 22, 24]. In two large recent series of patients with ectopic ACTH syndrome, the rate of curative resection was only 12–29% [24, 25]. Despite these discouraging figures overall, higher rates of cure have been observed in selected patient populations. In a review of 44 patients with ectopic ACTH syndrome cause by tumors other than small-cell lung cancer, operative cure was reported in 76% of patients with localized disease [163]. In another series, curative surgery attempted in 12 patients with ectopic ECTH syndrome caused by bronchial carcinoid was successful in 11 patients (83%) [23]. In addition to its effect on oncologic outcome, complete resection of the causative lesion should also induce remission of Cushing's syndrome [22, 24].

Patients with ectopic ACTH syndrome from an unmanageable primary source require an alternative modality to address their hypercortisolism [116]. Such a situation can be encountered if resection of the primary tumor is technically unfeasible or oncologically inadvisable, if sequelae of uncontrolled hypercortisolism prohibit highly stressful treatments for tumor control (e.g., definitive surgery, or chemotherapy), or if the ACTH-secreting lesion is occult [24, 116]. In these cases, medical management with steroidogenesis inhibition is an important adjunctive treatment, normalizing cortisol levels in about half of patients and relieving symptoms of hypercortisolism in approximately one-third [164]. When steroidogenesis inhibitors are not tolerated or ineffective, consideration should be given to bilateral adrenalectomy in patients with reasonable life expectancy [116, 165]. Due to physiologic compromise related to underlying malignancy and often severe hypercortisolism, morbidity and mortality rates for patients undergoing bilateral adrenalectomy for ectopic ACTH syndrome are higher than those reported in patients undergoing this procedure for other indications [122]. In a review of 23 studies of patients undergoing bilateral adrenalectomy for Cushing's syndrome, operative mortality was 4% among 130 patients with ectopic ACTH secretion, and overall median rate of surgical morbidity was 18% (range 6–31%) [122]. In 10 studies reporting long-term outcomes among 132 patients with ectopic ACTH syndrome undergoing bilateral adrenalectomy, median mortality rate was 39% (range 15–85%) at a median follow-up of 35 months, likely reflecting progression of underlying malignancy for these patients [122]. Despite the overall unfavorable prognosis for these patients, bilateral adrenalectomy can provide effective palliation by rapidly and definitively controlling life-threatening hypercortisolism with acceptable perioperative morbidity and mortality and is an important consideration for selected patients [112, 166]. A thoughtful assessment of clinical response must be made soon after the initiation of medical management for patients with severe disease, and early involvement of the surgical team is necessary because delay in definitive surgical treatment with bilateral adrenalectomy can lead to further decompensation and loss of treatment opportunity [116, 166]. Moreover, appropriate control of severe hypercortisolism may occasionally convert patients with ectopic ACTH syndrome who are otherwise at prohibitive risk for definitive management of their underlying tumor into candidates for curative treatment [116].

Management of Primary Adrenal Hyperplasia

Surgical management is indicated for both macronodular and micronodular forms of primary adrenal hyperplasia [8]. For patients with PPNAD, bilateral adrenalectomy is typically preferred [29, 167, 168]. In a retrospective review of 34 patients with PPNAD, those undergoing laparoscopic bilateral adrenalectomy had a complication rate of 7% and no reported perioperative mortality [167]. Long-term follow-up ranging 1–27 years was available in 25 patients, all of whom reported sustained improvement in symptoms of Cushing's syndrome. In addition to undergoing definitive surgical treatment for Cushing's syndrome, patients with PPNAD should be screened for other manifestations of Carney complex, especially cardiac myxoma, which may be present in over 50% of patients with this disorder and is an important cause of mortality [10, 26, 29, 167].

Bilateral adrenalectomy has also historically been the preferred approach for AIMAH because of the high likelihood of recurrence following unilateral resection [167, 169–172]. Whether the optimal initial approach should be bilateral or unilateral adrenalectomy has recently been contested however [8]. Several authors have recently reported long intervals of eucortisolemia following unilateral resection in patients with AIMAH, and therefore advocate a staged strategy in selected patients [169, 173–175]. Potential advantages of unilateral surgery including a reduced risk of adrenal insufficiency must be weighed against the likelihood of recurrence, factoring in patient preferences and values. In addition, particular subtypes of AIMAH with aberrant hormone receptors may respond to medical therapy, avoiding the need for surgery in certain situations [26]. The exceedingly rare nature of the primary adrenal hyperplasia syndromes precludes rigorous analysis to determine the optimal choice, and decision-making should therefore be individualized [8]. Patients with AIMAH undergoing unilateral adrenalectomy should be closely monitored for recurrence of Cushing's syndrome and offered staged contralateral adrenalectomy when it is encountered [8, 26, 169, 173–175].

Surgical Approach to Cortisol-Secreting Adrenocortical Tumors

Unilateral adrenalectomy is indicated for benign cortisol-secreting adrenal tumors unless perioperative risks are prohibitive [8, 176]. The rate of biochemical remission following unilateral adrenalectomy for cortisol-secreting adenoma has been reported at nearly 100% [8, 97]. Morbidity and mortality are favorable, particularly with minimally invasive approaches, which have essentially supplanted open surgery for benign-appearing adrenal lesions since the introduction of laparoscopic adrenalectomy in 1992 [10, 177–183]. Minimally invasive approaches include laparoscopic transperitoneal adrenalectomy, which is usually performed with the patient in a lateral decubitus position, and posterior retroperitoneoscopic adrenalectomy, performed with the patient in a modified prone position [184–186]. In the laparoscopic transperitoneal approach, access to the right adrenal gland is obtained by partial mobilization of the right lobe of the liver, and access to the left adrenal gland is obtained by a partial left-sided medial visceral rotation including the spleen, pancreas, and splenic flexure of the colon [184, 185]. Robotic assisted variations on either transperitoneal or retroperitoneal techniques may offer technical advantages in specific situations, but there is currently no compelling evidence demonstrating improved outcomes with these approaches [187].

Retrospective studies comparing outcomes of laparoscopic transperitoneal adrenalectomy to open approaches demonstrate decreased blood loss and transfusion requirement, lower utilization of parenteral pain medication, more rapid resumption of normal diet, shorter hospital length of stay, and more rapid return to work [19, 188–191]. In addition, postoperative pulmonary and wound infection are less commonly reported following laparoscopy compared with open approaches to adrenalectomy [188, 192]. Reported operative times in early studies were notably longer for laparoscopy compared with open approaches but decreased with experience, suggesting a measurable learning curve effect for the first 20–30 cases [181, 182, 190–192]. For patients with Cushing's syndrome undergoing open adrenalectomy, an increase in splenic injury and susceptibility to infectious and venous thromboembolism was historically reported [193]. By contrast, no increase in perioperative complications or mortality was demonstrated for the subset of patients with Cushing's syndrome (15–33%) among three recent 10-year retrospective studies of patients undergoing laparoscopic adrenalectomy for a variety of indications [179, 181, 182, 194].

Prior to the widespread adoption of laparoscopic adrenalectomy, the open posterior retroperitoneal approach was a preferred technique for resection of well-localized benign adrenal tumors [10, 189, 193, 195]. Posterior retroperitoneoscopic adrenalectomy, the minimally invasive analog to the posterior approach, was introduced by Walz in 1996 and has gained popularity after encouraging outcomes from several large series were reported [196–201]. In 2006, Walz et al. reported favorable operative results in a series of 560 posterior retroperitoneoscopic adrenalectomies for diverse indications, demonstrating no operative mortality, and a low rate of major complications (1.3%) [199]. Mean operative time was 67 ± 40 min, with significantly improved times later in the series consistent with a learning curve effect [199]. This group later reported no mortality and no major complications among 99 patients undergoing this procedure specifically for Cushing's syndrome, with a cure rate of 99% at a mean follow-up of 71 months [200]. Other series have also demonstrated low mortality and morbidity with this technique, and showed improved outcomes with increasing experience [45, 196–198, 202]. Posterior retroperitoneoscopic adrenalectomy can offer technical advantages in situations where peritoneal access and visceral mobilization may be hazardous, as may be the case for patients with numerous prior abdominal operations. In addition, transperitoneal laparoscopy may be somewhat less convenient compared to the posterior retroperitoneoscopic technique for bilateral adrenalectomy, as labor-intensive repositioning to the contralateral decubitus position is required during the procedure for access to the opposite adrenal gland [116, 198, 203]. Despite these advantages, several limitations are noteworthy. First, this procedure has historically been avoided in severely obese patients due to technical challenges with exposure and dissection. Although two recent series included a substantial proportion of patients with BMI in excess of 30 and reported favorable outcomes, the additional technical challenge is nonetheless an important consideration, particularly for surgeons on the earlier side of the learning curve [196, 200]. Second, surgeons with significant expertise in this technique have recommended its use be avoided in tumors exceeding 7 or 8 cm in diameter, in part because tumors above this threshold are difficult to manipulate [196, 199, 201]. In addition, the likelihood of malignancy increases substantially in tumors of this size, and capsular rupture of adrenocortical carcinoma has devastating consequences [40]. Finally, posterior retroperitoneoscopy may be an unfamiliar approach even to highly skilled laparoscopic surgeons accustomed to transperitoneal abdominal surgery, and formal training in this technique may be necessary prior to its adoption into practice to optimize outcome [45, 116, 196].

Robotically assisted techniques can be utilized for minimally invasive adrenalectomy via either transperitoneal or retroperitoneal approach [187, 204]. Advantages of robotically assisted procedures include magnified stereoscopic vision, improved ergonomics, instrument wrist articulation, and filtration of physiologic tremor [187]. However, two important drawbacks are loss of haptic feedback and cost [205]. Although numerous studies comparing robotically assisted techniques to conventional laparoscopy have been published, the quality of evidence remains low due to sample size, heterogeneity, and lack of randomization [205]. A recent meta-analysis of nine studies including 600 patients reported a statistically significant decrease in blood loss (25 cc), and hospital stay (0.5 days) for patients undergoing robotically assisted adrenalectomy compared to those undergoing conventional laparoscopy [206]. Transperitoneal and posterior retroperitoneoscopic approaches were considered together within each comparative arm, and accounted for approximately 75% and 25% of cases, respectively. The authors conclude that the clinical impact of these small differences in blood loss and hospital stay is unlikely to be significant [205, 206]. Currently, no compelling data justify widespread adoption of robotically assisted minimally invasive adrenalectomy in favor of conventional transperitoneal laparoscopy or posterior retroperitoneoscopic approaches, and additional study of this technique is necessary before definitive recommendations can be made.

Significant controversy surrounds the use of minimally invasive approaches in the surgical management of adrenocortical carcinoma. Adrenocortical carcinoma is a notoriously aggressive malignancy with poor survival in advanced disease [39, 207]. It is established that outcomes following resection of adrenocortical carcinoma depend on the oncologic quality of initial resection, and it is generally accepted that open adrenalectomy is the most appropriate approach for large or locoregionally advanced disease, assuming that resection is technically feasible [8, 40]. In such situations, the practical advantages of open surgery are wide exposure of the entire peritoneal cavity for examination, enhanced ability to mobilize the adrenal gland and perform a regional lymphadenectomy utilizing a no-touch technique, and facilitation of *en bloc* multivisceral resection when necessary to achieve an R0 resection without disturbing the tumor capsule [40, 208]. Smaller, localized adrenocortical carcinomas, while potentially amenable to minimally invasive approaches from a purely technical perspective, still pose significant risk of recurrence and mortality, and mandate an oncologically optimal operation [209, 210]. Concerns that the numerous practical challenges of minimally invasive surgery could increase the chance of an oncologically inferior operation, coupled with alarming reports of recurrence following laparoscopic resections of adrenocortical cancer led many experts to choose only open surgery for this difficult disease [208]. Retrospective analyses from large referral centers and multiple individual reports initially alerted investigators to devastating cases of peritoneal carcinomatosis following laparoscopic resections of adrenocortical carcinomas which occurred even after operations in which no intraoperative tumor spillage or capsular rupture was reported [209–211]. Among six patients with adrenocortical carcinoma resected laparoscopically and subsequently referred to MD Anderson Cancer Center, all either died of their disease or suffered recurrence, and four developed peritoneal carcinomatosis. In four of these patients no intraoperative adverse events were reported and in five patients tumor size was less than or equal to 6 cm, although all tumors were reported to have atypical radiographic features [210]. Likewise, Leboulleux et al. reported peritoneal carcinomatosis occurring in three of five patients undergoing laparoscopic adrenalectomy for adrenocortical carcinoma despite R0 resection [209]. Although both studies reported much higher rates of peritoneal carcinomatosis after laparoscopic adrenalectomy compared to open resection, inherent referral biases preclude definitive clinical conclusions based on these data alone despite statistical significance [209, 210]. Miller et al. reported a rate of margin positivity or tumor spillage of 50% in 17 patients undergoing laparoscopic adrenalectomy at outside institutions, compared to 18% for those undergoing open resection at the University of Michigan, despite larger tumor size for the latter group [211]. In addition, significantly shorter mean time to recurrence was demonstrated in patients treated with laparoscopic adrenalectomy compared to open resection, a surprising result given their smaller tumor size on averages. These findings underscore the challenges of achieving an adequate resection laparoscopically, as well as the consequences for failing to do so [208]. By contrast, more recent studies have reported statistically equivalent oncologic outcomes following resection of adrenocortical carcinoma via laparoscopic or open technique, but must be interpreted with great caution in light of methodological flaws and limited sample size [208, 212–217]. This debate is likely to continue as the rare nature of this malignancy has prevented large, randomized studies from definitively addressing this question to date. In the meantime, although minimally invasive adrenalectomy does offer substantial short-term benefits in morbidity and is an optimal approach for benign lesions, the potential tradeoff against the fatal consequences of an oncologically inadequate resection must be carefully considered.

Subclinical Cushing's Syndrome

Subclinical Cushing's syndrome is a pathologic state of mild hypercortisolism lacking clinically apparent features of Cushing's syndrome, with an estimated overall prevalence of 0.2–2% in adults [3, 66, 218, 219]. In early reports, subclinical Cushing's syndrome was considered "preclinical," although the rate of progression to fully developed Cushing's syndrome is now known to be less than 1% [220–224]. This syndrome is typically identified in the biochemical evaluation of patients with incidentally identified adrenal nodules (adrenal incidentalomas), which are found with increasing frequency due to improvements in cross-sectional imaging [36, 225]. Adrenal incidentalomas are reported at a rate of 4–7% in modern series, with a higher rate in the elderly (up to 10%) [36, 220, 222, 225–228]. These rates of detection match the prevalence reported in autopsy series from the 1960s to 1990s [225]. Reported rates of cortisol secretion attributed to adrenal incidentalomas are highly variable, ranging from 5 to 48% of cases [36, 64, 73, 221, 227, 229–235]. A recent meta-analysis of 1298 patients with adrenal incidentalomas reported a prevalence of apparent Cushing's syndrome in 0.7%, whereas subclinical Cushing's syndrome was reported in 6.3% [226].

A major limitation in the study of subclinical Cushing's syndrome has been the lack of consensus regarding its precise definition. The diagnosis hinges on demonstration of some degree of HPA axis suppression despite the absence of overt signs or symptoms of Cushing's syndrome [3, 66]. The inherent subjectivity in the clinical assessment for features of Cushing's syndrome produces significant diagnostic challenges however, as such cases are by their nature borderline, and some inter-observer variability between treating physicians is therefore expected [66]. The 1 mg DST is the most commonly used laboratory study for demonstrating HPA axis suppression in this setting, although the threshold for morning cortisol level has been the subject of ongoing discussion [231, 236, 237]. Recent series utilize a heterogeneous range from 1 to 5 mcg/dL [64, 67], with higher thresholds sacrificing sensitivity for specificity [3]. A variety of other criteria including suppression of ACTH, low DHEA-S, elevated 24-h urinary free cortisol, and several other clinical and laboratory criteria are used as adjuncts [64, 65, 67, 238–240].

Despite some of the diagnostic challenges, the clinical impact of subclinical Cushing's syndrome is increasingly recognized, with multiple retrospective studies reporting higher rates of metabolic syndrome, osteoporosis, and decreased quality of life in patients with this condition [232, 236, 239, 241–247]. In a recent study of 198 patients, investigators demonstrated that those with a morning cortisol level exceeding 1.8 mcg/dL after 1 mg DST had a higher prevalence of diabetes, osteoporosis, and fractures, as well as an increase in all-cause and cardiovascular mortality compared to patients with a nonfunctioning adrenal incidentaloma [236, 248].

The benefits of definitive surgical treatment for such patients are not yet fully understood [3, 64, 66]. Available studies aimed at addressing outcomes following unilateral adrenalectomy for subclinical Cushing's syndrome in the setting of an adrenal incidentaloma are small in size and mostly retrospective in nature [65, 67, 238, 249–251]. The only prospective, randomized study evaluating outcomes of adrenalectomy in this population included only 45 patients overall, of whom 23 were randomized for surgery by a single surgeon. Patients undergoing surgery demonstrated improvements in diabetes (63%), hypertension (67%), obesity (50%), and hyperlipidemia (38%), whereas none of those undergoing aggressive conservative management experienced any improvement [65]. These data were included as part of a meta-analysis of ten studies comparing unilateral adrenalectomy for subclinical Cushing's syndrome to conservative management, in which Bancos et al. reported a hazard ratio of 11.0 (95% CI 4.3–27.8) for improvement in hypertension, and a hazard ratio of 3.9 (95% CI 1.5–9.9) for improvement in diabetes. Trends for improvement in dyslipidemia and obesity were observed but did not achieve statistical significance [64].

Box 26.1
Available evidence suggests favorable outcomes following laparoscopic adrenalectomy for many patients with subclinical Cushing's syndrome. Based on the retrospective nature of most available studies and limitations of the only available RCT in this domain, the Sackett level of evidence is currently limited to 3a-2b. Establishing consensus criteria for the diagnosis of subclinical Cushing's syndrome will facilitate the collection of larger scale multi-institution data and the design of randomized studies to improve the strength of recommendations for patients with this condition.

Medical Management of Cushing's Syndrome

Medical therapy is an important component of the overall treatment strategy for many patients with Cushing's syndrome. A variety of medications may be considered for either their ability to directly lower cortisol levels or their effects on cortisol-related risk factors for morbidity or mortality [252]. Agents directed at lowering cortisol levels may be necessary for control of severe hypercortisolemia preoperatively or as definitive management for those who have failed surgery or whose perioperative risk profile is prohibitive [8, 26, 116]. Several glucocorticoid-directed medications that can be useful in these settings include ketoconazole, metyrapone, mifepristone, and occasionally etomidate or mitotane [164]. Medications acting on the pituitary that have been useful in Cushing's disease include cabergoline and pasireotide [5].

Ketoconazole is one of the commonly used inhibitors of steroidogenesis and is generally well tolerated, although hepatotoxicity may limit its use in some patients and careful monitoring during treatment is necessary [8, 252]. Ketoconazole requires stomach acidity for absorption and should not be used with proton pump inhibitors [5]. Efficacy is variable and may exceed 50% in patients with Cushing's disease, although results in patients with ectopic ACTH syndrome may be less satisfactory [8, 252]. Metyrapone is another steroidogenesis inhibitor which has demonstrated biochemical control and clinical improvement in over 50% of patients with Cushing's syndrome. Side effects of metyrapone are mostly gastrointestinal and are less common when taken with food, but due to its short half-life frequent dosing is necessary [8, 252]. Mitotane is both a steroidogenesis inhibitor and an adrenolytic agent that is used primarily for the treatment of advanced adrenocortical cancer [8]. It has been used in combination with other steroidogenesis inhibitors in severe situations as an alternative to bilateral adrenalectomy, but is highly teratogenic and may be stored for prolonged periods of time in adipose [8, 252]. Mifepristone is a glucocorticoid receptor antagonist and antiprogestin [5]. Mifepristone appears especially effective in improving blood glucose control due to hypercortisolism, but may be difficult to monitor as neither cortisol levels nor symptoms of adrenal insufficiency can be used to guide dosing, and titration must be performed instead of the basis of glucose control and weight loss [8, 253]. In addition, mineralocorticoid effects of mifepristone may lead to serious side effects such as worsening hypertension and hypokalemia, as well as endometrial hyperplasia in females [5]. Finally, etomidate is the only steroidogenesis inhibitor available as an infusion, and can be an ideal choice in rare situations of severe hypercortisolism in acutely ill patients in an ICU setting [5].

Cabergoline and pasireotide act directly on corticotroph tumors to decrease production of ACTH and their use is therefore limited to patients specifically with Cushing's disease [8]. Cabergoline is a dopamine agonist that has demonstrated a biochemical response in up to 40% of patients [8]. However, response may not be durable in a significant proportion of patients, and calcification of the cardiac valves may be observed as a side effect of this medication [252]. Pasireotide has been shown in large, randomized studies to normalize urinary cortisol in up to 26% of patients with sustained clinical responses. Side effects of pasireotide include hyperglycemia and suppression of growth hormone, which may worsen the overall catabolic state of nonresponders in particular [252].

Successful combination therapy utilizing a variety of these medications has been reported with potential pharmacologic advantages including synergy in mechanism of action and decrease in dosages of individual agents necessary to achieve clinical effect [252, 254]. Combination therapy may be used temporarily with down-titration of dose or discontinuation of agents following response [252]. Patients undergoing any treatment regimen directed at reducing cortisol levels should be monitored carefully for adrenal insufficiency and may require dose reduction, interruption, or initiation of glucocorticoid replacement depending on the clinical circumstances [8].

Patients with Cushing's syndrome often require medications directed at their numerous glucocorticoid-related comorbidities, an important consideration since many of these conditions may persist despite curative treatment as previously discussed [8]. Antihypertensives to consider include spironolactone (for its anti-mineralocorticoid effect), and angiotensin-converting enzyme inhibitors or angiotensin-receptor blockers given the prevalence of diastolic dysfunction and left ventricular hypertrophy in patients with Cushing's syndrome [252]. Additional medications may be necessary for glucose intolerance, dyslipidemia, osteoporosis, or psychiatric disorders [8].

Cushing's Syndrome in Children

Children account for only 7–10% of new cases of endogenous Cushing's syndrome, and most present before they are 5 years old [28, 31]. The most commonly reported features of Cushing's syndrome in children are weight gain with decreased linear growth trajectory [8, 28]. Plethora, headaches, delayed sexual development, and virilization may also be commonly reported; however, muscular weakness, insomnia, and memory impairment are less typical in children [28]. As in the adult population, pituitary causes of Cushing's syndrome are more common than primary adrenal lesions in children older than 7 years of age. In younger children, however, primary adrenal lesions are the more frequent etiology [28, 255]. The rate of adrenocortical malignancy in young children presenting with Cushing's syndrome and unilateral adrenal mass reportedly exceeds 65–70%, although the most common reasons children with adrenocortical malignancies come to clinical attention are abdominal mass and virilization [26, 256–259]. Macronodular adrenal hyperplasia and occasionally adrenal adenomas can be seen in association with McCune–Albright syndrome, a congenital disorder characterized by fibrous bony dysplasia, café-au-lait spots, and endocrine dysfunction usually consisting of precocious puberty. Although rarely described, the development of Cushing's syndrome in patients with McCune–Albright usually occurs before 6 months of age [260, 261].

A 24-h urine collection may be a challenging study to obtain in children, but 24-h urinary free cortisol has a sensitivity of 89% for Cushing's syndrome in this population [262]. Late-night salivary cortisol may be especially helpful in differentiating Cushing's syndrome from childhood obesity [8]. Results in children with Cushing's disease undergoing TSS are generally more favorable than for adults, with median remission of 80% (range 69–100%), and median recurrence of 6% [21, 33, 255, 263, 264]. Data on children undergoing surgery for primary adrenal lesions are limited, but as in adults indications for unilateral adrenalectomy include adrenocortical adenoma and carcinoma. Likewise, bilateral adrenalectomy is indicated for children with either micronodular or macronodular adrenal hyperplasia, selected patients with refractory Cushing's disease, or extremely rare cases of ectopic ACTH syndrome in children [256, 259, 265, 266]. Mean time to recovery of the HPA axis in a large series of children undergoing curative surgery for Cushing's syndrome was 12.6 ± 3.3 months [32]. In addition to suppression of pituitary gonadotropins, hypercortisolism in children may also lead to growth hormone deficiency, which may persist over a year after curative surgery and lead to missed growth targets [8, 267–269].

Cushing's Syndrome in Pregnancy

Hypercortisolism inhibits normal ovarian follicular development and ovulation, and can lead to amenorrhea and infertility [4, 8, 9, 270]. As a result of reproductive dysfunction associated with hypercortisolism, Cushing's syndrome is uncommon in pregnancy, with fewer than 150 cases reported, but carries significant risk of maternal and fetal morbidity and mortality [270, 271]. Cushing's syndrome in pregnancy presents unique diagnostic and management challenges despite presenting with many of the same features of hypercortisolism discussed previously [270, 271]. Expected physiologic changes of pregnancy such as weight gain, and pregnancy-related complications such as glucose intolerance, hypertension, and preeclampsia, can overlap with features of Cushing's syndrome [270]. Moreover, the accuracy of screening tests for Cushing's syndrome can be profoundly affected by several specific physiologic changes in pregnancy [2]. Increased production of CBG due to placental estrogens impairs the reliability of assays measuring total cortisol [2, 9]. Urine free cortisol excretion increases throughout the second and third trimesters, and levels up to threefold above the upper limit of normal can be seen in the absence of pathologic hypercortisolism [272]. In addition, poorly understood alterations in HPA axis function occur during normal gestation that result in a steady increase in plasma ACTH and blunted cortisol suppression after dexamethasone testing [272]. Safety concerns regarding the use of gadolinium, ionizing radiation, and MRI in early pregnancy also contribute to challenges in evaluating the pregnant patient with Cushing's syndrome [273, 274].

The distribution of etiologies accounting for Cushing's syndrome among pregnant patients differs from nonpregnant adults [272, 275]. In particular, the rate of adrenocortical adenomas appears to be 4–5-fold higher [10, 271]. In a review of 136 pregnancies occurring in patients with Cushing's syndrome, the most commonly reported etiologies were adrenocortical adenoma (41%), Cushing's disease (29%), and adrenocortical carcinoma (9%) [271]. Although supporting evidence is limited, surgical management (with either TSS or adrenalectomy as indicated by etiology) is generally recommended as first-line treatment in such cases [275]. Laparoscopic adrenalectomy is considered a safe operation in pregnancy; however, current guidelines recommend that pregnant patients be positioned in a modified left lateral decubitus position to reduce compression on the inferior vena cava, and that abdominal access technique and trocar placement be adjusted to accommodate fundal height [273, 275]. Although recently debated, the optimal timing of surgery for pregnant patients has traditionally been between the end of the first trimester up to the first half of the second trimester [270, 271, 273]. Medical therapy is an alternative modality, although available agents have important limitations [270, 271]. Mitotane is a powerful teratogen and should never be used in the setting of pregnancy [274]. Ketoconazole has reported teratogenic effects in animal studies accounting for its FDA category C classification, although its successful use has been reported in several cases of pregnant patients with Cushing's syndrome without observable adverse effect [271, 276]. By contrast, metyrapone is a generally well-tolerated agent with no known teratogenic effects, but its use in pregnancy may be limited by worsening hypertension leading to preeclampsia in some cases [176, 270]. In pregnant patients with Cushing's syndrome undergoing primary medical therapy, metyrapone has been advocated as a first-line agent, with ketoconazole reserved for refractory cases [271].

Summary

Cushing's syndrome is a rare state of pathologic cortisol excess that may result from a number of underlying etiologies and cause widespread clinical manifestations. Early recognition, accurate diagnosis, and effective management are essential to decreasing morbidity and mortality, but require significant clinical expertise and often multidisciplinary assessment.

References

1. Sharma ST, Nieman LK. Cushing's syndrome: all variants, detection, and treatment. Endocrinol Metab Clin North Am. 2011;40(2):379–91, viii–ix
2. Nieman LK, Biller BM, Findling JW, et al. The diagnosis of Cushing's syndrome: an Endocrine Society Clinical Practice Guideline. J Clin Endocrinol Metab. 2008;93:1526–40.
3. Nieman LK. Update on subclinical Cushing's syndrome. Curr Opin Endocrinol Diabetes Obes. 2015;22(3):180–4.
4. Juszczak A, Morris DG, Grossman AB, Nieman LK. Cushing's syndrome. In: Endocrinology: adult and pediatric. p. 227–255.e11.
5. Sharma ST, Nieman LK, Feelders RA. Cushing's syndrome: epidemiology and developments in disease management. Clin Epidemiol. 2015;7:281–93.
6. Nieman LK. Cushing's syndrome: update on signs, symptoms and biochemical screening. Eur J Endocrinol. 2015;173(4):M33–8.
7. Biller BM, Grossman AB, Stewart PM, et al. Treatment of adrenocorticotropin-dependent Cushing's syndrome: a consensus statement. J Clin Endocrinol Metab. 2008;93(7):2454–62.
8. Nieman LK, Biller BM, Findling JW, et al. Treatment of Cushing's syndrome: an endocrine society clinical practice guideline. J Clin Endocrinol Metab. 2015;100(8):2807–31.
9. Hall JE. Adrenocortical hormones. In: Guyton and Hall textbook of medical physiology. p. 965–82.
10. Porterfield JR, Thompson GB, Young WF Jr, Chow JT, Fryrear RS, van Heerden JA, et al. Surgery for Cushing's syndrome: an historical review and recent ten-year experience. World J Surg. 2008;32:659–77.
11. Mengden T, Hubmann P, Müller J, Greminger P, Vetter W. Urinary free cortisol versus 17-hydroxycorticosteroids: a comparative study of their diagnostic value in Cushing's syndrome. Clin Investig. 1992;70(7):545–8.
12. Evans PJ, Peters JR, Dyas J, Walker RF, Riad-fahmy D, Hall R. Salivary cortisol levels in true and apparent hypercortisolism. Clin Endocrinol (Oxf). 1984;20(6):709–15.
13. Nieman LK. Update in the medical therapy of Cushing's disease. Curr Opin Endocrinol Diabetes Obes. 2013;20(4):330–4.
14. Cidlowski JA, Malchoff CD, Malchoff DM. Glucocorticoid receptors, their mechanisms of action, and glucocorticoid resistance in endocrinology: adult and pediatric. p. 1718–26.e4.
15. Wei L, Macdonald TM, Walker BR. Taking glucocorticoids by prescription is associated with subsequent cardiovascular disease. Ann Intern Med. 2004;141(10):764–70.
16. Isidori AM, Graziadio C, Paragliola RM, et al. The hypertension of Cushing's syndrome: controversies in the pathophysiology and focus on cardiovascular complications. J Hypertens. 2015;33(1):44–60.
17. Scheffel RS, Dora JM, Weinert LS, et al. Invasive fungal infections in endogenous Cushing's syndrome. Infect Dis Rep. 2010;2(1):e4.
18. Chrousos GP. The hypothalamic-pituitary-adrenal axis and immunemediated inflammation. N Engl J Med. 1995;332:1351–62.
19. Van der pas R, Leebeek FW, Hofland LJ, De herder WW, Feelders RA. Hypercoagulability in Cushing's syndrome: prevalence, pathogenesis and treatment. Clin Endocrinol (Oxf). 2013;78(4):481–8.
20. van der Pas R, de Bruin C, Lee Beek FW, et al. The hypercoagulable state in Cushing's disease is associated with increased levels of procoagulant factors and impaired fibrinolysis, but is not reversible after short-term biochemical remission induced by medical therapy. J Clin Endocrinol Metab. 2012;97:1303–10.
21. Pivonello R, De Leo M, Cozzolino A, Colao A. The treatment of Cushing's disease. Endocr Rev. 2015;36(4):385–486.
22. Ejaz S, Vassilopoulou-Sellin R, Busaidy NL, et al. Cushing syndrome secondary to ectopic adrenocorticotropic hormone secretion: the University of Texas MD Anderson Cancer Center Experience. Cancer. 2011;117:4381–9.
23. Isidori AM, Kaltsas GA, Pozza C, et al. The ectopic adrenocorticotropin syndrome: clinical features, diagnosis, management, and long-term follow-up. J Clin Endocrinol Metab. 2006;91(2):371–7.

24. Ilias I, Torpy DJ, Pacak K, Mullen N, Wesley RA, Nieman LK. Cushing's syndrome due to ectopic corticotropin secretion: twenty years' experience at the National Institutes of Health. J Clin Endocrinol Metab. 2005;90(8):4955–62.
25. Aniszewski JP, Young WF, Thompson GB, Grant CS, Van Heerden JA. Cushing syndrome due to ectopic adrenocorticotropic hormone secretion. World J Surg. 2001;25(7):934–40.
26. Lacroix A, Bourdeau I. Bilateral adrenal Cushing's syndrome: macronodular adrenal hyperplasia and primary pigmented nodular adrenocortical disease. Endocrinol Metab Clin North Am. 2005;34:441–58.
27. Horvath A, Stratakis C. Primary pigmented nodular adrenocortical disease and Cushing's syndrome. Arq Bras Endocrinol Metabol. 2007;51(8):1238–44.
28. Stratakis CA. Cushing syndrome in pediatrics. Endocrinol Metab Clin North Am. 2012;41(4):793–803.
29. Correa R, Salpea P, Stratakis CA. Carney complex: an update. Eur J Endocrinol. 2015;173(4):M85–97.
30. Courcoutsakis N, Prassopoulos P, Stratakis CA. CT findings of primary pigmented nodular adrenocortical disease: Rare cause of ACTH-independent Cushing syndrome. Am J Roentgenol. 2010;194:W541.
31. James BC, Aschebrook-kilfoy B, Cipriani N, Kaplan EL, Angelos P, Grogan RH. The incidence and survival of rare cancers of the thyroid, parathyroid, adrenal, and pancreas. Ann Surg Oncol. 2016;23(2):424–33.
32. Lodish M, Dunn SV, Sinaii N, Keil MF, Stratakis CA. Recovery of the hypothalamic-pituitary-adrenal axis in children and adolescents after surgical cure of Cushing's disease. J Clin Endocrinol Metab. 2012;97(5):1483–91.
33. Storr HL, Alexandraki KI, Martin L, et al. Comparisons in the epidemiology, diagnostic features and cure rate by transsphenoidal surgery between paediatric and adult-onset Cushing's disease. Eur J Endocrinol. 2011;164(5):667–74.
34. Fassnacht M, Arlt W, Bancos I, et al. Management of adrenal incidentalomas: European Society of Endocrinology Clinical Practice Guideline in collaboration with the European Network for the Study of Adrenal Tumors. Eur J Endocrinol. 2016;175(2):G1–G34.
35. Nieman LK. Approach to the patient with an adrenal incidentaloma. J Clin Endocrinol Metab. 2010;95(9):4106–13.
36. Lee JM, Kim MK, Ko SH, et al. Clinical guidelines for the management of adrenal incidentaloma. Endocrinol Metab (Seoul). 2017;32(2):200–18.
37. Thiel A, Reis AC, Haase M, et al. PRKACA mutations in cortisol-producing adenomas and adrenal hyperplasia: a single-center study of 60 cases. Eur J Endocrinol. 2015;172(6):677–85.
38. Amini N, Margonis GA, Kim Y, et al. Curative resection of adrenocortical carcinoma: rates and patterns of postoperative recurrence. Ann Surg Oncol. 2016;23(1):126–33.
39. Chagpar R, Siperstein AE, Berber E. Adrenocortical cancer update. Surg Clin North Am. 2014;94(3):669–87.
40. Else T, Kim AC, Sabolch A, et al. Adrenocortical carcinoma. Endocr Rev. 2014;35(2):282–326.
41. Findling JW, Raff H. Cushing's syndrome: important issues in diagnosis and management. J Clin Endocrinol Metab. 2006;91(10):3746–53.
42. Etxabe J, Vazquez JA. Morbidity and mortality in Cushing's disease: an epidemiological approach. Clin Endocrinol (Oxf). 1994;40(4):479–84.
43. Lindholm J, Juul S, Jørgensen JO, et al. Incidence and late prognosis of Cushing's syndrome: a population-based study. J Clin Endocrinol Metab. 2001;86(1):117–23.
44. Faggiano A, Pivonello R, Spiezia S, et al. Cardiovascular risk factors and common carotid artery caliber and stiffness in patients with Cushing's disease during active disease and 1 year after disease remission. J Clin Endocrinol Metab. 2003;88(6):2527–33.
45. Lee CR, Walz MK, Park S, et al. A comparative study of the transperitoneal and posterior retroperitoneal approaches for laparoscopic adrenalectomy for adrenal tumors. Ann Surg Oncol. 2012;19(8):2629–34.
46. Arnaldi G, Scandali VM, Trementino L, Cardinaletti M, Appolloni G, Boscaro M. Pathophysiology of dyslipidemia in Cushing's syndrome. Neuroendocrinology. 2010;92(Suppl 1):86–90.
47. Friedman TC, Mastorakos G, Newman TD, et al. Carbohydrate and lipid metabolism in endogenous hypercortisolism: shared features with metabolic syndrome X and NIDDM. Endocr J. 1996;43(6):645–55.
48. Pivonello R, De leo M, Vitale P, et al. Pathophysiology of diabetes mellitus in Cushing's syndrome. Neuroendocrinology. 2010;92(Suppl 1):77–81.
49. Hudson JI, Hudson MS, Griffing GT, Melby JC, Pope HG. Phenomenology and family history of affective disorder in Cushing's disease. Am J Psychiatry. 1987;144(7):951–3.
50. Haskett RF. Diagnostic categorization of psychiatric disturbance in Cushing's syndrome. Am J Psychiatry. 1985;142(8):911–6.
51. Starkman MN, Schteingart DE. Neuropsychiatric manifestations of patients with Cushing's syndrome. Relationship to cortisol and adrenocorticotropic hormone levels. Arch Intern Med. 1981;141(2):215–9.
52. Dorn LD, Burgess ES, Dubbert B, et al. Psychopathology in patients with endogenous Cushing's syndrome: 'atypical' or melancholic features. Clin Endocrinol (Oxf). 1995;43(4):433–42.
53. Ross EJ, Linch DC. Cushing's syndrome—killing disease: discriminatory value of signs and symptoms aiding early diagnosis. Lancet. 1982;2(8299):646–9.
54. Pecori giraldi F, Pivonello R, Ambrogio AG, et al. The dexamethasone-suppressed corticotropin-releasing hormone stimulation test and the desmopressin test to distinguish Cushing's syndrome from

pseudo-Cushing's states. Clin Endocrinol (Oxf). 2007;66(2):251–7.
55. Kaltsas G, Manetti L, Grossman AB. Osteoporosis in Cushing's syndrome. Front Horm Res. 2002;30:60–72.
56. Pecori giraldi F, Moro M, Cavagnini F. Gender-related differences in the presentation and course of Cushing's disease. J Clin Endocrinol Metab. 2003;88(4):1554–8.
57. Clayton RN, Raskauskiene D, Reulen RC, et al. Mortality and morbidity in Cushing's disease over 50 years in Stokeon-Trent, UK: audit and meta-analysis of literature. J Clin Endocrinol Metabol. 2011;96:632–42.
58. Stuijver DJ, van Zaane B, Feelders RA, et al. Incidence of venous thromboembolism in patients with Cushing's syndrome: a multicenter cohort study. J Clin Endocrinol Metab. 2011;96:3525–32.
59. Domi R. Cushing's surgery: role of the anesthesiologist. Indian J Endocrinol Metab. 2011;15(Suppl 4):S322–8.
60. Sarlis NJ, Chanock SJ, Nieman LK. Cortisolemic indices predict severe infections in Cushing syndrome due to ectopic production of adrenocorticotropin. J Clin Endocrinol Metab. 2000;85:42–7.
61. Bakker RC, Gallas PR, Romijn JA, Wiersinga WM. Cushing's syndrome complicated by multiple opportunistic infections. J Endocrinol Invest. 1998;21(5):329–33.
62. Petersenn S, Newell-price J, Findling JW, et al. High variability in baseline urinary free cortisol values in patients with Cushing's disease. Clin Endocrinol (Oxf). 2014;80(2):261–9.
63. Lee SH, Song KH, Kim J, et al. New diagnostic criteria for subclinical hypercortisolism using postsurgical hypocortisolism: the Co-work of Adrenal Research study. Clin Endocrinol (Oxf). 2017;86(1):10–8.
64. Bancos I, Alahdab F, Crowley RK, et al. Therapy of endocrine disease: improvement of cardiovascular risk factors after adrenalectomy in patients with adrenal tumors and subclinical Cushing's syndrome: a systematic review and meta-analysis. Eur J Endocrinol. 2016;175(6):R283–95.
65. Boscaro M, Sonino N, Scarda A, et al. Anticoagulant prophylaxis markedly reduces thromboembolic complications in Cushing's syndrome. J Clin Endocrinol Metab. 2002;87:3662–6.
66. Iacobone M, Citton M, Scarpa M, Viel G, Boscaro M, Nitti D. Systematic review of surgical treatment of subclinical Cushing's syndrome. Br J Surg. 2015;102(4):318–30.
67. Iacobone M, Citton M, Viel G, et al. Adrenalectomy may improve cardiovascular and metabolic impairment and ameliorate quality of life in patients with adrenal incidentalomas and subclinical Cushing's syndrome. Surgery. 2012;152(6):991–7.
68. Akaza I, Yoshimoto T, Iwashima F, et al. Clinical outcome of subclinical Cushing's syndrome after surgical and conservative treatment. Hypertens Res. 2011;34(10):1111–5.
69. Nieman L. Pitfalls in the diagnosis and differential diagnosis of Cushing's syndrome. Clin Endocrinol (Oxf). 2014;80(3):333–4.
70. Arnaldi G, Angeli A, Atkinson AB, Bertagna X, Cavagnini F, Chrousos GP, et al. Diagnosis and complications of Cushing's syndrome: a consensus statement. J Clin Endocrinol Metab. 2003;88:5593–602.
71. Budyal S, Jadhav SS, Kasaliwal R, et al. Is it worthwhile to screen patients with type 2 diabetes mellitus for subclinical Cushing's syndrome? Endocr Connect. 2015;4(4):242–8.
72. Sturgeon C, Shen WT, Clark OH, Duh QY, Kebebew E. Risk assessment in 457 adrenal cortical carcinomas: how much does tumor size predict the likelihood of malignancy? J Am Coll Surg. 2006;202(3):423–30.
73. NIH state-of-the-science statement on management of the clinically inapparent adrenal mass ("incidentaloma"). NIH Consens State Sci Statements. 2002;19(2):1–25.
74. Slattery JM, Blake MA, Kalra MK, et al. Adrenocortical carcinoma: contrast washout characteristics on CT. AJR Am J Roentgenol. 2006;187:W21–4.
75. Korobkin M, Brodeur FJ, Yutzy GG, et al. Differentiation of adrenal adenomas from nonadenomas using CT attenuation values. Am J Roentgenol. 1996;166:531–6.
76. Caoili EM, Korobkin M, Francis IR, Cohan RH, Dunnick NR. Delayed enhanced CT of lipid-poor adrenal adenomas. AJR Am J Roentgenol. 2000;175:1411–5.
77. Haider MA, Ghai S, Jhaveri K, Lockwood G. Chemical shift MR imaging of hyperattenuating (>10 HU) adrenal masses: does it still have a role? Radiology. 2004;231:711–6.
78. Rockall AG, Babar SA, Sohaib SA, et al. CT and MR imaging of the adrenal glands in ACTH-independent cushing syndrome. Radiographics. 2004;24(2):435–52.
79. Johnson PT, Horton KM, Fishman EK. Adrenal mass imaging with multidetector CT: pathologic conditions, pearls, and pitfalls. Radiographics. 2009;29:1333–51.
80. Bharwani N, Rockall AG, Sahdev A, et al. Adrenocortical carcinoma: the range of appearances on CT and MRI. AJR Am J Roentgenol. 2011;196:W706–14.
81. Williams AR, Hammer GD, Else T. Transcutaneous biopsy of adrenocortical carcinoma is rarely helpful in diagnosis, potentially harmful, but does not affect patient outcome. Eur J Endocrinol. 2014;170(6):829–35.
82. Hall WA, Luciano MG, Doppman JL, Patronas NJ, Oldfield EH. Pituitary magnetic resonance imaging in normal human volunteers: occult adeno-

mas in the general population. Ann Intern Med. 1994;120(10):817–20.
83. Newell-price J, Trainer P, Besser M, Grossman A. The diagnosis and differential diagnosis of Cushing's syndrome and pseudo-Cushing's states. Endocr Rev. 1998;19(5):647–72.
84. Wind JJ, Lonser RR, Nieman LK, Devroom HL, Chang R, Oldfield EH. The lateralization accuracy of inferior petrosal sinus sampling in 501 patients with Cushing's disease. J Clin Endocrinol Metab. 2013;98(6):2285–93.
85. Valassi E, Swearingen B, Lee H, et al. Concomitant medication use can confound interpretation of the combined dexamethasone-corticotropin releasing hormone test in Cushing's syndrome. J Clin Endocrinol Metab. 2009;94(12):4851–9.
86. Isidori AM, Sbardella E, Zatelli MC, et al. Conventional and nuclear medicine imaging in ectopic Cushing's syndrome: a systematic review. J Clin Endocrinol Metab. 2015;100(9):3231–44.
87. Dunnick NR, Avram A, Mendiratta-lala M, Turcu AF. Adrenal Imaging. Endocrinol Metab Clin North Am. 2017;46(3):741–59.
88. Masciocchi M. Pancreatic Imaging. Endocrinol Metab Clin North Am. 2017;46(3):761–81.
89. Plotz CM, Knowlton AI, Ragan C. The natural history of Cushing's syndrome. Am J Med. 1952;13:597–614.
90. Ntali G, Asimakopoulou A, Siamatras T, et al. Mortality in Cushing's syndrome: systematic analysis of a large series with prolonged follow-up. Eur J Endocrinol. 2013;169(5):715–23.
91. Dekkers OM, Horváth-puhó E, Jørgensen JO, et al. Multisystem morbidity and mortality in Cushing's syndrome: a cohort study. J Clin Endocrinol Metab. 2013;98(6):2277–84.
92. Bolland MJ, Holdaway IM, Berkeley JE, et al. Mortality and morbidity in Cushing's syndrome in New Zealand. Clin Endocrinol (Oxf). 2011;75:436–42.
93. Lindsay JR, Nansel T, Baid S, Gumowski J, Nieman LK. Long-term impaired quality of life in Cushing's syndrome despite initial improvement after surgical remission. J Clin Endocrinol Metab. 2006;91(2):447–53.
94. Hammer GD, Tyrrell JB, Lamborn KR, et al. Transsphenoidal microsurgery for Cushing's disease: initial outcome and long-term results. J Clin Endocrinol Metab. 2004;89(12):6348–57.
95. Swearingen B, Biller BM, Barker FG, et al. Long-term mortality after transsphenoidal surgery for Cushing disease. Ann Intern Med. 1999;130(10):821–4.
96. Pikkarainen L, Sane T, Reunanen A. The survival and well-being of patients treated for Cushing's syndrome. J Intern Med. 1999;245(5):463–8.
97. Iacobone M, Mantero F, Basso SM, Lumachi F, Favia G. Results and long-term follow-up after unilateral adrenalectomy for ACTH-independent hypercortisolism in a series of fifty patients. J Endocrinol Invest. 2005;28(4):327–32.
98. Graversen D, Vestergaard P, Stochholm K, Gravholt CH, Jørgensen JO. Mortality in Cushing's syndrome: a systematic review and meta-analysis. Eur J Intern Med. 2012;23(3):278–82.
99. Arnaldi G, Mancini T, Polenta B, Boscaro M. Cardiovascular risk in Cushing's syndrome. Pituitary. 2004;7(4):253–6.
100. Colao A, Pivonello R, Spiezia S, et al. Persistence of increased cardiovascular risk in patients with Cushing's disease after five years of successful cure. J Clin Endocrinol Metab. 1999;84(8):2664–72.
101. Mishra AK, Agarwal A, Gupta S, Agarwal G, Verma AK, Mishra SK. Outcome of adrenalectomy for Cushing's syndrome: experience from a tertiary care center. World J Surg. 2007;31:142532.
102. Fallo F, Sonino N, Barzon L, et al. Effect of surgical treatment on hypertension in Cushing's syndrome. Am J Hypertens. 1996;9(1):77–80.
103. Hermus AR, Smals AG, Swinkels LM, et al. Bone mineral density and bone turnover before and after surgical cure of Cushing's syndrome. J Clin Endocrinol Metab. 1995;80(10):2859–65.
104. Sippel RS, Elaraj DM, Kebebew E, Lindsay S, Tyrrell JB, Duh QY. Waiting for change: symptom resolution after adrenalectomy for Cushing's syndrome. Surgery. 2008;144(6):1054–60.
105. Ragnarsson O, Berglund P, Eder DN, Johannsson G. Long-term cognitive impairments and attentional deficits in patients with Cushing's disease and cortisol-producing adrenal adenoma in remission. J Clin Endocrinol Metab. 2012;97(9):E1640–8.
106. Van aken MO, Pereira AM, Biermasz NR, et al. Quality of life in patients after long-term biochemical cure of Cushing's disease. J Clin Endocrinol Metab. 2005;90(6):3279–86.
107. Yaneva M, Kalinov K, Zacharieva S. Mortality in Cushing's syndrome: data from 386 patients from a single tertiary referral center. Eur J Endocrinol. 2013;169(5):621–7.
108. Imai T, Funahashi H, Tanaka Y, Tobinaga J, Wada M, Morita-Matsuyama T, et al. Adrenalectomy for treatment of Cushing syndrome: results in 122 patients and long-term followup studies. World J Surg. 1996;20:7816.
109. Di dalmazi G, Berr CM, Fassnacht M, Beuschlein F, Reincke M. Adrenal function after adrenalectomy for subclinical hypercortisolism and Cushing's syndrome: a systematic review of the literature. J Clin Endocrinol Metab. 2014;99(8):2637–45.
110. Kulshreshtha B, Arora A, Aggarwal A, Bhardwaj M. Prolonged adrenal insufficiency after unilateral adrenalectomy for Cushing's Syndrome. Indian J Endocrinol Metab. 2015;19(3):430–2.
111. Kissane NA, Cendan JC. Patients with Cushing's syndrome are care-intensive even in the era of laparoscopic adrenalectomy. Am Surg. 2009;75:279–83.
112. Prajapati OP, Verma AK, Mishra A, Agarwal G, Agarwal A, Mishra SK. Bilateral adrenalectomy

for Cushing's syndrome: pros and cons. Indian J Endocrinol Metab. 2015;19(6):834–40.
113. Berruti A, Fassnacht M, Haak H, et al. Prognostic role of overt hypercortisolism in completely operated patients with adrenocortical cancer. Eur Urol. 2014;65(4):832–8.
114. Park HS, Roman SA, Sosa JA. Outcomes from 3144 adrenalectomies in the United States: which matters more, surgeon volume or specialty? Arch Surg. 2009;144:1060–7.
115. Abiven G, Coste J, Groussin L, et al. Clinical and biological features in the prognosis of adrenocortical cancer: poor outcome of cortisol-secreting tumors in a series of 202 consecutive patients. J Clin Endocrinol Metab. 2006;91(7):2650–5.
116. Morris LF, Harris RS, Milton DR, et al. Impact and timing of bilateral adrenalectomy for refractory adrenocorticotropic hormone-dependent Cushing's syndrome. Surgery. 2013;154(6):1174–83.
117. Small M, Lowe GD, Forbes CD, Thomson JA. Thromboembolic complications in Cushing's syndrome. Clin Endocrinol (Oxf). 1983;19(4):503–11.
118. Patil CG, Lad SP, Harsh GR, Laws ER, Boakye M. National trends, complications, and outcomes following transsphenoidal surgery for Cushing's disease from 1993 to 2002. Neurosurg Focus. 2007;23(3):E7.
119. Sackett DL, Straus SE, Richardson WS, et al. Evidence-based medicine: how to practice and teach EBM. 2nd ed. Edinburgh: Churchill Livingstone; 2000. p. 173–7.
120. Katznelson L. Bilateral adrenalectomy for Cushing's disease. Pituitary. 2015;18(2):269–73.
121. Charmandari E, Nicolaides NC, Chrousos GP. Adrenal insufficiency. Lancet. 2014;383(9935):2152–67.
122. Ritzel K, Beuschlein F, Mickisch A, Osswald A, Schneider HJ, Schopohl J, et al. Clinical review: outcome of bilateral adrenalectomy in Cushing's syndrome: a systematic review. J Clin Endocrinol Metab. 2013;98:3939–48.
123. Yakushiji F, Kita M, Hiroi N, Ueshiba H, Monma I, Miyachi Y. Exacerbation of rheumatoid arthritis after removal of adrenal adenoma in Cushing's syndrome. Endocr J. 1995;42(2):219–23.
124. Takasu N, Komiya I, Nagasawa Y, Asawa T, Yamada T. Exacerbation of autoimmune thyroid dysfunction after unilateral adrenalectomy in patients with Cushing's syndrome due to an adrenocortical adenoma. N Engl J Med. 1990;322(24):1708–12.
125. Raccah D, Zeitoun C, Lafforgue P, et al. [Inflammatory rheumatism flare-up after surgical treatment of Cushing's disease: two cases]. Rev Med Interne. 1992;13(4):302–4.
126. Walmsley D, Bevan JS. Suppression of medical conditions by Cushing's syndrome. BMJ. 1995;310(6993):1537.
127. Steuer A, Cavan DA, Lowy C. Sarcoidosis presenting after resection of an adrenocortical adenoma. BMJ. 1995;310(6979):567–8.
128. Berker M, Işikay I, Berker D, Bayraktar M, Gürlek A. Early promising results for the endoscopic surgical treatment of Cushing's disease. Neurosurg Rev. 2013;37:105–14.
129. Starke RM, Reames DL, Chen CJ, Laws ER, Jane JA. Endoscopic transsphenoidal surgery for Cushing disease: techniques, outcomes, and predictors of remission. Neurosurgery. 2013;72(2):240–7.
130. Alahmadi H, Cusimano MD, Woo K, et al. Impact of technique on Cushing disease outcome using strict remission criteria. Can J Neurol Sci. 2013;40(3):334–41.
131. Wagenmakers MA, Boogaarts HD, Roerink SH, et al. Endoscopic transsphenoidal pituitary surgery: a good and safe primary treatment option for Cushing's disease, even in case of macroadenomas or invasive adenomas. Eur J Endocrinol. 2013;169(3):329–37.
132. Dehdashti AR, Gentili F. Current state of the art in the diagnosis and surgical treatment of Cushing disease: early experience with a purely endoscopic endonasal technique. Neurosurg Focus. 2007;23(3):E9.
133. Petersenn S, Beckers A, Ferone D, et al. Therapy of endocrine disease: outcomes in patients with Cushing's disease undergoing transsphenoidal surgery: systematic review assessing criteria used to define remission and recurrence. Eur J Endocrinol. 2015;172(6):R227–39.
134. Ramm-pettersen J, Halvorsen H, Evang JA, et al. Low immediate postoperative serum-cortisol nadir predicts the short-term, but not long-term, remission after pituitary surgery for Cushing's disease. BMC Endocr Disord. 2015;15:62.
135. Bertagna X, Guignat L. Approach to the Cushing's disease patient with persistent/recurrent hypercortisolism after pituitary surgery. J Clin Endocrinol Metab. 2013;98(4):1307–18.
136. Zada G, Governale LS, Laws ER. Intraoperative conversion from endoscopic to microscopic approach for the management of sellar pathology: incidence and rationale in a contemporary series. World Neurosurg. 2010;73(4):334–7.
137. Blevins LS, Christy JH, Khajavi M, Tindall GT. Outcomes of therapy for Cushing's disease due to adrenocorticotropin-secreting pituitary macroadenomas. J Clin Endocrinol Metab. 1998;83(1):63–7.
138. Ciric I, Ragin A, Baumgartner C, Pierce D. Complications of transsphenoidal surgery: results of a national survey, review of the literature, and personal experience. Neurosurgery. 1997;40(2):225–36.
139. Laws ER. Pituitary surgery. Endocrinol Metab Clin North Am. 1987;16(3):647–65.
140. Hofmann BM, Hlavac M, Martinez R, Buchfelder M, Müller OA, Fahlbusch R. Long-term results after microsurgery for Cushing disease: experience with 426 primary operations over 35 years. J Neurosurg. 2008;108(1):9–18.
141. Yap LB, Turner HE, Adams CB, Wass JA. Undetectable postoperative cortisol does not always predict long-term remission in Cushing's disease: a single centre audit. Clin Endocrinol (Oxf). 2002;56(1):25–31.

142. Rees DA, Hanna FW, Davies JS, Mills RG, Vafidis J, Scanlon MF. Long-term follow-up results of transsphenoidal surgery for Cushing's disease in a single centre using strict criteria for remission. Clin Endocrinol (Oxf). 2002;56(4):541–51.
143. Mampalam TJ, Tyrrell JB, Wilson CB. Transsphenoidal microsurgery for Cushing disease. A report of 216 cases. Ann Intern Med. 1988;109(6):487–93.
144. Fahlbusch R, Buchfelder M, Müller OA. Transsphenoidal surgery for Cushing's disease. J R Soc Med. 1986;79(5):262–9.
145. Boggan JE, Tyrrell JB, Wilson CB. Transsphenoidal microsurgical management of Cushing's disease. Report of 100 cases. J Neurosurg. 1983;59(2):195–200.
146. Locatelli M, Bertani G, Carrabba G, et al. The trans-sphenoidal resection of pituitary adenomas in elderly patients and surgical risk. Pituitary. 2013;16(2):146–51.
147. Ammini AC, Bhattacharya S, Sahoo JP, et al. Cushing's disease: results of treatment and factors affecting outcome. Hormones (Athens). 2011;10(3):222–9.
148. Jagannathan J, Smith R, Devroom HL, et al. Outcome of using the histological pseudocapsule as a surgical capsule in Cushing disease. J Neurosurg. 2009;111(3):531–9.
149. Esposito F, Dusick JR, Cohan P, et al. Clinical review: Early morning cortisol levels as a predictor of remission after transsphenoidal surgery for Cushing's disease. J Clin Endocrinol Metab. 2006;91(1):7–13.
150. Bakiri F, Tatai S, Aouali R, et al. Treatment of Cushing's disease by transsphenoidal, pituitary microsurgery: prognosis factors and long-term follow-up. J Endocrinol Invest. 1996;19(9):572–80.
151. Salassa RM, Laws ER, Carpenter PC, Northcutt RC. Transsphenoidal removal of pituitary microadenoma in Cushing's disease. Mayo Clin Proc. 1978;53(1):24–8.
152. Kelly DF. Transsphenoidal surgery for Cushing's disease: a review of success rates, remission predictors, management of failed surgery, and Nelson's Syndrome. Neurosurg Focus. 2007;23(3):E5.
153. Liu JK, Fleseriu M, Delashaw JB, Ciric IS, Couldwell WT. Treatment options for Cushing disease after unsuccessful transsphenoidal surgery. Neurosurg Focus. 2007;23(3):E8.
154. Ram Z, Nieman LK, Cutler GB, Chrousos GP, Doppman JL, Oldfield EH. Early repeat surgery for persistent Cushing's disease. J Neurosurg. 1994;80(1):37–45.
155. Friedman RB, Oldfield EH, Nieman LK, et al. Repeat transsphenoidal surgery for Cushing's disease. J Neurosurg. 1989;71(4):520–7.
156. Reincke M, Ritzel K, Oßwald A, et al. A critical reappraisal of bilateral adrenalectomy for ACTH-dependent Cushing's syndrome. Eur J Endocrinol. 2015;173(4):M23–32.
157. Smith PW, Turza KC, Carter CO, Vance ML, Laws ER, Hanks JB. Bilateral adrenalectomy for refractory Cushing disease: a safe and definitive therapy. J Am Coll Surg. 2009;208(6):1059–64.
158. Thompson SK, Hayman AV, Ludlam WH, Deveney CW, Loriaux DL, Sheppard BC. Improved quality of life after bilateral laparoscopic adrenalectomy for Cushing's disease: a 10-year experience. Ann Surg. 2007;245(5):790–4.
159. Hawn MT, Cook D, Deveney C, Sheppard BC. Quality of life after laparoscopic bilateral adrenalectomy for Cushing's disease. Surgery. 2002;132(6):1064–8.
160. Gil-Cárdenas A, Herrera MF, Díaz-Polanco A, Rios JM, Pantoja JP. Nelson's syndrome after bilateral adrenalectomy for Cushing's disease. Surgery. 2007;141:147–52.
161. Neary NM, Lopez-chavez A, Abel BS, et al. Neuroendocrine ACTH-producing tumor of the thymus--experience with 12 patients over 25 years. J Clin Endocrinol Metab. 2012;97(7):2223–30.
162. Barbosa SL, Rodien P, Leboulleux S, et al. Ectopic adrenocorticotropic hormone-syndrome in medullary carcinoma of the thyroid: a retrospective analysis and review of the literature. Thyroid. 2005;15(6):618–23.
163. Zeiger MA, Pass HI, Doppman JD, et al. Surgical strategy in the management of non-small cell ectopic adrenocorticotropic hormone syndrome. Surgery. 1992;112(6):994–1000.
164. Valassi E, Crespo I, Gich I, Rodríguez J, Webb SM. A reappraisal of the medical therapy with steroidogenesis inhibitors in Cushing's syndrome. Clin Endocrinol (Oxf). 2012;77(5):735–42.
165. Chow JT, Thompson GB, Grant CS, Farley DR, Richards ML, Young WF. Bilateral laparoscopic adrenalectomy for corticotrophin-dependent Cushing's syndrome: a review of the Mayo Clinic experience. Clin Endocrinol (Oxf). 2008;68(4):513–9.
166. Chand G, Agarwal AK, Agarwal GK, Verma AK, Mishra A, Mishra SK. Improved quality of life after bilateral laparoscopic adrenalectomy for Cushing's disease. Ann Surg. 2008;247(5):906.
167. Powell AC, Stratakis CA, Patronas NJ, et al. Operative management of Cushing syndrome secondary to micronodular adrenal hyperplasia. Surgery. 2008;143(6):750–8.
168. Tiyadatah BN, Kalavampara SV, Sukumar S, et al. Bilateral simultaneous laparoscopic adrenalectomy in Cushing's syndrome. J Endourol. 2012;26(2):157–63.
169. Xu Y, Rui W, Qi Y, et al. The role of unilateral adrenalectomy in corticotropin-independent bilateral adrenocortical hyperplasias. World J Surg. 2013;37(7):1626–32.
170. Kumorowicz-czoch M, Dolezal-oltarzewska K, Roztoczynska D, et al. Causes and consequences of abandoning one-stage bilateral adrenalectomy recommended in primary pigmented nodular

adrenocortical disease—case presentation. J Pediatr Endocrinol Metab. 2011;24(7-8):565–7.

171. Guanà R, Gesmundo R, Morino M, et al. Laparoscopic unilateral adrenalectomy in children for isolated primary pigmented nodular adrenocortical disease (PPNAD): case report and literature review. Eur J Pediatr Surg. 2010;20(4):273–5.
172. Storr HL, Mitchell H, Swords FM, et al. Clinical features, diagnosis, treatment and molecular studies in paediatric Cushing's syndrome due to primary nodular adrenocortical hyperplasia. Clin Endocrinol (Oxf). 2004;61(5):553–9.
173. Debillon E, Velayoudom-cephise FL, Salenave S, et al. Unilateral adrenalectomy as a first-line treatment of Cushing's syndrome in patients with primary bilateral macronodular adrenal hyperplasia. J Clin Endocrinol Metab. 2015;100(12):4417–24.
174. Albiger NM, Ceccato F, Zilio M, et al. An analysis of different therapeutic options in patients with Cushing's syndrome due to bilateral macronodular adrenal hyperplasia: a single-centre experience. Clin Endocrinol (Oxf). 2015;82(6):808–15.
175. Ito T, Kurita Y, Shinbo H, et al. Successful treatment for adrenocorticotropic hormone-independent macronodular adrenal hyperplasia with laparoscopic adrenalectomy: a case series. J Med Case Reports. 2012;6:312.
176. Sarkar R, Thompson NW, Mcleod MK. The role of adrenalectomy in Cushing's syndrome. Surgery. 1990;108(6):1079–84.
177. Romiti C, Baldarelli M, Cappelletti Trombettoni M, Budassi A, Ghiselli R, Guerrieri M. Laparoscopic adrenalectomy for Cushing's syndrome: a 12-year experience. Minerva Chir. 2013;68(4):377–84.
178. Hirano D, Hasegawa R, Igarashi T, et al. Laparoscopic adrenalectomy for adrenal tumors: a 21-year single-institution experience. Asian J Surg. 2015;38(2):79–84.
179. Sommerey S, Foroghi Y, Chiapponi C, et al. Laparoscopic adrenalectomy—10-year experience at a teaching hospital. Langenbecks Arch Surg. 2015;400(3):341–7.
180. Kang T, Gridley A, Richardson WS. Long-term outcomes of laparoscopic adrenalectomy for adrenal masses. J Laparoendosc Adv Surg Tech A. 2015;25(3):182–6.
181. Conzo G, Pasquali D, Della pietra C, et al. Laparoscopic adrenal surgery: ten-year experience in a single institution. BMC Surg. 2013;13(Suppl 2):S5.
182. Ali JM, Liau SS, Gunning K, et al. Laparoscopic adrenalectomy: auditing the 10 year experience of a single centre. Surgeon. 2012;10(5):267–72.
183. Gagner M, Lacroix A, Bolté E. Laparoscopic adrenalectomy in Cushing's syndrome and pheochromocytoma. N Engl J Med. 1992;327(14):1033.
184. Chai YJ, Kwon H, Yu HW, et al. Systematic review of surgical approaches for adrenal tumors: lateral transperitoneal versus posterior retroperitoneal and laparoscopic versus robotic adrenalectomy. Int J Endocrinol. 2014;2014:918346.
185. Jacobs JK, Goldstein RE, Geer RJ. Laparoscopic adrenalectomy. A new standard of care. Ann Surg. 1997;225(5):495–501.
186. Gagner M, Lacroix A, Bolte E, Pomp A. Laparoscopic adrenalectomy. The importance of a flank approach in the lateral decubitus position. Surg Endosc. 1994;8(2):135–8.
187. Morris LF, Perrier ND. Advances in robotic adrenalectomy. Curr Opin Oncol. 2012;24(1):1–6.
188. Dudley NE, Harrison BJ. Comparison of open posterior versus transperitoneal laparoscopic adrenalectomy. Br J Surg. 1999;86(5):656–60.
189. Thompson GB, Grant CS, Van heerden JA, et al. Laparoscopic versus open posterior adrenalectomy: a case-control study of 100 patients. Surgery. 1997;122(6):1132–6.
190. Brunt LM, Doherty GM, Norton JA, Soper NJ, Quasebarth MA, Moley JF. Laparoscopic adrenalectomy compared to open adrenalectomy for benign adrenal neoplasms. J Am Coll Surg. 1996;183(1):1–10.
191. Guazzoni G, Montorsi F, Bocciardi A, et al. Transperitoneal laparoscopic versus open adrenalectomy for benign hyperfunctioning adrenal tumors: a comparative study. J Urol. 1995;153(5):1597–600.
192. Bulus H, Uslu HY, Karakoyun R, Koçak S. Comparison of laparoscopic and open adrenalectomy. Acta Chir Belg. 2013;113(3):203–7.
193. Mcleod MK. Complications following adrenal surgery. J Natl Med Assoc. 1991;83(2):161–4.
194. Kiernan CM, Shinall MC, Mendez W, Peters MF, Broome JT, Solorzano CC. Influence of adrenal pathology on perioperative outcomes: a multi-institutional analysis. Am J Surg. 2014;208(4):619–25.
195. Russell CF, Hamberger B, Van heerden JA, Edis AJ, Ilstrup DM. Adrenalectomy: anterior or posterior approach? Am J Surg. 1982;144(3):322–4.
196. Dickson PV, Jimenez C, Chisholm GB, et al. Posterior retroperitoneoscopic adrenalectomy: a contemporary American experience. J Am Coll Surg. 2011;212(4):659–65.
197. Schreinemakers JM, Kiela GJ, Valk GD, Vriens MR, Rinkes IH. Retroperitoneal endoscopic adrenalectomy is safe and effective. Br J Surg. 2010;97(11):1667–72.
198. Berber E, Tellioglu G, Harvey A, Mitchell J, Milas M, Siperstein A. Comparison of laparoscopic transabdominal lateral versus posterior retroperitoneal adrenalectomy. Surgery. 2009;146(4):621–5.
199. Walz MK, Alesina PF, Wenger FA, et al. Posterior retroperitoneoscopic adrenalectomy—results of 560 procedures in 520 patients. Surgery. 2006;140(6):943–8.
200. Alesina PF, Hommeltenberg S, Meier B, et al. Posterior retroperitoneoscopic adrenalectomy for clinical and subclinical Cushing's syndrome. World J Surg. 2010;34(6):1391–7.

201. Walz MK, Peitgen K, Hoermann R, Giebler RM, Mann K, Eigler FW. Posterior retroperitoneoscopy as a new minimally invasive approach for adrenalectomy: results of 30 adrenalectomies in 27 patients. World J Surg. 1996;20(7):769–74.
202. Chai YJ, Woo JW, Kwon H, Choi JY, Kim SJ, Lee KE. Comparative outcomes of lateral transperitoneal adrenalectomy versus posterior retroperitoneoscopic adrenalectomy in consecutive patients: A single surgeon's experience. Asian J Surg. 2016;39(2):74–80.
203. Agarwal S, Chand G, Agarwal A. Posterior retroperitoneoscopic adrenalectomy for clinical and subclinical Cushing's syndrome. World J Surg. 2011;35(1):237.
204. Dickson PV, Alex GC, Grubbs EG, Jimenez C, Lee JE, Perrier ND. Robotic-assisted retroperitoneoscopic adrenalectomy: making a good procedure even better. Am Surg. 2013;79(1):84–9.
205. Pahwa M. Robot assisted adrenalectomy: a handy tool or glorified obsession? Gland Surg. 2015;4(4):279–82.
206. Brandao LF, Autorino R, Laydner H, et al. Robotic versus laparoscopic adrenalectomy: a systematic review and meta-analysis. Eur Urol. 2014;65(6):1154–61.
207. Schteingart DE, Doherty GM, Gauger PG, et al. Management of patients with adrenal cancer: recommendations of an international consensus conference. Endocr Relat Cancer. 2005;12(3):667–80.
208. Porpiglia F, Miller BS, Manfredi M, Fiori C, Doherty GM. A debate on laparoscopic versus open adrenalectomy for adrenocortical carcinoma. Horm Cancer. 2011;2(6):372–7.
209. Leboulleux S, Deandreis D, Al ghuzlan A, et al. Adrenocortical carcinoma: is the surgical approach a risk factor of peritoneal carcinomatosis? Eur J Endocrinol. 2010;162(6):1147–53.
210. Gonzalez RJ, Shapiro S, Sarlis N, et al. Laparoscopic resection of adrenal cortical carcinoma: a cautionary note. Surgery. 2005;138:1078–85; discussion 1085–6
211. Miller BS, Ammori JB, Gauger PG, Broome JT, Hammer GD, Doherty GM. Laparoscopic resection is inappropriate in patients with known or suspected adrenocortical carcinoma. World J Surg. 2010;34(6):1380–5.
212. Lee CW, Salem AI, Schneider DF, et al. Minimally invasive resection of adrenocortical carcinoma: a multi-institutional study of 201 patients. J Gastrointest Surg. 2017;21(2):352–62.
213. Machado NO, Al qadhi H, Al wahaibi K, Rizvi SG. Laparoscopic adrenalectomy for large adrenocortical carcinoma. JSLS. 2015;19(3):e201500036.
214. Pędziwiatr M, Wierdak M, Natkaniec M, et al. Laparoscopic transperitoneal lateral adrenalectomy for malignant and potentially malignant adrenal tumours. BMC Surg. 2015;15:101.
215. Donatini G, Caiazzo R, Do cao C, et al. Long-term survival after adrenalectomy for stage I/II adrenocortical carcinoma (ACC): a retrospective comparative cohort study of laparoscopic versus open approach. Ann Surg Oncol. 2014;21(1):284–91.
216. Brix D, Allolio B, Fenske W, et al. Laparoscopic versus open adrenalectomy for adrenocortical carcinoma: surgical and oncologic outcome in 152 patients. Eur Urol. 2010;58(4):609–15.
217. Porpiglia F, Fiori C, Daffara F, et al. Retrospective evaluation of the outcome of open versus laparoscopic adrenalectomy for stage I and II adrenocortical cancer. Eur Urol. 2010;57(5):873–8.
218. Giordano R, Guaraldi F, Berardelli R, et al. Glucose metabolism in patients with subclinical Cushing's syndrome. Endocrine. 2012;41(3):415–23.
219. Reincke M. Subclinical Cushing's syndrome. Endocrinol Metab Clin North Am. 2000;29(1):43–56.
220. Arnaldi G, Boscaro M. Adrenal incidentaloma. Best Pract Res Clin Endocrinol Metab. 2012;26(4):405–19.
221. Terzolo M, Stigliano A, Chiodini I, et al. AME position statement on adrenal incidentaloma. Eur J Endocrinol. 2011;164(6):851–70.
222. Barzon L, Sonino N, Fallo F, Palu G, Boscaro M. Prevalence and natural history of adrenal incidentalomas. Eur J Endocrinol. 2003;149(4):273–85.
223. Young WF. Management approaches to adrenal incidentalomas. A view from Rochester, Minnesota. Endocrinol Metab Clin North Am. 2000;29(1):159–85.
224. Barzon L, Scaroni C, Sonino N, Fallo F, Paoletta A, Boscaro M. Risk factors and long-term follow-up of adrenal incidentalomas. J Clin Endocrinol Metab. 1999;84(2):520–6.
225. Bovio S, Cataldi A, Reimondo G, et al. Prevalence of adrenal incidentaloma in a contemporary computerized tomography series. J Endocrinol Invest. 2006;29(4):298–302.
226. Loh HH, Yee A, Loh HS, Sukor N, Kamaruddin NA. The natural progression and outcomes of adrenal incidentaloma: a systematic review and meta-analysis. Minerva Endocrinol. 2017;42(1):77–87.
227. Mantero F, Terzolo M, Arnaldi G, et al. A survey on adrenal incidentaloma in Italy. Study Group on Adrenal Tumors of the Italian Society of Endocrinology. J Clin Endocrinol Metab. 2000;85(2):637–44.
228. Grumbach MM, Biller BM, Braunstein GD, et al. Management of the clinically inapparent adrenal mass ("incidentaloma"). Ann Intern Med. 2003;138(5):424–9.
229. Terzolo M, Pia A, Reimondo G. Subclinical Cushing's syndrome: definition and management. Clin Endocrinol (Oxf). 2012;76(1):12–8.
230. Chiodini I. Clinical review: diagnosis and treatment of subclinical hypercortisolism. J Clin Endocrinol Metab. 2011;96(5):1223–36.

231. Stewart PM. Is subclinical Cushing's syndrome an entity or a statistical fallout from diagnostic testing? Consensus surrounding the diagnosis is required before optimal treatment can be defined. J Clin Endocrinol Metab. 2010;95(6):2618–20.
232. Terzolo M, Reimondo G, Bovio S, Angeli A. Subclinical Cushing's syndrome. Pituitary. 2004;7(4):217–23.
233. Sippel RS, Chen H. Subclinical Cushing's syndrome in adrenal incidentalomas. Surg Clin North Am. 2004;84(3):875–85.
234. Bülow B, Jansson S, Juhlin C, et al. Adrenal incidentaloma—follow-up results from a Swedish prospective study. Eur J Endocrinol. 2006;154(3):419–23.
235. Libè R, Dall'asta C, Barbetta L, Baccarelli A, Beck-peccoz P, Ambrosi B. Long-term follow-up study of patients with adrenal incidentalomas. Eur J Endocrinol. 2002;147(4):489–94.
236. Di dalmazi G, Vicennati V, Garelli S, et al. Cardiovascular events and mortality in patients with adrenal incidentalomas that are either non-secreting or associated with intermediate phenotype or subclinical Cushing's syndrome: a 15-year retrospective study. Lancet Diabetes Endocrinol. 2014;2(5):396–405.
237. Barzon L, Fallo F, Sonino N, Boscaro M. Overnight dexamethasone suppression of cortisol is associated with radiocholesterol uptake patterns in adrenal incidentalomas. Eur J Endocrinol. 2001;145(2):223–4.
238. Chiodini I, Morelli V, Salcuni AS, et al. Beneficial metabolic effects of prompt surgical treatment in patients with an adrenal incidentaloma causing biochemical hypercortisolism. J Clin Endocrinol Metab. 2010;95(6):2736–45.
239. Erbil Y, Ademoğlu E, Ozbey N, et al. Evaluation of the cardiovascular risk in patients with subclinical Cushing syndrome before and after surgery. World J Surg. 2006;30(9):1665–71.
240. Giordano R, Marinazzo E, Berardelli R, et al. Long-term morphological, hormonal, and clinical follow-up in a single unit on 118 patients with adrenal incidentalomas. Eur J Endocrinol. 2010;162(4):779–85.
241. Chiodini I, Morelli V, Masserini B, et al. Bone mineral density, prevalence of vertebral fractures, and bone quality in patients with adrenal incidentalomas with and without subclinical hypercortisolism: an Italian multicenter study. J Clin Endocrinol Metab. 2009;94(9):3207–14.
242. Tsuiki M, Tanabe A, Takagi S, Naruse M, Takano K. Cardiovascular risks and their long-term clinical outcome in patients with subclinical Cushing's syndrome. Endocr J. 2008;55(4):737–45.
243. Mitchell IC, Auchus RJ, Juneja K, et al. "Subclinical Cushing's syndrome" is not subclinical: improvement after adrenalectomy in 9 patients. Surgery. 2007;142(6):900–5.
244. Tauchmanovà L, Rossi R, Biondi B, et al. Patients with subclinical Cushing's syndrome due to adrenal adenoma have increased cardiovascular risk. J Clin Endocrinol Metab. 2002;87(11):4872–8.
245. Rossi R, Tauchmanova L, Luciano A, et al. Subclinical Cushing's syndrome in patients with adrenal incidentaloma: clinical and biochemical features. J Clin Endocrinol Metab. 2000;85(4):1440–8.
246. Debono M, Bradburn M, Bull M, Harrison B, Ross RJ, Newell-Price J. Cortisol as a marker for increased mortality in patients with incidental adrenocortical adenomas. J Clin Endocrinol Metab. 2014;99(12):4462–70.
247. Terzolo M, Pia A, Alì A, et al. Adrenal incidentaloma: a new cause of the metabolic syndrome? J Clin Endocrinol Metab. 2002;87(3):998–1003.
248. Di dalmazi G, Vicennati V, Rinaldi E, et al. Progressively increased patterns of subclinical cortisol hypersecretion in adrenal incidentalomas differently predict major metabolic and cardiovascular outcomes: a large cross-sectional study. Eur J Endocrinol. 2012;166(4):669–77.
249. Ricciato MP, Di donna V, Perotti G, Pontecorvi A, Bellantone R, Corsello SM. The role of adrenal scintigraphy in the diagnosis of subclinical Cushing's syndrome and the prediction of post-surgical hypoadrenalism. World J Surg. 2014;38(6):1328–35.
250. Perysinakis I, Marakaki C, Avlonitis S, et al. Laparoscopic adrenalectomy in patients with subclinical Cushing syndrome. Surg Endosc. 2013;27(6):2145–8.
251. Maehana T, Tanaka T, Itoh N, Masumori N, Tsukamoto T. Clinical outcomes of surgical treatment and longitudinal non-surgical observation of patients with subclinical Cushing's syndrome and nonfunctioning adrenocortical adenoma. Indian J Urol. 2012;28(2):179–83.
252. Feelders RA, Hofland LJ. Medical treatment of Cushing's disease. J Clin Endocrinol Metab. 2013;98:425–38.
253. Debono M, Chadarevian R, Eastell R, Ross RJ, Newell-Price J. Mifepristone reduces insulin resistance in patient volunteers with adrenal incidentalomas that secrete low levels of cortisol: a pilot study. PLoS One. 2013;8(4):e60984.
254. Corcuff JB, Young J, Masquefa-Giraud P, Chanson P, Baudin E, Tabarin A. Rapid control of severe neoplastic hypercortisolism with metyrapone and ketoconazole. Eur J Endocrinol. 2015;172:473–48.
255. Lonser RR, Wind JJ, Nieman LK, Weil RJ, Devroom HL, Oldfield EH. Outcome of surgical treatment of 200 children with Cushing's disease. J Clin Endocrinol Metab. 2013;98(3):892–901.
256. Lin X, Wu D, Chen C, Zheng N. Clinical characteristics of adrenal tumors in children: a retrospective review of a 15-year single-center experience. Int Urol Nephrol. 2017;49(3):381–5.
257. Cecchetto G, Ganarin A, Bien E, et al. Outcome and prognostic factors in high-risk childhood adrenocortical carcinomas: a report from the European Cooperative Study Group on Pediatric Rare Tumors (EXPeRT). Pediatr Blood Cancer. 2017;64(6)

258. Lalli E, Figueiredo BC. Pediatric adrenocortical tumors: what they can tell us on adrenal development and comparison with adult adrenal tumors. Front Endocrinol (Lausanne). 2015;6:1–9.
259. Kundel A, Thompson GB, Richards ML, et al. Pediatric endocrine surgery: a 20-year experience at the Mayo Clinic. J Clin Endocrinol Metab. 2014;99(2):399–406.
260. Brown RJ, Kelly MH, Collins MT. Cushing syndrome in the McCune-Albright syndrome. J Clin Endocrinol Metab. 2010;95(4):1508–15.
261. Kirk JM, Brain CE, Carson DJ, Hyde JC, Grant DB. Cushing's syndrome caused by nodular adrenal hyperplasia in children with McCune-Albright syndrome. J Pediatr. 1999;134(6):789–92.
262. Rodriguez-galindo C, Figueiredo BC, Zambetti GP, Ribeiro RC. Biology, clinical characteristics, and management of adrenocortical tumors in children. Pediatr Blood Cancer. 2005;45(3):265–73.
263. Batista DL, Oldfield EH, Keil MF, Stratakis CA. Postoperative testing to predict recurrent Cushing disease in children. J Clin Endocrinol Metab. 2009;94(8):2757–65.
264. Magiakou MA, Mastorakos G, Oldfield EH, et al. Cushing's syndrome in children and adolescents. Presentation, diagnosis, and therapy. N Engl J Med. 1994;331(10):629–36.
265. Yankovic F, Undre S, Mushtaq I. Surgical technique: retroperitoneoscopic approach for adrenal masses in children. J Pediatr Urol. 2014;10(2):400.e1–2.
266. Stanford A, Upperman JS, Nguyen N, Barksdale E, Wiener ES. Surgical management of open versus laparoscopic adrenalectomy: outcome analysis. J Pediatr Surg. 2002;37(7):1027–9.
267. Carroll PV, Monson JP, Grossman AB, et al. Successful treatment of childhood-onset Cushing's disease is associated with persistent reduction in growth hormone secretion. Clin Endocrinol (Oxf). 2004;60(2):169–74.
268. Magiakou MA, Mastorakos G, Gomez MT, Rose SR, Chrousos GP. Suppressed spontaneous and stimulated growth hormone secretion in patients with Cushing's disease before and after surgical cure. J Clin Endocrinol Metab. 1994;78(1):131–7.
269. Magiakou MA, Mastorakos G, Chrousos GP. Final stature in patients with endogenous Cushing's syndrome. J Clin Endocrinol Metab. 1994;79:1082–5.
270. Nassi R, Ladu C, Vezzosi C, Mannelli M. Cushing's syndrome in pregnancy. Gynecol Endocrinol. 2015;31(2):102–4.
271. Lindsay JR, Jonklaas J, Oldfield EH, Nieman LK. Cushing's syndrome during pregnancy: personal experience and review of the literature. J Clin Endocrinol Metab. 2005;90(5):3077–83.
272. Lindsay JR, Nieman LK. The hypothalamic-pituitary-adrenal axis in pregnancy: challenges in disease detection and treatment. Endocr Rev. 2005;26(6):775–99.
273. Pearl JP, Price RR, Tonkin AE, Richardson WS, Stefanidis D. SAGES guidelines for the use of laparoscopy during pregnancy. Surg Endosc. 2017;31(10):3767–82.
274. Leiba S, Weinstein R, Shindel B, et al. The protracted effect of o,p'-DDD in Cushing's disease and its impact on adrenal morphogenesis of young human embryo. Ann Endocrinol (Paris). 1989;50(1):49–53.
275. Eschler DC, Kogekar N, Pessah-pollack R. Management of adrenal tumors in pregnancy. Endocrinol Metab Clin North Am. 2015;44(2):381–97.
276. Zieleniewski W, Michalak R. A successful case of pregnancy in a woman with ACTH-independent Cushing's syndrome treated with ketoconazole and metyrapone. Gynecol Endocrinol. 2017;33(5):349–52.
277. Faucz FR, Zilbermint M, Lodish MB, et al. Macronodular adrenal hyperplasia due to mutations in an armadillo repeat containing 5 (ARMC5) gene: a clinical and genetic investigation. J Clin Endocrinol Metab. 2014;99(6):E1113–9.
278. Rockall AG, Sohaib SA, Evans D, et al. Computed tomography assessment of fat distribution in male and female patients with Cushing's syndrome. Eur J Endocrinol. 2003;149(6):561–7.
279. Van zaane B, Nur E, Squizzato A, et al. Hypercoagulable state in Cushing's syndrome: a systematic review. J Clin Endocrinol Metab. 2009;94(8):2743–50.
280. Guilhaume B, Bertagna X, Thomsen M, et al. Transsphenoidal pituitary surgery for the treatment of Cushing's disease: results in 64 patients and long term follow-up studies. J Clin Endocrinol Metab. 1988;66(5):1056–64.
281. Gagner M, Pomp A, Heniford BT, Pharand D, Lacroix A. Laparoscopic adrenalectomy: lessons learned from 100 consecutive procedures. Ann Surg. 1997;226(3):238–46.
282. Toniato A, Merante-boschin I, Opocher G, Pelizzo MR, Schiavi F, Ballotta E. Surgical versus conservative management for subclinical Cushing syndrome in adrenal incidentalomas: a prospective randomized study. Ann Surg. 2009;249(3):388–91.

Conn's Syndrome

27

Lip Min Soh

Introduction

Primary aldosteronism was first described by Dr. Jerome Conn in 1955 as a clinical entity of potassium depletion and hypertension caused by an adrenocortical adenoma [1]. Patients often had episodes of severe muscle weakness and paralysis, tetany and paraesthesias, and hypertension was the rule. At that time, it was believed that it accounted for <1% of hypertension cases [2].

The understanding of primary aldosteronism has since grown over the years, and we now know that it is not solely due to an adrenocortical adenoma, but a group of disorders with aldosterone production in excess and autonomous from the renin-angiotensin system. Its detrimental effects also go beyond simply that of hypertension and hypokalaemia. Aldosterone excess has a direct impact on end-organ damage, particularly in cardiovascular events, increasing the relative risks of atrial fibrillation, myocardial infarction and stroke at 12, 6 and 4, respectively, compared to age-, gender- and blood pressure-matched essential hypertensives [3].

Early identification of the condition, followed by accurate classification of the subtype and underlying cause, will allow appropriate treatment whether medical or surgical, to ameliorate these deleterious complications.

L. M. Soh
Endocrinology, National University Hospital, Singapore, Singapore
e-mail: lip_min_soh@nuhs.edu.sg

Case Detection

The causes of primary aldosteronism (PA) can be divided into two main groups, those with unilateral disease which can be surgically curable and those with bilateral disease which should be medically treated (Table 27.1) [4]. The first large prospective study, the Primary Aldosteronism Prevalence in Hypertensives (PAPY) study published in 2006, found that 11.2% of 1125 patients with newly diagnosed hypertension referred to hypertensive centres had PA, and 4.8% had a surgically curable subtype [5].

The Endocrine Society clinical practice guidelines on management of primary aldosteronism advocate screening in the following patient populations [6]:

1. Sustained blood pressure (BP) >150/100 mmHg on three measurements on separate days.
2. BP >140/90 mmHg resistant to three conventional antihypertensive drugs including a diuretic.
3. Controlled BP <140/90 mmHg on four or more antihypertensive drugs.
4. Hypertension with hypokalaemia (both spontaneous and diuretic induced).

R. Parameswaran, A. Agarwal (eds.), *Evidence-Based Endocrine Surgery*,
https://doi.org/10.1007/978-981-10-1124-5_27

Table 27.1 Causes of primary aldosteronism

Surgically remediable (unilateral disease)	Not surgically remediable (bilateral disease)
Aldosterone-producing adenoma (APA)—35%	
Primary (unilateral) idiopathic hyperplasia—2%	Bilateral idiopathic hyperplasia (BAH)—60%
Aldosterone-producing adrenocortical carcinoma	
Familial type II hyperaldosteronism	Familial type I hyperaldosteronism (glucocorticoid-remediable aldosteronism)
Ectopic aldosterone-producing adenoma/ carcinoma	

5. Hypertension and adrenal incidentaloma.
6. Hypertension and obstructive sleep apnoea.
7. Hypertension and a family history of early-onset hypertension or cerebrovascular accident at young age <40 years old.
8. First-degree relatives of patients with primary aldosteronism.

Compared to the earlier edition of the guidelines published in 2008 [7], the main differences are (a) lowering of blood pressure threshold (previously >160/100 mmHg), as well as (b) the incorporation of patients with obstructive sleep apnoea (OSA) for screening.

There is growing evidence that there is a high prevalence of PA in patients with OSA [8]. Calhoun et al. reported a PA prevalence of 36% among subjects at high risk of OSA using the Berlin questionnaire, compared to 19% of those at low risk [9]. Di Murro et al. found similar results, 25.4% vs. 9.8%, this time using the overnight polysomnography for the diagnosis of OSA [10]. In addition, there is strong positive association of plasma aldosterone levels with the severity of OSA [11–13]. In small studies, the addition of spironolactone reduced the severity of OSA and blood pressure in resistant hypertension patients with moderate-to-severe OSA [14, 15]. The mechanism has been postulated to be related to diuresis and a consequent reduction of pharyngeal oedema and upper airway resistance.

Screening of PA should be done by measuring the plasma aldosterone concentration (PAC) and renin (plasma renin activity PRA or direct renin concentration DRC), and calculating the aldosterone-renin ratio (ARR). However, there are numerous technical aspects and patient preparation that need to take place to allow accurate interpretation of the results (Table 27.2).

Different cut-off values for the interpretation of PAC, PRA/ DRC as well as ARR will result in different sensitivities and specificities. A commonly used threshold is when PAC is >415 pmol/L (15 ng/dL), and the ARR is >750 (equivalent to 27 when PAC is measured in ng/dL). The lowest renin value that can be used in calculation is 0.2 ng/mL/h for PRA and 0.36 ng/mL for DRA to avoid overinflation of the ARR [16]. This threshold would result in a sensitivity of 80.5% and a specificity of 84.5% when compared to the gold standard diagnosis of APA [5]. With a sensitivity of only 80.5%, one must therefore be aware that milder cases of PA, particularly those with BAH, can have aldosterone levels lower than 415 pmol/L and/ or ARRs lower than 750.

Case Confirmation

Using a low threshold to define positive screening results errs on the side of caution of not missing any cases of primary aldosteronism while recognising that there will be cases of false positivity. Hence, it is important to subject these patients to further testing for case confirmation. On the other hand, in cases where the clinical presentation is already indicative of PA (i.e. hypertension with spontaneous hypokalaemia, a high PAC >550 pmol/L and ARR >750), no further confirmatory testing may be necessary.

Several tests have been described and there is currently no gold standard for comparison. The five most common are the saline infusion test, oral sodium loading test, fludrocortisone suppression test, captopril challenge test and furosemide upright test. In my institution, we employ

Table 27.2 Patient preparation and interpretation of ARR

	Effect on aldosterone	Effect on renin	Effect on ARR
1. Patient preparation			
Correct hypokalaemia	↓ (Low K)	↔/↑	↓ (FN)
Liberal salt intake	↓	↓↓	↑ (FP)
2. Withdraw interfering medications (switch to non-interfering drugs such as verapamil, hydralazine, or alpha-blockers—prazosin, terazosin, doxazosin)			
Withdraw at least 4 weeks			
Spironolactone, eplerenone, amiloride, triamterene	↑	↑↑	↓ (FN)
K+-wasting diuretics	↔/↑	↑↑	↓ (FN)
Licorice products	↓	↔/↓	↓ (FN)
Withdraw at least 2 weeks			
Beta-blockers	↓	↓↓	↑ (FP)
Central agonists (methyldopa, clonidine)	↓	↓↓	↑ (FP)
NSAIDS	↓	↓↓	↑ (FP)
ACEI inhibitors	↓	↑↑	↓ (FN)
ARBs	↓	↑↑	↓ (FN)
Calcium channel blockers	↔/↓	↑	↓ (FN)
Renin inhibitors	↓	↓/↑[a]	↑ (FP)/↓ (FN)[a]
3. Day of blood collection			
1. Collect in the morning, after patients have been out of bed for at least 2 h 2. Sit patient for 5–15 min before sampling blood 3. Maintain blood sample at room temperature			
4. Other conditions			
Renal impairment	↔	↓	↑ (FP)
Premenopausal women (vs. males)	↔/↑ (luteal phase)	↓ (when using DRC[b])	↑ (FP)
Pregnancy	↑	↑↑	↓ (FN)
Malignant hypertension	↑	↑↑	↓ (FN)

Adapted from JW Funder et al.: An Endocrine Society Clinical Practice Guideline on the Management of Primary Aldosteronism [6]

FN false negative and *FP* false positive

[a]Renin inhibitors can cause false-positive results when renin is measured by PRA, and false-negative results when measured by DRC

[b]Measurement of ARR for premenopausal women should be done in the follicular phase where possible

the saline infusion test (SIT), which can be performed in the outpatient setting. Patients are given an intravenous infusion of 2 l of 0.9% saline. Blood samples for aldosterone, renin, potassium and cortisol are taken at 0 min and 4 h post-infusion. A post-infusion aldosterone level >170 pmol (6 ng/dL) in the seated position, or >280 pmol/L (10 ng/dL) in the recumbent position, confirms the diagnosis of primary aldosteronism [17]. It is important that the corresponding cortisol level is lower than baseline to exclude a confounding ACTH effect.

Subtype Classification

All patients confirmed to have PA should undergo high-resolution computed tomography (CT) scan of the adrenal glands to determine if they are normal, or characterise the presence of unilateral or bilateral hyperplasia and micro- or macro-adenomas, and exclude larger adrenal masses suggestive of carcinoma. Magnetic resonance imaging has no advantage over CT as it has lower spatial resolution, is subject to motion artefacts and is more expensive [6, 18].

CT appearances of hyperplasia or small nodules do not immediately confirm the diagnosis of adrenal hyperplasia versus aldosterone-producing adenomas. Seemingly hyperplastic glands may hide small hyperfunctioning nodules and small microadenomas seen on CT may actually be areas of hyperplasia. In addition, adrenal nodules seen on CT imaging may be incidental, non-functioning adenomas, and not the source of PA [19]. Distinguishing unilateral from bilateral disease is critical to guide appropriate management of PA.

Currently, the test widely considered to be the gold standard test for lateralisation is adrenal vein sampling [6, 20]. An expert consensus statement of the use of adrenal vein sampling (AVS) has been published by Rossi et al. [21]. Mineralocorticoid antagonists must be withdrawn for at least 4–6 weeks prior to AVS. For patients with resistant hypertension who require multiple antihypertensives for blood pressure control, other agents such as ACE inhibitors and beta-blockers are permissible, as long as the renin is still suppressed prior to the procedure. The low renin level obviates the possibility of stimulation of the contralateral gland, which can result in the false impression of bilateral disease.

A common protocol is done under continuous cosyntropin infusion 50 mcg/h starting 30 min before and continued throughout the procedure. This helps to (a) minimise stress-induced fluctuations in aldosterone secretion, (b) increase aldosterone secretion from an APA and (c) maximise the cortisol gradient from the adrenal vein to peripheral vein to confirm successful cannulation. When successful, the adrenal/peripheral vein cortisol ratio is typically >5:1, and should minimally be >3:1 to allow interpretation of the results [21–23]. To determine lateralisation, the aldosterone levels should be divided by the cortisol levels in the respective veins to account for dilutional effects from the inferior phrenic or accessory hepatic veins [24, 25]. A cortisol-corrected aldosterone ratio >4:1 is indicative of unilateral disease, while that of <3:1 is suggestive of bilateral disease [6, 20, 21, 23].

The success rate of AVS is often limited by inadequate cannulation of the right adrenal vein due to its small calibre and variable anatomic course. Measures that can improve this include (a) having an experienced radiologist dedicated to AVS, (b) using contrast-enhanced multidetector CT to guide the localisation of the right adrenal vein prior to the procedure [26, 27] and (c) having rapid intraprocedural cortisol assay to guide repositioning of the catheter and confirm successful cannulation [28–30]. The Adrenal Vein Sampling International Study found that it is generally safe, and the rate of major complications is low at 0.61% in experienced hands [31].

Nonetheless, as AVS is invasive, is available only in few centres and has variable success rates, there is continued interest in looking for alternative ways to accurately predict subtype classification. A clinical scoring system based on the radiographic appearance of the adrenal glands, potassium level and estimated glomerular filtration rate was first proposed by Küpers et al. [32]. It reported a remarkable 100% specificity, but such optimistic results have been dampened by data from other centres [33–35], showing that the scoring system was not sufficiently robust to be applied to larger populations.

One promising modality is ^{12}C-metomidate positron emission tomography-computed tomography (PET-CT) [36]. Metomidate is a potent inhibitor of adrenal steroidogenic enzymes CYP11B1 and CYP 11B2. Low-dose dexamethasone is given for 3 days prior to the scan to suppress normal adrenal cortex. A pilot study of 44 patients showed that it was non-inferior to AVS [37]. The standardised uptake value (SUV) was higher in APA compared to non-functioning adenomas. The specificity was 87% if SUV_{max} ratio was >1.25, and increased to 100% if the absolute tumour SUV_{max} was >17.

Management (Medical and Surgical) and Long-Term Outcome

Once subtype classification has been attained, typical management strategy would be surgery for unilateral disease (such as aldosterone-producing adenoma and primary idiopathic hyperplasia), and medical therapy for bilateral disease (bilateral idiopathic hyperplasia and familial type I hyperaldosteronism).

Laparoscopic adrenalectomy is preferred to an open approach, and is associated with low complication rate, lesser post-operative pain, shorter hospitalisation and faster functional recovery [38–41]. Potassium levels will normalise rapidly following surgery without the use of potassium supplementation. Hypertension is cured in approximately 40% of patients (BP defined <140/90 mmHg), but even for those who are not cured the pill burden for antihypertensive medication is reduced [42, 43].

Medical treatment is achieved with mineralocorticoid receptor (MR) antagonists with spironolactone or eplerenone (Table 27.3). Spironolactone is the preferred agent for many years, and several studies have shown reduction of systolic BP by 25% and diastolic BP of 22% in patients with BAH [6]. For patients with APA, 48% achieved a BP <140/90 mmHg [44]. Two studies have done head-to-head comparison of these two agents with conflicting results. In 141 patients with PA randomised to spironolactone versus eplerenone, spironolactone appeared to reduce BP more effectively [45]. However, in this trial eplerenone was given as a once-daily dosing which may have been inadequate due to the short half-life of 4–6 h. In contrast, in 34 patients with BAH, eplerenone appeared to be more effective, with 82.4% versus 76.5% reaching the target BP <140/90 mmHg [46].

Caution must be taken when initiating MR antagonists in patients with stage III chronic kidney disease (CKD) (decreased glomerular filtration rate, GFR <60 mL/min/1.73 m^2), and even more so in stage IV CKD (GFR <30 mL/min/1.73 m^2) where the medications may be contraindicated. It is important to also recognise that hyperaldosteronism causes a state of glomerular hyperfiltration. With treatment, whether medical or surgical, the creatinine level often rises, revealing the underlying degree and actual severity of renal impairment.

Long-Term Outcomes

The goal of treatment is not just to normalise the blood pressure and potassium levels. More importantly, it is aimed at reducing the long-term end-organ complications, which include that of cardiovascular, renal and glucose metabolism.

Data from the German Conn's study revealed a high prevalence of cardiovascular events (angina, myocardial infarction, chronic cardiac insufficiency and angioplasty) at 16.3% in patients with PA [47]. Milliez et al. were the first to show that there was a striking increase in the relative risks of myocardial infarction, atrial fibrillation and stroke in PA compared to age-, gender- and blood pressure-matched essential hypertensives at 12.1, 6.5 and 4.2, respectively [3]. Other large studies with case-control-matched patients with essential hypertension (EH) have corroborated these findings [48, 49].

With medical or surgical treatment, the cardiovascular event rate is reduced, and becomes comparable to that of patients with EH. Long-term data with an average follow-up of 7.4 years

Table 27.3 Medical treatment

	Dose titration	Considerations
Spironolactone	Starting dose 12.5–25 mg daily Doses as high as 400 mg/day have been given	Dose-dependant side effects include gynaecomastia, sexual dysfunction and irregular menses
Eplerenone	Starting dose 25 mg bd Doses as high as 300 mg/ day have been given	Short half-like requiring twice daily dosing. Less side effects than spironolactone Less side effects than spironolactone
Steroids for patients with GRA Dexamethasone Prednisolone	0.125–0.25 mg/day 2.5–5 mg/day	Lowest possible dose to avoid iatrogenic Cushing's syndrome Take at bedtime to suppress early-morning ACTH surge

from Catena et al. have shown that the occurrence of a combined cardiovascular end point (myocardial infarction, coronary revascularisation, stroke and sustained arrhythmia) was comparable in both groups [50]. A meta-analysis looking at the reduction of left ventricular mass following medical or surgical treatment also showed no significant difference between the two groups [51].

For renal outcomes, data from a large multicentre Italian PAPY study showed that the prevalence of 24-h microalbuminuria in patients with PA was twice that of patients with EH [52]. Following treatment, restoration of microalbuminuria was more common in the PA group [53]. With both medical and surgical treatment, there is an early decline of eGFR in the first year due to the reversal of abnormal intrarenal haemodynamics [54], but subsequent declines were comparable in both groups within an average follow-up duration of 6.4 years [53].

For metabolic sequelae, Fallo et al. found a much higher prevalence of metabolic syndrome in PA patients compared to essential hypertensives (41.1% vs. 29.6%), and that of hyperglycaemia was 27.0% versus 15.2% [55]. Treatment in a 6-year study restored insulin sensitivity in 54 patients with PA [56].

Newer Agents

Mineralocorticoid receptor antagonists (MRA) have shown to be effective in treating PA and preventing long-term complications. However, the use of spironolactone is often limited by the adverse effects of non-selective binding to androgen and progesterone receptors which results in painful gynaecomastia, sexual dysfunction and menstrual irregularities. This has prompted the search for newer agents, and the development has followed two main strategies, the first in developing a non-steroidal MRA that retains the pharmacologic benefits but avoids having the steroidal side effects. The forerunner in this group is a derivative of a dihydropyridine calcium channel blocker which has similar efficacy as spironolactone, but has no effect on other steroid receptors and the L-type calcium channel [57].

The second strategy is focused on the development of selective aldosterone synthase inhibitors. However, the compounds investigated in phase II trials have shown some non-selectivity and also decreased cortisol levels. It also failed to decrease the blood pressure consistently in all patients despite decreasing aldosterone levels, presumably due to the accumulation of precursors with mineralocorticoid activity [58]. It also remains to be seen if any new drugs developed will be as effective as spironolactone in preventing long-term complications.

A Word on Genetics

In the initial years, the genetic basis of PA was understood only for familial hyperaldosteronism type I where a chimeric gene of CYP11B2 and CYP11B1 leads to ACTH stimulation of aldosterone production. From 2011, the understanding of genetics in the pathogenesis of PA has progressed rapidly, and somatic mutations have been identified in key membrane proteins which affect potassium, calcium channels and ion pumps. Choi et al. first detected mutations in KCNJ5 using whole genomic sequencing [59]. Subsequently mutations in genes encoding Na/K--ATPase (ATP1A), Ca-ATPase (ATP2B3) [60, 61] as well as Ca1.3 (CACNA1D) [62] were also described. The end point of these mutations all led to calcium influx, membrane depolarisation and aldosterone hypersecretion. However, the type of mutations appears to affect the severity of the clinical phenotype, hyperplasia or size of adenomas [63].

Future Direction

In the early years, when hypokalaemia and hypertension were considered sine qua non for the diagnosis of PA, the condition was thought to be uncommon, with a prevalence of 1% [2]. In the 1990s, there was recognition that many patients with PA may be normokalaemic. ARR was more widely applied as a screening tool to hypertensive populations, and the prevalence of PA increased 5–10-fold [64]. In 2005, Stowasser et al. reported eight patients with genetically proven familial hyperaldosteronism type I who were normotensive, with comparable ambulatory blood pressures in age- and sex-matched normal controls. However, echocardiography revealed evidence of increased left ventricular wall thickness and reduced diastolic function [65].

At present, there is no gold standard test to screen or confirm the diagnosis of PA, and diagnostic thresholds are somewhat arbitrary, sometimes based on normotensive controls with no previous adrenal imaging who may not be entirely "normal". Piaditis et al. have reported variations of the confirmatory tests by adding dexamethasone to suppress ACTH, low-dose dexamethasone suppression saline infusion test (PD-SIT) and fludrocortisone dexamethasone suppression test (FDST). With the FDST, in a control group of 72 normotensives with normal adrenals on imaging, he found that the 97.5% upper limit of normal for PAC was 74 pmol/L, and ARR 32 pmol/mU. In comparison, in a group of 180 patients with unselected hypertension, 31% showed values exceeding both thresholds [66]. The higher levels corresponded with both the systolic and diastolic blood pressure. If the basal ARR was used, only 7.2% of the patients would have been diagnosed with PA. In a similar fashion, when thresholds for PD-SIT established using normal controls were applied to 151 patients with single adrenal adenomas, 24% had evidence of aldosterone excess. This was doubled compared to statistics generated by the classic SIT [67].

In summary, the disease epidemiology of primary aldosteronism appears to span from classic hypokalaemic hypertensive PA, normokalaemic low-renin hypertension and even subclinical normokalaemic normotensive PA, where aldosterone excess is already quietly mediating cardiovascular damage. There are numerous screening and confirmatory tests that one can employ, but one needs to bear in mind the clinical context and suspicion to determine the appropriate application and diagnostic thresholds. We can only presume that the true prevalence of PA is yet unknown, but is certainly likely to be much higher than that currently reported. It will be both our challenge to screen and manage and our conundrum if we should.

References

1. Conn JW, Louis LH. Primary aldosteronism, a new clinical entity. Ann Intern Med. 1956;44(1):1–15.
2. Ganguly A. Primary aldosteronism. N Engl J Med. 1998;339(25):1828–34.
3. Milliez P, Girerd X, Plouin PF, Blacher J, Safar ME, Mourad JJ. Evidence for an increased rate of cardiovascular events in patients with primary aldosteronism. J Am Coll Cardiol. 2005;45(8):1243–8.
4. Chao C-T, Wu V-C, Kuo C-C, Lin Y-H, Chang C-C, Chueh SJ, et al. Diagnosis and management of primary aldosteronism: An updated review. Annals of Medicine 2013;45(4):375–383.
5. Rossi GP, Bernini G, Caliumi C, Desideri G, Fabris B, Ferri C, et al. A prospective study of the prevalence of primary aldosteronism in 1,125 hypertensive patients. J Am Coll Cardiol. 2006;48(11):2293–300.
6. Funder JW, Carey RM, Mantero F, Murad MH, Reincke M, Shibata H, et al. The management of primary aldosteronism: case detection, diagnosis, and treatment: an Endocrine Society Clinical Practice Guideline. J Clin Endocrinol Metab. 2016;101(5):1889–916.
7. Funder JW, Carey RM, Fardella C, Gomez-Sanchez CE, Mantero F, Stowasser M, et al. Case detection, diagnosis, and treatment of patients with primary aldosteronism: an endocrine society clinical practice guideline. J Clin Endocrinol Metab. 2008;93(9):3266–81.
8. Monticone S, Viola A, Tizzani D, Crudo V, Burrello J, Galmozzi M, et al. Primary aldosteronism: who should be screened? Horm Metab Res. 2012;44(3):163–9.
9. Calhoun DA, Nishizaka MK, Zaman MA, Harding SM. Aldosterone excretion among subjects with resistant hypertension and symptoms of sleep apnea. Chest. 2004;125(1):112–7.
10. Di Murro A, Petramala L, Cotesta D, Zinnamosca L, Crescenzi E, Marinelli C, et al. Renin-angiotensin-aldosterone system in patients with sleep apnoea: prevalence of primary aldosteronism. J Renin-Angiotensin-Aldosterone Syst. 2010;11(3):165–72.
11. Gonzaga CC, Gaddam KK, Ahmed MI, Pimenta E, Thomas SJ, Harding SM, et al. Severity of obstructive sleep apnea is related to aldosterone status in subjects with resistant hypertension. J Clin Sleep Med. 2010;6(4):363–8.
12. Pratt-Ubunama MN, Nishizaka MK, Boedefeld RL, Cofield SS, Harding SM, Calhoun DA. Plasma aldosterone is related to severity of obstructive sleep apnea in subjects with resistant hypertension. Chest. 2007;131(2):453–9.

13. Sim JJ, Yan EH, Liu IL, Rasgon SA, Kalantar-Zadeh K, Calhoun DA, et al. Positive relationship of sleep apnea to hyperaldosteronism in an ethnically diverse population. J Hypertens. 2011;29(8):1553–9.
14. Yang L, Zhang H, Cai M, Zou Y, Jiang X, Song L, et al. Effect of spironolactone on patients with resistant hypertension and obstructive sleep apnea. Clin Exp Hypertens. 2016;38(5):464–8.
15. Gaddam K, Pimenta E, Thomas SJ, Cofield SS, Oparil S, Harding SM, et al. Spironolactone reduces severity of obstructive sleep apnoea in patients with resistant hypertension: a preliminary report. J Hum Hypertens. 2010;24(8):532–7.
16. Rossi GP. A comprehensive review of the clinical aspects of primary aldosteronism. Nat Rev Endocrinol. 2011;7(8):485–95.
17. Ahmed AH, Cowley D, Wolley M, Gordon RD, Xu S, Taylor PJ, et al. Seated saline suppression testing for the diagnosis of primary aldosteronism: a preliminary study. J Clin Endocrinol Metab. 2014;99(8):2745–53.
18. Magill SB, Raff H, Shaker JL, Brickner RC, Knechtges TE, Kehoe ME, et al. Comparison of adrenal vein sampling and computed tomography in the differentiation of primary aldosteronism. J Clin Endocrinol Metab. 2001;86(3):1066–71.
19. Kloos RT, Gross MD, Francis IR, Korobkin M, Shapiro B. Incidentally discovered adrenal masses. Endocr Rev. 1995;16(4):460–84.
20. Young WF, Stanson AW, Thompson GB, Grant CS, Farley DR, van Heerden JA. Role for adrenal venous sampling in primary aldosteronism. Surgery. 2004;136(6):1227–35.
21. Rossi GP, Auchus RJ, Brown M, Lenders JW, Naruse M, Plouin PF, et al. An expert consensus statement on use of adrenal vein sampling for the subtyping of primary aldosteronism. Hypertension. 2014;63(1):151–60.
22. Webb R, Mathur A, Chang R, Baid S, Nilubol N, Libutti SK, et al. What is the best criterion for the interpretation of adrenal vein sample results in patients with primary hyperaldosteronism? Ann Surg Oncol. 2012;19(6):1881–6.
23. Young WF, Stanson AW. What are the keys to successful adrenal venous sampling (AVS) in patients with primary aldosteronism? Clin Endocrinol. 2009;70(1):14–7.
24. Miotto D, De Toni R, Pitter G, Seccia TM, Motta R, Vincenzi M, et al. Impact of accessory hepatic veins on adrenal vein sampling for identification of surgically curable primary aldosteronism. Hypertension. 2009;54(4):885–9.
25. Matsuura T, Takase K, Ota H, Yamada T, Sato A, Satoh F, et al. Radiologic anatomy of the right adrenal vein: preliminary experience with MDCT. AJR Am J Roentgenol. 2008;191(2):402–8.
26. Ota H, Seiji K, Kawabata M, Satani N, Omata K, Ono Y, et al. Dynamic multidetector CT and non-contrast-enhanced MR for right adrenal vein imaging: comparison with catheter venography in adrenal venous sampling. Eur Radiol. 2016;26(3):622–30.
27. Omura K, Ota H, Takahashi Y, Matsuura T, Seiji K, Arai Y, et al. Anatomical variations of the right adrenal vein: concordance between multidetector computed tomography and catheter venography. Hypertension. 2017;69:428.
28. Reardon MA, Angle JF, Abi-Jaoudeh N, Bruns DE, Haverstick DM, Matsumoto AH, et al. Intraprocedural cortisol levels in the evaluation of proper catheter placement in adrenal venous sampling. J Vasc Interv Radiol. 2011;22(11):1575–80.
29. Rossi E, Regolisti G, Perazzoli F, Negro A, Grasselli C, Santi R, et al. Intraprocedural cortisol measurement increases adrenal vein sampling success rate in primary aldosteronism. Am J Hypertens. 2011;24(12):1280–5.
30. Stowasser M. Improving the success and reliability of adrenal venous sampling: focus on intraprocedural cortisol measurement. Clin Chem. 2012;58(9):1275–7.
31. Rossi GP, Barisa M, Allolio B, Auchus RJ, Amar L, Cohen D, et al. The Adrenal Vein Sampling International Study (AVIS) for identifying the major subtypes of primary aldosteronism. J Clin Endocrinol Metab. 2012;97(5):1606–14.
32. Kupers EM, Amar L, Raynaud A, Plouin PF, Steichen O. A clinical prediction score to diagnose unilateral primary aldosteronism. J Clin Endocrinol Metab. 2012;97(10):3530–7.
33. Riester A, Fischer E, Degenhart C, Reiser MF, Bidlingmaier M, Beuschlein F, et al. Age below 40 or a recently proposed clinical prediction score cannot bypass adrenal venous sampling in primary aldosteronism. J Clin Endocrinol Metab. 2014; 99(6):E1035–9.
34. Sze WC, Soh LM, Lau JH, Reznek R, Sahdev A, Matson M, et al. Diagnosing unilateral primary aldosteronism—comparison of a clinical prediction score, computed tomography and adrenal venous sampling. Clin Endocrinol. 2014;81(1):25–30.
35. Venos ES, So B, Dias VC, Harvey A, Pasieka JL, Kline GA. A clinical prediction score for diagnosing unilateral primary aldosteronism may not be generalizable. BMC Endocr Disord. 2014;14:94.
36. Mendichovszky IA, Powlson AS, Manavaki R, Aigbirhio FI, Cheow H, Buscombe JR, et al. Targeted molecular imaging in adrenal disease—an emerging role for metomidate PET-CT. Diagnostics (Basel). 2016;6(4):42.
37. Burton TJ, Mackenzie IS, Balan K, Koo B, Bird N, Soloviev DV, et al. Evaluation of the sensitivity and specificity of (11)C-metomidate positron emission tomography (PET)-CT for lateralizing aldosterone secretion by Conn's adenomas. J Clin Endocrinol Metab. 2012;97(1):100–9.
38. Duncan JL 3rd, Fuhrman GM, Bolton JS, Bowen JD, Richardson WS. Laparoscopic adrenalectomy is superior to an open approach to treat primary

hyperaldosteronism. Am Surg. 2000;66(10):932–5; discussion 5–6
39. Haveran LA, Novitsky YW, Czerniach DR, Kaban GK, Kelly JJ, Litwin DE. Benefits of laparoscopic adrenalectomy: a 10-year single institution experience. Surg Laparosc Endosc Percutan Tech. 2006;16(4):217–21.
40. Meria P, Kempf BF, Hermieu JF, Plouin PF, Duclos JM. Laparoscopic management of primary hyperaldosteronism: clinical experience with 212 cases. J Urol. 2003;169(1):32–5.
41. Lubikowski J, Uminski M, Andrysiak-Mamos E, Pynka S, Fuchs H, Wojcicki M, et al. From open to laparoscopic adrenalectomy: thirty years' experience of one medical centre. Endokrynol Pol. 2010;61(1):94–101.
42. Muth A, Ragnarsson O, Johannsson G, Wangberg B. Systematic review of surgery and outcomes in patients with primary aldosteronism. Br J Surg. 2015;102(4):307–17.
43. Steichen O, Amar L, Chaffanjon P, Kraimps JL, Menegaux F, Zinzindohoue F. SFE/SFHTA/AFCE consensus on primary aldosteronism, part 6: adrenal surgery. Ann Endocrinol (Paris). 2016;77(3):220–5.
44. Lim PO, Jung RT, MacDonald TM. Raised aldosterone to renin ratio predicts antihypertensive efficacy of spironolactone: a prospective cohort follow-up study. Br J Clin Pharmacol. 1999;48(5):756–60.
45. Parthasarathy HK, Menard J, White WB, Young WF Jr, Williams GH, Williams B, et al. A double-blind, randomized study comparing the antihypertensive effect of eplerenone and spironolactone in patients with hypertension and evidence of primary aldosteronism. J Hypertens. 2011;29(5):980–90.
46. Karagiannis A, Tziomalos K, Papageorgiou A, Kakafika AI, Pagourelias ED, Anagnostis P, et al. Spironolactone versus eplerenone for the treatment of idiopathic hyperaldosteronism. Expert Opin Pharmacother. 2008;9(4):509–15.
47. Born-Frontsberg E, Reincke M, Rump LC, Hahner S, Diederich S, Lorenz R, et al. Cardiovascular and cerebrovascular comorbidities of hypokalemic and normokalemic primary aldosteronism: results of the German Conn's Registry. J Clin Endocrinol Metab. 2009;94(4):1125–30.
48. Mulatero P, Monticone S, Bertello C, Viola A, Tizzani D, Iannaccone A, et al. Long-term cardio- and cerebrovascular events in patients with primary aldosteronism. J Clin Endocrinol Metab. 2013;98(12):4826–33.
49. Savard S, Amar L, Plouin PF, Steichen O. Cardiovascular complications associated with primary aldosteronism: a controlled cross-sectional study. Hypertension. 2013;62(2):331–6.
50. Catena C, Colussi G, Nadalini E, Chiuch A, Baroselli S, Lapenna R, et al. Cardiovascular outcomes in patients with primary aldosteronism after treatment. Arch Intern Med. 2008;168(1):80–5.
51. Marzano L, Colussi G, Sechi LA, Catena C. Adrenalectomy is comparable with medical treatment for reduction of left ventricular mass in primary aldosteronism: meta-analysis of long-term studies. Am J Hypertens. 2015;28(3):312–8.
52. Rossi GP, Bernini G, Desideri G, Fabris B, Ferri C, Giacchetti G, et al. Renal damage in primary aldosteronism: results of the PAPY Study. Hypertension. 2006;48(2):232–8.
53. Sechi LA, Novello M, Lapenna R, Baroselli S, Nadalini E, Colussi GL, et al. Long-term renal outcomes in patients with primary aldosteronism. JAMA. 2006;295(22):2638–45.
54. Catena C, Colussi G, Sechi LA. Mineralocorticoid receptor antagonists and renal involvement in primary aldosteronism: opening of a new era. Eur J Endocrinol. 2013;168(1):C1–5.
55. Fallo F, Pilon C, Urbanet R. Primary aldosteronism and metabolic syndrome. Horm Metab Res. 2012;44(3):208–14.
56. Catena C, Lapenna R, Baroselli S, Nadalini E, Colussi G, Novello M, et al. Insulin sensitivity in patients with primary aldosteronism: a follow-up study. J Clin Endocrinol Metab. 2006;91(9):3457–63.
57. Fagart J, Hillisch A, Huyet J, Barfacker L, Fay M, Pleiss U, et al. A new mode of mineralocorticoid receptor antagonism by a potent and selective nonsteroidal molecule. J Biol Chem. 2010; 285(39):29932–40.
58. Colussi G, Catena C, Sechi LA. Spironolactone, eplerenone and the new aldosterone blockers in endocrine and primary hypertension. J Hypertens. 2013;31(1):3–15.
59. Choi M, Scholl UI, Yue P, Bjorklund P, Zhao B, Nelson-Williams C, et al. K+ channel mutations in adrenal aldosterone-producing adenomas and hereditary hypertension. Science. 2011; 331(6018):768–72.
60. Beuschlein F, Boulkroun S, Osswald A, Wieland T, Nielsen HN, Lichtenauer UD, et al. Somatic mutations in ATP1A1 and ATP2B3 lead to aldosterone-producing adenomas and secondary hypertension. Nat Genet. 2013;45(4):440–4. 444e1–2
61. Tauber P, Aichinger B, Christ C, Stindl J, Rhayem Y, Beuschlein F, et al. Cellular pathophysiology of an adrenal adenoma-associated mutant of the plasma membrane Ca(2+)-ATPase ATP2B3. Endocrinology. 2016;157(6):2489–99.
62. Scholl UI, Goh G, Stolting G, de Oliveira RC, Choi M, Overton JD, et al. Somatic and germline CACNA1D calcium channel mutations in aldosterone-producing adenomas and primary aldosteronism. Nat Genet. 2013;45(9):1050–4.
63. Piaditis G, Markou A, Papanastasiou L, Androulakis II, Kaltsas G. Progress in aldosteronism: a review of the prevalence of primary aldosteronism in pre-hypertension and hypertension. Eur J Endocrinol. 2015;172(5):R191–203.
64. Mulatero P, Stowasser M, Loh KC, Fardella CE, Gordon RD, Mosso L, et al. Increased diagnosis of

primary aldosteronism, including surgically correctable forms, in centers from five continents. J Clin Endocrinol Metab. 2004;89(3):1045–50.

65. Stowasser M, Sharman J, Leano R, Gordon RD, Ward G, Cowley D, et al. Evidence for abnormal left ventricular structure and function in normotensive individuals with familial hyperaldosteronism type I. J Clin Endocrinol Metab. 2005;90(9):5070–6.

66. Gouli A, Kaltsas G, Tzonou A, Markou A, Androulakis II, Ragkou D, et al. High prevalence of autonomous aldosterone secretion among patients with essential hypertension. Eur J Clin Investig. 2011;41(11):1227–36.

67. Piaditis GP, Kaltsas GA, Androulakis II, Gouli A, Makras P, Papadogias D, et al. High prevalence of autonomous cortisol and aldosterone secretion from adrenal adenomas. Clin Endocrinol. 2009;71(6):772–8.

28 Phaeochromocytoma

Anand Kumar Mishra, Kulranjan Singh,
Pooja Ramakant, and Amit Agarwal

Introduction

Phaeochromocytomas (PCCs) are tumours that synthesize, store and secrete catecholamines and arise from chromaffin cells of adrenal medulla and extra-adrenal sympathetic ganglia cells. Embryologically, the paraganglia system originates from the neural crest cells, which can differentiate and migrate to form the adrenal medullary chromaffin cells, autonomic ganglion cells and extra-adrenal paraganglionic cells. These cells belong to the amine precursor uptake decarboxylase(APUD)cells. Phaeochromocytoma derives its name from phaios (dusky), chroma (colour) and cytoma (tumour). The term phaeochromocytoma was coined by Pick in 1912. Fränkel was first to report a phaeochromocytoma during autopsy in 1886. The first successful operations for phaeochromocytomas were first reported in 1926 by Cesar Roux in Lausanne, Switzerland, and C.H. Mayo in the United States; but in neither case was the diagnosis established before the operation.

A. K. Mishra · K. Singh · P. Ramakant
Department of Endocrine Surgery, King George's Medical University, Lucknow, India

A. Agarwal (✉)
Department of Endocrine Surgery, Sanjay Gandhi Post Graduate Institute of Medical Sciences, Lucknow, India

Aetiology

Phaeochromocytomas occur with a prevalence of approximately 1–2 per 100,000 adults. The overall prevalence of phaeochromocytoma is 0.05% in autopsy series and 0.1–0.6% in hypertensive patients. Approximately 4% of incidentalomas are phaeochromocytomas. They occur equally in men and women, with approximately equal frequency in both adrenal glands. Sporadic phaeochromocytomas usually present in fourth decade whereas hereditary forms earlier. Phaeochromocytoma was initially classified as a '10% tumour' but now recent evidence suggests that it is more likely to be a 20% tumour because:

- 20% are extra-adrenal, are most often located within the abdomen (mostly in the renal hilum or organ of Zuckerkandl) and carry a poorer prognosis.
- 20% are multifocal.
- 20% are malignant.
- 20% are bilateral.
- 25% are familial.
- 20% occur in children, are characterized by a slight male predominance and are less likely malignant than adult tumours. Approximately 30% of paediatric phaeochromocytomas are bilateral, extra-adrenal, multiple or familial.

The incidence of synchronous or metachronous phaeochromocytomas is more common in

R. Parameswaran, A. Agarwal (eds.), *Evidence-Based Endocrine Surgery*,
https://doi.org/10.1007/978-981-10-1124-5_28

Table 28.1 Genetic syndromes associated with phaeochromocytoma

Syndrome	Gene affected	Components
MEN2A (Sipple's syndrome)	Germline missense mutations in extracellular cysteine codons of *RET*	Medullary carcinoma of thyroid Phaeochromocytoma Hyperparathyroidism
MEN2B	Germline missense mutation in tyrosine kinase domain of *RET*	Medullary carcinoma of the thyroid Phaeochromocytoma Mucosal neuroma Marfanoid habitus Ganglioneuromas of the gastrointestinal tract
Neurofibromatosis (von Recklinghausen's disease) type I	NF1 gene	Cafe-au-lait spots Axillary freckling Multiple freckling Multiple neurofibromas Phaeochromocytoma
Von Hippel-Lindau disease	VHL gene	Retinal hemangiomatosis Cerebellar hemangioblastoma Phaeochromocytoma Renal cell tumours
Familial paraganglioma (PG) syndrome	Germline mutations within the succinate dehydrogenase complex subunit B (SDHB) SDHD and SDHC genes	Glomus tumours of the carotid body and extra-adrenal paraganglioma

patients with familial forms of phaeochromocytomas. The genetic syndromes having phaeochromocytomas are listed in Table 28.1.

Risk Factors

- *Strong*
  1. **Multiple endocrine neoplasia (MEN) syndrome type 2A and B:** The lifetime risk is 50%. Tumours are frequently bilateral but symptomatic in only 50% and only one-third have hypertension. The implicated gene in both MEN2A and -2B is the RET proto-oncogene.
  2. **Von Hippel-Lindau (VHL) disease:** The lifetime risk is 10–20%. These patients will have other manifestations including renal cell carcinoma and cerebellar haemangioblastomas, as well as renal and pancreatic cysts. This results from a germline mutation in the VHL suppressor gene.
  3. **Succinate dehydrogenase (SDH) subunit B, C and D gene mutations:** There is germline mutations in the SDH-B, -C and -D genes responsible for mitochondrial succinate dehydrogenase. Patients with these germline mutations are predisposed to phaeochromocytomas, as well as head and neck paragangliomas. Carriers of the SDH-B or -D gene mutations are more likely to have malignant disease.
- *Weak*

  Neurofibromatosis type 1 (NF1): The lifetime risk is 1% and up to 5% of patients with phaeochromocytomas have been found to have NF1. Other manifestations include benign tumours of the skin, nervous system and bone.

Familial and Hereditary Phaeochromocytomas

Literature suggests that phaeochromocytomas up to 35% in adults and up to 40% in children are hereditary, associated with neuroectodermal disorders (von Hippel-Lindau disease, tuberous sclerosis, Sturge-Weber syndrome or Carney's syndrome) or multiple endocrine neoplasia type 2, neurofibromatosis type 1 (von Recklinghausen's disease) and paraganglioma syndromes (germline mutations in the succinate dehydrogenase SDH-B, -C or -D genes).

Mutations of genes encoding the SDH complex assembly factor 2 (SDHAF2), transmembrane protein 127 (TMEM 127), SDH subunit A, MYC-associated factor X (MAX) and hypoxia-inducible factor 2-alpha (HIF2A) have now been described.

In MEN2, bilateral adrenal medullary hyperplasia (diffuse or nodular) is almost always present and precedes phaeochromocytoma, and develops in 30–50% of patients. Phaeochromocytomas are usually multicentric and bilateral in up to 50–80% of cases with long-term follow-up. They are rarely extra-adrenal or malignant. The incidence of clinically significant adrenal medullary disease is greater in MEN2B. In up to 25% of cases, the diagnosis of phaeochromocytoma precedes that of C-cell disease. Therefore, mutation analyses of the RET proto-oncogene on exons 10 and 11 should be performed in all patients with phaeochromocytoma to screen for MEN2.

Extra-Adrenal Phaeochromocytomas

Extra-adrenal phaeochromocytomas account for approximately 10% of phaeochromocytomas in adults and 30% in children. These are often multicentric and are more likely to be malignant than adrenal phaeochromocytomas (36% vs. 10%). They are rarely associated with familial and hereditary phaeochromocytoma, except in Carney's syndrome, which is associated with functioning extra-adrenal paraganglioma, pulmonary chondroma and gastric epithelioid leiomyosarcoma. Extra-adrenal phaeochromocytomas are most commonly found in the organ of Zuckerkandl at the distal aorta and aortic bifurcation, but can also be found between the base of the skull and the spermatic cords, with 85% of these extra-adrenal tumours located below the diaphragm. Bladder phaeochromocytomas are usually located at the trigone or dome of the bladder and patients may present with haematuria or micturition-induced symptoms. Extra-adrenal phaeochromocytoma locations are listed in Table 28.2.

Table 28.2 Extra-adrenal locations of phaeochromocytoma

Organ of Zuckerkandl
Urinary bladder
Liver hilum
Renal hilum
Posterior mediastinum
Intrapericardial
Neck

Pathophysiology and Symptomatology

Phaeochromocytomas secrete predominantly norepinephrine. Phenylethanolamine N-methyltransferase enzyme, which converts norepinephrine to epinephrine, is present primarily in the adrenal medulla and organ of Zuckerkandl. Therefore, high levels of epinephrine are suggestive of phaeochromocytoma of adrenal origin. Rarely, phaeochromocytomas secrete other neurohormones such as dopamine, VIP, adrenocorticotrophic hormones, beta-endorphins and a variety of other substances that can complicate the clinical manifestations and the differential diagnosis.

Phaeochromocytomas are the cause of hypertension in about 0.1% of hypertensive patients. The cardiovascular pathophysiology of phaeochromocytoma is characterized by:

- Lack of correlation between plasma concentration of catecholamine and haemodynamic profile or heart disease, and blood pressure.
- The haemodynamic features of hypertension are characterized by vasoconstriction, increased peripheral vascular resistance and left ventricular hypertrophy.
- Orthostatic hypotension, with an average decrease of 14 mmHg in systolic pressure, and orthostatic tachycardia commonly occur in phaeochromocytoma (71% and 58%, respectively) due to failure of increased peripheral vascular resistance.
- 50% of patients with phaeochromocytoma exhibit sustained hypertension, 45% are normotensive between paroxysms of hypertension and approximately 5% are normotensive.

Table 28.3 Signs and symptoms of phaeochromocytoma

Symptoms	Incidence (%)	Signs	Incidence (%)
Headache	76–100	Hypertension	76–100
Palpitations	51–75	Tachycardia or reflex bradycardia	51–75
Sweating	51–75	Postural hypotension	51–75
Anxiety/nervousness	26–50	Hypertension, paroxysmal	26–50
Nausea	26–50	Weight loss	26–50
Pain abdomen, chest	26–50	Hypermetabolism	26–50
Fatigue or weakness	26–50	Fasting hyperglycaemia	26–50
Dizziness	1–25	Tremor	26–50
Heat intolerance	1–25	Increased respiratory rate	26–50
Constipation	1–25	Decreased gastrointestinal motility	26–50
Breathlessness	1–25	Psychosis	1–25
Visual disturbances	1–25	Flushing, paroxysmal	1–25
Seizures, grand mal	1–25		

Hypertension is more often sustained rather than paroxysmal in 90% of children with phaeochromocytoma.

- 20% of patients with phaeochromocytoma will have essential hypertension.

Clinical Features

About 90% of patients present with episodes of classical triad of symptoms: headache, palpitations and sweating. It is called "classic triad" in phaeochromocytoma. Patients can have paroxysmal spells (five Ps—pressure: sudden increase in blood pressure; pain: headache, chest of cardiac origin and abdominal pain; perspiration; palpitations; and pallor). Profuse sweating is common in children (Table 28.3).

Hypertension: Elevation of blood pressure either continuous or paroxysmal is the most consistent presentation especially in a young patient. About half the patients show paroxysmal hypertension with symptom-free intervals between attacks (episodic hypertension). Sometimes, excessive fluctuations in blood pressure may be seen in patients who otherwise are normotensive. Orthostatic hypotension is frequently present and is probably due to reduced intravascular volume following chronic adrenergic stimulation (Figs. 28.1 and 28.2).

Other symptoms: A patient can present with anxiety or fear attacks, stroke in young or congestive heart failure. Less commonly, severe hypertensive reactions may occur during incidental surgery, following trauma, exercise, drug intake or micturition (in the setting of bladder phaeochromocytoma) when the diagnosis is unsuspected. An unrecognized phaeochromocy-

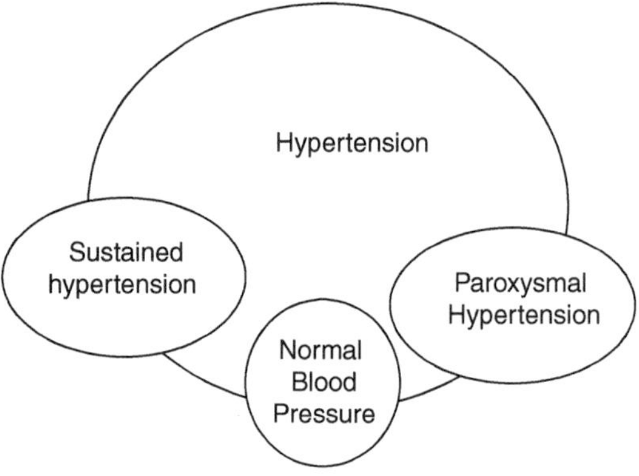

Fig. 28.1 Clinical features of phaeochromocytoma

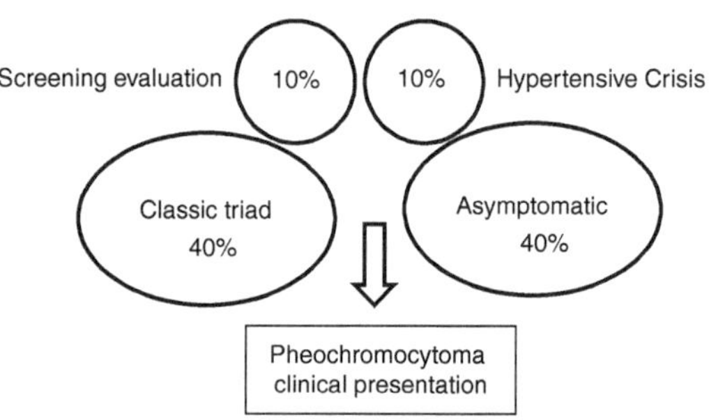

Fig. 28.2 Clinical features of phaeochromocytoma

toma may lead to death because of a hypertensive crisis, arrhythmia, myocardial infarction or multisystem crisis.

The symptoms mentioned above may be constant or intermittent. Duration and frequency of intermittent symptoms are variable, ranging from a few seconds to several days and from several times daily to once every few weeks. There may be precipitating factors for symptoms (postural changes, increase in intra-abdominal pressure, exertion, trauma, emotional stress, urination for bladder phaeochromocytoma, anaesthesia and tumour manipulation, tyramine-containing foods in the presence of monoamine oxidase inhibitors (MAOIs), drugs (corticosteroids, antibiotics—linezolid, glucagon, radiographic contrast dye, tricyclic antidepressants, metoclopramide, contrast agents, chemotherapeutic agents) and childbirth.

Pathology

PCCs are highly vascularized, greyish-pink on the cut surface and have areas of haemorrhage or necrosis. Microscopically, tumour cells are polygonal, but the configuration varies considerably. The differentiation between malignant and benign tumours is difficult like any endocrine malignancy. The following features suggest malignancy on histopathology:

- High PASS (phaeochromocytoma of the adrenal gland scale score)
- High number of Ki-67-positive cells
- Vascular invasion
- Capsular invasion

Diagnosis

Phaeochromocytoma is known as the great mimic as it can have diverse clinical manifestations. However, there are ten clinical situations in which it is appropriate to screen for a phaeochromocytoma:

- Symptomatic episodes, especially when paroxysmal and accompanied by hypertension
- Refractory hypertension
- Accelerated hypertension or malignant hypertension, especially in children and during the first two trimesters of pregnancy
- Paradoxical hypertensive response to beta-blockers
- Hypertensive crisis during anaesthesia, intubation, manipulation of any abdominal tumour, labour or angiography
- Patients with unexplained heart failure
- Patients with a family history of von Hippel-Lindau (VHL) syndrome, multiple endocrine neoplasia (MEN) 2A or 2B, type 1 neurofibromatosis (NF1) or inherited paraganglioma syndrome (due to mutation in one of the succinate dehydrogenase (*SDH*) genes)
- Marked labile hypertension or blood pressure resistant to standard multidrug therapeutic regimen
- Orthostatic hypotension in the absence of anti-hypertension therapy
- Incidentally discovered adrenal tumour, regardless of size, especially before resection or needle biopsy
- Children and young individuals with new onset of hypertension or seizures

Phaeochromocytoma diagnosis is based on elevated levels of catecholamines or products of catecholamine metabolism, either in the urine or serum (Table 28.4). The traditional diagnostic standard is a 24-h collection of urine for determination of catecholamines, vanillylmandelic acid and metanephrine levels. The key points in

Table 28.4 Sensitivity/specificity for catecholamines and metabolites

Investigation	Sensitivity (%)	Specificity (%)
Urinary catecholamines	86	83
Urinary metanephrines	97	72
Plasma catecholamines	84	88
Plasma metanephrines	98	89
Urinary VMA	64	95
Dopamine	7	99
Serum chromogranin A	86	74

relation to biochemical evaluation of PCCs include the following:

- Biochemical diagnosis is made by measurement of plasma or 12–24-h urinary metanephrines (99 and 97% sensitive), plasma or 12–24-h urinary catecholamines (86 and 84% sensitive) and urinary vanillylmandelic acid (72% sensitive).
- Urinary metanephrines often are the first-line screening test and in typical phaeochromocytoma levels are usually at least twice the upper limit of normal. Total metanephrine is less than 1.3 mg in 24 h; however, refer to reference ranges in individual laboratories
- Urinary vanillylmandelic acid (VMA) also may be useful but has a low sensitivity.
- At least two measurements may be required because of intermittent tumour secretion.
- False-positive results can occur with sympathomimetics, phenoxybenzamine, tricyclic antidepressants and other drugs (paracetamol).
- Chromogranin A has a sensitivity of 86% but poor diagnostic specificity for phaeochromocytoma. Chromogranin A is an acidic, monomeric protein stored and released with catecholamines from storage vesicles in the adrenal medulla.

Generally, biochemical levels of at least twofold above the normal range are regarded as diagnostic whereas lower values should be repeated. High-performance liquid chromatography (HPLC) appears to be the most sensitive and specific method for the measurement of fractionated catecholamines and metanephrines.

Provocative testing to diagnose phaeochromocytomas by histamine, tyramine and glucagon, which was used in previous decades, is now never used as it is dangerous. Clonidine, a central agonist, normally decreases plasma catecholamines by reducing sympathetic tone, so a clonidine suppression test may be useful to distinguish phaeochromocytoma from the patient with essential hypertension and elevated catecholamine levels. Two to three hours after clonidine administration, patients with essential hypertension should have a decrease in resting catecholamine levels (less than 500 pg/mL). Usually single dose of clonidine does not show response in phaeochromocytomas as they are not innervated and secrete catecholamines in an autonomous manner.

Genetics

Various genetic mutation tests for phaeochromocytoma include RET, VHL and SDH-B/C/D. This helps to screen the index case for other components of syndrome and also to screen the first-degree relatives. A simple way to do these tests in different settings is described in Table 28.5.

If mutation is identified at any point in the testing algorithm, no further testing should be performed.

Differential diagnosis: Thyrotoxicosis, acute clonidine withdrawal, hypoglycaemia, anxiety disorders or panic attacks, renovascular hypertension, menopause, migraines, carcinoid syndrome, pre-eclampsia, neuroblastoma and insulinoma.

Localization: After clinical and biochemical diagnosis, PCC may be located by magnetic resonance imaging (MRI), computerized tomography (CT) or radionuclide scanning with 123I-metaiodobenzylguanidine (MIBG), octreotide scintigraphy and positron emission imaging (PET). At least 85% of extra-adrenal and 98% of all phaeochromocytomas occur below the diaphragm, 2–3% are found in thorax and 1% are found in the neck. Most often the disease is localized in the abdomen (97%), the thorax (2–3%) and the neck (1%). The initial imaging test of choice is CT or MRI of the abdomen/adrenals.

Table 28.5 Simplified way of genetic testing in phaeochromocytoma

Paragangliomas	SDHB ⇨ SDHD ⇨ VHL
Bilateral phaeochromocytoma	VHL ⇨ RET
Sporadic unilateral phaeochromocytoma <20 years of age	VHL ⇨ RET ⇨ SDHB ⇨ SDHD
Sporadic unilateral phaeochromocytoma >20 years of age	SDHB ⇨ SDHD

The catecholamine profile may suggest the anatomic location. Urinary sample with high levels of epinephrine suggests an adrenal phaeochromocytoma; however exceptions have been reported. Norepinephrine-secreting tumours may be either in the adrenal gland or in an extra-adrenal location. MEN2- and NF-1-related phaeochromocytomas classically secrete epinephrine. VHL and SDHB-related phaeochromocytomas secrete norepinephrine.

CT scan: It can detect up to lesions >1 cm in size. Phaeochromocytomas are typically homogenous (40–50 Hounsfield units) with IV contrast enhancement. There may be areas of cystic necrosis, haemorrhage or calcification in larger tumours that may give a heterogenous appearance. The newer non-ionic contrast media usually do not pose a significant risk of hypertensive crisis and therefore CT scan is safe in a non-blocked patient.

MRI: MRI assesses the liver and retroperitoneum for possible metastatic disease besides providing anatomic detail. It also provides a functional imaging on T2. The hypervascularity of phaeochromocytomas gives an intermediate-to-high signal intensity with T2-weighted imaging. It does not have radiation exposure and IV contrast is not required. Therefore, it becomes radiological investigation of choice for pregnant women, children, annual screening examinations (for patients with high-risk germline mutations) and any patient with a contrast allergy. The greater resolution for different tissue types provides slighter superior sensitivity for extra-adrenal lesions compared with CT.

MIBG: MIBG is a norepinephrine analogue which accumulates in hyperfunctioning chromaffin tissue. I^{123} is better than I^{131} (90% vs. 77%). MIBG single-photon emission computed tomography (MIBG SPECT) or MIBG SPECT/CT will further improve the sensitivity over planar MIBG imaging. It is for the detection of multifocal or metastatic disease. Prior to MIBG imaging, oral iodine must be administered to avoid uptake of radioactive iodine by the thyroid gland. MIBG scans are negative in around 15% of phaeochromocytomas and in up to 50% of malignant tumours because of relatively lower affinity of MIBG to the norepinephrine transporters, lack of storage granules or loss of transporters by tumour cell dedifferentiation.

Octreotide Scintigraphy: ^{111}In-diethylenetriaminepentaacetic acid (DTPA)-octreotide and ^{121}I-DTPA-octreotide are radiolabelled analogue of somatostatin that are used to have a functional image of phaeochromocytomas because of high density of somatostatin receptors in them.

PET Imaging: PET imaging with 18F-fluorodopamine, 18F-fluorodopa, 18F-dihydroxy phenylalanine, 11C-hydroxy ephedrine and 11C-epinephrine is highly specific for phaeochromocytoma.

Preoperative Preparation

The perioperative blockade and intraoperative management are discussed in detail in chapter on perioperative management of endocrine hypertension. After biochemical diagnosis, all patients are prepared with alpha-blockade to block the catecholamine excess and their consequences during surgery. The main goals in preoperative preparation are:

- Normalize blood pressure and heart rate
- Restore volume depletion
- Prevent any intraoperative hypertensive crisis and arrhythmia

Medications used intraoperatively to control blood pressure surges include:

1. Sodium nitroprusside—reduces preload and afterload and has immediate onset and recovery in 1 min.
2. Calcium channel blockers—powerful arterial vasodilators.
3. Magnesium sulphate.
4. Esmolol—ultra-short-acting cardio selective beta-blocker: Esmolol hydrochloride, an intravenously administered selective beta-1 receptor antagonist, is used when beta-blockade of rapid onset and short duration is desired, or in critically ill patients in whom

adverse effects of bradycardia, heart failure or hypotension may necessitate rapid withdrawal of the drug.
5. Nitrogylcerin—rapidly acting venodilator.

Surgery of Phaeochromocytoma

Surgical excision of the tumour is the first-choice treatment for phaeochromocytoma. Surgery is planned only after selective alpha-adrenergic blocker (usually 7–14 days). A robust perioperative regime in a multidisciplinary setting results in remarkably safe surgical outcome with almost no mortality and minimal morbidity if any compared to the 30–40% mortality reported few decades ago. The principles of surgery in phaeochromocytoma are:

1. Complete tumour resection.
2. Minimal tumour manipulation in avoidance of tumour seeding and hypertensive crisis.
3. Control of vascular supply.
4. Adequate exposure to avoid another organ injury.
5. In MEN-associated adrenal medullary disease, surgical options include bilateral adrenalectomy or cortical-sparing subtotal adrenalectomy for adrenal medullary hyperplasia.

Numerous approaches can be made to the phaeochromocytoma. The proper approach depends on:

- Size of the tumour
- Side of the lesion
- Habitus of the patient
- Experience and preference of the surgeon

In today's era, laparoscopic approach if feasible is the approach of choice. Minimal manipulation of the tumour along with early ligation of outflow venous channels is desirable irrespective of the approach. The approach to the gland may be different; however certain concepts warrant attention:

- The adrenal glands lie high in the retroperitoneum and are located quite posterior, so adequate visualization is a must for a safe operation. Haemostasis should be rigorously maintained.
- The adrenal gland should be brought down by initially exposing the cranial attachments and dividing the rich blood supply between either right-angled clips or utilizing a forceps cautery.
- The principle is to work around tumour and early identification of the vascular supply and working around the cranial edge of the gland. It may be termed as lateral dissection. Initial aim is to make gland free superiorly. Now apply gentle traction on the kidney down and gland can be brought inferiorly for control of the adrenal vein and this is important to stabilize the patient from a burst of catecholamine release during manipulation.
- The posterior surface is generally devoid of vasculature, so it can be dissected by fingers.
- Phaeochromocytomas are extremely friable and fracture easily which can cause troublesome bleeding. Therefore, tension or traction should be maintained on the kidney or surrounding structures and not on the adrenal itself. The concept is that the "patient should be dissected from the tumour", a view which is particularly true in patients for a phaeochromocytoma in which the glands should not be manipulated.

Open Surgical Approaches

The following approaches are generally indicated for excision.

1. **Anterior trans-abdominal approach:** The anterior abdominal transperitoneal approach by subcostal incision for unilateral tumours is the most common approach. A bucket handle incision or the Chevron incision or midline incision is indicated mainly for patients with bilateral phaeochromocytoma or extra-adrenal or multiple adrenal tumours. This ensures an unhindered access to tumour site and also permits a thorough exploration of the entire abdominal cavity if needed as in multicentric/ectopic lesions.

2. **Lateral flank approach:** Well-localized unilateral tumours can also be approached through the flank approach using an incision through the bed of the 11th or 12th rib. Larger tumours should preferably be approached by an anterior abdominal or a thoracoabdominal incision.
3. **Thoracoabdominal approach:** It is indicated for large tumours or malignant phaeochromocytoma involving adjacent organs, such as the kidney, pancreas, spleen or inferior vena cava.

Laparoscopic Adrenalectomy: Laparoscopic adrenalectomy (LA) first described by Gagner in 1992 is currently considered the gold standard even though no randomized trails have ever been carried out between open and laparoscopic methods. LA can be achieved via a trans-abdominal/retroperitoneoscopic approach depending upon the surgeon's training and experience. LA is the preferred option in sporadic and majority of syndromic phaeochromocytomas (VHL, MEN, NF 1) in both unilateral and bilateral lesions. However, open adrenalectomy may be the preferred option in phaeochromocytomas associated with phaeochromocytoma—paraganglioma syndrome (SDH-B/C/D). *The technique of LA is described in detail in later chapter.*

Advantages:

- Less operative and perioperative morbidity with early recovery and less pain for the patient.
- No significant increase in cardiac index or left ventricular work has been noticed in spite of increased intraoperative hypertensive during LA when compared to open methods.

Robotic adrenalectomy: Robotic adrenalectomy was first performed in 1999 by Piazza et al. which has minimized many of the drawbacks of the laparoscopic surgery like compromised depth perception and camera syncing. It has been proposed as a safe, feasible and effective approach more so in obese, larger lesions and when contemplating cortical sparing surgery. However, cost implications, loss of haptic feedback and anaesthetic perspective are some of the drawbacks. In spite of its many advantages till date robotic adrenalectomy has not provided any distinct benefit over laparoscopy in terms of patient outcome and comfort.

Bilateral adrenalectomy: Bilateral adrenalectomy results in lifelong corticosteroid replacement with a high probability of imminent morbidity and mortality. Partial adrenalectomy performed first in 1996 via open method and 1998 via laparoscopy avoids complications by removing the tumour as well as presumably circumventing post-operative supplementation therapy. For the remnant gland to retain corticotropic function, at least 1/3rd of the adrenal grand with intact vascularity has to be preserved. The risk of recurrence should be kept in mind, which ranges between 0 and 21%. Endoscopic procedures result in better results, probably because of magnification. Cortical-sparing surgery has been advocated as the preferred method in MEN2/VHL-associated unilateral phaeochromocytoma because of high risk of contralateral metachronous phaeochromocytoma.

Complications

The complications which can happen during surgery of phaeochromocytoma are summarized in Table 28.6 and discussed in detail in the chapter on *complications in adrenal surgery*.

Post-operative Care

1. Fluid replacement, preferably with colloids to prevent hypotension—replace 1.5 times the blood volume for 24–48 h.
2. Central venous pressure and blood pressure monitoring
3. Blood glucose monitoring for 24 h

Persistent hypertension in the post-operative period can be because of the residual tumour, autonomic instability, pain and volume overload. Coexisting essential hypertension may also be a factor if it persists longer. One-fourth of patients may remain hypertensive after phaeochromocytoma

Table 28.6 Complications following adrenal surgery

Intraoperative complications	Post-operative complications following surgery
Haemorrhage	*Generic complications*
Inferior vena cava	Haemorrhage from adrenal arteries, inferior vena cava
Adrenal vein	Pneumothorax
Lumbar vein	Pancreatitis
Hepatic vein	Pneumonia
Vascular	Hiccoughs
Ligation of renal artery branch	*Specific:*
Ligation of mesenteric artery	Hypotension
IVC involvement	Hypertension
Adjacent organ injury	Hypoglycaemia
Pneumothorax	
Pancreas, liver, spleen	
Stomach, colon, kidney	
Complications related to HTN crisis	
Myocardial infarction	
Pulmonary oedema	
Acute heart failure	
Cerebral stroke	

removal. Biochemical testing should be repeated approximately 14 days following surgery to check for remaining disease. These patients require life-long follow-up.

Post-operative hypoglycaemia can occur due to relative increase in sensitivity to insulin after sudden withdrawal of the catecholamines. Therefore, blood sugar should be monitored hourly for the first 3 or 4 h after surgery. Patients with operation of bilateral phaeochromocytoma will develop adrenal insufficiency and will require steroid replacement therapy. Glucocorticoid preparations should be administered preoperatively when bilateral adrenalectomy is contemplated, especially in patients with bilateral tumours or in familial phaeochromocytoma.

Follow-Up

Repeat evaluations are done annually thereafter or recurrence of symptoms whichever is early. Ten to twenty per cent of patients will continue to be hypertensive and require long-term treatment following operation. Metastatic disease may be seen after several years in a rare patient. Metastatic disease is defined as presence of catecholamine secreting tissue in non-chromaffin-bearing organs. Recurrences are more likely in patients with MEN type 2A. Recurrences may also occur in patients who do not have any evidence of capsular or vascular invasion on histopathology. In the absence of distant disease, the pathologic diagnosis of malignancy of phaeochromocytoma is very difficult.

Phaeochromocytoma Crisis: Phaeochromocytoma crisis has been defined as acute severe presentation of catecholamine-induced hemodynamic instability causing end-organ damage or dysfunction. The reported incidence is up to 18% and it is ten times more frequently related to phaeochromocytoma compared to paraganglioma (Table 28.7). It is often reversible with appropriate treatment. It is described of two types:

Table 28.7 Emergency situations associated with phaeochromocytoma

Clinical setting	Symptoms
Phaeochromocytoma crisis	Hypertension and/or hypotension, multiple-organ failure, temperature of 40 °C, encephalopathy
Cardiovascular (on induction of anaesthesia, medication-induced or other mechanisms)	Collapse, hypertensive crisis, shock or profound hypotension, acute heart failure, myocardial infarction, arrhythmia, cardiomyopathy, myocarditis, dissecting aortic aneurysm, limb ischaemia, digital necrosis or gangrene
Respiratory	Adult respiratory distress syndrome, acute pulmonary oedema
Abdominal	Abdominal bleeding, acute intestinal obstruction, severe enterocolitis and peritonitis, colon perforation, bowel ischaemia plus generalized peritonitis, mesenteric vascular occlusion, acute pancreatitis, cholecystitis, megacolon
Neurological	Hemiplegia, limb weakness
Renal	Severe haematuria, acute pyelonephritis, acute renal failure
Metabolic	Diabetic ketoacidosis, lactic acidosis

Type A crisis: A more limited crisis without sustained hypotension
Type B crisis: Severe presentation with sustained hypotension, shock and multi-organ dysfunction

Malignant Phaeochromocytoma: About 10% of adrenal phaeochromocytomas are malignant and rates are higher in extra-adrenal sites. To establish the malignancy in phaeochromocytoma is difficult like any endocrine disease and preoperatively the criteria for malignancy are invasion into adjacent tissue or distant metastases. However, elevated urinary dopamine may be suggestive of a malignant phaeochromocytoma. Complete surgical excision is the only potentially curative therapy for malignant phaeochromocytoma and aggressive surgical resection is indicated in all patients who can tolerate the procedure. It is difficult to demonstrate malignancy in the surgical specimen also so long-term follow-up is required in all patients of phaeochromocytoma. It is well established that apparently benign, completely excised, well-encapsulated tumours can develop distant metastases after years of treatment.

Phaeochromocytoma in Pregnancy

Clinically PCCs in pregnancy mimic an amnion infection syndrome or pre-eclampsia and both mother and unborn child are threatened by hypertensive crisis during delivery. After adequate alpha-blockade laparoscopic adrenalectomy can be done in the first and second trimesters while in the third trimester elective caesarean together with consecutive adrenalectomy should be planned.

Conclusion

Phaeochromocytomas carry significant morbidity and mortality if untreated. Biochemical diagnosis and precise tumour localization are mandatory. Though at present preoperative blockade is the standard of care, few reports have questioned this approach. Complete surgical excision is the definitive treatment for benign and malignant phaeochromocytoma with low morbidity and mortality. Though laparoscopic adrenalectomy has become the standard of care for phaeochromocytomas, retroperitoneal approach is rapidly becoming an attractive option. Phaeochromocytoma and paraganglioma are now known to be associated with 16 susceptibility genes; hence it is important to have a high suspicion for familial phaeochromocytoma and the clinician should triage the genetic testing based on individual clinical features. As in many endocrine tumours, there are no uniform definitive or accurate histological criteria to distinguish malignancy, which is dependent on the clinical behaviour of the tumour. Over the last few decades, worldwide phaeochromocytomas have been operated with significantly reduced morbidity and mortality due to judicious use of alpha-blockade, beta-blockade and advances in intraoperative drug management of haemodynamic instability.

Bibliography

1. Manger WM, Gifford RW. Pheochromocytoma. J Clin Hypertens. 2002;4:62–72.
2. Manger WM. An overview of pheochromocytoma: history, current concepts, vagaries, and diagnostic challenges. Ann N Y Acad Sci. 2006;1073:1–20.
3. Pacak K. Preoperative management of the pheochromocytoma patient. J Clin Endocrinol Metab. 2007;92:4069–79.
4. Thomas RM, Ruel E, Shantavasinkul PC, Corsino L. Endocrine hypertension: an overview on the current etiopathogenesis and management options. World J Hypertens. 2015;5(2):14–27.
5. Lentschener C, Gaujoux S, Tesniere A, Dousset B. Point of controversy: perioperative care of patients undergoing pheochromocytoma removal-time for a reappraisal? Eur J Endocrinol. 2011;165(3):365–73.
6. Ramakrishna H. Pheochromocytoma resection: current concepts in anesthetic management. J Anaesthesiol Clin Pharmacol. 2015;31(3):317–23.
7. Goldstein RE, O'Neill JA Jr, Holcomb GW 3rd, Morgan WM 3rd, Neblett WW 3rd, Oates JA, Brown N, Nadeau J, Smith B, Page DL, Abumrad NN, Scott HW Jr. Clinical experience over 48 years with pheochromocytoma. Ann Surg. 1999;229(6):755–64; discussion 764–6
8. Groeben H, Nottebaum BJ, Alesina PF, Traut A, Neumann HP, Walz MK. Perioperative α-receptor

blockade in phaeochromocytoma surgery: an observational case series. Br J Anaesth. 2017;118(2):182–9.
9. Bruynzeel H, Feelders RA, Groenland TH, van den Meiracker AH, van Eijck CH, Lange JF, de Herder WW, Kazemier G. Risk factors for hemodynamic instability during surgery for pheochromocytoma. J Clin Endocrinol Metab. 2010;95(2):678–85.
10. Bravo E. Evolving concepts in the pathophysiology, diagnosis, and treatment of pheochromocytoma. Endocr Rev. 1994;15(3):356–68.
11. Pacak K, et al. Recent advances in genetics, diagnosis, localization, and treatment of pheochromocytoma. Ann Intern Med. 2001;134(4):315–29.
12. Manger WM, Gifford RW. Clinical and experimental pheochromocytoma. 2nd ed. Cambridge, MA: Blackwell Science; 1996.
13. Plouin PF, Degoulet P, Tugaye A, et al. Screening for phaeochromocytoma: in which hypertensive patients? A semilogical study of 2585 patients, including 11 with phaeochromcytoma. Nouv Press Med. 1981;10(11):869–72.
14. Brouwers FM, Lenders JW, Eisenhofer G, Pacak K. Pheochromocytoma as an endocrine emergency. Rev Endocr Metab Disord. 2003;4:121–8.
15. Jafri M, Maher ER. The genetics of phaeochromocytoma: using clinical features to guide genetic testing. Eur J Endocrinol. 2012;166:151–8.
16. Havekes B, King K, Lai EW, Romijn JA, Corssmit EP, Pacak K. New imaging approaches to pheochromocytomas and paragangliomas. Clin Endocrinol. 2010;72:137–45.
17. Brandao LF, Autorino R, Laydner H, Haber G-P, Ouzaid I, Sio MD, Perdona S, Stein RJ, Porpiglia F, Kaouk JH. Robotic versus laparoscopic adrenalectomy: a systematic review and meta-analysis. Eur Urol. 2014;65:1154–61.
18. Golden SH, Robinson KA, Saldanha I, et al. Clinical review: prevalence and incidence of endocrine and metabolic disorders in the United States: a comprehensive review. J Clin Endocrinol Metab. 2009;94:1853–78.
19. Lenders J, Eisenhofer G, Mannelli M, Pacak K. Phaeochromo cytoma. Lancet. 2005;366:665–75.
20. Gimenez-Roqueplo A, Dahia P, Robledo M. An update on the genetics of paraganglioma, pheochromocytoma, and associated hereditary syndromes. Horm Metab Res. 2012;44:328–33.
21. Scholz T, Eisenhofer G, Pacak K, et al. Clinical review: current treatment of malignant pheochromocytoma. J Clin Endocrinol Metab. 2007;92:1217–25.
22. Galan R, Kann H. Genetics and molecular pathogenesis of pheochromocytoma and paraganglioma. Clin Endocrinol. 2013;78:165–75.
23. Pacak K, Eisenhofer G, Ahlman H, et al. International symposium on pheochromocytoma: recommendations for clinical practice from the First International Symposium. Nat Clin Pract Endocrinol Metab. 2007;3:92102.
24. Eisenhofer G, Goldstein DS, Walther MM, et al. Biochemical diagnosis of pheochromocytoma: how to distinguish true from false positive test results. J Clin Endocrinol Metab. 2003;88:2656–66.
25. Goldstein DS, Eisenhofer G, Flynn JA, Wand G, Pacak K. Diagnosis and localization of pheochromocytoma. Hypertension. 2004;43:90710.
26. Agrawal R, Mishra SK, Bhatia E, Mishra A, Chand G, Agarwal G, Agarwal A, Verma AK. Prospective study to compare peri-operative hemodynamic alterations following preparation for pheochromocytoma surgery by phenoxybenzamine or prazosin. World J Surg. 2014;38(3):716–23.
27. Agarwal A, Mehrotra PK, Jain M, Gupta SK, Mishra A, Chand G, Agarwal G, Verma AK, Mishra SK, Singh U. Size of the tumour and Pheochromocytoma of the Adrenal Gland Scaled Score (PASS): can they predict malignancy? World J Surg. 2010;34(12):3022–8.
28. Bhargava PR, Mishra A, Agarwal G, Agarwal A, Verma AK, Mishra SK. Adrenal incidentalomas: experience from a developing country. World J Surg. 2008;32(8):1802–8.

Surgery for Adrenocortical Cancer: Evidence-Based Recommendations

29

Radu Mihai

Adrenocortical carcinoma (ACC) is an exceedingly rare tumour associated with poor survival for which radical surgical excision remains the only potentially curative treatment. This chapter is based on data collected by the author during publication of a systematic review of this topic published in the *British Journal of Surgery* [1] and during work as a senior author of guidelines for perioperative care of ACC patients published through a collaboration between the *European Society of Endocrine Surgeons* (ESES) and the *European Network for the Study of Adrenal Tumours* (ENSAT) [2].

Epidemiology of ACC

With an estimated annual incidence of 1–2 patients per million individuals ACC is frequently referred to as an *orphan disease*, i.e. a condition that affects fewer than 200,000 people nationwide in the USA. In the USA, the National Cancer Database recorded 4275 patients with ACC from 1985 to 2007 [3]. The Netherlands Cancer Registry [4] included 359 patients between 1993 and 2010 and demonstrated an increase in the percentage of patients receiving treatment within 6 months after diagnosis related to an increase in surgery for patients with advanced disease. The German ACC registry comprised 492 patients diagnosed between 1986 and 2007 [5]. The registry created by the European Network for Study of Adrenal Tumours (ENSAT; http://www.ensat.org) already contains clinical data on over 2000 patients.

Women appear to be more commonly affected, with a median female-to-male ratio of 1.6 in a population of 6658 women and 4865 men collected from 14 recent publications [1] . Left-sided tumours seem to be more common (2607 left-sided and 2169 right-sided tumours were reported in several recent series) [1].

Preoperative Assessment

Clinical Presentation

Two-thirds of patients present with symptoms or signs of excessive hormone secretion. One-third of patients have large non-secreting tumours and present with symptoms related to the size of the tumour. Clinical history and examination should assess:

- Signs/symptoms related to excess hormone production (e.g. Cushing's syndrome, virilization in females; feminization in males)
- Local compressive symptoms of a large intra-abdominal mass (e.g. pain, abdominal distension, early satiety, nausea/vomiting, weight loss, leg oedema)

R. Mihai
Department of Endocrine Surgery, Churchill Cancer Centre, Oxford University Hospitals NHS Foundation Trust, Oxford, UK
e-mail: radumihai@doctors.org.uk

R. Parameswaran, A. Agarwal (eds.), *Evidence-Based Endocrine Surgery*,
https://doi.org/10.1007/978-981-10-1124-5_29

- Genetic/familial context (Li-Fraumeni, multiple endocrine neoplasia type 1, Lynch syndrome, familial adenomatous polyposis, Gardner syndrome and Beckwith-Wiedemann syndrome)

Biochemical Assessment

Before operating on a suspected ACC it is imperative to exclude the diagnosis of phaeochromocytoma by measuring 24-h urinary metanephrines or plasma metanephrines. Excessive secretion of steroids/precursors should be assessed by dexamethasone suppression test in order to identify patients who need postoperative steroid replacement. A new promising approach for differentiating adenomas from ACCs uses mass spectrometry-based steroid profiling of 24-h urine samples [6] and this approach is under evaluation in a prospective multicentre trial EURINE-ACT (see www.ensat.org).

Radiological Assessment

Computed tomography (CT scan) provides information regarding the size, shape, margins, internal structure, vascular distribution, venous thrombus, lymph node involvement, adjacent organ invasion (i.e. invasion of the kidney, distal pancreas, spleen, liver or diaphragm), presence of intravascular thrombus and distant spread of tumour.

Most ACCs are large at presentation, with a diameter of >6 cm in more than 90% of cases [7, 8]. The median size reported in large series is 10–11 cm (range 2–40 cm) [7]. In an analysis of 457 patients with ACC recorded in the Surveillance, Epidemiology, and End Results (SEER) database [9] the risk of malignancy increased from 52% to 80%, 95% and 98%, and likelihood ratios for tumour size predicting malignancy were 2, 4, 16 and 24, respectively, for tumours <4 cm, >6 cm, >8 cm and >10 cm. This is the basis of recommending adrenalectomy for non-functional incidentalomas larger than 4 cm. In our own experience we found that at 8 cm threshold 1:6 tumours are benign and 5:6 tumours are malignant [10].

On non-enhanced CT scan a spontaneous density of >10 HU has a high sensitivity, but relatively low specificity to define an adrenal mass as malignant [7, 8, 11].

Metastases are frequently found at presentation and the most common sites are regional lymph nodes (25–46%), lungs (45–97%), liver (48–96%) and bones (11–33%) [12].

On MRI imaging the appearance of ACCs compared with the liver is iso/hypointense on T1-weighted and hyperintense on T2-weighted imaging [7, 13]. The chemical shift on contrast-enhanced MRI can identify the lipid-rich adenomas that have a very low risk of malignancy [14].

[^{18}F]fluorodeoxyglucose (FDG) PET–CT has 95% sensitivity and specificity for the diagnosis of ACC [15]. An adrenal-to-liver standardized uptake value (SUV) ratio above 1.6 provides 100% sensitivity and 100% negative predictive value for the diagnosis of ACC [16]. Similar appearance can occur in adrenal metastases; hence the scans should be interpreted with caution in patients with a previous diagnosis of malignancy [17]. Secondly, FDG-PET uptake values have limited prognostic value and do not correlate with survival [18].

Imaging with metomidate labelled with I^{123} (iodometomidate, [^{123}I]IMTO) can diagnose adrenocortical lesions with high specificity. In a prospective study of 58 patients with metastatic ACC, of 430 lesions detected by conventional imaging, 30% showed strong tracer accumulation [19]. Availability of this tracer is currently limited.

Preoperative Biopsy

The ESES-ENSAT guidelines recommend against preoperative biopsy of suspected ACC if surgical radical excision is feasible [2]. Biopsy is reasonable only in case of suspicion of primary adrenal lymphoma or when trying to demonstrate metastatic disease.

Staging

The ENSAT classification (Table 29.1) is currently used worldwide. It was originally based on data derived form 492 patients from the German ACC registry [5], it was validated in a North American population-based cohort of 573 patients, and it showed high accuracy in predicting recurrence and survival rates [20].

Genetic Analysis in Patients with ACC

Because ACC is a hallmark tumour in families with Li–Fraumeni syndrome caused by mutations in the tumour protein P53 (TP53) gene, some advocate TP53 testing in all patients with ACC regardless of age at diagnosis [21]. Others consider this test justified in all young adults with ACC as one in ten of them might carry such mutations [22]. In a study of 114 patients with confirmed ACC evaluated in the University of Michigan 53 completed TP53 testing, of whom 4 (8%) had a TP53 mutation even though none of them met the clinical diagnostic criteria for Li–Fraumeni syndrome [23].

Table 29.1 Staging systems for adrenocortical cancer

	Description
TNM [32]	
T1	≤5 cm, no local invasion
T2	>5 cm, no local invasion
T3	Any size, extension into periadrenal fat
T4	Any size, invasion into neighbouring organs
N1	Metastases into local lymph nodes
M1	Metastatic disease
AJCC/UICC [32]	
Stage I	T1 N0 M0
Stage II	T2 N0 M0
Stage III	T1–2 N1 M0 or T3 N0 M0
Stage IV	T3 N1 M0 or T4 any N M0 or any T any N M1
ENSAT [7]	
Stage I	T1 N0 M0
Stage II	T2 N0 M0
Stage III	T3–T4 N0 M0 or any T N1 M0
Stage IV	Any T any N M1 (distant metastases)

AJCC American Joint Committee on Cancer, *UICC* International Union Against Cancer, *ENSAT* European Network for Study of Adrenal Tumours

Radical Open Adrenalectomy for Adrenocortical Carcinoma

Complete tumour resection is the only curative treatment for ACC. Patients with locally advanced disease treated without surgery have poor survival. In a cohort of 320 patients registered in the SEER database the 1-year survival rate for stage III was only 13% if not operated and 77% after surgical treatment. For stage IV disease these figures were 16% and 54%, respectively [24].

There are several separate issues to be addressed:

Extent of the Initial Surgery for Locally Invasive Tumours

The radical surgical approach to locally invasive tumours should include a multivisceral resection. *En bloc* resections are done to prevent breaching of the tumour capsule with control of the large vessels, even through direct invasion into adjacent organs is rare. There are no published data demonstrating improved survival or lower local recurrence rates, but multivisceral resection allows safer vascular control and potentially complete venous tumour thrombus resection that could improve long-term disease-free survival [25].

Need for adjacent organ resection or extended resection. The upper limit of the perirenal space is not covered by Gerota's fascia, explaining the clinical finding that right-sided ACCs may invade the liver and/or diaphragm and left-sided ACCs may invade the spleen, pancreas and/or diaphragm [26, 27]. Although the published data offers scarce details about such intraoperative findings, it is generally agreed that adjacent organs should be resected *en bloc* if they are suspected to be invaded. This includes the spleen, distal pancreas, stomach, kidney, right liver, colon, diaphragm and wall of the vena cava or the left renal vein. The threshold for *en bloc* resection of adjacent organs, if they are suspected to be invaded, should be low.

To avoid the risk of capsular damage when dissecting the tumour from the kidney, some surgeons have advocated performing an *en bloc* resection of the retroperitoneal space including the kidney [28], although a survival benefit of this radical approach has not been proven [29, 30]. A retrospective study compared the oncological results of patients with stage II ACC treated by radical adrenalectomy alone or by nephro-adrenalectomy. The results did not support the hypothesis that nephrectomy improved the oncologic outcome [31]. Combined nephrectomy, however, offers a lower risk of capsular rupture and can facilitate a complete lymphadenectomy of the renal hilum. In a multicentre European study on surgery for ACC, a pathological invasion of the kidney was observed in only 30% of the cases with combined nephrectomy [28].

Regional Lymphadenectomy During Adrenalectomy for ACC

Retrospective data suggest that regional lymph node involvement in ACC has a negative impact on overall survival [32] and is frequently the cause of locoregional recurrence [33–35]. As recently reported by Fassnacht et al. [5] and independently validated in North America in the Surveillance, Epidemiology, and End Results (SEER) registries [20], patients with stage III tumours and positive lymph nodes have a 10-year overall survival of up to 40% after resection, although this finding has recently been challenged [36–38]. It is not yet decided whether a modified ENSAT classification should consider node-positive ACC as stage IV disease [36].

Reported rates of lymph node involvement range from 4 to 73% [5, 28, 32, 39–41] suggesting that formal regional lymphadenectomy is neither formally performed by surgeons nor accurately assessed or reported by pathologists. According to large American and French series, approximately one-third of patients with ACC had formal lymphadenectomy as part of the tumour resection, reflecting the heterogeneity of operative management [28, 41]. However, pathological postmortem studies of patients with ACC exhibited an involvement of lymph nodes in approximately 70% of patients [40]. The data from the German Adrenocortical Cancer registry suggest a reduced risk of local recurrence and disease-related death if more than five lymph nodes are removed [42]. In addition, lymph node dissection contributes to more accurate tumour staging, but its influence on overall and disease-free survival is uncertain [38]. The precise determination of which lymphatic fields and how many nodes should be dissected remains to be elucidated.

Management of Tumours with IVC Extension

Involvement of the IVC is a major challenge for surgical treatment of ACC. A first report [43] from Cochin Hospital, Paris, was based on 15 patients, in whom the upper limit of extension was the intrahepatic IVC in 2 patients, retrohepatic IVC in 6 and suprahepatic IVC in 7 patients, including 4 with extension into the right atrium. The operative technique was thrombectomy (13 patients), partial resection with direct closure (1) and total resection with replacement of the IVC (1). Median survival time was 8 months. Three patients were still alive after 24–45 months of follow-up, one of whom was reoperated for local recurrence at 17 months.

A subsequent publication from New York reported the outcome of 57 patients undergoing resection with curative intent for ACC, and for whom large-vessel extension was defined as vascular wall invasion or intraluminal extension of the neoplasm into the IVC or renal vein [44]. Compared with those without large-vessel extension, patients with such extension had a higher rate of tumour-positive surgical margins, shorter median overall survival (18 vs. 111 months) and shorter median recurrence-free survival (11 vs. 64 months).

A survey of members of ESES received replies from 18 centres in 9 countries and reported the outcome of 38 patients with ACC invading the IVC [45]. Open adrenalectomy was associated with resection of surrounding viscera in 24 patients. Complete resection (R0) was achieved in 20 patients, 7 patients had persistent microscopic disease (R1) and 4 had macroscopic residual disease (R2). Five patients died within 30 days, 25 died after a median of 5 (range 2–61) months after surgery and 13 patients were alive at a median of 16 (2–58) months, 6 of whom had no signs of distant disease.

Neoadjuvant Therapy for Potentially Unresectable Tumours

A recent publication from MD Anderson Cancer Center introduced the concept of '*borderline resectable adrenal tumours*' [46]. The authors compared 38 patients with ACC considered for immediate surgery with 15 patients who had borderline resectable ACC and received neoadjuvant therapy (mitotane and etoposide or cisplatin-based chemotherapy). Thirteen patients with borderline resectable ACC underwent surgical resection, of whom five had a partial response, seven had stable disease and one had progressive disease. Median disease-free survival for patients with borderline resectable ACC was 28 months, compared with 13 months for those who had initial surgery. Five-year overall survival rates were similar at 65% and 50%, respectively.

Palliative Surgery for ACC

The benefit of R2 resection of the primary ACC in the case of non-resectable metastatic or locally recurrent disease has not been well studied. Studies of other cancers such as renal carcinoma [47] cannot be extrapolated to ACC. In this setting, resection of primary ACC in the case of non-resectable metastatic disease or palliative (R2) resection cannot be recommended. Patients with incomplete resection (R2 or debulking surgery) and non-surgical patients had similar progression-free survival [34], even though anecdotal series have reported favourable outcome following surgery [48]. However, debulking surgery may be considered for large, symptomatic and/or oversecreting ACC resistant to medical treatment if at least 80% of the tumour is removable with a minimal/acceptable morbidity.

Laparoscopic Surgery for Adrenocortical Carcinomas

Some experienced surgeons have proposed a laparoscopic approach as a valuable alternative to open adrenalectomy, even for large tumours with malignant potential. This remains a controversial issue because operating on tumours with a diameter over 6–8 cm creates significant technical challenges in not breaching the tumour capsule and fracturing the tumour. Outcomes reported from large units might not be easy for the 'occasional' adrenal surgeon to match.

A systematic review [49] of 23 publications described 673 patients with localized ACC, of whom 112 had laparoscopic surgery. For tumours smaller than 10 cm in size without evidence of invasiveness, laparoscopic adrenalectomy did not seem to be oncologically inferior to open surgery when the operation was performed in a specialized centre. The main recommendation was that open adrenalectomy should still be regarded as standard treatment for ACC and that laparoscopic surgery should be performed within a clinical trial [49].

The published literature was also reviewed at the ESES 2012 symposium. In the absence of any randomized trial there was only qualitative evidence and the data were summarized as follows [50]. The comparison of oncological outcomes remains equivocal as there is an increased risk of local recurrence and peritoneal carcinomatosis when surgery is carried out by the laparoscopic route, although survival and recurrence rates appear to be similar. The conclusion was that laparoscopic resection may be performed in patients with stage I–II ACCs with a diameter smaller than 10 cm, with the aim of including removal of surrounding periadrenal fat to achieve R0 resection without tumour capsule rupture.

Most recent publications continue to be divided on whether or not laparoscopic adrenalectomy provides equivalent oncological outcomes, at least for smaller tumours without local invasion.

Surgery for Recurrent Disease

In 1999, a median survival of 74 months and a 5-year survival rate of 57% were reported in patients undergoing complete second resections for recurrent disease, compared with 16 months and zero, respectively, in those who had incomplete second resection (discussed by Else and colleagues [51]). In a retrospective analysis from the German ACC registry of 154 patients with first recurrence after initial radical resection, 101 patients underwent repeat surgery, with radical resection in 78; 99 patients received additional non-surgical therapy. After a median of 6 (range 1–221) months, 144 patients experienced progression. The best predictors of prolonged survival after first recurrence were time to first recurrence over 12 months and R0 resection. These data suggest that radical reoperation should only be offered to patients with delayed recurrence.

Surgeons at the Mayo Clinic reported recurrence in 93 of 125 patients who had an initial R0 resection [48]. The median time to recurrence was 15 (range 2–150) months. Of the 67 patients who underwent reoperation for recurrence, 48 had R0 resection. Median survival was 179 days for those who had no therapy, 226 days for patients managed without surgery and 1272 days for those who had debulking surgery. Radical resection (R0) for recurrence and a disease-free interval longer than 6 months were associated with survival after operation. Based on these data, patients with recurrent ACC may benefit from operative intervention, with improvement in survival and symptoms.

Surgery for Metastatic Disease

Radical surgery for metastatic disease is seldom reported as the number of such patients referred for surgery in each centre remains low. In a retrospective cohort study of 124 consecutive patients with metastatic ACC from the Gustave Roussy Institute and Cochin Hospital, Paris, the presence of hepatic and bone metastases, number of metastatic lesions, number of organs that are the site of metastasis, a high mitotic rate (more than 20 per 50 high-power fields) and atypical mitoses in the primary tumour were predictors of survival. Similarly, a report from the National Cancer Institute included over 100 procedures in 57 patients over three decades (1977–2009); there were 23 resections for liver metastases, 48 for pulmonary metastases, 22 for abdominal disease including local recurrences and 13 for metastases at other sites. Median and 5-year survival from time of first metastasectomy were 2.5 years and 41%, respectively. Patients with a disease-free interval of more than 1 year had better survival (median 6.6 vs. 1.7 years).

Surgery for liver metastases from ACC is rarely considered. A review published in 2006 identified only 48 reports, with complete clinical data available for analysis in only nine patients [52]. Based on this limited information, the impression was that metachronous metastases that developed after a minimum of 1 year following resection of the primary tumour, and were completely removable, may represent an indication for surgery. A series from the US National Cancer Institute reported only 19 liver resections from 1979 to 2009 [53]. Of the 19 patients, 13 had synchronous extrahepatic disease. The status 'disease in the liver only' was reached in 18 of 19 patients after surgery, and in 6 of 17 patients after a median follow-up of 6 years. A disease-free interval greater than 9 months after primary resection was associated with longer survival (median 4 vs. 1 year). The median overall survival (1.9 years) and 5-year survival rate (29%) were encouraging.

Similar outcomes were reported from Memorial Sloan–Kettering Cancer Center [29] in 28 patients with liver metastases who had surgery between 1978 and 2009. The median disease-free and overall survival after hepatectomy were 7 and 32 months, respectively, with a 5-year survival rate of 39%. Even though it is rarely curative, liver resection appears to be justified if it can be done with minimal morbidity.

Pulmonary metastasectomy for primary ACC was performed in only 24 patients recorded in the

German national registry (1989–2009) [54]. The 5-year survival rate was 25%, with median survival of 50 months. Age younger than 41 years at the time of first pulmonary metastasectomy was associated with improved survival. The data also showed that recurrence of pulmonary metastases should not preclude repeated surgical resection of these lesions.

Similar results were reported from US National Institutes of Health following analysis of 26 patients who underwent 60 pulmonary metastasectomies over three decades (1979–2010) [55]. After resection of a median of six metastases, 23 patients were rendered free from disease in the lung and 14 patients became completely disease free. Median overall and 5-year actuarial survival from initial pulmonary metastasectomy were 40 months and 41%, respectively. Time to first recurrence after adrenalectomy and T category of the primary tumour were associated with increased overall survival after pulmonary metastasectomy.

The most recent publication on this topic summarizes the experience of the Mayo Clinic and MD Anderson Cancer Centre over a decade (2000–2012) [56]. Synchronous resection of the primary ACC and metastatic disease was performed in 27 patients with lung (19 patients), liver (11) and brain (1) metastases. Complete resection (R0) was achieved in 11 patients. Median overall survival was improved in patients with R0 resection compared with those who had R2 resection (860 vs. 390 days). Patients undergoing neoadjuvant therapy had a trend towards better survival than those who had no neoadjuvant therapy. Adjuvant therapy was associated with improved recurrence-free survival at 6 months and 1 year, but not improved overall survival. The authors emphasized that the response to neoadjuvant chemotherapy may be of use in defining which patients benefit from surgical intervention.

The Need to Centralize Surgery for ACC

The rarity of the disease, the challenges raised by individual cases in deciding the extent of surgical resection, the need for multidisciplinary involvement for cases with IVC invasion and the clinical experience of allied specialties (pathology, oncology) make it mandatory to centralize the care of patients with ACC in a small number of centres so that the accumulated experience can improve the quality of care provided to such patients. This debate continues [57].

The national audit maintained by the British Association of Endocrine and Thyroid Surgeons (BAETS) recorded only 81 adrenalectomies for ACC during 2005–2012 among over 1700 adrenalectomies performed in the same interval. Based on the estimated incidence of ACC, it was predicted that over 500 patients should have been diagnosed during this time interval. Further proof of a lack of centralization of care of patients with ACC in the UK is shown by the publication of the joint experience of managing 30 patients with ACC over a decade at three large centres for endocrine surgery [58]. The number of patients in this report reinforces the hypothesis that most patients with ACC remain unknown to those with an expressed interest and confirmed expertise in the management of this condition. Several studies have demonstrated that patients operated in a referral centre have better outcomes. For example, disease-free survival was superior in patients who underwent primary resection at the MD Anderson Cancer Center, USA, compared with patients operated outside this institution, with a median survival of 25 versus 12 months, and also better overall survival (median not reached vs. 44 months) [59]. Similar data from the Netherlands showed that patients operated on in a Dutch Adrenal Network centre had significantly longer overall survival [60].

Management of ACCs in referral centres. For adrenal surgery, surgeons with a higher case load have a higher rate of R0 resection [61], and studies have highlighted the value of hospital or surgeon volume and the need for centralization irrespective of specialty practice [62–64]. This is especially important because the widespread use of laparoscopic adrenalectomy has made surgical indications more liberal [65, 66]. For ACC surgery [60, 67], the expertise of dedicated centres appears to have a positive impact on outcome, at least attributable to a multidisciplinary approach [68], even though a recent large American series failed to demonstrate improved overall survival in patients treated more aggressively in high-volume centres [69].

Various cut-offs have been proposed to define expert centres, from 4 to 10 adrenalectomies for ACC [67, 69], or 10 laparoscopic adrenalectomies [70] to 20 adrenalectomies per year [49], but no strong conclusion can be drawn from the available evidence, and the definition of a high-volume centre is often controversial and culturally oriented.

The minimal consensus reached was that referral centres can be defined as centres with surgeons that perform at least 15 adrenal procedures a year. A referral centre should at least have surgeons with expertise in both open and laparoscopic adrenal surgery and with expertise (or available help if required) in vascular, hepatic or pancreatic resection. Within the referral centre, all patients should be discussed preoperatively by a multidisciplinary team including surgeons, endocrinologists, oncologists, radiologists, pathologists, nuclear medicine physicians, biologists and geneticists.

Post-operative Considerations: Prognostic Markers

Stage of Disease at Presentation

The most important factor in determining survival is the stage of disease at presentation [5]. The widely used ENSAT staging system introduced in 2009 [20] cannot differentiate enough between patients who might benefit (or not) of adjuvant treatment; hence new prognostic markers/models are being sought.

Hormonal Activity of the Tumour

Cortisol secretion was reported to be independently associated with shorter recurrence-fee survival [71]. In an analysis of 234 patients who underwent surgery for ACC at 13 major cancer centres in the USA over two decades, patients with cortisol-secreting tumours had worse recurrence-free survival (10 months vs. 26 months in non-cortisol secreting) and worse overall survival (18 months vs. 50 months in non-cortisol-secreting patients) [71].

Surgical Margin Status

As expected, R0 resection (margin >1 mm) is associated with more favourable outcomes. Analysis of 165 patients from a multi-institutional database showed that 126 patients (76%) with R0 resection had median and 5-year overall survival of 96 months and 65% versus 25 months and 34% for patients who underwent R1 resection [72]. Recurrence-free survival at 5 years post-op was 30% after R0 resection and 14% after R1 resection [72]. Such data reinforce the hypothesis that selection of surgical technique should emphasize the need to achieve R0 margins in order to improve the outcome of these patients.

Histological Assessment of Adrenocortical Carcinoma

The Weiss scoring system remains the standard for differentiating adrenocortical adenomas from ACC. This score is based on the assessment at light microscopy of nine morphological parameters (Table 29.2). A score of less than 3 defines benign adenomas, a score of greater than 6 is associated with ACC and a score of 3–6 raises suspicion of malignancy [73]. Though widely used, this scoring system has significant limitations as it is observer dependent and has low reproducibility, and its applicability is low among non-expert pathologists.

Ki-67 Proliferation Index

Risk stratification based on whether Ki-67 is <10%, 10–19% or >20% was suggested by a retrospective analysis of 569 patients in whom the risk of recurrence and the overall survival after complete resection were influenced by Ki-67 [74]. Potentially this risk model will be implemented

Table 29.2 Weiss score

	Comments
Nuclear grade	
Mitotic rate	>5 per 50 HPFs (×40 objective, counting the greatest numbers of mitotic figures in areas with greatest number of mitoses)
Atypical mitotic figures	Abnormal distribution of chromosomes, excessive number of mitotic spindles
Cytoplasm	Presence of clear or vacuolated cells resembling normal zona fasciculata
Diffuse architecture	Over one-third of the tumour forms patternless sheets of cells; trabecular, columnar, alveolar or nesting patterns are regarded as non-diffuse
Necrosis	
Venous invasion	Tumour cells within endothelium-lined vessel, with smooth muscle as a component of the wall
Sinusoid invasion	Tumour cells within endothelium-lined vessel in adrenal gland with little supportive tissue
Invasion of tumour capsule	

Nine parameters are assessed on haematoxylin and eosin-stained sections from representative areas of the tumour. *HPF* high-power field

once automated software analysis for Ki-67 will resolve the current problems related to inter-observer variability in assessing Ki-67 staining.

Survival Nomograms

A nomogram predicting cancer-specific and all-cause mortality was developed in 205 patients with ACC using three variables (age, stage and surgical status), and provided 72–80% accuracy for prediction of cancer-specific or all-cause mortality at 1–5 years [75]. A prognostic score with five co-variables (hormone status other than isolated hyperandrogenism, tumour size larger than 75 mm, primary tumour classified as T3/T4, presence of microscopic venous invasion and a mitotic index of more than 5 per 50 high-power fields) has also been proposed for estimating the risk of metastasis and recurrence [76]. To date, neither of these prognostic models has been reproduced or tested by any other research group.

Genomics

miRNA expression profile, chromosomal and methylation alterations, and pattern of expression of main ACC driver genes can reveal subtypes of malignant tumours with different outcomes [77]. As most of these techniques are restricted to highly specialized laboratories, their translation in routine clinical practice is lagging. There is however a potential to the use of various molecular tools to classify ACCs and guide patient management in the era of 'personalized precision medicine'.

Adjuvant Therapies

The role of adjuvant mitotane and radiotherapy is above the scope of this chapter but represents a very important issue to be discussed as part of the multidisciplinary input that is crucial for ensuring an acceptable post-operative progression in patients with such aggressive disease.

Conclusion

Adrenocortical carcinoma remains a very challenging surgical condition. Despite significant progress in basic research it remains unclear how to implement in routine clinical practice the vast amount of information from -omics studies. International collaborative studies should address the open questions related to volume-outcome and need to centralise the care of such patients, the extent and indication for regional lymphadenectomy during surgery for ACC and the role of surgery in patients presenting with metastatic disease. The role of adjuvant mitotane treatment and the ongoing efforts to identify new drugs would need multidisciplinary input. Improving the long term outcome of patients with ACC should be a top priority for the research agenda in endocrinology in 2020s.

Acknowledgement Disclosure: The author declares no conflict of interest.

References

1. Mihai R. Diagnosis, treatment and outcome of adrenocortical cancer. Br J Surg. 2015;102(4):291–306.
2. Gaujoux S, et al. European Society of Endocrine Surgeons (ESES) and European Network for the Study of Adrenal Tumours (ENSAT) recommendations for the surgical management of adrenocortical carcinoma. Br J Surg. 2017;104(4):358–76.
3. Kutikov A, et al. Effects of increased cross-sectional imaging on the diagnosis and prognosis of adrenocortical carcinoma: analysis of the National Cancer Database. J Urol. 2011;186(3):805–10.
4. Kerkhofs TM, et al. Surgery for adrenocortical carcinoma in The Netherlands: analysis of the national cancer registry data. Eur J Endocrinol. 2013;169(1):83–9.
5. Fassnacht M, et al. Limited prognostic value of the 2004 International Union Against Cancer staging classification for adrenocortical carcinoma: proposal for a Revised TNM Classification. Cancer. 2009;115(2):243–50.
6. Arlt W, et al. Urine steroid metabolomics as a biomarker tool for detecting malignancy in adrenal tumors. J Clin Endocrinol Metab. 2011;96(12):3775–84.
7. Zini L, Porpiglia F, Fassnacht M. Contemporary management of adrenocortical carcinoma. Eur Urol. 2011;60(5):1055–65.
8. Zhang HM, et al. CT features and quantification of the characteristics of adrenocortical carcinomas on unenhanced and contrast-enhanced studies. Clin Radiol. 2012;67(1):38–46.
9. Sturgeon C, et al. Risk assessment in 457 adrenal cortical carcinomas: how much does tumor size predict the likelihood of malignancy? J Am Coll Surg. 2006;202(3):423–30.
10. Abdel-Aziz TE, et al. Risk of adrenocortical carcinoma in adrenal tumours greater than 8 cm. World J Surg. 2015;39(5):1268–73.
11. Petersenn S, et al. Computed tomography criteria for discrimination of adrenal adenomas and adrenocortical carcinomas: analysis of the German ACC registry. Eur J Endocrinol. 2015;172(4):415–22.
12. Libe R, Fratticci A, Bertherat J. Adrenocortical cancer: pathophysiology and clinical management. Endocr Relat Cancer. 2007;14(1):13–28.
13. Ilias I, et al. The optimal imaging of adrenal tumours: a comparison of different methods. Endocr Relat Cancer. 2007;14(3):587–99.
14. Harrison B. The indeterminate adrenal mass. Langenbeck's Arch Surg. 2012;397(2):147–54.
15. Gust L, et al. Preoperative 18F-FDG uptake is strongly correlated with malignancy, Weiss score, and molecular markers of aggressiveness in adrenal cortical tumors. World J Surg. 2012;36(6):1406–10.
16. Nunes ML, et al. 18F-FDG PET for the identification of adrenocortical carcinomas among indeterminate adrenal tumors at computed tomography scanning. World J Surg. 2010;34(7):1506–10.
17. Watanabe H, et al. Adrenal-to-liver SUV ratio is the best parameter for differentiation of adrenal metastases from adenomas using 18F-FDG PET/CT. Ann Nucl Med. 2013;27(7):648–53.
18. Tessonnier L, et al. (18)F-FDG uptake at initial staging of the adrenocortical cancers: a diagnostic tool but not of prognostic value. World J Surg. 2013;37(1):107–12.
19. Kreissl MC, et al. [(1)(2)(3)I]Iodometomidate imaging in adrenocortical carcinoma. J Clin Endocrinol Metab. 2013;98(7):2755–64.
20. Lughezzani G, et al. The European Network for the Study of Adrenal Tumors staging system is prognostically superior to the international union against cancer-staging system: a North American validation. Eur J Cancer. 2010;46(4):713–9.
21. Waldmann J, et al. Clinical impact of TP53 alterations in adrenocortical carcinomas. Langenbeck's Arch Surg. 2012;397(2):209–16.
22. Herrmann LJ, et al. TP53 germline mutations in adult patients with adrenocortical carcinoma. J Clin Endocrinol Metab. 2012;97(3):E476–85.
23. Raymond VM, et al. Prevalence of germline TP53 mutations in a prospective series of unselected patients with adrenocortical carcinoma. J Clin Endocrinol Metab. 2013;98(1):E119–25.
24. Tran TB, et al. Surgical management of advanced adrenocortical carcinoma: a 21-year population-based analysis. Am Surg. 2013;79(10):1115–8.
25. Gaujoux S, Brennan MF. Recommendation for standardized surgical management of primary adrenocortical carcinoma. Surgery. 2012;152(1):123–32.
26. Lim JH, Auh YH. Anatomic relation between the bare area of the liver and the right perirenal space. AJR Am J Roentgenol. 1994;162(3):733–4.
27. Lim JH, Kim B, Auh YH. Continuation of gas from the right perirenal space into the bare area of the liver. J Comput Assist Tomogr. 1997;21(4):667–70.
28. Icard P, et al. Adrenocortical carcinomas: surgical trends and results of a 253-patient series from the French Association of Endocrine Surgeons study group. World J Surg. 2001;25(7):891–7.
29. Gaujoux S, et al. Resection of adrenocortical carcinoma liver metastasis: is it justified? Ann Surg Oncol. 2012;19(8):2643–51.
30. Bellantone R, et al. Role of reoperation in recurrence of adrenal cortical carcinoma: results from 188 cases collected in the Italian National Registry for Adrenal Cortical Carcinoma. Surgery. 1997;122(6):1212–8.
31. Fiori C, Daffara F, Defrancia S. Does nephrectomy during adrenalectomy for adrenal cancer improve oncological results? Eur Urol. 2012;11(1):e1105.
32. Bilimoria KY, et al. Adrenocortical carcinoma in the United States: treatment utilization and prognostic factors. Cancer. 2008;113(11):3130–6.
33. Fassnacht M, et al. Efficacy of adjuvant radiotherapy of the tumor bed on local recurrence of adre-

nocortical carcinoma. J Clin Endocrinol Metab. 2006;91(11):4501–4.
34. Erdogan I, et al. The role of surgery in the management of recurrent adrenocortical carcinoma. J Clin Endocrinol Metab. 2013;98(1):181–91.
35. Kendrick ML, et al. Adrenocortical carcinoma: surgical progress or status quo? Arch Surg. 2001;136(5):543–9.
36. Libe R, et al. Prognostic factors in stage III-IV adrenocortical carcinomas (ACC): an European Network for the Study of Adrenal Tumor (ENSAT) study. Ann Oncol. 2015;26(10):2119–25.
37. Nilubol N, Patel D, Kebebew E. Does lymphadenectomy improve survival in patients with adrenocortical carcinoma? A population-based study. World J Surg. 2016;40(3):697–705.
38. Saade N, Sadler C, Goldfarb M. Impact of regional lymph node dissection on disease specific survival in adrenal cortical carcinoma. Horm Metab Res. 2015;47(11):820–5.
39. Soreide JA, Brabrand K, Thoresen SO. Adrenal cortical carcinoma in Norway, 1970–1984. World J Surg. 1992;16(4):663–7; discussion 668
40. King DR, Lack EE. Adrenal cortical carcinoma: a clinical and pathologic study of 49 cases. Cancer. 1979;44(1):239–44.
41. Harrison LE, Gaudin PB, Brennan MF. Pathologic features of prognostic significance for adrenocortical carcinoma after curative resection. Arch Surg. 1999;134(2):181–5.
42. Reibetanz J, et al. Impact of lymphadenectomy on the oncologic outcome of patients with adrenocortical carcinoma. Ann Surg. 2012;255(2):363–9.
43. Chiche L, et al. Adrenocortical carcinoma extending into the inferior vena cava: presentation of a 15-patient series and review of the literature. Surgery. 2006;139(1):15–27.
44. Turbendian HK, et al. Adrenocortical carcinoma: the influence of large vessel extension. Surgery. 2010;148(6):1057–64; discussion 1064.
45. Mihai R, et al. Outcome of operation in patients with adrenocortical cancer invading the inferior vena cava--a European Society of Endocrine Surgeons (ESES) survey. Langenbeck's Arch Surg. 2012;397(2):225–31.
46. Bednarski BK, et al. Borderline resectable adrenal cortical carcinoma: a potential role for preoperative chemotherapy. World J Surg. 2014;38(6):1318–27.
47. Flanigan RC, et al. Nephrectomy followed by interferon alfa-2b compared with interferon alfa-2b alone for metastatic renal-cell cancer. N Engl J Med. 2001;345(23):1655–9.
48. Dy BM, et al. Operative intervention for recurrent adrenocortical cancer. Surgery. 2013;154(6):1292–9; discussion 1299
49. Jurowich C, et al. Is there a role for laparoscopic adrenalectomy in patients with suspected adrenocortical carcinoma? A critical appraisal of the literature. Horm Metab Res. 2013;45(2):130–6.
50. Carnaille B. Adrenocortical carcinoma: which surgical approach? Langenbeck's Arch Surg. 2012;397(2):195–9.
51. Else T, et al. Adrenocortical carcinoma. Endocr Rev. 2014;35(2):282–326.
52. Di Carlo I, et al. Liver resection for hepatic metastases from adrenocortical carcinoma. HPB (Oxford). 2006;8(2):106–9.
53. Ripley RT, et al. Liver resection and ablation for metastatic adrenocortical carcinoma. Ann Surg Oncol. 2011;18(7):1972–9.
54. op den Winkel J, et al. Metastatic adrenocortical carcinoma: results of 56 pulmonary metastasectomies in 24 patients. Ann Thorac Surg. 2011;92(6):1965–70.
55. Kemp CD, et al. Pulmonary resection for metastatic adrenocortical carcinoma: the National Cancer Institute experience. Ann Thorac Surg. 2011;92(4):1195–200.
56. Dy BM, et al. Surgical resection of synchronously metastatic adrenocortical cancer. Ann Surg Oncol. 2015;22(1):146–51.
57. Porpiglia F, et al. A debate on laparoscopic versus open adrenalectomy for adrenocortical carcinoma. Horm Cancer. 2011;2(6):372–7.
58. Aspinall SR, et al. How is adrenocortical cancer being managed in the UK? Ann R Coll Surg Engl. 2009;91(6):489–93.
59. Grubbs EG, et al. Recurrence of adrenal cortical carcinoma following resection: surgery alone can achieve results equal to surgery plus mitotane. Ann Surg Oncol. 2010;17(1):263–70.
60. Hermsen IG, et al. Surgery in adrenocortical carcinoma: importance of national cooperation and centralized surgery. Surgery. 2012;152(1):50–6.
61. Ip JC, et al. Improving outcomes in adrenocortical cancer: an Australian perspective. Ann Surg Oncol. 2015;22(7):2309–16.
62. Bergamini C, et al. Complications in laparoscopic adrenalectomy: the value of experience. Surg Endosc. 2011;25(12):3845–51.
63. Park HS, Roman SA, Sosa JA. Outcomes from 3144 adrenalectomies in the United States: which matters more, surgeon volume or specialty? Arch Surg. 2009;144(11):1060–7.
64. Simhan J, et al. Trends in regionalization of adrenalectomy to higher volume surgical centers. J Urol. 2012;188(2):377–82.
65. Gallagher SF, et al. Trends in adrenalectomy rates, indications, and physician volume: a statewide analysis of 1816 adrenalectomies. Surgery. 2007;142(6):1011–21. discussion 1011-21
66. Saunders BD, et al. Trends in utilization of adrenalectomy in the United States: have indications changed? World J Surg. 2004;28(11):1169–75.
67. Lombardi CP, et al. Adrenocortical carcinoma: effect of hospital volume on patient outcome. Langenbeck's Arch Surg. 2012;397(2):201–7.
68. Fassnacht M, et al. Improved survival in patients with stage II adrenocortical carcinoma followed up pro-

spectively by specialized centers. J Clin Endocrinol Metab. 2010;95(11):4925–32.
69. Gratian L, et al. Treatment patterns and outcomes for patients with adrenocortical carcinoma associated with hospital case volume in the United States. In: Ann Surg Oncol, vol. 21; 2014. p. 3509.
70. Greco F, et al. Laparoscopic adrenalectomy in urological centres—the experience of the German Laparoscopic Working Group. BJU Int. 2011;108(10):1646–51.
71. Margonis GA, et al. Outcomes after resection of cortisol-secreting adrenocortical carcinoma. Am J Surg. 2016;211(6):1106–13.
72. Margonis GA, et al. Adrenocortical carcinoma: impact of surgical margin status on long-term outcomes. Ann Surg Oncol. 2016;23(1):134–41.
73. Papotti M, et al. Pathology of the adrenal cortex: a reappraisal of the past 25 years focusing on adrenal cortical tumors. Endocr Pathol. 2014;25(1):35–48.
74. Beuschlein F, et al. Major prognostic role of Ki67 in localized adrenocortical carcinoma after complete resection. J Clin Endocrinol Metab. 2015;100(3):841–9.
75. Zini L, et al. External validation of a nomogram predicting mortality in patients with adrenocortical carcinoma. BJU Int. 2009;104(11):1661–7.
76. Freire DS, et al. Development and internal validation of an adrenal cortical carcinoma prognostic score for predicting the risk of metastasis and local recurrence. Clin Endocrinol. 2013;79(4):468–75.
77. de Krijger RE, Bertherat J. 5th international ACC symposium: classification of adrenocortical cancers from pathology to integrated genomics: real advances or lost in translation? Horm Cancer. 2016;7(1):3–8.

Paragaglioma

30

Toni Beninato and Quan-Yang Duh

Introduction

Paragangliomas are tumors derived from extra-adrenal chromaffin cells of the sympathetic and parasympathetic ganglia. Sympathetic paraganglioma arises from the paravertebral ganglia of the thorax, abdomen, and pelvis and produces catecholamines. In contrast, parasympathetic paraganglioma rises from the parasympathetic ganglia along the glossopharyngeal and vagal nerves in the neck and at the base of the skull. These do not produce catecholamines. Paraganglioma comprises about 15–20% of chromaffin-cell tumors, the other 80–85% being pheochromocytoma which arises from the adrenal medulla [1]. When compared to pheochromocytoma, paraganglioma is more likely to be part of a hereditary syndrome and be diagnosed at a younger age, has noradrenergic phenotype, and has multifocal or metastatic disease [2]. In this chapter, we will focus on the diagnosis, evaluation, and management of paraganglioma, which includes extra-adrenal tumors of the sympathetic and parasympathetic ganglia. Pheochromocytoma will be covered elsewhere.

T. Beninato
Weill Cornell Medicine, New York, NY, USA

Q.-Y. Duh (✉)
University of California, San Francisco, CA, USA
e-mail: quan-yang.duh@va.gov

Background and Etiology

The term "paragangliome" was used by Alezais and Pyron in 1908 to describe all chromaffin tumors [3]. Eventually, the terminology was adjusted to call chromaffin tumors of the adrenal gland "pheochromocytoma" and tumors arising from all other paraganglia "paraganglioma." Using the terminology "chromaffin tumors" to describe paraganglioma is also misleading, as chromaffin staining is present in the adrenal medulla and sympathetic paraganglia but absent in parasympathetic ganglia of the head and neck, from which a subset of paragangliomas arise [4]. Paraganglioma cells derive from the neural crest and are located in the paravertebral or para-aortic region from the base of the skull to the pelvic floor. Sympathetic paraganglioma occurs most commonly around the inferior mesenteric artery or at the aortic bifurcation in the organ of Zuckerkandl but can arise from any sympathetic ganglia in the chest, abdomen, and pelvis [5].

The overall prevalence of pheochromocytoma and paraganglioma in adult patients with hypertension ranges from 0.2 to 0.6% [1]. In the pediatric population, these tumors are even more rare with an incidence of 0.2–0.3 cases per million [6]. The most common age at presentation is in the third to the fifth decade, with up to 50% of tumors found incidentally on imaging studies done for another reason [7, 8]. At least one third of patients with paraganglioma have germline mutations that lead to disease; these patients are

R. Parameswaran, A. Agarwal (eds.), *Evidence-Based Endocrine Surgery*,
https://doi.org/10.1007/978-981-10-1124-5_30

more likely to present at a younger age and with multifocal tumors [9, 10].

Paraganglioma has a higher incidence of malignancy than pheochromocytoma: as many as 33% of extra-adrenal tumors are malignant [11]. In a review of patients with malignant paraganglioma, these patients were more likely to be diagnosed at a younger age, have noradrenergic phenotype, and have multifocal disease and synchronous metastases. Five- and 10-year survival for malignant paraganglioma was 88.9% and 77.3%, respectively [2].

Presentation, Investigation, and Treatment Options

Presentation

As stated earlier, as many as 50% of paraganglioma are found in patients who are asymptomatic and are discovered incidentally on imaging studies performed for another reason [7, 8]. Patients may also present with classic symptoms of catecholamine excess, such as sustained or cyclical hypertension, anxiety, weakness, or vomiting. Catecholamine excess can also result in decreased circulating blood volume, tachycardia, hyperglycemia, and diabetes. Extreme catecholamine excess can result in crisis causing stress-induced Takotsubo cardiomyopathy, multisystem organ failure, fever, encephalopathy, myocardial infarction, and stroke [1, 5, 11, 12].

Biochemical Testing

Paraganglioma in the chest, abdomen, and pelvis is derived from sympathetic ganglia and secreted catecholamines. Paraganglioma in the neck is derived from parasympathetic ganglia and is not biochemically active. If a sympathetic paraganglioma is suspected, patients should undergo biochemical testing for plasma-free metanephrines or 24-h collection of urinary fractionated metanephrines [1]. Metanephrines are metabolites of catecholamines produced by O-methyltransferase, an enzyme specific to adrenal chromaffin cells or other chromaffin-derived tumors [13]. Testing for metanephrines therefore has been found to be superior to testing for catecholamines or vanillylmandelic acid (VMA) as they are more specific to these tumors [14, 15]. Paraganglioma in particular has often been found to have an increase in noradrenergic metabolites compared to pheochromocytoma [16].

It is recommended that plasma metanephrines be drawn with the patient in the supine position (for at least 30 min prior to drawing blood) rather than the seated position [1]. The seated posture results in an increased release of norepinephrine and therefore metabolism to normetanephrine in patients without tumors, but this response is not seen in patients with tumors [17]. Therefore, patients without tumors who have their blood taken in the seated position may have similar values to those with tumors, resulting in an increased possibility of false-negative tests [18]. For this reason, the supine position has been shown to be superior.

Elevation in metanephrines should be at least three times the upper limit of the diagnostic range to be considered a positive test [12, 19]. Lower levels of elevation should either undergo repeat blood testing or 24-h urine testing or consideration of the clonidine suppression test [20]. The clonidine suppression test is considered positive if norepinephrine levels are elevated 2 h after clonidine is given at a dose of 300 μg/70 kg body weight [1]. It should be noted that several medications can cause false-positive results for plasma and urinary metanephrines [1, 19]. These medications are listed in Table 30.1.

Table 30.1 Medications that may interfere with testing for plasma or urinary metanephrines

Medication
Acetaminophen
Labetalol
Sotalol
α-Methyldopa
Tricyclic antidepressants
Buspirone
Phenoxybenzamine
MAO-inhibitors
Sulphasalazine
Mesalamine
Levodopa

Imaging

Cross-sectional imaging is an essential part of the workup of paraganglioma as it provides valuable information for operative planning. Computerized tomography (CT) scanning is usually the first-line imaging modality used and has a sensitivity ranging from 88 to 100% [21–23] (Fig. 30.1). Paraganglioma often appears homo- or heterogeneous and may have necrotic centers. They may contain calcifications and may also be either solid or cystic. They often have an attenuation of greater than 20 Hounsfield units, which differentiates them from adenomas, and often have slower washout of contrast on delayed imaging [24]. MRI (Fig. 30.2) has a similar sensitivity (up to 100%) and is often used in patients with metastatic disease and skull base and neck tumors, in those with surgical clips or other artifact-producing metallic objects in their body, in patients with allergy to CT contrast agents, and in patients in whom there is a need to limit radiation exposure [1, 25]. Paraganglioma enhances on T2-weighted imaging and also may appear heterogeneous due to internal hemorrhage or necrosis [26].

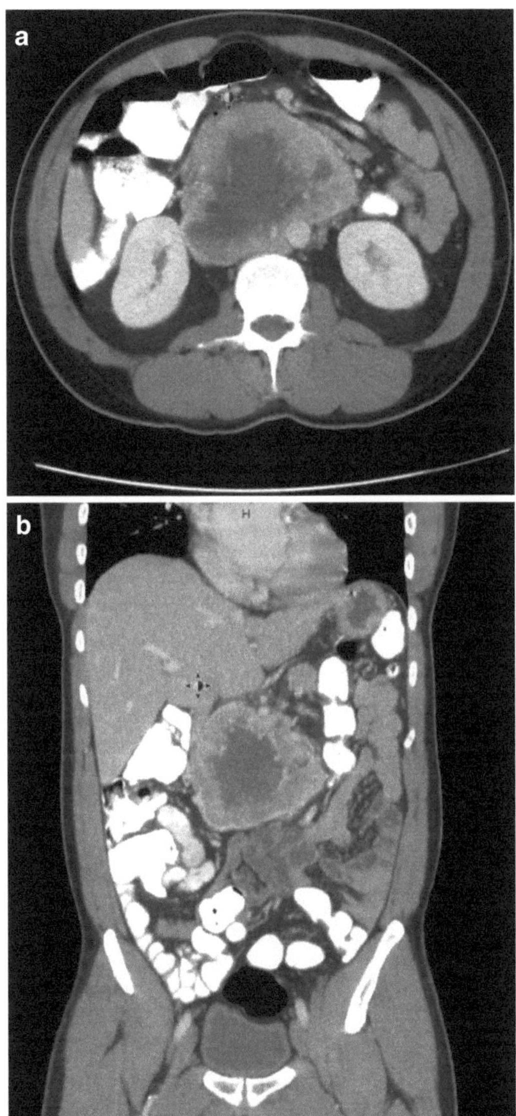

Fig. 30.1 CT scan, (**a**) axial view and (**b**) coronal view of an intra-abdominal paraganglioma

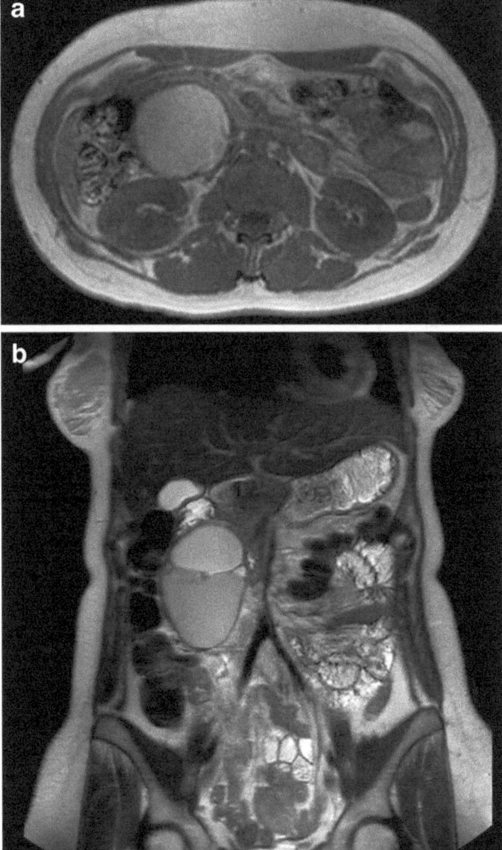

Fig. 30.2 T2-weighted imaging MRI, demonstrating (**a**) axial view and (**b**) coronal view of an intra-abdominal paraganglioma

Metaiodobenzylguanidine (MIBG) scanning was classically used for the localization of pheochromocytoma and paraganglioma but is used less frequently with the improvement in resolution of cross-sectional imaging. The sensitivity and specificity of MIBG imaging for paraganglioma are 56–75% and 84–100%, respectively [27–30]. The sensitivity decreases in patients with metastatic paraganglioma and in those with SDH-related disease [31]. Up to 50% of normal adrenal glands have physiologic uptake of ^{123}I-MIBG which can result in false-positive results [32, 33]. ^{123}I-MIBG functional imaging is recommended in patients with metastatic paraganglioma in whom ^{131}I-MIBG treatment is planned as treatment for avid metastases [1].

PET/CT imaging is being used increasingly over MIBG scanning in patients with known or suspected metastatic disease. Several studies have demonstrated the superiority of ^{18}F-FDG PET over ^{131}I-MIBG in patients with metastatic disease or in patients with certain genetic mutations, such as *SDHB* [34, 35]. More recently, radiolabeled DOTA peptides that target somatostatin receptors expressed on paraganglioma have shown promise in diagnostic imaging and treatment. ^{68}Ga-DOTATATE (^{68}gallium 1,4,7,10-teraazacyclododecane-1,4,5,10-teraacetic acid octreotate) is the most commonly used of these peptides. In a study comparing the performance of ^{68}Ga-DOTATATE PET/CT, ^{18}F-FDG PET/CT, and ^{131}I-MIBG scintigraphy in mapping metastatic pheochromocytoma and paraganglioma, Tan et al. found that ^{68}Ga-DOTATATE PET/CT had a superior sensitivity and accuracy on a per-patient and per-lesion basis compared to the other imaging modalities [36]. Similarly, in a cohort of patients with *SDHB* mutations by Janssen et al., ^{68}Ga-DOTATATE was found to have a lesion-based detection rate of 98.6%, superior to that of ^{18}F-FDG, ^{18}F-FDOPA, ^{18}F-FDa PET/CT, and CT/MRI [37]. Functional imaging with these peptides is not yet widely available, but as its accessibility increases, it is likely to become the preferred modality in patients with metastatic or *SDH*-related disease.

Genetic Testing

It is recommended that all patients with pheochromocytoma and paraganglioma be considered for genetic testing [1]. As many as one third of patients with pheochromocytoma or paraganglioma will have a germline mutation; however, if patients with a family history, other syndromic features, and bilateral or metastatic disease are excluded, the number drops to about 12% [38–42]. In younger patients, the yield is much higher, with up to 80% having a germline mutation [43]. Paraganglioma specifically has a fourfold higher risk of germline mutation than adrenal locations of tumor, mostly confined to the SDH genes [44]. We refer all patients with pheochromocytoma or paraganglioma for consultation with a genetic counselor for an evaluation of the patients' individualized risks of germline mutations and appropriate testing accordingly.

Pheochromocytoma and paraganglioma may be diagnosed as part of a syndromic presentation for which genetic testing is required for conformation of the syndrome and delineation of the specific type of mutation. Neurofibromatosis type 1 (mutation in *NF1)* and multiple endocrine neoplasia type 2 (*RET*) are almost always associated with adrenal tumors [1, 5]. Von Hippel-Lindau syndrome (*VHL*) is usually associated with adrenal tumors, but some patients may have extra-adrenal paragangliomas [45]. These are usually parasympathetic tumors of the head and neck. Carney triad (paraganglioma, gastric stromal tumors, and pulmonary chondroma) and Carney-Stratakis syndrome (paraganglioma and gastric stromal sarcomas) also present as syndromes [46].

The majority of hereditary paraganglioma fall into the succinate dehydrogenase (SDH) family of mutations, also known as hereditary paraganglioma syndromes 1–5 (PGL1–5). SDH is a protein located on the inner mitochondrial membrane and functions in the mitochondrial respiratory chain and the Krebs cycle [47]. SDH mutations are thought to be responsible for up to 25% of all paraganglioma [9, 48]. The various SDH subtype mutations result in distinct phenotypes.

PGL1–3 are mostly limited to nonfunctioning head and neck tumors; sympathetic paraganglioma is rarely seen. PGL1 is from a variety of mutations in SDHD [49]. These mutations are maternally imprinted, so are often seen to skip generations [50, 51]. Patients with SDHD mutations usually present at around age 30 with multiple parasympathetic skull base and neck paraganglioma [38, 52]. PGL2 is a rare mutation in SDH-AF2 that was mostly characterized in a single family [53, 54]. Patients present with head and neck paraganglioma with 70% of tumors arising from the carotid body [45]. PGL3 is from mutations in SDHC. SDHC mutations also result in head and neck tumors, 70% of which are from the carotid body. In contrast to SDHD mutations, SDHC mutations usually result in solitary tumors [55].

PGL4 is due to mutations in the SDHB subunit. Penetrance of this mutation varies from 14–77% in the literature [52, 56, 57]. These patients are most likely to present with thoracoabdominal sympathetic paraganglioma and are also at risk for head and neck parasympathetic paraganglioma, renal cell carcinoma, and gastrointestinal stromal tumors (GIST) [38, 49]. This is the most common of the SDH subtypes to have a mutation and is found in 30% of patients with metastatic paraganglioma [58]. Finally, PGL5 is due to mutations in the SDHA subunit. SDHA mutations are rare and have an overall low likelihood of abdominal paraganglioma but can be associated with GIST tumors [59, 60].

Treatment Options

For the majority of patients who present with solitary, extra-adrenal sympathetic paraganglioma, surgical excision is the mainstay of treatment. Patients with functional tumors must undergo preoperative alpha-blockade prior to surgery. Further details on blockade and surgical technique will be discussed in the next section.

The management of patients with metastatic disease is challenging. In these patients, the goals of therapy are twofold: to reduce tumor burden and also manage the biochemical impact of the disease. Treatment options for metastatic disease include surgical debulking, local ablative therapy, chemotherapy, and targeted radiolabeled therapies [61].

If surgical resection is feasible, metastasectomy should be considered as the first-line treatment in patients with metastatic or recurrent paraganglioma. In a series of 34 patients undergoing surgery for metastatic pheochromocytoma or paraganglioma, 41% were able to achieve an R0 resection, with a median disease-free survival of 4.6 years. Additionally, 56% of patients with biochemically active disease achieved normalization of fractionated metanephrines or catecholamines, with a significant reduction in number of antihypertensive medications [62]. Another recent series compared 89 patients undergoing surgery for metastatic pheochromocytoma or paraganglioma to 24 who did not, using propensity score matching to adjust for selection bias. Patients treated with surgery had improved overall survival over those who did not have surgery regardless of age, primary tumor size and location, number of metastatic sites, and genetic background. Furthermore, 70% of patients with hormonally active tumors had an improvement in their symptoms after surgery [63].

Radiolabeled therapies also play a role in the management of metastatic paraganglioma. In patients who have tumors that take up ^{123}I-MIBG on imaging, ^{131}I-MIBG can be used for treatment [64]. Therapy is usually not curative, but can result in partial tumor response and reduction in biochemical markers of disease [65]. Similarly, the presence of somatostatin receptors on the surface of the tumor can allow for targeting with peptide receptor radionuclide therapies. A study by Kong et al. treated 20 patients with ^{177}Lu-DOTA-octreotate with a median progression-free survival of 39 months and reduced antihypertensive dosing in 8/14 patients on these medications [66]. Although still experimental, targeted somatostatin therapies may offer options in the future for patients whose disease is not amenable to surgery.

More traditional therapies can also be attempted in patients with metastatic disease. Chemotherapy using cyclophosphamide, vincristine, and dacarbazine is often used but with early relapse in most patients [67]. External beam radiation can be considered for management of osseous metastases or other inoperable tumors [68]. Finally, arterial embolization or chemoembolization may be useful in patients with hepatic metastases [69].

Surgical Technique

The most common procedure for paraganglioma encountered by the endocrine surgeon is excision of intra-abdominal sympathetic paraganglioma. Similar to pheochromocytoma, adequate preoperative preparation is essential for a successful operation. Hormonally functional paraganglioma needs preoperative blockade with either alpha-blocking agents or calcium channel blockers, with the addition of beta-blockade as needed to control tachycardia. Concurrently with blockade, the patient must undergo salt and volume loading to address volume contraction.

We use phenoxybenzamine for preoperative alpha-blockade. The medication is started at least 10–14 days before surgery, with most patients receiving blockade over several weeks preoperatively. The starting dose is 10 mg twice per day and titrated up every 1–2 days as tolerated. Patients are asked to record their blood pressure (seated and standing), heart rate, and weight daily to monitor tolerance as the dose is increased. The goal blood pressure is <140/90 mm Hg seated, while maintaining the standing systolic blood pressure at >100 mm Hg for younger patients and 110 mm Hg for older patients. Patients' weight is monitored as a surrogate for fluid status: patients will often gain 10 pounds of water weight during preoperative blockade. Patients are encouraged to liberalize their salt intake to encourage fluid retention and are given salt tablets if they are averse to salty foods. Patients with congestive heart failure or renal failure will have less aggressive fluid and salt administration than healthy patients. Beta-blockade is added in patients after alpha-blockade if there is tachycardia >90–100 beats per minute. Patients are also counseled on the side effects of phenoxybenzamine including fatigue, nasal congestion, and dizziness, the presence of which is often used as weak surrogates for adequate alpha-blockade. Alpha- and (if taking) beta-blockade are continued to the morning of the operation.

The operative technique must be tailored to the individual patient's tumor and the surgeon's comfort with the various approaches. While laparoscopic resection has become the standard for most pheochromocytomas, many paraganglioma still require open resection. Since paraganglioma may arise in any of the para-aortic sympathetic ganglia, the location of the tumor plays a large role in the feasibility of laparoscopic resection. Paraganglioma that is located in the vicinity of the adrenal glands may be amenable to a traditional laparoscopic approach, but many inferiorly located, retroperitoneal tumors that require extensive visceral rotation may require an open resection. Compared to pheochromocytomas, paragangliomas tend to have multiple short feeding arteries that can cause significant bleeding that are difficult to control. Some surgeons may employ a laparoscopic approach initially to facilitate the initial dissection and then open through a smaller incision for removal of the tumor. Regardless of the technique employed, the main goals of the procedure are to completely excise the tumor without breaching the tumor capsule. Tumor disruption may lead to seeding of disease and local tumor recurrence ("paragangliomatosis" or "pheochromocytomatosis") which is very challenging to manage. Care must also be taken to avoid complications, which include massive hemorrhage due to proximity to the large vessels and injury to nearby organs. Paraganglioma, in contrast to pheochromocytoma, often has dense adhesions to surrounding structures that may make dissection more difficult and increases the risk of injury to the adherent structures. The Endocrine Society Clinical Practice Guidelines released in 2014 recommend open resection of paraganglioma, although laparoscopic resection can be performed for "small, non-invasive tumors in surgically favorable locations" [1].

Intraoperatively, it is essential to have an anesthesia team that is knowledgeable about the physiology of these tumors and their preoperative blockade. In the initial phases of the operation, the patient may become hypertensive during dissection or manipulation of the tumor, requiring interruption of dissection and administration of rapid-acting vasodilators by the anesthesia team. Monitoring of the patients' fluid status is also important, as inadequate fluid repletion can contribute to postoperative hypotension. After the blood supply to the tumor is ligated, hypotension can occur due to decreasing levels of circulating catecholamines. Vasopressor support may be required after the blood supply is taken but can often be titrated off in the operating room depending on the adequacy of preoperative alpha-blockade and the patients' fluid status.

Postoperatively, we routinely observe the patient in the post-anesthesia recovery unit for 4 h. The patients' hemodynamic status is monitored closely, as occasionally vasopressor support that was stopped in the operating room may need to be restarted. Patients' blood glucose is also monitored, as postoperative hypoglycemia can occur as the circulating catecholamines decline. If patients are hemodynamically normal and off of vasopressor agents after 4 h of observation, they can be safely transferred to the surgical floor. If vasopressor support is still required, or if there are other concerns, the patient is transferred to the ICU, where vasopressors can usually be stopped on the first postoperative day after volume resuscitation. Patients who undergo laparoscopic resection can often be discharged the next day. However, if open resection or extensive laparoscopic dissection is required, patients may need more time as an inpatient.

Results

After discharge from the hospital, patients are seen for follow-up 2 weeks after surgery. Metanephrines are assessed at this visit and then usually monitored annually. Patients who did not undergo consultation with a genetic counselor preoperatively are encouraged to do so. Currently, there is no way to distinguish histopathologically whether the tumor has the propensity to metastasize or recur, so patients must be monitored with yearly history and physical exam and plasma or urinary metanephrines [70, 71]. Patients who test positive for a predisposing mutation may need to be monitored more closely. One retrospective study showed an overall risk of recurrence of pheochromocytoma and paraganglioma at 5 and 10 years of 6% and 16%, respectively [72].

When paragangliomas are malignant, the course can be variable and often depends on the number of metastatic sites, biochemical activity of the tumors, presence or absence of a genetic syndrome, and the patients' overall health. In a review of over 300 patients with pheochromocytoma and paraganglioma, Choi et al. found that 13% of patients with paraganglioma had malignant disease. The median survival in patients with both malignant pheochromocytoma and paraganglioma was 7.2 years, and the 5-year survival was 75.4%. They found that older age and synchronous presentation of metastases were independently associated with poor survival [73]. Another study by Hamidi et al. reviewed 272 patients with malignant pheochromocytoma and paraganglioma. They found that metastases developed at a median of 5.5 years from the initial diagnosis and that median overall and disease-specific survival were 24.6 and 33.7 years, respectively. Shorter survival was seen in patients who were men, were older at diagnosis, and presented with synchronous metastasis, in those with large primary tumors and elevated dopamine, and in those who did not undergo resection of the primary tumor [2]. Patients with metastatic disease may be subject to a variety of different treatments, as discussed earlier, and response to treatment can be variable. Patel et al. reviewed 17 patients with metastatic pheochromocytoma and paraganglioma who underwent a variety of procedures and found that low total metabolic tumor volume calculated on 18F-FDG PET/CT scanning was predictive of a biochemical response [74]. When selecting treatment options for patients with malignant disease, it is important to consider the goals of treatment of reducing tumor burden and controlling symptoms from excess catecholamines.

Complications

Complications from surgery are similar to those of any surgical procedure, including bleeding, infection, and injury to nearby structures. In patients with paraganglioma, the location of the tumor dictates the structures that are at risk, in particular the large blood vessels that may supply the tumor. As mentioned previously, paraganglioma often has dense adhesions to nearby structures which may be at risk for injury during dissection.

The other complications from surgery that must be recognized are those from inadequate preoperative blockade. Insufficient alpha-blockade can result in hemodynamic lability and potential catecholamine crisis during surgery that could be catastrophic. Similarly, patients need to be adequately monitored and fluid resuscitated postoperatively to prevent hypotension. Blood glucose must also be monitored so that hypoglycemia is recognized if it occurs [75]. It is important to note that even when these patients present in crisis, surgical treatment is not an emergency, and appropriate planning and medical stabilization can help ensure a good outcome [76].

Conclusion

Although paraganglioma is a rare tumor, it is one that the endocrine surgeon should be prepared to treat. Preoperative alpha-blockade is an important part of the management and can be undertaken in cooperation with an endocrinologist familiar with these tumors. Surgeons should be prepared to perform an open resection of paraganglioma and only attempt a minimally invasive approach if they are extremely comfortable with the technique. Patients usually do well if adequate preoperative planning is undertaken. All patients should be referred for genetic counseling, preferably preoperatively, to better risk-stratify them and their family members. Patients with recurrence or metastatic tumors should be managed by a multidisciplinary team that is comfortable treating this disease.

References

1. Lenders JW, Duh QY, Eisenhofer G, et al. Pheochromocytoma and paraganglioma: an endocrine society clinical practice guideline. J Clin Endocrinol Metab. 2014;99:1915–42.
2. Hamidi O, Young WF Jr, Iniguez-Ariza NM, et al. Malignant pheochromocytoma and paraganglioma: 272 patients over 55 years. J Clin Endocrinol Metab. 2017;102:3296–305.
3. Alezais H, Peyron A. Un groupe nouveau de tumeurs epitheliliale: les paragangliomes. Compte Rend Soc Biol. 1908;65:745–7.
4. Else T. 15 YEARS OF PARAGANGLIOMA: pheochromocytoma, paraganglioma and genetic syndromes: a historical perspective. Endocr Relat Cancer. 2015;22:T147–59.
5. Kiernan CM, Solorzano CC. Pheochromocytoma and paraganglioma: diagnosis, genetics, and treatment. Surg Oncol Clin N Am. 2016;25:119–38.
6. Waguespack SG, Rich T, Grubbs E, et al. A current review of the etiology, diagnosis, and treatment of pediatric pheochromocytoma and paraganglioma. J Clin Endocrinol Metab. 2010;95:2023–37.
7. Baguet JP, Hammer L, Mazzuco TL, et al. Circumstances of discovery of phaeochromocytoma: a retrospective study of 41 consecutive patients. Eur J Endocrinol. 2004;150:681–6.
8. Kopetschke R, Slisko M, Kilisli A, et al. Frequent incidental discovery of phaeochromocytoma: data from a German cohort of 201 phaeochromocytoma. Eur J Endocrinol. 2009;161:355–61.
9. Neumann HP, Bausch B, McWhinney SR, et al. Germ-line mutations in nonsyndromic pheochromocytoma. N Engl J Med. 2002;346:1459–66.
10. Gimenez-Roqueplo AP, Dahia PL, Robledo M. An update on the genetics of paraganglioma, pheochromocytoma, and associated hereditary syndromes. Horm Metab Res. 2012;44:328–33.
11. Lenders JW, Eisenhofer G, Mannelli M, et al. Phaeochromocytoma. Lancet. 2005;366:665–75.
12. Chen H, Sippel RS, O'Dorisio MS, et al. The North American Neuroendocrine Tumor Society consensus guideline for the diagnosis and management of neuroendocrine tumors: pheochromocytoma, paraganglioma, and medullary thyroid cancer. Pancreas. 2010;39:775–83.
13. Eisenhofer G, Keiser H, Friberg P, et al. Plasma metanephrines are markers of pheochromocytoma produced by catechol-O-methyltransferase within tumors. J Clin Endocrinol Metab. 1998;83:2175–85.
14. Manu P, Runge LA. Biochemical screening for pheochromocytoma. Superiority of urinary metanephrines measurements. Am J Epidemiol. 1984;120:788–90.
15. Lenders JW, Keiser HR, Goldstein DS, et al. Plasma metanephrines in the diagnosis of pheochromocytoma. Ann Intern Med. 1995;123:101–9.

16. Eisenhofer G, Lenders JW, Linehan WM, et al. Plasma normetanephrine and metanephrine for detecting pheochromocytoma in von Hippel-Lindau disease and multiple endocrine neoplasia type 2. N Engl J Med. 1999;340:1872–9.
17. Lenders JW, Willemsen JJ, Eisenhofer G, et al. Is supine rest necessary before blood sampling for plasma metanephrines? Clin Chem. 2007;53:352–4.
18. Raber W, Raffesberg W, Bischof M, et al. Diagnostic efficacy of unconjugated plasma metanephrines for the detection of pheochromocytoma. Arch Intern Med. 2000;160:2957–63.
19. Eisenhofer G, Goldstein DS, Walther MM, et al. Biochemical diagnosis of pheochromocytoma: how to distinguish true- from false-positive test results. J Clin Endocrinol Metab. 2003;88:2656–66.
20. Darr R, Lenders JW, Stange K, et al. Diagnosis of pheochromocytoma and paraganglioma: the clonidine suppression test in patients with borderline elevations of plasma free normetanephrine. Dtsch Med Wochenschr. 2013;138:76–81.
21. Lumachi F, Tregnaghi A, Zucchetta P, et al. Sensitivity and positive predictive value of CT, MRI and 123I-MIBG scintigraphy in localizing pheochromocytomas: a prospective study. Nucl Med Commun. 2006;27:583–7.
22. Berglund AS, Hulthen UL, Manhem P, et al. Metaiodobenzylguanidine (MIBG) scintigraphy and computed tomography (CT) in clinical practice. Primary and secondary evaluation for localization of phaeochromocytomas. J Intern Med. 2001;249:247–51.
23. Maurea S, Cuocolo A, Reynolds JC, et al. Iodine-131-metaiodobenzylguanidine scintigraphy in preoperative and postoperative evaluation of paragangliomas: comparison with CT and MRI. J Nucl Med. 1993;34:173–9.
24. Caoili EM, Korobkin M, Francis IR, et al. Adrenal masses: characterization with combined unenhanced and delayed enhanced CT. Radiology. 2002;222:629–33.
25. Pacak K, Eisenhofer G, Carrasquillo JA, et al. Diagnostic localization of pheochromocytoma: the coming of age of positron emission tomography. Ann N Y Acad Sci. 2002;970:170–6.
26. Baez JC, Jagannathan JP, Krajewski K, et al. Pheochromocytoma and paraganglioma: imaging characteristics. Cancer Imaging. 2012;12:153–62.
27. Bhatia KS, Ismail MM, Sahdev A, et al. 123I-metaiodobenzylguanidine (MIBG) scintigraphy for the detection of adrenal and extra-adrenal phaeochromocytomas: CT and MRI correlation. Clin Endocrinol (Oxf). 2008;69:181–8.
28. Wiseman GA, Pacak K, O'Dorisio MS, et al. Usefulness of 123I-MIBG scintigraphy in the evaluation of patients with known or suspected primary or metastatic pheochromocytoma or paraganglioma: results from a prospective multicenter trial. J Nucl Med. 2009;50:1448–54.
29. Fiebrich HB, Brouwers AH, Kerstens MN, et al. 6-[F-18]Fluoro-L-dihydroxyphenylalanine positron emission tomography is superior to conventional imaging with (123)I-metaiodobenzylguanidine scintigraphy, computer tomography, and magnetic resonance imaging in localizing tumors causing catecholamine excess. J Clin Endocrinol Metab. 2009;94:3922–30.
30. Milardovic R, Corssmit EP, Stokkel M. Value of 123I-MIBG Scintigraphy in Paraganglioma. Neuroendocrinology. 2010;91:94–100.
31. van der Horst-Schrivers AN, Kerstens MN, Wolffenbuttel BH. Preoperative pharmacological management of phaeochromocytoma. Neth J Med. 2006;64:290–5.
32. Furuta N, Kiyota H, Yoshigoe F, et al. Diagnosis of pheochromocytoma using [123I]-compared with [131I]-metaiodobenzylguanidine scintigraphy. Int J Urol. 1999;6:119–24.
33. Mozley PD, Kim CK, Mohsin J, et al. The efficacy of iodine-123-MIBG as a screening test for pheochromocytoma. J Nucl Med. 1994;35:1138–44.
34. Timmers HJ, Chen CC, Carrasquillo JA, et al. Staging and functional characterization of pheochromocytoma and paraganglioma by 18F-fluorodeoxyglucose (18F-FDG) positron emission tomography. J Natl Cancer Inst. 2012;104:700–8.
35. Timmers HJ, Kozupa A, Chen CC, et al. Superiority of fluorodeoxyglucose positron emission tomography to other functional imaging techniques in the evaluation of metastatic SDHB-associated pheochromocytoma and paraganglioma. J Clin Oncol. 2007;25:2262–9.
36. Tan TH, Hussein Z, Saad FF, et al. Diagnostic performance of (68)Ga-DOTATATE PET/CT, (18)F-FDG PET/CT and (131)I-MIBG scintigraphy in mapping metastatic pheochromocytoma and paraganglioma. Nucl Med Mol Imaging. 2015;49:143–51.
37. Janssen I, Blanchet EM, Adams K, et al. Superiority of [68Ga]-DOTATATE PET/CT to other functional imaging modalities in the localization of SDHB-associated metastatic pheochromocytoma and paraganglioma. Clin Cancer Res. 2015;21:3888–95.
38. Benn DE, Robinson BG. Genetic basis of phaeochromocytoma and paraganglioma. Best Pract Res Clin Endocrinol Metab. 2006;20:435–50.
39. Fishbein L, Merrill S, Fraker DL, et al. Inherited mutations in pheochromocytoma and paraganglioma: why all patients should be offered genetic testing. Ann Surg Oncol. 2013;20:1444–50.
40. Gimenez-Roqueplo AP, Favier J, Rustin P, et al. Mutations in the SDHB gene are associated with extra-adrenal and/or malignant phaeochromocytomas. Cancer Res. 2003;63:5615–21.
41. Pacak K. Preoperative management of the pheochromocytoma patient. J Clin Endocrinol Metab. 2007;92:4069–79.
42. Brito JP, Asi N, Bancos I, et al. Testing for germline mutations in sporadic pheochromocytoma/paraganglioma: a systematic review. Clin Endocrinol (Oxf). 2015;82:338–45.

43. Babic B, Patel D, Aufforth R, et al. Pediatric patients with pheochromocytoma and paraganglioma should have routine preoperative genetic testing for common susceptibility genes in addition to imaging to detect extra-adrenal and metastatic tumors. Surgery. 2017;161:220–7.
44. Erlic Z, Rybicki L, Peczkowska M, et al. Clinical predictors and algorithm for the genetic diagnosis of pheochromocytoma patients. Clin Cancer Res. 2009;15:6378–85.
45. Rednam SP, Erez A, Druker H, et al. Von Hippel-Lindau and hereditary pheochromocytoma/paraganglioma syndromes: clinical features, genetics, and surveillance recommendations in childhood. Clin Cancer Res. 2017;23:e68–75.
46. Stratakis CA, Carney JA. The triad of paragangliomas, gastric stromal tumours and pulmonary chondromas (Carney triad), and the dyad of paragangliomas and gastric stromal sarcomas (Carney-Stratakis syndrome): molecular genetics and clinical implications. J Intern Med. 2009;266:43–52.
47. Benn DE, Robinson BG, Clifton-Bligh RJ. 15 YEARS OF PARAGANGLIOMA: clinical manifestations of paraganglioma syndromes types 1-5. Endocr Relat Cancer. 2015;22:T91–103.
48. Baysal BE, Willett-Brozick JE, Lawrence EC, et al. Prevalence of SDHB, SDHC, and SDHD germline mutations in clinic patients with head and neck paragangliomas. J Med Genet. 2002;39:178–83.
49. Ricketts CJ, Forman JR, Rattenberry E, et al. Tumor risks and genotype-phenotype-proteotype analysis in 358 patients with germline mutations in SDHB and SDHD. Hum Mutat. 2010;31:41–51.
50. Taschner PE, Jansen JC, Baysal BE, et al. Nearly all hereditary paragangliomas in the Netherlands are caused by two founder mutations in the SDHD gene. Genes Chromosomes Cancer. 2001;31:274–81.
51. Neumann HP, Erlic Z. Maternal transmission of symptomatic disease with SDHD mutation: fact or fiction? J Clin Endocrinol Metab. 2008;93:1573–5.
52. Neumann HP, Pawlu C, Peczkowska M, et al. Distinct clinical features of paraganglioma syndromes associated with SDHB and SDHD gene mutations. JAMA. 2004;292:943–51.
53. van Baars F, Cremers C, van den Broek P, et al. Genetic aspects of nonchromaffin paraganglioma. Hum Genet. 1982;60:305–9.
54. Hao HX, Khalimonchuk O, Schraders M, et al. SDH5, a gene required for flavination of succinate dehydrogenase, is mutated in paraganglioma. Science. 2009;325:1139–42.
55. Schiavi F, Boedeker CC, Bausch B, et al. Predictors and prevalence of paraganglioma syndrome associated with mutations of the SDHC gene. JAMA. 2005;294:2057–63.
56. Eijkelenkamp K, Osinga TE, de Jong MM, et al. Calculating the optimal surveillance for head and neck paraganglioma in SDHB-mutation carriers. Fam Cancer. 2017;16:123–30.
57. Jafri M, Whitworth J, Rattenberry E, et al. Evaluation of SDHB, SDHD and VHL gene susceptibility testing in the assessment of individuals with non-syndromic phaeochromocytoma, paraganglioma and head and neck paraganglioma. Clin Endocrinol (Oxf). 2013;78:898–906.
58. Brouwers FM, Eisenhofer G, Tao JJ, et al. High frequency of SDHB germline mutations in patients with malignant catecholamine-producing paragangliomas: implications for genetic testing. J Clin Endocrinol Metab. 2006;91:4505–9.
59. Boikos SA, Pappo AS, Killian JK, et al. Molecular subtypes of KIT/PDGFRA wild-type gastrointestinal stromal tumors: a report from the National Institutes of Health Gastrointestinal Stromal Tumor Clinic. JAMA Oncol. 2016;2:922–8.
60. Korpershoek E, Favier J, Gaal J, et al. SDHA immunohistochemistry detects germline SDHA gene mutations in apparently sporadic paragangliomas and pheochromocytomas. J Clin Endocrinol Metab. 2011;96:E1472–6.
61. Chrisoulidou A, Kaltsas G, Ilias I, et al. The diagnosis and management of malignant phaeochromocytoma and paraganglioma. Endocr Relat Cancer. 2007;14:569–85.
62. Strajina V, Dy BM, Farley DR, et al. Surgical treatment of malignant pheochromocytoma and paraganglioma: retrospective case series. Ann Surg Oncol. 2017;24:1546–50.
63. Roman-Gonzalez A, Zhou S, Ayala-Ramirez M, et al. Impact of surgical resection of the primary tumor on overall survival in patients with metastatic pheochromocytoma or sympathetic paraganglioma. Ann Surg. 2018;268(1):172–178
64. Bomanji J, Britton KE, Ur E, et al. Treatment of malignant phaeochromocytoma, paraganglioma and carcinoid tumours with 131I-metaiodobenzylguanidine. Nucl Med Commun. 1993;14:856–61.
65. Loh KC, Fitzgerald PA, Matthay KK, et al. The treatment of malignant pheochromocytoma with iodine-131 metaiodobenzylguanidine (131I-MIBG): a comprehensive review of 116 reported patients. J Endocrinol Invest. 1997;20:648–58.
66. Kong G, Grozinsky-Glasberg S, Hofman MS, et al. Efficacy of peptide receptor radionuclide therapy for functional metastatic paraganglioma and pheochromocytoma. J Clin Endocrinol Metab. 2017;102:3278–87.
67. Averbuch SD, Steakley CS, Young RC, et al. Malignant pheochromocytoma: effective treatment with a combination of cyclophosphamide, vincristine, and dacarbazine. Ann Intern Med. 1988;109:267–73.
68. Teno S, Tanabe A, Nomura K, et al. Acutely exacerbated hypertension and increased inflammatory signs due to radiation treatment for metastatic pheochromocytoma. Endocr J. 1996;43:511–6.
69. Kebebew E, Duh QY. Benign and malignant pheochromocytoma: diagnosis, treatment, and follow-up. Surg Oncol Clin N Am. 1998;7:765–89.
70. Eisenhofer G, Bornstein SR, Brouwers FM, et al. Malignant pheochromocytoma: current status and

initiatives for future progress. Endocr Relat Cancer. 2004;11:423–36.
71. Parenti G, Zampetti B, Rapizzi E, et al. Updated and new perspectives on diagnosis, prognosis, and therapy of malignant pheochromocytoma/paraganglioma. J Oncol. 2012;2012:872713.
72. Amar L, Servais A, Gimenez-Roqueplo AP, et al. Year of diagnosis, features at presentation, and risk of recurrence in patients with pheochromocytoma or secreting paraganglioma. J Clin Endocrinol Metab. 2005;90:2110–6.
73. Choi YM, Sung TY, Kim WG, et al. Clinical course and prognostic factors in patients with malignant pheochromocytoma and paraganglioma: a single institution experience. J Surg Oncol. 2015;112:815–21.
74. Patel D, Mehta A, Nilubol N, et al. Total 18F-FDG PET/CT metabolic tumor volume is associated with postoperative biochemical response in patients with metastatic pheochromocytomas and paragangliomas. Ann Surg. 2016;263:582–7.
75. Chen Y, Hodin RA, Pandolfi C, et al. Hypoglycemia after resection of pheochromocytoma. Surgery. 2014;156:1404–8; discussion 1408–1409.
76. Scholten A, Cisco RM, Vriens MR, et al. Pheochromocytoma crisis is not a surgical emergency. J Clin Endocrinol Metab. 2013;98:581–91.

Perioperative Management of Endocrine Hypertension

31

Peter Hambly

Introduction

Many endocrine disorders are recognised causes of hypertension (Fig. 31.1). In terms of perioperative management, such conditions fall into two groups:

1. Those in which hypertension is managed with a standard approach, as used for patients with non-endocrine hypertension.
2. Those in which special interventions are required.

Hyperaldosteronism (Conn's Syndrome)
Cushing's Syndrome
Phaeochromocytoma/Paraganglionoma
Acromegaly
Hyperthyroidism
Hypothyroidism

Fig. 31.1 Endocrine Causes Of Hypertension

The first group includes patients with Cushing's syndrome, acromegaly and thyroid disorders. Control and management of hypertension in these cases is usually straightforward. The second group includes patients with Conn's syndrome and phaeochromocytoma/paraganglioma.

Because of its complexity and the risks of hypertension-related morbidity, the majority of this chapter concerns the management of phaeochromocytoma.

Perioperative Hypertension: Standard Approach

Hypertension is common in the surgical population. There is high-quality evidence that medical management of hypertension significantly reduces the long-term incidence of stroke, coronary artery disease and heart failure, and control of blood pressure is a desirable objective for this reason alone. It is beyond the scope of this chapter to give a comprehensive account of the general management of hypertension, which depends on a wide range of patient factors, but modern

P. Hambly
Oxford University Hospitals NHS Trust, Oxford, UK

R. Parameswaran, A. Agarwal (eds.), *Evidence-Based Endocrine Surgery*,
https://doi.org/10.1007/978-981-10-1124-5_31

management usually comprises treatment with one or more of the following drugs: calcium channel blockers, angiotensin-converting enzyme inhibitors, angiotensin receptor blockers, diuretics or beta-blockers.

In the short term, it is widely accepted that inadequate preoperative treatment of hypertension leads to increased haemodynamic instability during and after surgery. It has long been assumed that this instability leads to an increase in perioperative cardiovascular events, though there is actually little evidence to support this belief. Nevertheless, it is common practice to postpone elective surgery in patients whose preoperative blood pressure is deemed excessive.

Given the uncertainties involved, the question of what exactly constitutes inadequate treatment of hypertension has become vexed. In the UK, this question has recently been addressed in guidelines issued by the Association of Anaesthetists of Great Britain and Ireland and the British Hypertension Society [1]. The guidelines state that elective noncardiac surgery may proceed if a patient has a documented blood pressure reading of less than 160 mmHg systolic and less than 100 mmHg diastolic, taken in the primary care setting, within the last 12 months. In the absence of such evidence of normotension from primary care, elective surgery may proceed provided readings taken in the preoperative clinic or admission ward are less than 180 mmHg systolic and 110 mmHg diastolic.

Conn's Syndrome

Conn's syndrome or primary hyperaldosteronism is the commonest endocrine cause of hypertension. Indeed, recent studies suggest that a significant proportion of patients with supposedly 'essential' hypertension may have an aldosterone-secreting adrenal adenoma. The hypertension is usually, but not always, accompanied by hypokalaemia. The preoperative management of hypertension in Conn's syndrome follows the basic principles outlined above but differs in the choice of antihypertensive agents. Specific aldosterone antagonists such as spironolactone are favoured as first-line interventions. It is important to ensure the correction of hypokalaemia before surgery, which may require the addition of oral potassium supplements.

Phaeochromocytoma and Paraganglioma

Background

Phaeochromocytomas are rare catecholamine-secreting tumours derived from chromaffin tissue. Paragangliomas are related neuroendocrine tumours of arising from extra-adrenal paraganglia. Though the surgical approach is obviously different for the two tumours, the perioperative management of blood pressure is the same, and the two conditions will considered together here.

Pathophysiology

The main clinical effects of phaeochromocytomas arise from raised levels of circulating catecholamines, principally adrenaline and noradrenaline, and in rare cases, dopamine. There is also an enhancement of the sympathetic nervous system by a number of mechanisms: increased production and storage of catecholamines in vesicles in sympathetic nerves, increased frequency of sympathetic neuronal impulse and selective desensitisation of presynaptic α-2 receptors which causes increased release of noradrenaline during stimulation [2]. This explains the severe hypertension that may result from relatively small increases in circulating noradrenaline. It is also important to understand that catecholamine release is not the whole story in phaeochromocytoma. Many other vasoactive substances may be produced in individual tumours including vasoactive intestinal peptide (VIP), calcitonin gene-related peptide and others [3].

In addition to the cardiovascular changes, the release of catecholamines exerts an important effect on glucose metabolism. Blood glucose tends to be elevated due to stimulation of lipolysis, inhibition of glucose uptake in muscle cells and increased gluconeogenesis and glycogenolysis.

Diagnosis

Phaeochromocytoma may present with symptoms such as headache, palpitations sweating, or anxiety. However, it is commonly asymptomatic. Up to half of cases are identified incidentally on abdominal imaging for an unrelated indication [4]. The diagnosis is confirmed by biochemical tests. Historically this was by 24-h urine vanillylmandelic acid (VMA) levels, though this has now given way to measurement of metanephrines, in either plasma or urine.

Preoperative Management

Historical Aspects

In early studies, adrenalectomy for phaeochromocytoma carried a mortality of up to 45% [5]. The intraoperative release of catecholamines caused dysrhythmias, myocardial ischaemia, left ventricular failure and strokes. Prolonged postoperative hypotension commonly followed resection and was deemed responsible for the majority of deaths. It was assumed at the time that vasoconstriction by circulating catecholamines led to a chronic reduction in blood volume, which led to profound hypotension once the pressor effects of the tumour were removed. This led to the assumption that optimal preoperative care should include treatment with vasodilating drugs and fluid administration. Although the evidence base has recently been questioned [5], the practice of preoperative vasodilation therapy persists to this day, and the operative mortality has fallen, to near zero in recent studies.

Arterial Pressure Control

Preoperative therapy with α-blocking medication is standard practice, and most authors recommend therapy for at least 2 weeks before surgery. As explained above, phaeochromocytoma causes a phenomenon of sympathetic upregulation, making the cardiovascular system more reactive to small increases in circulating catecholamines. It is likely that preoperative α-blockade helps to reverse this effect. Hence the aim of preoperative blockade is not simply to block circulating vasopressor, but also to dampen the responses of the sympathetic nervous system to it. To this end, the duration of therapy is probably as important as the dosage. In the author's unit, we occasionally postpone surgery to allow for an extra week of therapy when the degree of blockade is not satisfactory.

Phenoxybenzamine

Phenoxybenzamine is a non-selective, non-competitive α-blocker with a long duration of action. It is probably the most commonly used drug for this indication. Its α_2 action causes blockade of presynaptic receptors responsible for the regulation of noradrenaline from sympathetic nerve terminals, which causes reflex tachycardia via increased stimulation of β_1 receptors. For this reason, the concomitant use of a β-blocker is required. Central α_2 effects cause side effects of somnolence, headache and nasal congestion. Its long duration of action may be implicated in postoperative hypotension, and some [4] have suggested it be stopped 48 h before surgery. This is not the practice in the author's unit.

Doxazosin

Doxazosin is a specific, competitive inhibitor at the α_1 receptor. Its lack of α_2 effects means that it causes no tachycardia or sedation. Some studies have shown a lower incidence of postoperative hypotension. Its efficacy in phaeochromocytoma is currently being compared with phenoxybenzamine in the PRESCRIPT trial [6]. On a practical level, phenoxybenzamine is an old drug with few other modern indications, which, in the author's experience, is becoming harder to obtain. It is likely that practice will change in favour of doxazosin in the future for this reason alone.

β-Blockade

Tachyarrhythmias may occur with adrenaline- or dopamine-secreting tumours or may be secondary to α-blockade. The non-selective β-blocker propranolol is commonly used, though there are theoretical reasons to prefer a selective β_1 antagonist such as atenolol or metoprolol, which do not oppose β_2-mediated vasodilation. In any event, β-blockade should be introduced after the commencement of α-blockade.

Calcium Channel Blockers

Calcium channel blockers inhibit noradrenaline-induced calcium influx and have been used in phaeochromocytoma, mainly as an adjunct to improve control in patients already receiving an α-blocker. They are not recommended as monotherapy [4] unless hypertension is very mild, or severe orthostatic hypotension occurs with α-blockade.

Metyrosine

Metyrosine (α-methyl-p-tyrosine) is a catecholamine synthesis inhibitor, which acts by inhibition of tyrosine hydroxylase. Phaeochromocytomas have significantly enhanced tyrosine hydroxylase activity compared with normal adrenal tissue. At least one study has shown greater haemodynamic stability with metyrosine compared with phenoxybenzamine, but its use is limited by a long list of side effects, which include extrapyramidal phenomena, sedation, depression and a potentially negative effect on cardiac function.

Titration of Antihypertensive Therapy

The overall aim of preoperative blockade is to minimise the haemodynamic disturbance that inevitably occurs during tumour resection. There is no evidence-based consensus on what should be considered adequate blockade for this purpose. In the author's unit, patients are commenced on modest doses of phenoxybenzamine and propranolol at the time of diagnosis. For logistic reasons this usually occurs much more than 2 weeks preoperatively. For 3–4 days before surgery, patients are assessed with frequent lying/standing pulse and blood pressure recordings. Medication is then titrated to achieve the following end points:

Systolic blood pressure >150 mmHg
Pulse <80 bpm
Significant postural drop in systolic pressure (>20 mmHg)
Standing systolic pressure >90 mmHg
No significant rise in pulse on standing

When a patient's recordings fail to meet these criteria, it is usually necessary to increase the dose of medication by at least 30–50% at a time to achieve an effect. As mentioned above, when the criteria are not met despite increases in dosage, postponing surgery to allow more time at the higher doses is often effective.

Is Preoperative Blockade Necessary?

It is clear that much of the usual preoperative management of phaeochromocytoma is based on historical custom and lacks firm evidence base. Although mortality has fallen dramatically since the 1950s, given the huge advances in anaesthetic and surgical techniques as well the improvements in postoperative care and monitoring that have occurred in the interim, it is unlikely that the use of preoperative α-blockade is solely responsible for this improvement in outcomes. Some authors have published series of phaeochromocytoma excision carried out in selected patients without perioperative, and this has led some to question the usual practice [5]. In one such series [7], 29 patients were operated on without preoperative blockade, without significant morbidity. However, arterial pressure during surgery was higher than those in the treated group, in some cases requiring treatment with sodium nitroprusside and glyceryl trinitrate simultaneously. The author has, to date, not experienced a case in which this combination of powerful antihypertensive agents was necessary to maintain control of arterial pressure and considers that these findings somewhat strengthen rather than weaken the case for preoperative blockade. In any event, there is not yet compelling evidence to abandon the assumption that preoperative blockade reduces intraoperative cardiovascular instability and that this is desirable outcome in its own right.

Fluid Volume

Early authors concluded that phaeochromocytoma was associated with chronic hypovolaemia secondary to vasoconstriction. However, this assumption has not been confirmed by subsequent research. Studies of plasma volume using I^{131}-labelled human albumin have failed to identify significant hypovolaemia in the great majority of patients. Even if it is true, the use of preoperative α-blockade should theoretically allow correction of any deficit. The routine use of intravenous fluid replacement before phaeochromocytoma excision is therefore not considered necessary.

Cardiac Function

Cardiac function may be impaired in phaeochromocytoma. Chronic hypertension can lead to ventricular hypertrophy, which commonly causes a degree of diastolic dysfunction. In other words, the stiffened ventricle fails to relax normally, and the filling of the ventricle in diastole is impaired. In addition, up to 10% of phaeochromocytoma patients have a form of catecholamine-related cardiomyopathy, and occasionally patients present in over cardiac failure. The condition appears to be similar to Takotsubo (or 'stress-related') cardiomyopathy. Cardiac assessment including echocardiography is therefore recommended. Patients with significant left ventricular impairment pose a difficult challenge and need to be managed in close consultation with cardiologists. The main fear is that catecholamine release during tumour handling will precipitate cardiac failure, and such patients need to be managed with appropriate backup facilities, including intraoperative transoesophageal echocardiography and cardiopulmonary bypass, readily available. Cardiac function tends to return to normal after excision of the tumour.

Intraoperative Management

Whatever regime of preoperative preparation employed, the excision of a phaeochromocytoma is inevitably associated with cardiovascular instability. The anaesthetist's job is to minimise the extent of the instability. To this end it is important to be aware of, and prepared for, the usual pattern of behaviour. A typical case involves intermittent 'surges' of arterial pressure, consistent with small intravenous increments of noradrenaline released from the tumour. Obviously, tumour manipulation is a likely cause of this, and surges tend to become more frequent and severe as the surgeon dissects closer to the gland, and especially once he or she has divided Gerota's fascia. Another important moment is during induction of anaesthesia (before intubation), when a paradoxical increase in arterial pressure may be observed. This may be the result of increased blood flow to the adrenal gland resulting from the vasodilatory effects of anaesthetic induction agents. In contrast, manoeuvres that normally cause hypertension, such as intubation, may have little effect in patients treated with significant α-blockade. Another piece of advice is to intervene early at the first sign of a surge in pressure. An approach that one might use in other circumstances, whereby a 'threshold' pressure (of say 150 mmHg) is chosen above which antihypertensive medication will be used, is not recommended. With this approach, arterial pressure is likely to be in the mid-200s before any intervention takes effect. A better strategy is to observe very carefully for any rise from the baseline and treat immediately. More than most procedures, phaeochromocytoma surgery benefits from close communication between surgeon and anaesthetist during the operation.

Monitoring

The rapid changes in arterial pressure that are more or less guaranteed to occur during phaeochromocytoma excision make an arterial cannula, inserted before induction of anaesthesia, an essential requirement. A central venous catheter is also required, mainly for the delivery of vasoactive medications. Though not in the author's routine practice, additional cardiovascular monitoring with oesophageal Doppler or other devices may be useful, particularly in large tumours or open procedures where significant blood loss may be anticipated.

Anaesthetic Technique

Many different techniques of anaesthesia are routinely employed for phaeochromocytoma surgery, and there is no evidence to point to the superiority of any individual regimen. Although it is technically possible to carry out the procedure under regional anaesthesia, it is difficult and offers no specific advantages. Therefore general anaesthesia is the standard approach. Because of the requirement of surgery, it is usually to maintain the airway with endotracheal tubes and to provide controlled ventilation during surgery. In the author's unit, anaesthesia is maintained with propofol and remifentanil, on the grounds that rapid offset of action is desirable particularly after the surgeon divides the adrenal vein. This may contribute to a lower incidence of postoperative hypotension. Some authors counsel against inadequate muscle relaxation, as a possible cause of intraoperative instability, but although coughing and movement are undesirable, there is no reason why muscle relaxants per se are essential, and a technique based on remifentanil can obviate their need for most of the procedure. Spinal or epidural analgesia may be a useful adjunct for open procedures and may contribute to control of arterial pressure but probably confer no benefit in laparoscopic surgery.

Antihypertensive Treatment

There is a wide range of antihypertensive agents used, and as is a common theme in phaeochromocytoma management, none has any evidence-based advantage over any other. However, although the choice of individual agents is open, a structured and planned approach is recommended. The author divides the agents chosen into five categories, in ascending order of potency, moving from one category to the next depending on the frequency and magnitude of blood pressure surges (see Table 31.1). At the first level, the haemodynamics can be influenced simply by adjusting anaesthetic depth or analgesia, as in any other case. As the case progresses, specific antihypertensives of ascending potency are employed, culminating in the most potent drugs such as sodium nitroprusside.

Table 31.1 Antihypertensive management during phaeochromocytoma surgery

Level 1	Adjustment of depth of anaesthesia
Level 2	Magnesium sulphate 1 g bolus
Level 3	Labetalol 5–20 mg bolus Nicardipine 1–2 mg bolus Phentolamine 1–2 mg bolus
Level 4	Glyceryl trinitrate (GTN) bolus 0.1 mg Clevidipine infusion
Level 5	GTN infusion Sodium nitroprusside infusion

Magnesium Sulphate

Though almost never adequate as a sole agent, magnesium sulphate is useful in the early stages of surgical excision. It inhibits adrenal catecholamine release, as well as reducing receptor sensitivity, and has a useful anti-dysrhythmic effect. It is given by bolus dose of 10–15 mg/kg, repeated up to a maximum of 60 mg/kg.

Labetalol

Labetalol is a drug with both α- and β-blocking properties. Its α-effects are greater when given IV, than when taken orally. It provides smooth and moderately potent antihypertensive actions when given in intravenous doses of 5–20 mg. Because of its β-action, there is a theoretical risk of paroxysmal hypertension, but this has never been observed by the author. It has a relatively long duration of action, with a biological half-life of 5–6 h, which may be implicated in postoperative hypertension.

Phentolamine

Another drug with a long history behind it, phentolamine is a reversible non-selective α-antagonist. It is given in intravenous dose of 1–2 mg. It has a relatively short duration of action, with a biological half-life of 20–30 min. Like phenoxybenzamine, it can cause reflex tachycardia, which is a consideration in patients who have not received preoperative β-blockade.

Nicardipine

Nicardipine is a calcium channel blocker and a potent arterial vasodilator. It has relatively little effect on venous tone, and hence cardiac preload and cardiac output are maintained. It does not cause reflex tachycardia. It can be given in boluses of 1–2 mg. It has an elimination half-life of 40–60 min.

Clevidipine

Clevidipine is a novel calcium channel blocker, which is metabolised by plasma esterases, and thus has a short half-life. Experience is limited in phaeochromocytoma, but it is theoretically promising. It is very lipid soluble and is presented in a lipid emulsion, giving it an identical appearance to propofol. Care needs to be taken not to confuse the two in the pressurised situation of phaeochromocytoma surgery.

Glyceryl Trinitrate (GTN)

GTN is a direct-acting vasodilator, which acts via production of nitric oxide in vascular smooth muscle. It is principally a venodilator. It is a highly potent antihypertensive which can be given by infusion or by small boluses. It has a rapid onset and offset of action, one which closely matches the timescale of a typical hypertensive surge. It may cause a reflex tachycardia.

Sodium Nitroprusside (SNP)

SNP is another nitric oxide-mediated smooth muscle relaxant, which acts principally on arterioles. It has a rapid onset of action and extreme potency, which means it can only safely be used by infusion. Although undeniably effective, it is better suited to treating sustained hypertension and is difficult to use in the episodic hypertension of phaeochromocytoma. There is a risk of severe hypotension if dosage is not judged accurately. The solution needs to be protected from light. Prolonged infusion can cause cyanide toxicity. It is another old-fashioned drug with few remaining modern indications and can be hard to obtain. The author has now abandoned its use in favour of GTN, by bolus and infusion.

Isolation of the Tumour

A key moment in the anaesthetic management of phaeochromocytoma is the point at which the surgeon divides the venous drainage of the gland, whereupon no further secretion of catecholamine occurs. This is usually followed by an abrupt fall in blood pressure. The adrenal gland typically has a single main vein, though there is often more than one. The abrupt cardiovascular response to isolating the tumour means that this event can be more obvious to the anaesthetist than to the surgeon. The benefit of short-acting antihypertensive agents is felt at this point, and if the anaesthetist is paying sufficient attention, hypotension is usually transient and mild, needing no treatment other than small doses of ephedrine or metaraminol.

Occasionally, hypotension is more severe and prolonged. There is much debate about the factors responsible for this complication, much of it centring on arguments about the best preoperative regimen. Given the large doses of antihypertensive medication administered before and during surgery, it is perhaps surprising that hypotension does not happen more often. Some authors have drawn a correlation between the incidence of hypotension and the levels of preoperative catecholamine secretion. In practice, most cases are readily treated with postoperative noradrenaline infusion, which is usually required for no longer than 12 h. Rarely, with massive tumours, a distinct phenomenon of catecholamine-resistant hypotension may occur (see below).

Postoperative Management

The postoperative course of a typical laparoscopic adrenalectomy for phaeochromocytoma is uncomplicated. It is sensible to monitor patients in a high-dependency setting, where invasive arterial monitoring can be used, but in practice postoperative problems are uncommon. In the absence of persistent hypertension, preoperative α-blockers can be stopped immediately. β-blockade is usually tapered off over a day or two to avoid rebound tachycardia.

Hypoglycaemia

Because of the effects of excess catecholamines on glucose metabolism, most patients with phaeochromocytoma have raised insulin levels. The abrupt removal of the tumour can lead to a period of hypoglycaemia, while insulin secretion is adjusted. Persistent β-blockade may also mask its symptoms. Frequent blood glucose estimations are advisable in the first few hours after surgery.

Persistent Hypertension

There are many reasons for hypertension to occur in the early postoperative phase, including usual causes such as pain, full bladder, etc. Hypertension requiring the continuance of intravenous antihypertensive drugs is a worrying sign that suggests incomplete resection or bilateral or metastatic disease. Even in those patients without recurrence, hypertension is a common finding on long-term follow-up.

Catecholamine-Resistant Hypotension

There are several case reports [8], as well as two cases within the author's experience in which excision of phaeochromocytoma leads to severe hypotension that fails to respond to catecholamine infusion. It appears to be a phenomenon associated with massive and/or malignant tumours, and in several cases profound shock responded readily to administration of arginine vasopressin. Although vasopressin is a vasoconstrictor that can be expected to treat hypotension, there may be specific reason why it is effective in massive phaeochromocytoma. Firstly, it does not act via α-receptors, which may be still blocked or downregulated because of preoperative management. Second, in some patients there is evidence of an oversecretion of vasopressin, and abrupt removal of this source may leave the hypophyseal-pituitary axis unable to immediately make up the shortfall. Finally, there is some evidence that chronic catecholamine excess may cause down-regulation of vasopressin synthesis and release in the hypothalamus and pituitary. Arginine vasopressin is given via initial bolus of 2 units and then followed by an infusion of up to 2.4 units per hour (adult dosage).

References

1. Hartle A, McCormack T, et al. The measurement of adult blood pressure and management of hypertension before elective surgery. Anaesthesia. 2016;71:326–37.
2. Ahmed I, Jepegnanam C. Recognition and management of Phaeochromocytoma. Anaesth Intens Care Med. 2015;10:465–9.
3. Herrera MF, Stone E, et al. Pheochromocytoma producing multiple vasoactive peptides. Archiv Surg. 1992;127(1):105–8.
4. Connor D, Boumphrey S. Perioperative care of phaeochromocytoma. BJA Educ. 2015;16(5):153–8.
5. Lentschener C, Gaujoux S, et al. Point of controversy: perioperative care of patients undergoing phaeochromocytoma removal – time for reappraisal? Eur J Endocrinol. 2011;165:365–73.
6. Phenoxybenzamine versus Doxazosin in PCC Patients (PRESCRIPT). http://clinicaltrials.gov/show/NCT01379898
7. Boutros AR, Bravo EL etc al. Perioperative management of 63 patients with phaeochromocytoma. Cleve Clin J Med 1990; 57: 613-617.
8. Roth JV. Use of vasopressin bolus and infusion to treat catecholamine-resistant hypotension during phaeochromocytoma resection. Anaesthesiology. 2007;106(4):883–4.

Laparoscopic Adrenalectomy

32

Jesse Shulin Hu and Wei Keat Cheah

Introduction

Since its first description in 1992, laparoscopic adrenalectomy has become the gold standard for the surgical treatment of most adrenal conditions. The benefits of a minimally invasive approach to adrenal resection include decreased length of stay, decreased analgesic use, lesser blood loss and shorter recovery time. In addition, difficulty with open surgical exposure and the small size of the adrenal gland make this organ particularly amenable to a minimally invasive technique. The anatomical location of the adrenal gland has led to a number of laparoscopic approaches, including lateral transperitoneal, retroperitoneal and robotic.

Background

The adrenal glands are retroperitoneal organs located superior to the kidneys. The adrenal glands have a golden orange colour distinct from the pale retroperitoneal fat they are embedded in. The glands are highly vascularized and derive their blood supply from branches of the inferior phrenic, aortic and renal arteries. Each gland has a single central vein which drains directly into the inferior vena cava on the right and into the left renal vein on the left.

Understanding the venous drainage and relations of the adrenal gland to its surrounding structures is key to learning adrenalectomy. The right adrenal gland is bordered inferiorly by the right kidney, supero-posterolaterally by the diaphragm, anteriorly by the liver and medially by the inferior vena cava. The left adrenal gland is bordered inferiorly by the left kidney and left renal vein, supero-posteriorly by the diaphragm and anteriorly by the tail of the pancreas (Fig. 32.1).

The adrenal gland is made up of the cortex and the medulla. The adrenal cortex produces glucocorticoids (cortisone), mineralocorticoids (aldosterone) and sex steroids. The adrenal medulla secretes epinephrine, norepinephrine and dopamine. The abnormal secretion of any of the hormones produced by the adrenal gland results in unique clinical presentations/syndromes and is an indication for surgical resection.

The history of adrenal surgery is longstanding. In 1889, Knowsley-Thornton [1] performed the first successful adrenalectomy when he removed a large, 20-pound, adrenal tumour with the left kidney in a 36-year-old woman. Subsequently, Perry Sargent [2] performed the first planned adrenalectomy in 1914. In 1927, Charles Mayo [1] was the first surgeon to use the flank approach when he performed adrenalectomy for pheochromocytoma. Through the early

J. S. Hu · W. K. Cheah (✉)
Department of Surgery, Ng Teng Fong General Hospital, National University Health System, Singapore, Singapore
e-mail: wei_keat_cheah@nuhs.edu.sg

R. Parameswaran, A. Agarwal (eds.), *Evidence-Based Endocrine Surgery*,
https://doi.org/10.1007/978-981-10-1124-5_32

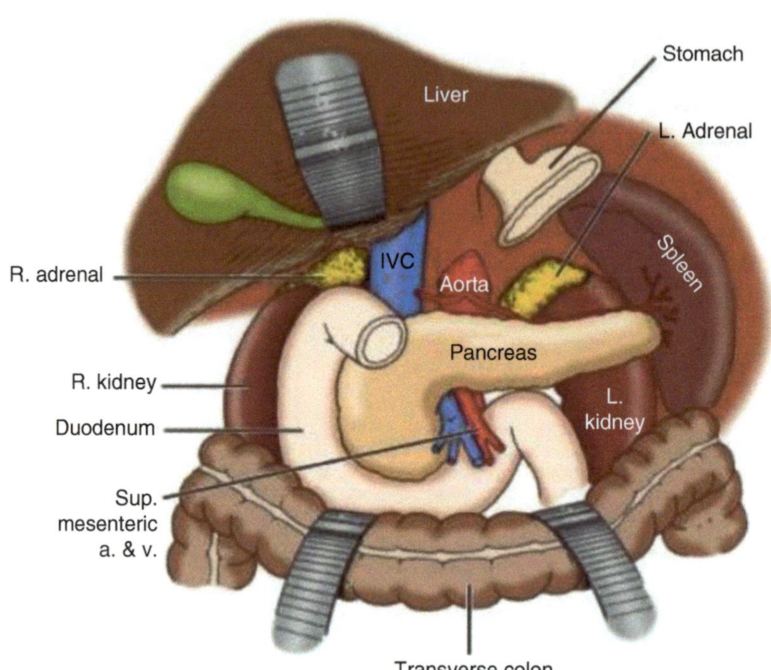

Fig. 32.1 Relations of adrenal gland

to mid-1900s, multiple changes in surgical approaches to the adrenal gland were developed to augment several posterior and anterior approaches. However, little change to adrenal surgery was seen for decades until the first laparoscopic adrenalectomy was described by Michael Gagner [3] in 1992. Since then, laparoscopic adrenalectomy [4] has become standard of care approach for the majority of benign adrenal tumours.

Presentations, Investigations and Treatment Options

Presentation

The most common presentation of a patient with adrenal tumour is that of an adrenal incidentaloma. An adrenal incidentaloma is defined [5, 6] as an adrenal mass greater than 1 cm which was unexpectedly detected through an imaging procedure performed for reasons unrelated to adrenal dysfunction. It is the result of advances in imaging technologies, in particular computed tomography and magnetic resonance imaging, and their widespread use in clinical practice.

The prevalence of adrenal incidentaloma is variable and has been reported [7–10] to be ranging from 0.4% to 4.4% of all CT scans. The prevalence is increased when higher resolution scanners are used and has been found in up to 10% in the elderly [11]. In autopsy studies [11–13], the prevalence of adrenal incidentaloma is reported to range from 1 to 9%.

The majority of adrenal incidentalomas are clinically non-functioning, benign adrenal cortical adenomas which do not need to be removed. The management of an adrenal incidentaloma requires the clinician to answer two pertinent questions that determine the need for the degree of evaluation and need for therapy.

Firstly, is it malignant?

Malignancy is an uncommon cause of adrenal incidentaloma in patients without a known diagnosis of cancer. Primary adrenal carcinoma is rare with an incidence of 1 per million. It is suspected when the mass is more than 4 cm in diameter when discovered [12], and hence most guidelines recommend the surgical excision of adrenal tumours which are larger than 4 cm in size. Other features such Hounsfield unit >10 and delayed contrast washout [14–16] and change in size over time have also a strong predictive value.

However, the adrenal gland is not an uncommon site of metastasis, with reported prevalence of 3.1% [17] in one large retrospective study. The primary malignancies that have known predilections for adrenal metastases are melanoma, renal cell carcinoma, lung cancer and breast cancer. The role of laparoscopic adrenalectomy in management of isolated adrenal metastasis at this point is still controversial.

Secondly, is it functional?

While most adrenal incidentalomas are nonfunctional, 10–15% secrete excess amounts of hormones [18, 19]. Hence, one should look out for clinical features suggestive of increased adrenal function and perform the necessary tests to rule out a functional tumour, in particular pheochromocytoma.

Other than presenting as an adrenal incidentaloma, the patient may present with clinical signs and symptoms of hormone hypersecretion.

The classical features of primary hyperaldosteronism (Conn syndrome) are hypertension and hypokalaemia. It is the most common cause of secondary hypertension and should be suspected in a patient with early-onset hypertension or hypertension that is difficult to control with medication [20].

Cushing's syndrome is the result of excessive cortisol secretion. It results in the characteristic features of moon facies, hirsutism, truncal obesity, abdominal straie and the "buffalo hump". Patients also commonly have hypertension and diabetes. Adrenalectomy is the treatment of choice in subclinical Cushing's or when Cushing's syndrome is due to an adrenocortical tumour (ACTH-independent Cushing's syndrome).

Pheochromocytomas are rare tumours arising from the chromaffin cells of the adrenal medulla which result in excessive production of catecholamines. The patient may complain of episodic headaches, diaphoresis, palpitations and marked or labile hypertension.

Rarely, the patient may present with an abdominal mass or pain due to a large mass/haemorrhage.

Investigations

The first step in the work-up of an adrenal tumour is to determine its functional status, in particular to rule out pheochromocytoma. This is because an undiagnosed pheochromocytoma can result in cardiovascular instability during surgery.

Initial screening tests and further confirmatory tests for the functional status of the adrenal tumour are listed in the Table 32.1.

The imaging modality of choice is CT or MRI with contrast which shows the characteristics of the adrenal tumour and its relations to the surrounding structures. Further imaging with positron emission tomography may be required in patients whom malignancy is suspected.

Preoperative biopsy of the adrenal mass should only be performed in patients with suspected metastasis causing the adrenal mass and if the biopsy findings would result in a change in management plan. It is pertinent to exclude pheochromocytoma before a biopsy is performed to avoid triggering a hypertensive crisis.

Adrenal venous sampling may be required in patients with Conn syndrome to determine if there's lateralizing source of increased aldosterone [20].

Table 32.1 Investigations for functional status of adrenal tumour

Diagnosis	Initial tests	Further tests (may or may not be required)
Conn syndrome	Plasma aldosterone concentration and plasma renin activity	Urinary aldosterone and potassium while on high-salt diet (salt loading test)
Cushing's syndrome	24-h urinary free cortisol level 1 mg overnight dexamethasone suppression test	Plasma ACTH level High-dose dexamethasone suppression test
Phaeochromocytoma	24-h urinary catecholamines and metanephrines	

Treatment Options

Adrenalectomy is indicated in patients with functional tumours, tumours suspicious of malignancy and solitary unilateral adrenal metastases. Laparoscopic adrenalectomy is the treatment of choice [21] for most adrenal lesions. Compared to the open approach, it is associated with less blood loss, less pain, shorter length of stay, faster return to normal activities and less morbidity.

Contraindications [22–25] to the laparoscopic approach are large tumours >8 cm and any tumour with extra-adrenal extension or local invasion. The worry is tumour spillage and the inability to achieve R0 resection. Although some papers [22, 24, 26] have suggested that laparoscopic adrenalectomy can be safely performed for adrenal cancers in experienced hands, the numbers are small due to the rarity of the disease.

Laparoscopic adrenalectomy can be performed via various approaches, transperitoneally, retroperitoneally or robotic. Many systematic reviews [27–29] have compared the various approaches and are inconclusive regarding the superiority of one approach to the others.

Since its introduction in 1995, posterior retroperitoneal adrenalectomy (PRA) [30–32] has been utilised more frequently and increasing in popularity. This approach allows direct access to the retroperitoneum and adrenal gland without breaching the peritoneum and avoiding the need for intra-abdominal organ mobilisation. The potential advantage of the retroperitoneal approach is the ability to perform a bilateral adrenalectomy without repositioning the patient and also avoiding entry into the abdominal cavity, in particular one that has previous abdominal surgery and its associated adhesions. Furthermore, CO_2 insufflation pressures in the retroperitoneum can be kept significantly higher without limiting cardiac filling pressures while limiting troublesome bleeding. Multiple retrospective series have demonstrated safety and efficacy of PRA. The largest series is by M. Walz [33] who published results of 560 PRA in 520 patients for neoplasms ranging from 0.5 to 10 cm. His results were equivalent to contemporary series of transperitoneal laparoscopic adrenalectomies, including a minor morbidity of 14.4% and conversion rate of 1.7%. In his series, conversion rate was defined by conversion to open approach or transperitoneal approach. Since then, more surgical units have started adopting the PRA approach.

However, the PRA approach is technically demanding and has a steeper learning curve as the anatomy is not familiar to most surgeons. The general principles of the PRA approach include:

- *Patient positioning*: The patient is placed in the prone position with the hips and knees flexed at approximately 90° and the adrenal gland being approached posteriorly beneath the 12th rib (Fig. 32.2).
- *Port placement sites:* Three incisions, one 12 mm and two 5 mm, are typically used for trocar placement. The initial trocar entry into the retroperitoneum is confirmed by direct vision. The first incision is placed approximately 1 cm inferior to the tip of the 12th rib, and the retroperitoneum is bluntly entered. With an index finger directly in the retroperitoneum, an incision is made laterally at the posterior axillary line and a blunt trocar inserted. Another trocar is inserted between the first trocar site and the spine, along the paraspinal muscles, approximately 4 cm from the inferior border of the 12th rib.
- *Exposure:* A critical step of the PRA procedure is exposure of the superior pole of the

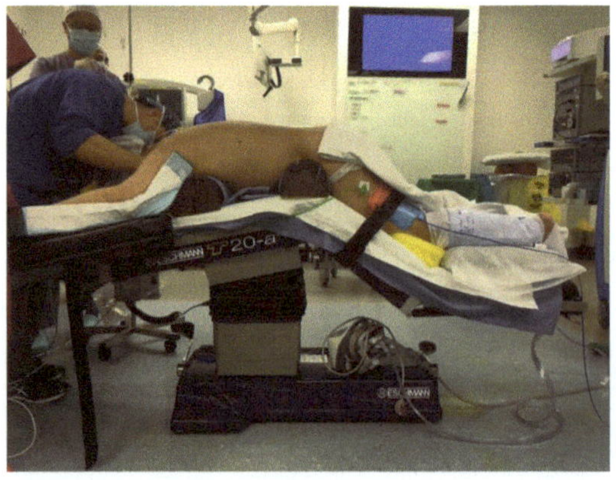

Fig. 32.2 Positioning for PRA approach

kidney by identifying and opening the overlying Gerota's fascia.
- *Resection*: This involves dissecting the adrenal gland and the surrounding perinephric fat from the kidney from laterally to medially. After complete mobilisation, the next critical step is to identify and secure the blood supply to the adrenal gland. The adrenal arteries are identified on the inferior and medial aspects of the adrenal gland and may be divided using electrocautery. The main adrenal vein is usually controlled with surgical clips.

Relative contraindications to PRA include tumours larger than 7 cm and patients with BMI > 40 kg/m2. The working space is considerably smaller with the RPA approach, and therefore neoplasms larger than 7 cm are difficult to dissect safely. In addition, the creation of the retroperitoneal working space can be limited by a large pannus in an obese patient.

Some papers have described robot-assisted adrenalectomy which is associated with increased cost while the potential added advantage remains to be seen.

The more widely practised approach is the transperitoneal approach which would be described in more details below.

Surgical Technique

In patients with functional tumours, preoperative consultation with an endocrinologist and an anaesthesiologist is crucial to adequately prepare the patient for surgery. All patients with pheochromocytoma require alpha blockade (preferably with phenoxybenzamine) for at least 7–10 days before surgery, followed by beta blockade if tachycardia is still present after alpha blockade is achieved. Those with Conn syndrome require hypokalaemia to be corrected and blood pressure adequately controlled, commonly with spironoloctone. Patients with Cushing's syndrome will require stress doses of steroids perioperatively and post-operatively.

Laparoscopic adrenalectomy is performed under general anaesthesia. Additional intraoperative monitoring such as the arterial line and urinary catheter is required in those with pheochromocytoma. In addition to diabetic patients, blood sugar monitoring is also required in those with pheochromocytoma and Cushing's syndrome. Nasogastric tube is typically inserted to allow decompression of the stomach. Antibiotic prophylaxis, usually a first-generation cephalosporin, is given prior to skin incision. Sequential compressive devices are placed for deep vein thrombosis prophylaxis.

For laparoscopic transperitoneal adrenalectomy, the patient is placed in the lateral decubitus position with the affected side facing upward and the operative table flexed just above the level of the iliac crest. (Fig. 32.3) Achieving a good positioning prior to incision is pertinent in ensuing success in surgery.

Laparoscopic access may be obtained by an open or closed technique based on the surgeon's preference. The authors prefer an open technique where an incision is made at the anterior axillary line, 2 fingerbreadths below the costal margin.

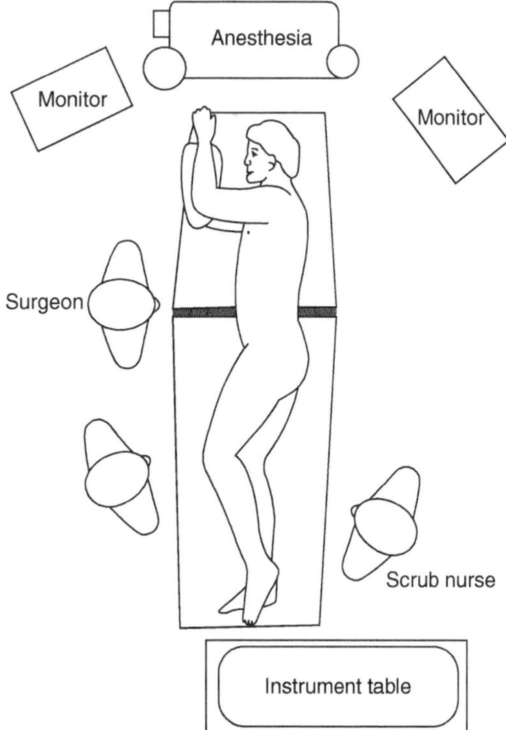

Fig. 32.3 Positioning of patient for laparoscopic adrenalectomy

This is for placement of the 10–12 mm trocar which acts as a camera port. If a closed technique is chosen, a Veress needle is placed just below the costal margin to insufflate the peritoneal cavity followed by insertion of a trocar at the midclavicular line, 2 fingerbreadths below the costal margin.

Typically, at least three ports are required, one for the camera and two acting as working ports. The port at the anterior axillary line is usually used as the camera port, while the ports at the midclavicular line and posterior axillary line are used as working ports. A fourth port is needed for the right side to retract the liver and occasionally on the left side to retract the spleen. It is typically placed 2 fingerbreadths below the xiphisternum.

After insertion of the first trocar, pneumoperitoneum is achieved using CO2 insufflation to a pressure of 10–12 mmHg. The laparoscopic camera is inserted and general laparoscopy is performed. Following which, the working ports are inserted under camera vision and mobilisation begins. The use of energy devices such as ultrasonic dissector help with the dissection. The mobilisation of the right and left adrenalectomy are described separately due to the differences in their relations to the surrounding organs. Once mobilisation is completed and the adrenal vein is identified, subsequent dissection is similar for both sides.

Mobilisation of the Right Side

The liver is retracted using a snake-type retractor or a Nathanson liver retractor. The liver is mobilised anteriorly by incising the retroperitoneal attachments towards the medial aspect and then the triangular ligament to the level of the diaphragm. Adequate mobilisation of the liver is crucial to allow cephalad retraction of the liver. The hepatic flexure may need to be mobilised inferiorly and medially.

At this point, the adrenal gland is usually visualised. If not, the inferior vena cava is a good landmark to starting our dissection. The dissection of the inferior vena cava starts at the level above the right renal vein and progresses superiorly towards the liver. Kocherization of the duodenum may be required to allow better visualisation of the inferior vena cava. Dissection of the vena cava allows visualisation and identification of the short adrenal vein which is located at the supero-medial edge of the adrenal gland as it enters the inferior vena cava.

Mobilisation of the Left Side

The splenic flexure and descending colon are mobilised medially, and the lateral attachments of the spleen are divided until the left crus of the diaphragm, taking care to avoid injury to the short gastric vessels. The spleen can be mobilised medially once the splenocolic and lienorenal ligaments are divided, allowing adequate exposure of the adrenal gland. The position of the patient and the mobilisation of the spleen usually allow the spleen to drop away from the operating field. Occasionally, a snake-type retractor is required for retraction of the spleen. Dissection is carried down from the superior to medial in the relatively avascular plane. Care is taken not to dissect in the plane between the spleen & the tail of the pancreas. Dissection lateral to the kidney should be avoided as it may allow the Gerota fascia to fall medially, making the adrenal dissection more difficult.

An incision is made into the Gerota fascia over the upper pole of the kidney. The incision is extended medially and dissected towards the renal vein. Once the renal vein is visualised, careful dissection along the superior border of the vein will allow for identification of the adrenal vein which is located in the inferio-medial edge of the adrenal gland as it enters the left renal vein.

Dissection of the Adrenal Vein

Once the adrenal vein is visualised, it is carefully dissected using gentle suction and the Maryland dissector. The right adrenal vein, compared to the left, is often short and broad as it drains directly into the vena cava. Therefore, great care must be taken during dissection to avoid injury to the adrenal vein and the inferior vena cava.

After the adrenal vein is dissected, clips are placed at the proximal and distal side. The adrenal vein is divided between clips. When performing adrenalectomy for pheochromocytoma, communication between the surgeon and anaesthesiologist is crucial to allow for IV fluid loading and even possible need for inotropic support as division of the adrenal vein can cause precipitous drop in blood pressure resulting in cardiovascular instability and even collapse.

After the adrenal vein is controlled and divided, the adrenal gland can be dissected free from its remaining attachments. Grasping of the adrenal gland must be avoided as it can result in disruption of the adrenal capsule. Instead, the peri-adrenal fat or overlying peritoneum can be grasped and blunt dissection performed to free the adrenal gland. The numerous small arterial branches that supply the adrenal gland encountered during dissection can be controlled by electrosurgical device.

The adrenal gland is placed in a specimen retrieval bag and removed through the trocar or after slight enlargement of the 10 mm port site. The operating field is inspected for bleeding and the clips are checked to ensure that they are in place. A drain is usually not necessary except in cases where pancreatic tail injury is suspected. The pneumoperitoneum is released and the trocars are removed. The fascia is closed in the larger ports, while skin closure is achieved using absorbable sutures.

Results

Postoperatively, the patient is usually monitored in a regular surgical ward or in the surgical high dependency ward if inotropic support was required in excision of phaeochromocytoma. The patient can be started on clear fluids and progress to regular diet as tolerated. Oral analgesia is usually adequate for pain control and early mobilisation is highly encouraged.

Blood pressure monitoring and titration of antihypertensive medications are required for those with functional tumours. Co-management with the endocrinologist is recommended for those with functional tumours, in particular steroid management for patients with Cushing's syndrome. Electrolytes, in particular potassium levels, should be monitored in those with Conn syndrome.

Most patients can be discharged 24–48 h after surgery. Follow-up in the surgical outpatient clinic usually takes place about 2–3 weeks after discharge where the wound and histology are reviewed.

Complications

The complications of laparoscopic adrenalectomy can be classified into general complications in relation to laparoscopic surgery, site specific (injury to surrounding organs) and functional.

General Complications

Bleeding

Wound infection especially in Cushing's syndrome.

Conversion to open (3–5%).

Risks in relation to general anaesthesia.

Site Specific (Injury to Adjacent Structures) – <3%

Right	Left
Colon—hepatic flexure	Spleen
Duodenum	Tail of pancreas
Liver	Diaphragm
Gallbladder	Colon—splenic flexure
Diaphragm	
Inferior vena cava	

Functional

Intraoperative hypertensive crisis and labile blood pressure in pheochromocytoma.

Postoperative adrenal insufficiency in Cushing's syndrome.

Conclusion

In conclusion, laparoscopic adrenalectomy is the preferred method for removing most adrenal tumours. It can be carried out safely with good surgical outcomes in experienced hands.

References

1. Welbourn RB. The history of endocrine surgery. Westport, CT: Greenwood Publishing Group; 1990.
2. Prager G, Heinz-Peer G, Passler C, Kaczirek K, Schindl M, Scheuba C, et al. Surgical strategy in adrenal masses. Eur J Radiol. 2002;41(1):70–7.
3. Gagner M, Lacroix A, Bolte E. Laparoscopic adrenalectomy in Cushing's syndrome and pheochromocytoma. N Engl J Med. 1992;327(14):1033.
4. Assalia A, Gagner M. Laparoscopic adrenalectomy. Br J Surg. 2004;91(10):1259–74.
5. Young WF Jr. Clinical practice. The incidentally discovered adrenal mass. N Engl J Med. 2007;356(6):601–10.
6. Terzolo M, Bovio S, Pia A, Reimondo G, Angeli A. Management of adrenal incidentaloma. Best Pract Res Clin Endocrinol Metab. 2009;23(2):233–43.
7. Aron DC. The adrenal incidentaloma: disease of modern technology and public health problem. Rev Endocr Metab Disord. 2001;2(3):335–42.
8. Bovio S, Cataldi A, Reimondo G, Sperone P, Novello S, Berruti A, et al. Prevalence of adrenal incidentaloma in a contemporary computerized tomography series. J Endocrinol Invest. 2006;29(4):298–302.
9. Herrera MF, Grant CS, van Heerden JA, Sheedy PF, Ilstrup DM. Incidentally discovered adrenal tumors: an institutional perspective. Surgery. 1991;110(6):1014–21.
10. Terzolo M, Ali A, Osella G, Mazza E. Prevalence of adrenal carcinoma among incidentally discovered adrenal masses. A retrospective study from 1989 to 1994. Gruppo Piemontese Incidentalomi Surrenalici. Arch Surg. 1997;132(8):914–9.
11. Terzolo M, Stigliano A, Chiodini I, Loli P, Furlani L, Arnaldi G, et al. AME position statement on adrenal incidentaloma. Eur J Endocrinol. 2011;164(6):851–70.
12. Angeli A, Osella G, Ali A, Terzolo M. Adrenal incidentaloma: an overview of clinical and epidemiological data from the National Italian Study Group. Horm Res. 1997;47(4-6):279–83.
13. Zeiger MA, Thompson GB, Duh QY, Hamrahian AH, Angelos P, Elaraj D, et al. American Association of Clinical Endocrinologists and American Association of Endocrine Surgeons Medical Guidelines for the Management of Adrenal Incidentalomas: executive summary of recommendations. Endocr Pract. 2009;15(5):450–3.
14. Grumbach MM, Biller BM, Braunstein GD, Campbell KK, Carney JA, Godley PA, et al. Management of the clinically inapparent adrenal mass ("incidentaloma"). Ann Intern Med. 2003;138(5):424–9.
15. Hamrahian AH, Ioachimescu AG, Remer EM, Motta-Ramirez G, Bogabathina H, Levin HS, et al. Clinical utility of noncontrast computed tomography attenuation value (hounsfield units) to differentiate adrenal adenomas/hyperplasias from nonadenomas: Cleveland Clinic experience. J Clin Endocrinol Metab. 2005;90(2):871–7.
16. Dunnick NR, Korobkin M, Francis I. Adrenal radiology: distinguishing benign from malignant adrenal masses. AJR Am J Roentgenol. 1996;167(4):861–7.
17. Lam KY, Lo CY. Metastatic tumours of the adrenal glands: a 30-year experience in a teaching hospital. Clin Endocrinol (Oxf). 2002;56(1):95–101.
18. Cawood TJ, Hunt PJ, O'Shea D, Cole D, Soule S. Recommended evaluation of adrenal incidentalomas is costly, has high false-positive rates and confers a risk of fatal cancer that is similar to the risk of the adrenal lesion becoming malignant; time for a rethink? Eur J Endocrinol. 2009;161(4):513–27.
19. Mantero F, Terzolo M, Arnaldi G, Osella G, Masini AM, Ali A, et al. A survey on adrenal incidentaloma in Italy. Study group on adrenal tumors of the Italian society of endocrinology. J Clin Endocrinol Metab. 2000;85(2):637–44.
20. Funder JW, Carey RM, Mantero F, Murad MH, Reincke M, Shibata H, et al. The Management of Primary Aldosteronism: Case Detection, Diagnosis, and Treatment: An Endocrine Society Clinical Practice Guideline. The Journal of Clinical Endocrinology & Metabolism 2016:101(5):1889–1916.
21. Thompson GB, Grant CS, van Heerden JA, Schlinkert RT, Young WF Jr, Farley DR, et al. Laparoscopic versus open posterior adrenalectomy: a case-control study of 100 patients. Surgery. 1997;122(6):1132–6.
22. Gonzalez RJ, Shapiro S, Sarlis N, Vassilopoulou-Sellin R, Perrier ND, Evans DB, et al. Laparoscopic resection of adrenal cortical carcinoma: a cautionary note. Surgery. 2005;138(6):1078–85. discussion 85–6
23. Saunders BD, Doherty GM. Laparoscopic adrenalectomy for malignant disease. Lancet Oncol. 2004;5(12):718–26.
24. Shen WT, Kebebew E, Clark OH, Duh QY. Reasons for conversion from laparoscopic to open or hand-assisted adrenalectomy: review of 261 laparoscopic adrenalectomies from 1993 to 2003. World J Surg. 2004;28(11):1176–9.
25. Shen ZJ, Chen SW, Wang S, Jin XD, Chen J, Zhu Y, et al. Predictive factors for open conversion of laparoscopic adrenalectomy: a 13-year review of 456 cases. J Endourol. 2007;21(11):1333–7.
26. Machado NO, Al Qadhi H, Al Wahaibi K, Rizvi SG. Laparoscopic adrenalectomy for large adrenocortical carcinoma. JSLS. 2015;19(3):e2015.00036.
27. Brandao LF, Autorino R, Laydner H, Haber GP, Ouzaid I, De Sio M, et al. Robotic versus laparoscopic adrenalectomy: a systematic review and meta-analysis. Eur Urol. 2014;65(6):1154–61.
28. Chai YJ, Kwon H, Yu HW, Kim SJ, Choi JY, Lee KE, et al. Systematic review of surgical approaches for

adrenal tumors: lateral transperitoneal versus posterior retroperitoneal and laparoscopic versus robotic adrenalectomy. Int J Endocrinol. 2014;2014:918346.
29. Constantinides VA, Christakis I, Touska P, Palazzo FF. Systematic review and meta-analysis of retroperitoneoscopic versus laparoscopic adrenalectomy. Br J Surg. 2012;99(12):1639–48.
30. Mercan S, Seven R, Ozarmagan S, Tezelman S. Endoscopic retroperitoneal adrenalectomy. Surgery. 1995;118(6):1071–5. discussion 5–6
31. Walz MK, Peitgen K, Krause U, Eigler FW. Dorsal retroperitoneoscopic adrenalectomy--a new surgical technique. Zentralblatt fur Chirurgie. 1995;120(1):53–8.
32. Walz MK, Peitgen K, Hoermann R, Giebler RM, Mann K, Eigler FW. Posterior retroperitoneoscopy as a new minimally invasive approach for adrenalectomy: results of 30 adrenalectomies in 27 patients. World J Surg. 1996;20(7):769–74.
33. Walz MK, Alesina PF, Wenger FA, Deligiannis A, Szuczik E, Petersenn S, et al. Posterior retroperitoneoscopic adrenalectomy—results of 560 procedures in 520 patients. Surgery. 2006;140(6):943–8. discussion 8–50

Complications of Adrenal Surgery 33

Rajeev Parameswaran

There has been a significant improvement in the understanding of adrenal disease over last ten decades, with better understanding of the physiology and biochemistry and imaging. Similarly, with the introduction of laparoscopy in the 1990s, adrenalectomy moved from a morbid open procedure to a less invasive and less morbid procedure. Despite the advances, complications do arise, and some are related to the disease process and others to the surgical approaches. These complications may be avoided by adequate vigilance and preparation and may be divided into preoperative, intraoperative and postoperative complications, which are addressed in this chapter.

Introduction

Adrenalectomy is performed for patients with tumours or disorders arising in the adrenal cortex or medulla and may present in three ways: (a) *those associated with hyperfunctioning adrenal lesions*, (b) *those associated with malignancy* and (c) *those with uncertain significance and picked up incidentally*. Where presenting with hormonal oversecretion, the symptoms are related to the excess of cortisol, mineralocorticoids, androgens and catecholamines or their metabolites. Adrenal malignancies may present with symptoms of hormone excess or pressure effects of the tumour especially when large. Secondary hypertension is a common feature seen in functioning adrenal neoplasms, along with metabolic problems such as hyperglycaemia, hypokalaemia and metabolic alkalosis. The various causes of adrenal masses are shown in Table 33.1.

Complication is defined as a condition or event leading to unfavourable patient health by causing irreversible damage and deviation in the normal postoperative course and resulting in prolonged hospital stay. Complications sustained following surgery may be classified based on the severity of injury as proposed by Dindo and Clavien [1] and is shown in Table 33.2. However, in this chapter complications will be classified as preoperative, intraoperative and postoperative. One of the key measures to prevent complications is to ensure that patients are selected appropriately for surgery. It is important that certain principles are followed to ascertain that both short-term and long-term outcomes are significantly better. The choice of type of surgery and indications depend on few factors, namely, tumour size, tumour function and imaging characteristics.

R. Parameswaran
Division of Endocrine Surgery, National University Hospital Singapore, Singapore, Singapore
e-mail: rajeev_parameswaran@nuhs.edu.sg

R. Parameswaran, A. Agarwal (eds.), *Evidence-Based Endocrine Surgery*,
https://doi.org/10.1007/978-981-10-1124-5_33

Table 33.1 Causes of adrenal masses

Due to hormone excess	Non-hormonal causes
Cushing's adenoma	Adenoma
Aldosteronoma	Angiomyolipoma
Pheochromocytoma	Neuroblastoma
Congenital adrenal hyperplasia	Ganglioneuroma
Macronodular adrenal disease	Carcinoma
	Cyst
	Metastasis
Uncommon causes	
Haemangioma Haemorrhage Amyloidosis Tuberculosis	

Table 33.2 Classification of Surgical Complications by Dindo and Clavien

Grade	Definition
Grade I	Any deviation from the normal postoperative course without the need for pharmacological treatment or surgical, endoscopic and radiological interventions
Grade II	Requiring pharmacological treatment with drugs other than such allowed for grade I complications
Grade III Grade IIIa Grade IIIb	Requiring surgical, endoscopic or radiological intervention Intervention not under general anaesthesia Intervention under general anaesthesia
Grade IV Grade IVa Grade IVb	Life-threatening complication (including CNS complications) * requiring IC/ICU management Single-organ dysfunction (including dialysis) Multiorgan dysfunction
Grade V	Death of a patient

Surgery for adrenal pathology is discussed in previous chapter. The choices of surgery are open and laparoscopic surgery, and in general patients with benign functioning or non-functioning adrenal tumours should be offered laparoscopic adrenalectomy either through an anterior or posterior retroperitoneal approach. However, in patients with adrenal cancers or large tumours where laparoscopic surgery is not feasible, an open approach is adopted.

Preoperative Complications

As with any major surgical procedure, patients would need assessment for cardiopulmonary issues, and this may guide as to whether the patient is likely to have a laparoscopic or open approach. Laparoscopic surgery is generally preferred for most cases due to less postoperative pain and impact on respiratory function when compared to open approach. The preoperative problems in adrenal surgery faced are usually related to the functioning adrenal nodules for which the patient is usually undergoing surgery. One of the preoperative issues faced with specific functioning adrenal tumours is *hypertension* and *electrolyte abnormalities*. The hypertension needs adequate control as inadequate control may lead to myocardial ischaemia, arrhythmias or congestive cardiac failure. The perioperative management of hypertension has been discussed in an earlier chapter. Some of the specific preoperative problems seen in functioning endocrine tumours is shown in Table 33.3. Briefly the principles of preoperative preparation for adrenalectomy include:

- Bowel preparation not necessary.
- Prophylaxis with low molecular weight is required especially in cancer.
- Adequate blockade with long-acting alpha-blockers followed by beta-adrenergic blockers to control hypertension.

Table 33.3 Preoperative complications in functioning adrenal tumours

Tumour	Complications
Pheochromocytoma	Hypertension Vasoconstriction Cardiac failure Myocardial ischaemia
Cushing's syndrome	Hypertension Hyperglycaemia Hypokalaemia Osteopenia Immunosuppression
Conn's syndrome	Hypertension Hypokalaemia

- Perioperative hydrocortisone followed by postoperative replacement with dose reduction strategy.
- Potassium replacement in patients with Conn's syndrome.

Intraoperative Complications

Intraoperative complications in adrenal surgery may be briefly divided into two: those related to the disease process and those relating to surgical access and conduct of surgery. The three common complications relating to the disease process include haemodynamic instability due to hypotension, hypertension and arrhythmias and are seen more during the resection of pheochromocytomas. It is therefore important to ensure that anaesthesia is smooth and should anticipate problems that may occur especially during tumour manipulation. Tumour manipulation results in significant catecholamine release leading to haemodynamic instability especially when performed by open approach in comparison to laparoscopic adrenalectomy [2, 3]. Some of the anaesthetic considerations for functional adrenal tumours include:

- Anxiolytics before surgery
- Intraarterial monitoring with placement before GA [4]
- Large bore peripheral and central intravenous catheters [5]
- Placement of urinary catheter [6]
- Appropriate control of intraoperative hypertension with nitroprusside and myocardial stabilization with intravenous magnesium sulphate [7]

Hypertensive episodes seen in pheochromocytomas during surgery may manifest at induction or events that cause sympathetic stimulation such as intubation or nasogastric intubation. Drugs used during peri- and intraoperative period are usually vagolytic agents such as ketamine, atropine, pancuronium and halothane [8]. Analgesics such as morphine and antiemetics can also cause release of catecholamines and thereby induce hypertension [8]. Surgical preparation in the form of positioning and placements of incisions without adequate analgesia can also induce hypertension. Most of the hypertension observed here can be managed with effective analgesia and increasing depth of anaesthesia.

The more dramatic effect of hypertension is seen in the actual surgical intervention with creation of pneumoperitoneum, direct manipulation of the gland or squeezing of the gland, and requires appropriate vasodilators for control of hypertension. Factors predictive of intraoperative hypertension during pheochromocytoma surgery include elevated preoperative plasma noradrenaline concentration, tumour size >4 cm, a higher BP before and after α-adrenergic receptor blockade (cut-off, 130/85 mmHg) and a pronounced preoperative postural BP fall (>10 mmHg) [9]. There is no difference in perioperative instability between patients with benign or malignant pheochromocytomas or those with inherited versus sporadic conditions [9]. The perioperative mortality of patients without adequate preparation may be as high as 30–45% [10].

Postoperative hypotension may occur after adrenalectomy for pheochromocytoma as a result of downregulation of α-adrenergic receptors, residual effects of long-acting α-blockers or vasodilators, contralateral adrenal suppression or hypovolemia [11]. Factors predictive of postoperative hypotension include large tumour size (more than 6 cm), significantly elevated urinary epinephrine and norepinephrine levels and use of doxazosin rather than phenoxybenzamine. The treatment of hypotension should be with large amounts of fluids after the resection of tumour [12], and this can range from 500 mL to 3 L preoperatively to about 1400 mL postoperatively [13]. The correction of hypovolemia is associated with reduced operative mortality after catecholamine resection [14]. Pressor agents may be used once the hypovolemia is corrected, and the agents used may be norepinephrine, epinephrine or vasopressin [15].

Role of Intravenous Magnesium Sulphate in the Management of Intraoperative Haemodynamics

Magnesium has important effects on the cardiovascular system through its modulatory effects on sodium and potassium currents on conducting system of the heart [16]. It also has vasodilator activity because of its action of catecholamine inhibition and function as a calcium antagonist [17, 18]. Magnesium has also an inhibitory activity on catecholamine release in response to noxious stimuli [19]. The abovementioned physiological effects make magnesium an attractive option for the treatment of pheochromocytomas and functioning paragangliomas, after the first description of its use by James in 1985 [20]. The therapeutic efficacy is also seen in children and pregnant women with pheochromocytoma or paraganglioma [21, 22]. Magnesium appears to have a stabilizing effect on patients who present with arrhythmias in pheochromocytomas [23, 24], and this is more so the case in tumours that secrete a high level of adrenaline [5].

Complications Relating to Surgical Access and Conduct of Surgery

The operative technique of adrenalectomy is discussed in another chapter. The indications and the use of a transperitoneal approach versus retroperitoneal or open are dependent on factors such as surgeon and operative experience [25], location and tumour size [26]. Generally, most surgeons are comfortable with an upper size of 6–8 cm when it comes to laparoscopic approach [27, 28]. Transperitoneal approach has the advantage of better orientation and visualization of key structures [29] and is the approach most surgeons favour. However, the popularity of retroperitoneal approach is increasing especially in small tumours and in bilateral pathology due to benefit of direct access to the adrenal gland and avoid potential injury to the visceral organs [30].

In the Swedish national cohort study of 659 patients who underwent adrenalectomy, the incidence of complications was about 5% and less than 2% requiring a reoperation [31]. The risk of conversion was about 6% in the study and this related to large tumour size and malignancy, with no observed perioperative and 30-day mortality [31]. Prolonged length of stay was seen in patients with left-sided tumours, bilateral tumours, open adrenalectomy and conversion of laparoscopic to open procedure [31]. The complications sustained during adrenalectomy irrespective of the approach are generally the same and are related to the anatomical topography and related to access in minimally invasive surgery. The most common major complications reported in the literature [32], include the following:

- Vascular injuries
- Bowel-related injuries
- Injuries to liver and spleen
- Pancreatic injury
- Diaphragm injury

Vascular Injuries

Vascular injuries represent the most common complication during laparoscopic adrenalectomy, and these are related to access problems or dissection of the vasculature [33, 34]. The reported incidence in the literature is low (0.7–5.4%) [35–37]. The vascular structures that are usually injured on the right side are the adrenal vein and inferior vena cava, which can result in severe bleeding and may be difficult to tackle [32, 38]. On the left side, the crucial step is the identification of the renal pedicle at the hilum which lends as the landmark to identify the left adrenal vein [39], and any injury may result in bleeding but not as catastrophic on the right side. The little veins encountered during adrenalectomy usually pose no major problems during surgery due to high pressure created by the pneumoperitoneum but when the pressure is released may lead to hematomas or postoperative hemodynamic instability requiring blood transfusions or reinterventions [36].

Strategies to Prevent Vascular Injuries

- Clear understating of the vascular anatomy, including variations.
- Evaluate imaging studies for the anatomy.
- Ensure correct instruments and applicators available (hemolock, energy device for dissection).
- In presence of bleeding, first apply gentle pressure with a tonsil strip or sponge gauze using a grasper.
- Increase pneumoperitoneum pressure up to 25 mmHg.
- Use of haemostatic agents such as fibrin glue or cellulose.
- If the bleeding vessel can be clearly identified, electrocautery or clips may be applied.
- Laparoscopic suturing if possible (need special expertise).
- Large vessel injury—convert to open procedure.

Visceral Injury

Visceral injury sustained during laparoscopic adrenalectomy includes—those to the bowel, on the right side—injury to the liver, gall bladder and bile ducts and on the left side injury to the pancreas and spleen. Injuries to the bowel can cause life-threatening complications and can occur during access for laparoscopic adrenal surgery; however only up to a third of them are recognized intraoperatively [40, 41]. Delayed recognition of bowel injuries can be fatal in up to 25% of patients and not acted upon [42, 43]. The risk of bowel injuries is not very well reported in the literature, but the incidence is reported to be about 1.5% following laparoscopic general surgical and urological procedures [33–35, 40]. The most common injured bit is the small bowel, and the most common cause for the injury is thermal damage by electrocautery [40].

On the right side, the liver, gall bladder and bile ducts may be injured rarely and are caused usually by excess traction and poor or difficult access [44]. The most common injury to the liver is usually laceration of the capsule during retraction especially in the presence of adhesions. It is essential that these be taken gently with an energy device such as harmonic scalpel or ligasure. Dissection of larger tumours carries a higher risk of laceration [45]. Retroperitoneal adrenalectomy may decrease the incidence of such injuries but may be an option only in smaller tumours.

Similarly, on the left side the spleen and pancreas are at risk of injury [46]. The injuries are due to excess traction, inadequate visualization or related to inappropriate movements and penetrating injury especially when the instrument is not in vision. Small lacerations on the spleen may be treated by compression with a laparoscopic gauze or application of adhesives such as oxidized cellulose, gelatin sponge and fibrin glue. Major bleeding or injuries that cannot be managed with laparoscopically need conversion to open procedure. Pancreatic injuries are less common and have been reported in about 2% of patients [33, 35]. Ductal injuries may be difficult to manage and may result in pancreatic fistulae.

Strategies to Prevent Visceral Injuries

- Proper visualization of structures
- Good technique and handling of instruments
- Avoid electrocautery to minimize thermal injuries
- Adequate exposure and reflection of colon and duodenum
- Use retroperitoneal approach if indicated

Diaphragmatic and Pleural Injury

Diaphragmatic injuries are rare in laparoscopic adrenalectomy but when they occur may lead to serious and severe complications. The reported incidence in the literature is about 0.6% [47]. The defect in the diaphragm may cause insulated air to create the pneumoperitoneum into the thorax leading to pneumothorax and pneumomediastinum. Small defects may go unnoticed and may be detected by the "floppy diaphragm sign" which refers to billowing of the diaphragm into the abdominal cavity because of the positive pressure in the pleural space [48]. The other way a diaphragmatic hole can be diagnosed is by the increase in airway pressure accompanied by increase in end-tidal carbon dioxide, hypoxia and hypotension. Defects that are small may be repaired laparoscopically, but for larger defects, an intercostal drain may need to be placed [49].

Other rare and major complications that have been reported include those of complete transection of the porta hepatis, ligation of the hepatic artery, ligation of the ureter, ligation of the renal artery and resection of the normal adrenal.

Postoperative Complications

The complications seen in patients following adrenal surgery depend on two factors: (a) the type of adrenal lesion being resected and (b) general complications following laparoscopic and open surgery. To minimize complications, it is important to institute adequate analgesia, incentive spirometry to reduce atelectasis and respiratory infections and early ambulation to reduce deep vein thrombosis. Electrolyte abnormalities are not uncommon and therefore require monitoring as well as close blood pressure monitoring. In this section, the commonly encountered postoperative complications are discussed.

The postoperative complications associated with specific adrenal tumours are shown in Table 33.4. Following resection of a Conn's adenoma, patients require close monitoring of blood pressure and potassium levels. Whilst hypokalaemia is corrected soon after surgery in most patients, some may experience salt wasting and hyperkalaemia from suppression of the contralateral gland [50]. Patients with pheochromocytomas should be monitored very closely as they are at increased risk of postoperative hypoglycaemia, hypertension and hypotension [51]. Hypoglycaemia usually results from rebound hyperinsulinemia after tumour removal [51], and hypotension from withdrawal of catecholamines which requires volume replacement [52].

Table 33.4 Specific complications associated with various adrenal tumours treated surgically

Primary aldosteronism	Hypokalaemia Hyperkalaemia
Cushing's syndrome	Hypocortisolism Osteoporotic fractures Hyperglycaemia Poor wound healing Wound infection
Pheochromocytoma	Hypotension

Following adrenalectomy for Cushing's disease especially bilateral adrenalectomy, patients require long-term steroid replacement. In the absence of steroids, they are at risk of Addisonian crisis and Nelson's syndrome [53]. Patients with Cushing's disease are also at increased risk of wound complications, infections and osteoporosis [54]. Patients undergoing bilateral adrenalectomy have a higher morbidity and mortality in comparison to those with unilateral surgery [53]. The 10-year mortality is higher in patients with an ectopic source for Cushing's (44%) versus primary adrenal disease (less than 3%) [53]. Most of the mortality occurs in the first year; hence close monitoring of cortisol-related morbidities is important [54].

The general complications following adrenal surgery include pneumonia, urinary tract infection, infections of the wound, abscess and collections in retroperitoneal area. Patients are also at risk of developing incisional hernia, especially in Cushing's patients [55]. Port site recurrences are not uncommon for resection of malignant tumours [56].

In summary, adrenal surgery is not without complications and is usually related to the underlying pathology that is being treated. The ways complications may be minimized include:

Adequate preoperative preparation
Good understanding of the disease being treated
Thorough knowledge of the anatomy of the adrenal and surrounding structures

Good surgical technique and choice of surgery
Knowledge of complications, early recognition and management

References

1. Dindo D, Demartines N, Clavien PA. Classification of surgical complications: a new proposal with evaluation in a cohort of 6336 patients and results of a survey. Ann Surg. 2004;240(2):205–13.
2. Weingarten TN, Welch TL, Moore TL, Walters GF, Whipple JL, Cavalcante A, et al. Preoperative levels of catecholamines and metanephrines and intraoperative hemodynamics of patients undergoing pheochromocytoma and paraganglioma resection. Urology. 2017;100:131–8.
3. Fernandez-Cruz L, Taura P, Saenz A, Benarroch G, Sabater L. Laparoscopic approach to pheochromocytoma: hemodynamic changes and catecholamine secretion. World J Surg. 1996;20(7):762–8. discussion 8
4. Ramakrishna H. Pheochromocytoma resection: current concepts in anesthetic management. J Anaesthesiol Clin Pharmacol. 2015;31(3):317–23.
5. Prys-Roberts C. Phaeochromocytoma--recent progress in its management. Br J Anaesth. 2000;85(1):44–57.
6. Inabnet WB, Pitre J, Bernard D, Chapuis Y. Comparison of the hemodynamic parameters of open and laparoscopic adrenalectomy for pheochromocytoma. World J Surg. 2000;24(5):574–8.
7. Phitayakorn R, McHenry CR. Perioperative considerations in patients with adrenal tumors. J Surg Oncol. 2012;106(5):604–10.
8. Memtsoudis SG, Swamidoss C, Psoma M. Anesthesia for adrenal surgery. In: Linos D, van Heerden JA, editors. Adrenal glands: diagnostic aspects and surgical therapy. Berlin, Heidelberg: Springer; 2005. p. 287–97.
9. Bruynzeel H, Feelders RA, Groenland THN, van den Meiracker AH, van Eijck CHJ, Lange JF, et al. Risk factors for hemodynamic instability during surgery for pheochromocytoma. J Clin Endocrinol Metabol. 2010;95(2):678–85.
10. Hull CJ. Phaeochromocytoma. Diagnosis, preoperative preparation and anaesthetic management. Br J Anaesth. 1986;58(12):1453–68.
11. Namekawa T, Utsumi T, Kawamura K, Kamiya N, Imamoto T, Takiguchi T, et al. Clinical predictors of prolonged postresection hypotension after laparoscopic adrenalectomy for pheochromocytoma. Surgery. 2016;159(3):763–70.
12. Bravo EL. Pheochromocytoma. Curr Ther Endocrinol Metab. 1997;6:195–7.
13. Desmonts JM, Le Houelleur J, Remond P, Duvaldestin P. Anaesthetic management of patients with phaeochromocytoma: a review of 102 cases. Br J Anaesth. 1977;49(10):991–8.
14. Desmonts JM, Marty J. Anaesthetic management of patients with phaeochromocytoma. Br J Anaesth. 1984;56(7):781–9.
15. Benumof J. Anesthesia & uncommon diseases. 4th ed. Philadelphia, PA: Saunders; 1998.
16. Bara M, Guiet-Bara A, Durlach J. Regulation of sodium and potassium pathways by magnesium in cell membranes. Magnes Res. 1993;6(2):167–77.
17. Houston M. The role of magnesium in hypertension and cardiovascular disease. J Clin Hypertens (Greenwich). 2011;13(11):843–7.
18. Iseri LT, French JH. Magnesium: nature's physiologic calcium blocker. Am Heart J. 1984;108(1):188–93.
19. James MF, Beer RE, Esser JD. Intravenous magnesium sulfate inhibits catecholamine release associated with tracheal intubation. Anesth Analg. 1989;68(6):772–6.
20. James MF. The use of magnesium sulfate in the anesthetic management of pheochromocytoma. Anesthesiology. 1985;62(2):188–90.
21. Golshevsky JR, Karel K, Teale G. Phaeochromocytoma causing acute pulmonary oedema during emergency caesarean section. Anaesth Intensive Care. 2007;35(3):423.
22. Duley L, Gülmezoglu AM, Henderson-Smart DJ, Chou D. Magnesium sulphate and other anticonvulsants for women with pre-eclampsia. Cochrane Database Syst Rev. 2010;(11):CD000025.
23. El-Sherif N, Turitto G. Electrolyte disorders and arrhythmogenesis. Cardiol J. 2011;18(3):233.
24. van der Heide K, de Haes A, Wietasch GJ, Wiesfeld AC, Hendriks HG. Torsades de pointes during laparoscopic adrenalectomy of a pheochromocytoma: a case report. J Med Case Rep. 2011;5(1):368.
25. Park HS, Roman SA, Sosa JA. Outcomes from 3144 adrenalectomies in the United States: which matters more, surgeon volume or specialty? Arch Surg. 2009;144(11):1060–7.
26. Gaujoux S, Bonnet S, Leconte M, Zohar S, Bertherat J, Bertagna X, et al. Risk factors for conversion and complications after unilateral laparoscopic adrenalectomy. Br J Surg. 2011;98(10):1392–9.
27. Zacharias M, Haese A, Jurczok A, Stolzenburg JU, Fornara P. Transperitoneal laparoscopic adrenalectomy: outline of the preoperative management, surgical approach, and outcome. Eur Urol. 2006;49(3):448–59.
28. McKinlay R, Mastrangelo MJ Jr, Park AE. Laparoscopic adrenalectomy: indications and technique. Curr Surg. 2003;60(2):145–9.
29. Brix D, Allolio B, Fenske W, Agha A, Dralle H, Jurowich C, et al. Laparoscopic versus open adrenalectomy for adrenocortical carcinoma: surgical and oncologic outcome in 152 patients. Eur Urol. 2010;58(4):609–15.
30. Guazzoni G, Cestari A, Montorsi F, Bellinzoni P, Centemero A, Naspro R, et al. Laparoscopic treatment of adrenal diseases: 10 years on. BJU Int. 2004;93(2):221–7.

31. Thompson LH, Nordenström E, Almquist M, Jacobsson H, Bergenfelz A. Risk factors for complications after adrenalectomy: results from a comprehensive national database. Langenbeck's Archiv Surg. 2017;402(2):315–22.
32. Strebel RT, Müntener M, Sulser T. Intraoperative complications of laparoscopic adrenalectomy. World J Urol. 2008;26(6):555–60.
33. Fahlenkamp D, Rassweiler J, Fornara P, Frede T, Loening SA. Complications of laparoscopic procedures in urology: experience with 2,407 procedures at 4 German centers. J Urol. 1999;162(3 Pt 1):765–70. discussion 70–1
34. Meraney AM, Samee AA, Gill IS. Vascular and bowel complications during retroperitoneal laparoscopic surgery. J Urol. 2002;168(5):1941–4.
35. Permpongkosol S, Link RE, Su LM, Romero FR, Bagga HS, Pavlovich CP, et al. Complications of 2,775 urological laparoscopic procedures: 1993 to 2005. J Urol. 2007;177(2):580–5.
36. Rosevear HM, Montgomery JS, Roberts WW, Wolf JS Jr. Characterization and management of postoperative hemorrhage following upper retroperitoneal laparoscopic surgery. J Urol. 2006;176(4 Pt 1):1458–62.
37. Walz MK, Alesina PF, Wenger FA, Deligiannis A, Szuczik E, Petersenn S, et al. Posterior retroperitoneoscopic adrenalectomy—results of 560 procedures in 520 patients. Surgery. 2006;140(6):943–8. discussion 8–50
38. Salomon L, Soulie M, Mouly P, Saint F, Cicco A, Olsson E, et al. Experience with retroperitoneal laparoscopic adrenalectomy in 115 procedures. J Urol. 2001;166(1):38–41.
39. Kalady MF, McKinlay R, Olson JA Jr, Pinheiro J, Lagoo S, Park A, et al. Laparoscopic adrenalectomy for pheochromocytoma. A comparison to aldosteronoma and incidentaloma. Surg Endosc. 2004;18(4):621–5.
40. Bishoff JT, Allaf ME, Kirkels W, Moore RG, Kavoussi LR, Schroder F. Laparoscopic bowel injury: incidence and clinical presentation. J Urol. 1999;161(3):887–90.
41. Brown JA, Canal D, Sundaram CP. Optical-access visual obturator trocar entry into desufflated abdomen during laparoscopy: assessment after 96 cases. J Endourol. 2005;19(7):853–5.
42. Chandler JG, Corson SL, Way LW. Three spectra of laparoscopic entry access injuries. J Am Coll Surg. 2001;192(4):478–90. discussion 90–1
43. O'Boyle CJ, Kapadia CR, Sedman PC, Brough WA, Royston CM. Laparoscopic transperitoneal adrenalectomy. Surg Endosc. 2003;17(12):1905–9.
44. Taneja SS, Smith RB, Ehrlich RM. Complications of urologic surgery: prevention and management. 3rd ed. Philadelphia, PA: W.B. Saunders; 2001.
45. Kim AW, Quiros RM, Maxhimer JB, El-Ganzouri AR, Prinz RA. Outcome of laparoscopic adrenalectomy for pheochromocytomas vs aldosteronomas. Arch Surg. 2004;139(5):526–9. discussion 9–31
46. Brunt LM. The positive impact of laparoscopic adrenalectomy on complications of adrenal surgery. Surg Endosc. 2002;16(2):252–7.
47. Del Pizzo JJ, Jacobs SC, Bishoff JT, Kavoussi LR, Jarrett TW. Pleural injury during laparoscopic renal surgery: early recognition and management. J Urol. 2003;169(1):41–4.
48. Voyles CR, Madden B. The "floppy diaphragm" sign with laparoscopic-associated pneumothorax. JSLS. 1998;2(1):71–3.
49. Aron M, Colombo JR Jr, Turna B, Stein RJ, Haber GP, Gill IS. Diaphragmatic repair and/or reconstruction during upper abdominal urological laparoscopy. J Urol. 2007;178(6):2444–50.
50. Al Fehaily M, Duh QY. Clinical manifestation of aldosteronoma. Surg Clin North Am. 2004;84(3):887–905.
51. Kinney MA, Narr BJ, Warner MA. Perioperative management of pheochromocytoma. J Cardiothorac Vasc Anesth. 2002;16(3):359–69.
52. Lenders JW, Eisenhofer G, Mannelli M, Pacak K. Phaeochromocytoma. Lancet. 2005;366(9486):665–75.
53. Osswald A, Plomer E, Dimopoulou C, Milian M, Blaser R, Ritzel K, et al. Favorable long-term outcomes of bilateral adrenalectomy in Cushing's disease. Eur J Endocrinol. 2014;171(2):209–15.
54. Nieman LK, Biller BMK, Findling JW, Murad MH, Newell-Price J, Savage MO, et al. Treatment of Cushing's Syndrome: an Endocrine Society Clinical Practice Guideline. J Clin Endocrinol Metabol. 2015;100(8):2807–31.
55. Gauger PG. Complications of adrenal surgery. 2012.
56. Gonzalez RJ, Shapiro S, Sarlis N, Vassilopoulou-Sellin R, Perrier ND, Evans DB, et al. Laparoscopic resection of adrenal cortical carcinoma: a cautionary note. Surgery. 2005;138(6):1078–85. discussion 85–6

34 Managing Adrenal Insufficiency and Crisis

Troy H. Puar and Kirthika Jeyaraman

Key Points

- Adrenal insufficiency can be classified as primary (adrenal failure commonly from Addison's disease or tuberculosis) or secondary (hypothalamic-pituitary disease from pituitary tumours or suppression from exogenous steroid use).
- The clinical presentation can be non-specific, leading to mortality from delayed diagnosis. Hence clinicians need to have a high index of suspicion.
- Adrenal crisis is often precipitated by an acute medical illness (e.g. gastroenteritis) or surgical stress.
- Adrenal crisis is a medical emergency, and empirical intravenous saline and glucocorticoids should be started immediately if suspected.

Introduction

Adrenal insufficiency is caused by deficient production or action of glucocorticoids and, in some cases, mineralocorticoids and androgens from the adrenal glands. Presenting symptoms can be non-specific such as fatigue, weight loss, weakness, anorexia, abdominal pain and vomiting. Although treatment (glucocorticoids) is readily available, studies show that patients with adrenal insufficiency continue to have increased mortality risk [1–4], likely from the risk of adrenal crisis [5, 6]. Adrenal crisis is an endocrine emergency caused by insufficient glucocorticoid levels and can be precipitated by acute illnesses or surgical procedures. Early recognition and prompt management of adrenal crisis with intravenous saline and glucocorticoids can avert further deterioration and mortality.

Background and Etiology

The adrenal glands are Y-shaped glands located at the upper poles of the kidneys. They consist of an outer cortex (90%) and inner medulla (10%). The adrenal medulla secretes catecholamines (adrenaline, noradrenaline and dopamine). The adrenal cortex consists of three layers, or zones, which secrete the following hormones:

- Zona glomerulosa—'mineralocorticoids' (aldosterone)
- Zona fasciculata—'glucocorticoids' (cortisol)
- Zona reticularis—androgens (mainly dehydroepiandrosterone, DHEA)

T. H. Puar (✉) · K. Jeyaraman
Department of Endocrinology, Changi General Hospital, Singapore, Singapore
e-mail: troy_puar@cgh.com.sg; kirthika_jeyaraman@cgh.com.sg

R. Parameswaran, A. Agarwal (eds.), *Evidence-Based Endocrine Surgery*,
https://doi.org/10.1007/978-981-10-1124-5_34

Adrenal insufficiency may be primary or secondary. Primary adrenal insufficiency is due to destruction of adrenal cortex. Secondary adrenal insufficiency is caused by hypothalamic-pituitary pathology or adrenal suppression from long-term exogenous steroid use. With widespread exogenous corticosteroid use, secondary adrenocortical insufficiency due to steroid withdrawal is the most common cause of adrenal insufficiency.

Primary Adrenal Insufficiency

The prevalence of primary adrenal insufficiency is around 93–140 per million [7]. Thomas Addison's monograph in 1855 focused on disease of the suprarenal capsules and contained the classic description of the endocrine disturbance known as "Addison's disease" [8]. Autoimmune adrenalitis (up to 80% of cases) is the most common cause of primary adrenal insufficiency in developed countries, while adrenal tuberculosis still remains a major factor in developing countries [7, 9]. Other causes of primary adrenal insufficiency are listed in Table 34.1.

In autoimmune primary adrenal insufficiency, humoral and cell-medicated immune mechanisms are directed at the adrenal cortex. Majority of these patients have antibodies against steroidogenic enzymes, most often 21-hydroxylase [13]. Adrenal insufficiency can be isolated or form part of an autoimmune polyglandular syndrome (APS) which is more common in females (60%) [7, 14].

- APS type 1 is an autosomal recessive disorder caused by mutations in the autoimmune regulator (AIRE) gene [15]. More than 75% of patients with APS type 1 develop hypoparathyroidism before the age of 10 years, followed by Addison's disease.
- APS type 2 is the more common type of APS and may be inherited in an autosomal recessive, autosomal dominant or polygenic manner and is characterized by multiple endocrinopathies including Addison's disease, autoimmune thyroid disease and type 1 diabetes mellitus [7, 15].

Secondary Adrenal Insufficiency

Secondary adrenal insufficiency occurs with hypothalamus or pituitary gland pathology. Lack of corticotropin-releasing hormone (CRH)/adrenocorticotropic hormone (ACTH) production from the hypothalamus/pituitary, respectively, leads to adrenal hypoplasia and atrophy, from absence of adrenal stimulation. This results in decreased glucocorticoid production. Any process that affects the hypothalamus and pituitary gland can lead to secondary adrenal insufficiency (Table 34.2). This can be an isolated hormone deficiency or associated with other pituitary hormone deficiencies.

Secondary adrenal insufficiency also occurs in patients who have been on long-term steroids after withdrawal of exogenous steroids. Both prolonged use and supraphysiological doses of glucocorticoid therapy may inhibit CRH production by the hypothalamus and cause adrenal suppression [16]. Paradoxically, these patients may have Cushingoid features (moon face, central adiposity, thin skin and easy bruising) due to long-term excessive exogenous steroid use.

Clinical Presentation

Primary vs. Secondary Adrenal Insufficiency

In primary adrenal insufficiency, ACTH levels are chronically elevated, as there is a lack of cortisol feedback to the pituitary gland. Chronically elevated ACTH then stimulates the melanocortin receptors. Hence, patients with primary adrenal insufficiency may have suggestive physical findings such as hyperpigmentation of the skin, palmar creases, scars and buccal mucosa (Fig. 34.1). This does not occur in patients with secondary adrenal insufficiency. Patients with an autoimmune cause of primary adrenal insufficiency may have other autoimmune conditions or vitiligo, which may predate the onset of adrenal insufficiency or occur after the diagnosis of Addison's.

Table 34.1 Causes of primary adrenal insufficiency

Condition	Associated features
Autoimmune adrenalitis	
• Isolated adrenal insufficiency	Hyperpigmentation, hyponatremia and hyperkalaemia
• Autoimmune polyglandular syndrome (APS)	APS (type 1): Hypoparathyroidism occurs before Addison's disease APS (type 2): Autoimmune thyroid disease, type 1 diabetes mellitus and Addison's disease
Infection	
• Tuberculosis • Fungal (cryptococcosis, histoplasmosis) • HIV (cytomegalovirus, mycobacterium) • Syphilis	Commonest cause of adrenal insufficiency in developing world Immunocompromised patients are at risk for either primary infection or disseminated infection involving the adrenal gland
Malignancy	
• Metastasis	Rare, usually bilateral with extensive damage of adrenal glands [10]. Common primary tumours include lungs, colon, breast, kidneys and pancreas
• Lymphoma	Adrenal involvement as a part of disseminated lymphoma is common, but it is a rare site for primary non-Hodgkin lymphoma
Infiltration	
• Amyloidosis • Hemochromatosis	
Adrenal haemorrhage	
• Meningococcal septicaemia	Waterhouse-Friderichsen syndrome, haemorrhagic adrenalitis caused by Neisseria meningitidis
• Anticoagulants • Trauma	Warfarin, heparin, aspirin or other non-steroidal anti-inflammatory drugs (NSAIDS)
Adrenal infarction	Risk factors include anti-phospholipid antibody syndrome, heparin induced thrombocytopenia, myelodysplastic syndrome
Iatrogenic	
• Ketoconazole, flucanozole, etomidate	Inhibit adrenal cortisol synthesis
• Rifampicin, phenytoin	Increases peripheral cortisol metabolism
• Bilateral adrenalectomy	
Others	
• Congenital adrenal hyperplasia	Autosomal recessive disorder with deficiency of enzymes involved in the synthesis of cortisol, aldosterone or both. Deficiency of 21-hydroxylase, resulting from mutations or deletions of *CYP21A*, is the most common form
• Adrenoleukodystrophy	X-linked disorder caused by mutations in ABCD gene Presents in males in childhood or early adulthood with neurological impairments. Adrenal insufficiency may precede neurological manifestations [12]
• Congenital adrenal hypoplasia	Familial failure of adrenal cortical development due to mutations/deletions of DAX1 gene
• Familial glucocorticoid deficiency/resistance	Rare familial or sporadic condition characterized by end-organ insensitivity to glucocorticoids [11]

Patients with primary adrenal insufficiency are at greater risk of salt and water depletion and, consequently, hypotension and adrenal crisis [17]. This is because they have concomitant mineralocorticoid deficiency due to destruction of the zona fasciculata. However, patients with secondary adrenal insufficiency, who have an intact renin-angiotensin-aldosterone axis, are still at risk of adrenal crisis [18–20]. The key points that differentiate them from primary adrenal insufficiency are listed in Table 34.3.

Table 34.2 Causes of secondary adrenal insufficiency

Hypothalamic/pituitary causes	
• Pituitary tumour, metastasis (rare), craniopharyngioma • Pituitary surgery, irradiation • Pituitary necrosis or bleed • Infection—tuberculosis • Infiltration—Wegner's, haemochromatosis, sarcoidosis	This can be isolated or associated with other pituitary hormone deficiencies, such as thyroid hormone, growth hormone and sex hormone deficiencies Space-occupying lesions can cause headaches, and cranial nerve palsies, such as bi-temporal hemianopia
Exogenous steroid use	Increased risk with • Systemic steroids • Potent steroids (e.g. prednisolone, methylprednisolone, dexamethasone) • Longer duration of use • Supraphysiological and higher doses

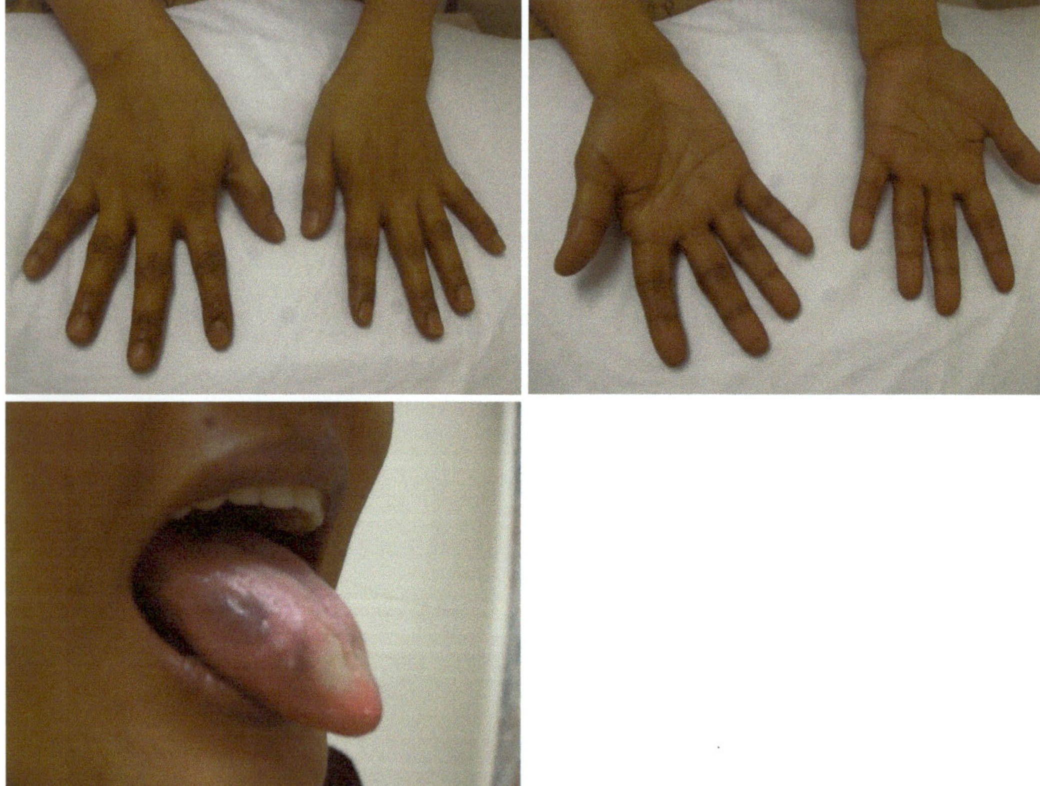

Fig. 34.1 Images of a patient with Addison's disease before treatment demonstrating hyperpigmentation noted over the skin creases of the hands (above) and tongue (below) (Courtesy of Dr. Soh Shui Boon)

Chronic Adrenal Insufficiency

Patients with either primary or secondary adrenal insufficiency may present chronically with complains of fatigue, lethargy, weakness, decrease in appetite and anorexia, which are non-specific, and this can lead to a delay in diagnosis. Other symptoms include nausea, vomiting and diarrhoea. Orthostatic hypotension may occur as cortisol is required to maintain vascular tone [21], and it potentiates catecholamine action [22].

Table 34.3 Clinical features of primary and secondary adrenal insufficiency

Primary adrenal insufficiency	Secondary adrenal insufficiency
Fatigue and loss of weight Hyperpigmentation Gastrointestinal symptoms (abdominal pain, diarrhoea, nausea and vomiting) Hypotension (postural) Salt craving Vitiligo Muscle spasms	Fatigue Gastrointestinal symptoms (abdominal pain, diarrhoea, nausea and vomiting) Symptoms of other anterior pituitary hormone deficiencies may occur Cushingoid features (moon face, thin skin and easy bruising) may be seen in patients on long-term or supraphysiological doses of exogenous steroids
Elevated ACTH Hyperkalaemia	Low/inappropriately normal ACTH Normokalemia

Acute Adrenal Insufficiency (Adrenal Crisis)

Acute adrenal insufficiency or adrenal crisis can be defined as "an acute deterioration in a patient with adrenal insufficiency", with "a principal manifestation of hypotension or hypovolemic shock" [23]. They may also have altered sensorium, such as confusion or even coma. In addition to symptoms of anorexia and fatigue as mentioned, gastrointestinal symptoms may be dominant, such as abdominal pain, nausea, vomiting and diarrhoea. Hence, patients may be misdiagnosed as an acute abdomen. Marked laboratory abnormalities may also be present. This is a medical emergency, and delay in treatment can lead to rapid deterioration and death.

Acute adrenal crisis may be the first presentation of a patient with undiagnosed adrenal insufficiency, occurring in up to 50% of patients with Addison's disease [24]. Hence, there is a need to have a high index of suspicion, particularly in patients with possible causes or associated conditions of adrenal insufficiency as shown in Tables 34.1 and 34.2.

Precipitants of an Adrenal Crisis

In addition to underlying chronic adrenal insufficiency, in more than 90% of cases, there is a precipitant for developing an adrenal crisis [19, 20, 25, 26]. Gastroenteritis is the most common precipitant of adrenal crisis, and this may be due to intestinal absorption of replacement exogenous glucocorticoids being directly affected [19, 20, 25, 26]. Other common precipitants include medical illness such as febrile illness and respiratory infections. Surgical stress can also lead to an adrenal crisis, and prophylactic glucocorticoid stress doses should be administered periprocedure (discussed later), with close monitoring thereafter. Psychological stress has also been implicated to precipitate adrenal crisis [26]. Sudden withdrawal of glucocorticoids contributed to a crisis in 10% of cases [20, 26], and this may not always be intentional, as some patients may be unaware that they are receiving glucocorticoid treatment. Omission of replacement steroids periprocedure for fasted patients can be another reason.

Risk Factors for Adrenal Crisis

Primary Adrenal Insufficiency and Comorbidities

Patients with primary adrenal insufficiency have concomitant mineralocorticoid deficiency and are at increased risk of adrenal crisis [18, 27]. Patients with other comorbidities, such as type 1 and type 2 diabetes mellitus, hypogonadism [19, 25] and diabetes insipidus [20], were also found to be associated with a higher risk of adrenal crisis.

Steroids and Other Drugs

The most common cause of adrenal insufficiency is exogenous steroid use, and these patients are also at risk of an adrenal crisis. Risk of adrenal suppression with exogenous steroids is higher with systemic steroids, more potent steroids (e.g. dexamethasone, prednisolone) and longer duration of use [16]. One study showed a correlation between adrenal suppression and the duration and cumulative doses of steroids, with 29 of 60 patients (48.3%) having adrenal insufficiency after prednisolone was withdrawn at an average dose of 7 mg [28]. Unfortunately, there is no single dose or duration at which adrenal suppression occurs, due to interindividual variability in sensitivity, and it can occur with prednisolone doses of less than 5 mg daily for 1–4 weeks [29].

Weak glucocorticoids like megestrol and medroxyprogesterone can cause adrenal suppression at therapeutic doses [16]. Topical or inhaled steroids may have adequate systemic absorption to cause adrenal suppression [16]. Co-treatment with itraconazole [30] or ritonavir [31], which impair hepatic CYP3A metabolism of steroids, will increase this risk. Other drugs may also precipitate adrenal crisis, by inhibiting adrenal steroid production (e.g. ketoconazole, fluconazole) [32] or increasing peripheral metabolism of circulating steroids, e.g. levothyroxine [33], phenytoin, rifampicin and phenobarbitone [34].

Previous Adrenal Crisis

Previous episodes of an adrenal crisis is another important risk factor [19, 26], although it is important to stress that in some patients, their first crisis is fatal [26]. Hence, adrenal crisis remains a serious problem facing these patients.

Investigations

Initial Biochemistry

Hyponatraemia is common in acute adrenal insufficiency and is contributed by unregulated antidiuretic hormone release, leading to impaired free water excretion from the kidneys [35, 36]. In addition, in primary adrenal insufficiency, mineralocorticoid deficiency leads to hyponatremia and concomitant hyperkalaemia. Other biochemistry findings include uraemia from dehydration, eosinophilia and hypoglycaemia. Hypercalcemia is uncommon, but has been described in several cases, and attributed to decreased renal calcium excretion and increased bone resorption [7, 9].

Diagnostic Tests

Patients with adrenal insufficiency have low cortisol levels, with either a high ACTH, above 22 pmol/L (in primary adrenal insufficiency) or inappropriately normal/low ACTH (in secondary adrenal insufficiency) [7, 9]. As ACTH and cortisol are secreted in a circadian manner, it is best to assess for inadequate cortisol levels in the early morning ~7–8 am, when levels are expected to be at its peak in normal physiological states. A low 8 am cortisol <138 nmol/L (<5 μg/dL) is strongly suggestive of adrenal insufficiency [37], while levels >550 nmol/L (>20 μg/dL) generally excludes the diagnosis of AI [38]. It should be noted that serum cortisol levels may be affected by differences in assays, protein or nutritional status [39], binding to cortisol-binding globulin [40] and cross reactivity to exogenous hydrocortisone and prednisolone. In patients with serum cortisol between these levels, a dynamic test to stimulate cortisol production can be done, in the form of a corticotropin stimulation test or insulin tolerance test.

In corticotropin stimulation test, baseline cortisol and ACTH levels are taken. Following which, 250 μg of corticotropin is administered intravenous or intramuscular, with cortisol levels taken 30 and 60 min after infusion. It is generally accepted that cortisol levels >550 nmol/L post-stimulation reflect an adequate adrenal response [41–43].

In patients with chronic hypothalamic-pituitary disease, there is decreased adrenal response to ACTH stimulation, leading to a blunted response [44]. Institution of corticotropin 250 μg leads to supraphysiological serum levels of synthetic corticotropin, which may be able to stimulate the intact but hypoplastic adrenals, producing a 'normal' result (false negative). An alternative is the low-dose 1 μg corticotropin stimulation test with evaluation of cortisol levels at 15 min and 30 min [37]. However, it remains controversial if it adds any value to the 250 μg test [45, 46]. More importantly, corticotropin stimulation test should not be conducted within the first 6 weeks after a pituitary insult or surgery. During this period, the adrenals may not have undergone atrophy yet and are still able to mount a normal response to exogenous corticotropin. This gives a false reassurance that the adrenals are functioning normally, when they may progressively lose function over time.

In an insulin tolerance test, intravenous insulin is administered to the patient to induce hypoglycaemia, which is a strong stimulus for CRH, ACTH and cortisol production and release. It evaluates the entire hypothalamic-pituitary-adrenal axis in contrast to corticotropin stimulation test which only evaluates the adrenal reserves. Similarly, peak cortisol levels >550 nmol/L excludes the diagnosis of adrenal insufficiency. However, this test requires close monitoring by a physician, and it is contraindicated in patients with a history of seizures or cardiovascular disease, elderly patients and those with established adrenal insufficiency (8 am cortisol <138 nmol/L) [47].

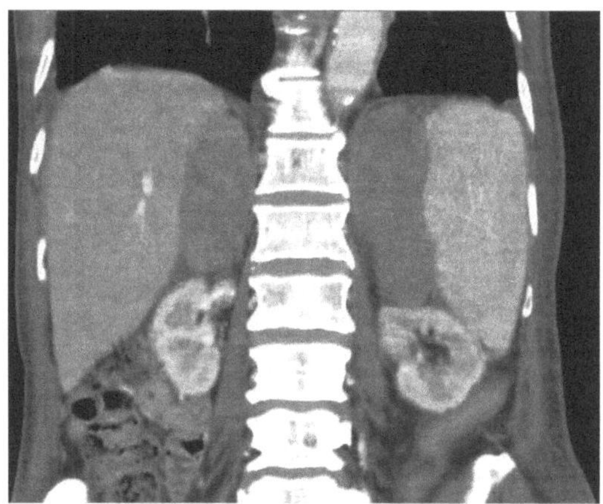

Fig. 34.2 Patient presented with symptoms of nausea and vomiting, and computed tomography of the abdomen showed bilateral adrenal infiltration. Patient had adrenal insufficiency from adrenal lymphoma (Courtesy of Dr. Tay Tunn Lin)

Further Investigations

Patients with secondary adrenal insufficiency should be assessed clinically for an underlying etiology. They may have hyperfunctioning pituitary tumours (acromegaly) or panhypopituitarism from surgery or a non-functioning pituitary adenoma. Further investigations may include assessing the other anterior pituitary hormones (prolactin, IGF-1, TSH, FSH, LH, free T4 and sex hormones) and a MRI of the pituitary gland.

Patients with primary adrenal insufficiency may also have low aldosterone and elevated renin. Adrenal autoantibodies to CYP21A2, if available, may be sent [48, 49]. A chest radiograph may reveal pulmonary tuberculosis. A computed tomography (CT) of the abdomen can be done to detect any adrenal pathology, such as tuberculosis, lymphoma or haemorrhage (Fig. 34.2). In patients with Addison's disease, one should consider screening for other autoimmune conditions, such as thyroid dysfunction and pernicious anaemia. An algorithm for the work-up of a patient with suspected adrenal insufficiency is provided in Fig. 34.3.

Treatment

Acute Adrenal Insufficiency (Adrenal Crisis)

Acute adrenal insufficiency (or Addisonian crisis) is a medical emergency. It is important to have a high index of suspicion. This includes suspecting the diagnosis in a patient with known chronic adrenal insufficiency, or with risk factors for AI (e.g. previous pituitary or adrenal surgery, chronic exogenous steroid use), who presents with symptoms and signs of acute adrenal insufficiency (nausea, vomiting, lethargy, hypotension). It is paramount that treatment is not delayed for the purpose of investigation [9, 23]. Baseline blood tests can be drawn (random cortisol, aldosterone, ACTH, renin) before empirical treatment is instituted immediately. Similar cut-offs for diagnosis as mentioned above may be used. Patients with equivocal results can be reassessed for adrenal insufficiency at a later point, after their acute illness has resolved.

The principals of treatment are fluid resuscitation and steroid replacement. Intravenous saline infusion should be given without delay (e.g. 1 L

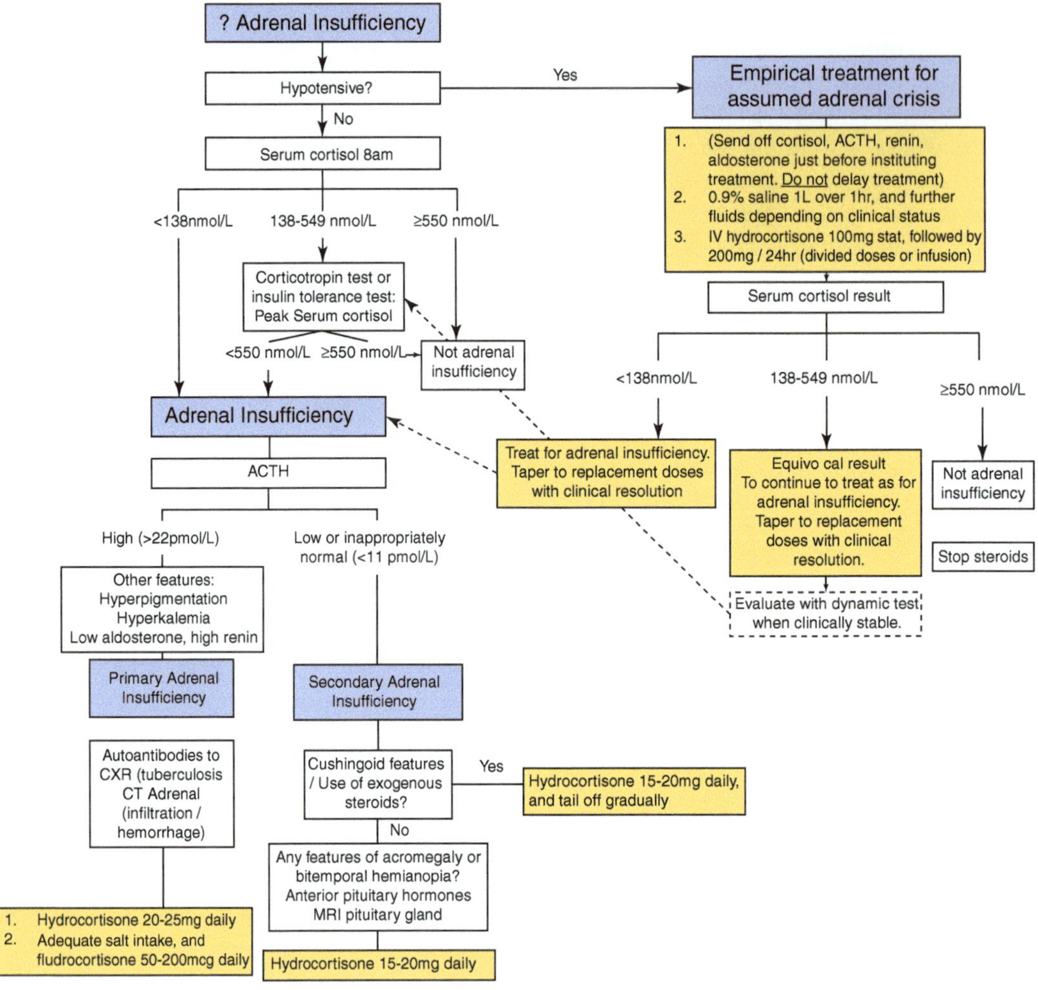

Fig. 34.3 Algorithm for the investigation and management of a patient with suspected adrenal insufficiency

saline 0.9% over 1 h) to replete the salt and water loss that has resulted from adrenal insufficiency [38, 50], with further fluids guided by clinical status. A dextrose-containing solution may be required to correct hypoglycaemia.

Parental glucocorticoids should be given, e.g. 100 mg hydrocortisone IV or IM bolus, followed by 200 mg hydrocortisone daily (in divided doses or infusion) [43, 50]. In some institutions, parental prednisolone has also been used. 50 mg or more of hydrocortisone per day contains adequate mineralocorticoid activity, and additional fludrocortisone is not required [38]. The underlying precipitant of acute AI should also be addressed, such as infection, anaemia or acute myocardial infarction. With appropriate treatment of hypocortisolism, there should be rapid improvement of hypotension within the first 1–2 h [17, 51]. Glucocorticoid replacement doses can be gradually tapered to physiological doses with clinical resolution.

Chronic Adrenal Insufficiency

Normal adrenals produce about 5–10 mg/m^2 body surface area of cortisol daily [52, 53], which works out to a daily dose of hydrocortisone 15–25 mg/day. Patients with primary adrenal insufficiency may require slightly higher doses

(20–25 mg/day) compared to those with secondary adrenal insufficiency (15–20 mg/day) [54]. Other glucocorticoids include prednisolone, prednisone and dexamethasone. They differ in their potency, duration of action and mineralocorticoid activity. 10 mg of hydrocortisone is roughly equivalent to about 2 mg prednisolone, or 0.25 mg dexamethasone [54]. Hydrocortisone has a short duration of action and is often given in two to three divided doses per day, e.g. 10 mg upon waking, 5 mg at midday and 5 mg at 4 pm, to mimic the normal circadian rhythm. Prednisolone is more potent and has longer duration of action. Prednisolone can be given as a single 3–5 mg dose in the morning, which is an alternative in patients with reduced compliance [43]. Dexamethasone is a potent glucocorticoid, with almost no mineralocorticoid activity and has a long duration of action, which can lead to suppression of the hypothalamus-pituitary axis. In patients with tertiary adrenal insufficiency from exogenous steroid use, there are no prospective trials assessing an optimal withdrawal method. However, hydrocortisone is generally preferred as it is the least potent and suppressive, and its shorter duration of action allows for axis recovery in between doses [16]. To monitor for adequate glucocorticoid replacement, patients should be assessed for resolution of symptoms (e.g. lethargy, orthostatic hypotension, hyponatraemia), as well as avoidance of overtreatment (Cushingoid effects like excessive weight gain, hypertension, hyperglycaemia).

Patients with primary adrenal insufficiency have concomitant mineralocorticoid deficiency. They should receive adequate salt intake from their diet and may also require additional mineralocorticoid replacement. Hydrocortisone 20 mg has about the same mineralocorticoid activity as 50 μg of fludrocortisone. Patients with primary adrenal insufficiency usually still require another 50–200 μg of fludrocortisone daily. Similarly, patients should be monitored for resolution of orthostatic hypertension and hyperkalaemia and avoidance of excessive replacement (e.g. peripheral oedema, hypokalaemia).

In women with primary and secondary adrenal insufficiency, DHEA levels are lower, as this is produced mainly from the adrenals. A trial of DHEA therapy (25–50 mg) given in the mornings may be considered in patients with primary adrenal insufficiency if symptoms of low libido, low energy levels or depression persist despite adequate glucocorticoid and mineralocorticoid replacement [7, 43]. The target will be a mid-normal DHEAS levels in the morning (pre-dose). However, if there is no clinical improvement after 6 months, this should be discontinued [43].

Prevention

In patients with an intact hypothalamic-pituitary-adrenal axis, there is a normal physiologic response to stress, with increased endogenous glucocorticoid production. However, patients with chronic adrenal insufficiency on replacement are reliant on exogenous steroids and need to increase their exogenous steroid intake in periods of physiological stress. Failure to do so can lead to acute adrenal crisis. Hence, it is paramount for patients to be well educated in managing their illness and crisis prevention.

Generally, with mild illness (e.g. non-febrile viral illness), patients do not require additional stress doses and should be advised as such. This is important as unnecessary additional glucocorticoids can also have adverse Cushingoid effects such as weight gain, increased risk of hypertension and diabetes mellitus.

Increased steroid requirements depend on the anticipated medical or surgical stress. In patients with minor febrile illness that can be managed at home, patients are advised to double their steroid intake during the period of fever and to revert to their usual doses after resolution of illness. In gastroenteritis, patients should exercise extra caution as persistent vomiting or diarrhoea reduces enteral absorption of glucocorticoid replacement. Patients may be required to do self-injection of intramuscular hydrocortisone and subsequently seek medical attention (Table 34.4).

Self-administration of intramuscular hydrocortisone should be taught to both patients and their family members. In an impending adrenal crisis, patients may have altered sensorium, and

Table 34.4 Sick day rules for patients with adrenal insufficiency and on long-term replacement steroids—during medical illness

Anyone who feels seriously unwell should take 'extra' hydrocortisone (as detailed below), even if they are not aware of fever or infection	
Medical illness with temperature more than 37.5 °C (99.5 °F)	• Double the normal daily steroid dose (no increase in fludrocortisone is required) • Seek medical help if the temperature reaches 40 °C (104 °F) • As soon as the temperature returns to normal, the steroid dose should be gradually tapered back to normal daily dose
In event of vomiting or diarrhoea	• Take an additional oral hydrocortisone 20 mg immediately and sip rehydration/electrolyte fluids
In event of repeated vomiting or diarrhoea	• Take intramuscular hydrocortisone 100 mg immediately and seek medical help

*Material reproduced with permission from the UK Addison's disease self-help group (ADSHG, UK), material formulated by the UK Addison's Clinical Advisory Panel (ACAP)

may not be able to do self-injections or seek help [55]. Hence, it is ideal that close family members or friends are aware of their illness and can take action when needed. Self-administration is particularly important if they live in places where emergency medical care may be hours away. There is hope that a hydrocortisone pen could be developed in the future, allowing easier delivery of subcutaneous hydrocortisone to avert an adrenal crisis [56–58]. In addition, all patients should be advised to carry a medic alert card or necklace on their bodies at all times, with information on their condition in cases of emergency [59].

The importance of education and repeatedly assessing for this at each visit cannot be overemphasized. Numerous studies have showed that patients may not be confident of self-injection despite keeping the injection kits at home [19, 60]. Patient support groups can be helpful [60]. Websites [61] and online educational videos [62] also serve as a useful aid for further information.

When travelling, patients should be advised to carry additional medication on their bodies at all times (not only in checked-in luggages) and include a doctor's prescription or letter when carrying injectables across immigration borders. A new European emergency card may be brought along on travels, which contains information of the patient's condition in English, as well as in various local languages [63]. Caution should be exercised when travelling to distant parts of the world where medical access may be difficult, and patients should avoid food sources that may increase their risk of gastroenteritis.

Managing Patients with Adrenal Insufficiency Perioperatively

When these patients undergo elective or emergency procedures, it is important that the surgeon and anaesthetist if present are aware that they are on chronic exogenous replacement steroids. Additional steroid cover is dependent on the expectant surgical stress (Table 34.5). For example, a patient going for elective colonoscopy should receive parental hydrocortisone 100 mg during the purgative preparation, another 100 mg at the start of procedure, and double their usual oral steroids doses after the procedure. They should then tail down the oral doses to their usual doses on the day after procedure. On the other hand, a patient undergoing a major surgery (e.g. coronary artery bypass) should receive parenteral hydrocortisone 100 mg just before anaesthesia, followed by 200 mg/day (in divided doses or infusion) on the first surgical day, with tapered doses subsequently depending on clinical status. Studies have shown that patients with intact adrenal glands produce increased glucocorticoids during acute surgical stress, but this reverts rapidly to normal physiological levels by the second to fourth postoperative day in uncomplicated cases [64, 65]. Hence, if patients have a normal postoperative recovery, steroid doses can be reduced by the second to fourth postoperative day. Patients who have recovered enteral function

Table 34.5 Recommendations prior to surgery and invasive procedures for patients with adrenal insufficiency and on long-term replacement steroids

Major surgery	• Any surgery will require intramuscular or intravenous steroid injection • Administer 100 mg IM or 50–100 mg IV hydrocortisone just before anaesthesia • Post procedure, continuous IV infusion 200 mg/24 h or 100 mg IM or IV every 6 h is given until able to eat and drink. Then double oral dose for 48+ h, then taper to normal dose
Minor surgery and major dental surgery	• 100 mg IV/ IM hydrocortisone just before anaesthesia • Post procedure, double oral dose for 24 h, then return to normal dose
Major dental surgery (under local anaesthesia)	• Double dose (up to 20 mg oral hydrocortisone) 1 h before surgery, or 50–100 mg IM hydrocortisone just before anaesthesia
Labour and vaginal birth	• 100 mg IM hydrocortisone at onset of labour and then 6 hourly until delivery • Double oral dose for vaginal birth for 24–48 h after delivery. If well, then return to normal dose
Invasive bowel procedures requiring laxatives (e.g. colonoscopy)	• Admission overnight with 100 mg IV/IM hydrocortisone and IV fluids during purgative preparation • 100 mg IV/IM hydrocortisone at commencement • Post procedure, double usual maintenance oral dose for 24 h, then return to normal dose
Other invasive procedures (e.g., gastroscopy)	• 100 mg IV/IM hydrocortisone at commencement • Post procedure, double oral dose for 24 h, then return to normal dose

*Material reproduced with permission from the UK Addison's disease self-help group (ADSHG, UK), material formulated by the UK Addison's Clinical Advisory Panel (ACAP)

and allowed oral diet can be given oral replacements. Concerns with prolonged excessive and unnecessary steroid replacement are that it can lead to metabolic complications such as increased glucose levels, poor wound healing. However, inadequate replacement must be avoided, as it can precipitate hypotension and adrenal crisis.

Replacement of steroids in medical stress is more controversial as often the illness may be more prolonged and the clinical course more unpredictable. Generally, in acutely ill patients who require intensive care management should also receive 200 mg /day of hydrocortisone, with subsequent tapered doses depending on the clinical condition.

Conclusion

Adrenal insufficiency remains an important diagnosis for physicians and surgeons to be aware of, as it can masquerade as various other conditions. Treatment is readily available, with good outcomes. Patients with adrenal insufficiency are always at risk of an acute adrenal crisis when they have an intercurrent illness or stressors such as surgery, which should be prevented with additional exogenous steroids. Patients should all be educated on intramuscular hydrocortisone self-injections to avert a crisis. Intravenous saline infusion and parenteral glucocorticoids are the mainstay of treatment for an adrenal crisis.

References

1. Rosén T, Bengtsson BA. Premature mortality due to cardiovascular disease in hypopituitarism. Lancet Lond Engl. 1990;336(8710):285–8.
2. Tomlinson JW, Holden N, Hills RK, Wheatley K, Clayton RN, Bates AS, et al. Association between premature mortality and hypopituitarism. West Midlands Prospective Hypopituitary Study Group. Lancet Lond Engl. 2001;357(9254):425–31.
3. Bensing S, Brandt L, Tabaroj F, Sjöberg O, Nilsson B, Ekbom A, et al. Increased death risk and altered cancer incidence pattern in patients with isolated or combined autoimmune primary adrenocortical insufficiency. Clin Endocrinol (Oxf). 2008;69(5):697–704.
4. Bergthorsdottir R, Leonsson-Zachrisson M, Odén A, Johannsson G. Premature mortality in patients with Addison's disease: a population-based study. J Clin Endocrinol Metab. 2006;91(12):4849–53.
5. Burman P, Mattsson AF, Johannsson G, Höybye C, Holmer H, Dahlqvist P, et al. Deaths among adult patients with hypopituitarism: hypocortisolism during acute stress, and de novo malignant brain tumors contribute to an increased mortality. J Clin Endocrinol Metab. 2013;98(4):1466–75.
6. Mills JL, Schonberger LB, Wysowski DK, Brown P, Durako SJ, Cox C, et al. Long-term mortality in the United States cohort of pituitary-derived growth hormone recipients. J Pediatr. 2004;144(4):430–6.

7. Arlt W, Allolio B. Adrenal insufficiency. Lancet Lond Engl. 2003;361(9372):1881–93.
8. Bishop PMF. The history of the discovery of Addison's disease. Proc R Soc Med. 1950;43(1):35–42.
9. Oelkers W. Adrenal insufficiency. N Engl J Med. 1996;335(16):1206–12.
10. Lutz A, Stojkovic M, Schmidt M, Arlt W, Allolio B, Reincke M. Adrenocortical function in patients with macrometastases of the adrenal gland. Eur J Endocrinol. 2000;143(1):91–7.
11. Charmandari E, Kino T, Chrousos GP. Familial/sporadic glucocorticoid resistance: clinical phenotype and molecular mechanisms. Ann N Y Acad Sci. 2004;1024:168–81.
12. Moser HW. Adrenoleukodystrophy: phenotype, genetics, pathogenesis and therapy. Brain J Neurol. 1997;120(Pt 8):1485–508.
13. Falorni A, Nikoshkov A, Laureti S, Grenbäck E, Hulting AL, Casucci G, et al. High diagnostic accuracy for idiopathic Addison's disease with a sensitive radiobinding assay for autoantibodies against recombinant human 21-hydroxylase. J Clin Endocrinol Metab. 1995;80(9):2752–5.
14. Betterle C, Dal Pra C, Mantero F, Zanchetta R. Autoimmune adrenal insufficiency and autoimmune polyendocrine syndromes: autoantibodies, autoantigens, and their applicability in diagnosis and disease prediction. Endocr Rev. 2002;23(3):327–64.
15. Nagamine K, Peterson P, Scott HS, Kudoh J, Minoshima S, Heino M, et al. Positional cloning of the APECED gene. Nat Genet. 1997;17(4):393–8.
16. Hopkins RL, Leinung MC. Exogenous Cushing's syndrome and glucocorticoid withdrawal. Endocrinol Metab Clin North Am. 2005;34(2):371–84. ix
17. Rushworth RL, Torpy DJ, Falhammar H. Adrenal crises: perspectives and research directions. Endocrine. 2017;55(2):336–45.
18. Smans LCCJ, Van der Valk ES, Hermus ARMM, Zelissen PMJ. Incidence of adrenal crisis in patients with adrenal insufficiency. Clin Endocrinol (Oxf). 2016;84(1):17–22.
19. White K, Arlt W. Adrenal crisis in treated Addison's disease: a predictable but under-managed event. Eur J Endocrinol. 2010;162(1):115–20.
20. Hahner S, Loeffler M, Bleicken B, Drechsler C, Milovanovic D, Fassnacht M, et al. Epidemiology of adrenal crisis in chronic adrenal insufficiency: the need for new prevention strategies. Eur J Endocrinol. 2010;162(3):597–602.
21. Allolio B, Ehses W, Steffen HM, Müller R. Reduced lymphocyte beta 2-adrenoceptor density and impaired diastolic left ventricular function in patients with glucocorticoid deficiency. Clin Endocrinol (Oxf). 1994;40(6):769–75.
22. Walker BR, Connacher AA, Webb DJ, Edwards CR. Glucocorticoids and blood pressure: a role for the cortisol/cortisone shuttle in the control of vascular tone in man. Clin Sci Lond Engl 1979. 1992;83(2):171–8.
23. Puar THK, Stikkelbroeck NMML, Smans LCCJ, Zelissen PMJ, Hermus ARMM. Adrenal crisis: still a deadly event in the 21st century. Am J Med. 2016;129(3):339.e1–9.
24. Zelissen PM. Addison patients in the Netherlands: medical report of the survey. Hague Neth Dutch Addison Soc. 1994;
25. Omori K, Nomura K, Shimizu S, Omori N, Takano K. Risk factors for adrenal crisis in patients with adrenal insufficiency. Endocr J. 2003;50(6):745–52.
26. Hahner S, Spinnler C, Fassnacht M, Burger-Stritt S, Lang K, Milovanovic D, et al. High incidence of adrenal crisis in educated patients with chronic adrenal insufficiency: a prospective study. J Clin Endocrinol Metab. 2015;100(2):407–16.
27. Meyer G, Badenhoop K, Linder R. Addison's disease with polyglandular autoimmunity carries a more than 2·5-fold risk for adrenal crises: German health insurance data 2010-2013. Clin Endocrinol (Oxf). 2016;85(3):347–53.
28. Sacre K, Dehoux M, Chauveheid MP, Chauchard M, Lidove O, Roussel R, et al. Pituitary-adrenal function after prolonged glucocorticoid therapy for systemic inflammatory disorders: an observational study. J Clin Endocrinol Metab. 2013;98(8):3199–205.
29. Schlaghecke R, Kornely E, Santen RT, Ridderskamp P. The effect of long-term glucocorticoid therapy on pituitary-adrenal responses to exogenous corticotropin-releasing hormone. N Engl J Med. 1992;326(4):226–30.
30. Bolland MJ, Bagg W, Thomas MG, Lucas JA, Ticehurst R, Black PN. Cushing's syndrome due to interaction between inhaled corticosteroids and itraconazole. Ann Pharmacother. 2004;38(1):46–9.
31. St Clair K, Maguire JD. Role of fluconazole in a case of rapid onset ritonavir and inhaled fluticasone-associated secondary adrenal insufficiency. Int J STD AIDS. 2012;23(5):371–2.
32. Shibata S, Kami M, Kanda Y, Machida U, Iwata H, Kishi Y, et al. Acute adrenal failure associated with fluconazole after administration of high-dose cyclophosphamide. Am J Hematol. 2001;66(4):303–5.
33. Graves L, Klein RM, Walling AD. Addisonian crisis precipitated by thyroxine therapy: a complication of type 2 autoimmune polyglandular syndrome. South Med J. 2003;96(8):824–7.
34. Bornstein SR. Predisposing factors for adrenal insufficiency. N Engl J Med. 2009;360(22):2328–39.
35. Oelkers W. Hyponatremia and inappropriate secretion of vasopressin (antidiuretic hormone) in patients with hypopituitarism. N Engl J Med. 1989;321(8):492–6.
36. Verbalis JG, Goldsmith SR, Greenberg A, Korzelius C, Schrier RW, Sterns RH, et al. Diagnosis, evaluation, and treatment of hyponatremia: expert panel recommendations. Am J Med. 2013;126(10 Suppl 1):S1–42.
37. Kazlauskaite R, Evans AT, Villabona CV, Abdu TAM, Ambrosi B, Atkinson AB, et al. Corticotropin tests for hypothalamic-pituitary- adrenal insufficiency: a metaanalysis. J Clin Endocrinol Metab. 2008;93(11):4245–53.

38. Bouillon R. Acute adrenal insufficiency. Endocrinol Metab Clin North Am. 2006;35(4):767–75. ix
39. Vincent RP, Etogo-Asse FE, Dew T, Bernal W, Alaghband-Zadeh J, le Roux CW. Serum total cortisol and free cortisol index give different information regarding the hypothalamus-pituitary-adrenal axis reserve in patients with liver impairment. Ann Clin Biochem. 2009;46(Pt 6):505–7.
40. Dhillo WS, Kong WM, Le Roux CW, Alaghband-Zadeh J, Jones J, Carter G, et al. Cortisol-binding globulin is important in the interpretation of dynamic tests of the hypothalamic—pituitary—adrenal axis. Eur J Endocrinol. 2002;146(2):231–5.
41. Oelkers W. The role of high- and low-dose corticotropin tests in the diagnosis of secondary adrenal insufficiency. Eur J Endocrinol. 1998;139(6):567–70.
42. May ME, Carey RM. Rapid adrenocorticotropic hormone test in practice. Retrospective review. Am J Med. 1985;79(6):679–84.
43. Bornstein SR, Allolio B, Arlt W, Barthel A, Don-Wauchope A, Hammer GD, et al. Diagnosis and treatment of primary adrenal insufficiency: an endocrine society clinical practice guideline. J Clin Endocrinol Metab. 2016;101(2):364–89.
44. Wood JB, Frankland AW, James VH, Landon J. A rapid test of adrenocortical function. Lancet Lond Engl. 1965;1(7379):243–5.
45. Mayenknecht J, Diederich S, Bähr V, Plöckinger U, Oelkers W. Comparison of low and high dose corticotropin stimulation tests in patients with pituitary disease. J Clin Endocrinol Metab. 1998;83(5):1558–62.
46. Dekkers OM, Timmermans JM, Smit JWA, Romijn JA, Pereira AM. Comparison of the cortisol responses to testing with two doses of ACTH in patients with suspected adrenal insufficiency. Eur J Endocrinol. 2011;164(1):83–7.
47. Grinspoon SK, Biller BM. Clinical review 62: laboratory assessment of adrenal insufficiency. J Clin Endocrinol Metab. 1994;79(4):923–31.
48. Conrad K, Roggenbuck D, Reinhold D, Sack U. Autoantibody diagnostics in clinical practice. Autoimmun Rev. 2012;11(3):207–11.
49. Winqvist O, Karlsson FA, Kämpe O. 21-hydroxylase, a major autoantigen in idiopathic Addison's disease. Lancet Lond Engl. 1992;339(8809):1559–62.
50. Husebye ES, Allolio B, Arlt W, Badenhoop K, Bensing S, Betterle C, et al. Consensus statement on the diagnosis, treatment and follow-up of patients with primary adrenal insufficiency. J Intern Med. 2014;275(2):104–15.
51. Andrews RC, Herlihy O, Livingstone DEW, Andrew R, Walker BR. Abnormal cortisol metabolism and tissue sensitivity to cortisol in patients with glucose intolerance. J Clin Endocrinol Metab. 2002;87(12):5587–93.
52. Esteban NV, Loughlin T, Yergey AL, Zawadzki JK, Booth JD, Winterer JC, et al. Daily cortisol production rate in man determined by stable isotope dilution/mass spectrometry. J Clin Endocrinol Metab. 1991;72(1):39–45.
53. Kerrigan JR, Veldhuis JD, Leyo SA, Iranmanesh A, Rogol AD. Estimation of daily cortisol production and clearance rates in normal pubertal males by deconvolution analysis. J Clin Endocrinol Metab. 1993;76(6):1505–10.
54. Reisch N, Arlt W. Fine tuning for quality of life: 21st century approach to treatment of Addison's disease. Endocrinol Metab Clin North Am. 2009;38(2):407–18, ix–x
55. Peacey SR, Pope RM, Naik KS, Hardern RD, Page MD, Belchetz PE. Corticosteroid therapy and intercurrent illness: the need for continuing patient education. Postgrad Med J. 1993;69(810):282–4.
56. Allolio B. Extensive expertise in endocrinology. Adrenal crisis. Eur J Endocrinol. 2015;172(3):R115–24.
57. Hahner S, Burger-Stritt S, Allolio B. Subcutaneous hydrocortisone administration for emergency use in adrenal insufficiency. Eur J Endocrinol. 2013;169(2):147–54.
58. Rushworth RL, Bischoff C, Torpy DJ. Preventing adrenal crises: home-administered subcutaneous hydrocortisone is an option. Intern Med J. 2017;47(2):231–2.
59. Wass JAH, Arlt W. How to avoid precipitating an acute adrenal crisis. BMJ. 2012;345:e6333.
60. Repping-Wuts HJWJ, Stikkelbroeck NMML, Noordzij A, Kerstens M, Hermus ARMM. A glucocorticoid education group meeting: an effective strategy for improving self-management to prevent adrenal crisis. Eur J Endocrinol. 2013;169(1):17–22.
61. National Adrenal Diseases Foundation. Website homepage. [Internet]. NADF. [cited 2017 Feb 24]. http://www.nadf.us/.
62. Dutch Adrenal Society. Animation Movies [Internet]. [cited 2017 Feb 24]. http://adrenals.eu/video/.
63. Grossman A, Johannsson G, Quinkler M, Zelissen P. Therapy of endocrine disease: perspectives on the management of adrenal insufficiency: clinical insights from across Europe. Eur J Endocrinol. 2013;169(6):R165–75.
64. Salem M, Tainsh RE, Bromberg J, Loriaux DL, Chernow B. Perioperative glucocorticoid coverage. A reassessment 42 years after emergence of a problem. Ann Surg. 1994;219(4):416–25.
65. Udelsman R, Norton JA, Jelenich SE, Goldstein DS, Linehan WM, Loriaux DL, et al. Responses of the hypothalamic-pituitary-adrenal and renin-angiotensin axes and the sympathetic system during controlled surgical and anesthetic stress. J Clin Endocrinol Metab. 1987;64(5):986–94.

Part IV

Neuroendocrine

Gastric and Duodenal Neuroendocrine Tumours

35

Asim Shabbir, Jimmy So, and Hrishikesh Salgaonkar

Gastric neuroendocrine tumours (GNETs) arise in enterochromaffin cells. They are rare neoplasms and account for 1% of all gastric neoplasms; however, the incidence has been increasing over the last decade. The increase in diagnosis is due to high incidence of chronic atrophic gastritis and intensive screening on endoscopy. Four types of GNETs have been identified: type 1 is well differentiated and is usually benign; type 2 is associated with multiple endocrine neoplasia (MEN1); type 3 is sporadic, well-differentiated neuroendocrine low-grade carcinoma with a high incidence of metastasis; and type 4 is poorly differentiated, high-grade carcinoma with the worst prognosis. The treatment of GNETs is dependent on the size of the lesion and type, with well-defined treatment strategies for types 2, 3 and 4. The treatment of type 1 GNET is controversial. In advanced inoperable disease treatment, choices are based on tumour factors and presence of symptoms.

Introduction

Neuroendocrine tumours were initially called as carcinoid tumours arising from enterochromaffin or Kulchitsky cells. The term carcinoid was first used by Oberdorfer in 1907 to describe a carcinoma-like tumour with less malignant potential with a broad spectrum of clinical behaviours [1, 2]. The neuroendocrine cells have a unique capacity to synthesize and secrete hormones and neuropeptides which play an important role in gastrointestinal physiology [3] and can be identified by specific markers such as chromogranin A and synaptophysin [4]. GNETs are heterogeneous tumours with unique clinical syndromes and symptoms but may be asymptomatic and discovered incidentally.

Epidemiology

The prevalence of GNETs has been estimated at 35 per 100,000 population [5] and incidence between 1.2 and 1.8 per 1,000,000 persons per year [6]. The incidence of gastric NETs has been shown to increase from 2% to 6% during the time period 1950 to 2007, based on figures from SEER data in the United States and Norway [7–9]. The increasing incidence could be explained by increased access to endoscopy through surveillance, increasing biopsies of polyps, enhanced imaging, improved immunohistochemistry and better understanding of the disease [3, 10–12]. The frequency of GNETs amongst all gastrointestinal NETs (GINETs) is about 5–15% [7, 9, 10, 13], and it is the most common of all GINETs, with majority of them being benign [13].

A. Shabbir (✉) · J. So · H. Salgaonkar
Division of Upper Gastrointestinal Surgery, National University Hospital Singapore, Singapore, Singapore
e-mail: asim_shabbir@nuhs.edu.sg

R. Parameswaran, A. Agarwal (eds.), *Evidence-Based Endocrine Surgery*,
https://doi.org/10.1007/978-981-10-1124-5_35

The increasing use of proton pump inhibitors has possibly also contributed to increase in GNETs, but the causality has not been proven [14, 15]. The mean age at which the disease presents is around 60–64 years [13, 16–18], with higher age in Asian population [19], and most frequent type is GNET type 1, with a predilection for women [20]. Variations in relation to race have also been described [5, 9].

Pathogenesis of GNETs

The gastric mucosa is divided into the proximal oxyntic gland area (the proximal 80% of the stomach that includes the body and fundus) and the distal antral or pyloric gland area which synthesizes, stores and secretes gastrin. Gastrin acts on enterochromaffin-like cells to regulate gastric acid production. The enterochromaffin (ECL) cells are seen in the fundus and are the principal endocrine cell type of the stomach, where they account for 35% of the total oxyntic endocrine cells in humans [21]. The proliferation and activation of the ECL cell are primarily regulated by the levels of gastrin concentration and initiation of signal transduction via the cholecystokinin 2 receptor in the gastric body and fundus [22]. Factors which can increase the serum gastrin level such as gastrin infusion, partial fundectomy, antral isolation from acid, inhibition of acid secretion by H2 receptor antagonists, or proton pump inhibitors have been shown to be associated with ECL cell hypertrophy [23] and hyperplasia [24–28]. The type 1 and 2 GNETs develop through the sequence of hyperplasia-dysplasia-neoplasia similar to the adenoma carcinoma sequence [29]. Type 3 and 4 GNETs do not have hypergastrinemia as the underlying cause and occur as sporadic tumours.

Types of Gastric NET

There are essentially four types of GNETs: type 1 which is well differentiated and is benign; type 2, associated with multiple endocrine neoplasia (MEN1); type 3, sporadic, well-differentiated neuroendocrine low-grade carcinoma with a high incidence of metastasis; and type 4, poorly differentiated, high-grade carcinoma associated with the worst prognosis [30]. The clinicopathological characteristics of four types of GNETs are shown in Table 35.1.

Type 1 GNET

Type 1 is the most frequent type of GNET and accounts for 75% of all GNETs [31]. They are generally benign and associated with chronic atrophic gastritis which may be immune or non-immune related. The tumours are often multiple, of a small size with median diameter of 5 mm and located at the gastric body or fundus [32]. The tumours may be broad based or polypoidal or

Table 35.1 Clinicopathological characteristics of GNETs

	Type 1	Type 2	Type 3	Type 4
Frequency	70–80%	5%	15–20%	Rare
Focality	Multifocal	Multifocal	Solitary	Solitary
Size	0.5–1 cm	Less than 1.5 cm	Variable	Large
Associated conditions	Chronic atrophic gastritis	MEN1 ZES	None	None
Histology	Well differentiated	Well differentiated	Well differentiated	Poorly differentiated
pH	Achlorhydria	Hyper acidic	Normal	Normal
Gastrin	Very high	Very high	Normal	Normal
Clinical behaviour	Benign	1/3rd risk of metastasis	2/3rd with invasion and lymph node metastasis	Metastasis common
Metastases	Less than 10%	10–30%	50–100%	80–100%
Mortality	Uncommon	Less than 10%	25–30%	More than 50%

flat. The broad based may present with ulceration or bleeding. The polypoid lesions may mimic hyperplastic polyps. The smaller GNETs are benign with very low risk of invasion beyond the submucosa. Larger lesions are also predominantly benign with risk of invasion into the muscularis propria in less than 10% of cases [33]. Chronic atrophic gastritis-associated GNETs are associated with lymph node metastasis in 5% and distant metastasis in around 2% [31, 33].

Type 2 GNET

Type 2 GNETs occur in patients with MEN1 and gastrin-producing tumours and constitute about 6–8% of all GNETs [34]. ECL cell hyperplasia is seen in about 80% of patients with MEN1 associated with ZES and usually seen in the fundus [33, 35]. The type 2 tumours develop in hyperplasia-dysplasia-neoplasia sequence and are usually associated with diffuse hyperplasia. The development of type 2 GNETs is not seen in patients with sporadic Zollinger-Ellison syndrome (ZES) and almost invariably seen in ZES associated with MEN1 [36]. They are usually multiple and smaller than 1.5 cm but larger than type 1 tumours. The risk of malignancy in type 2 tumours is intermediate between type 1 and sporadic NETs, with only 10% of cases infiltrating beyond the submucosa. Lymph node metastasis is seen in up to a third of patients and distant metastasis in about 10–20% of patients [33].

Type 3 GNETs

Type 3 GNETs are distinct to type 1 and 2 tumours in that they are sporadic and solitary and account for 15–20% of all GNETs. They have no association with hypergastrinemia and occur without the presence of endocrine cell proliferation [37]. Clinically the tumours may present with bleeding, obstruction or metastasis. These tumours are much more aggressive and a good proportion of patients present with disseminated disease [37]. The sporadic variants are generally large with more than 70% having a mean size of about 3 cm [33]. Majority of the tumours are in the body and fundus of the stomach and are likely to show invasion beyond the muscularis propria and involve all the layers of the gastric wall. Lymph node metastasis is seen in about two third of patients at the time of diagnosis.

Type 4 GNETs

The type 4 GNETs are also known as poorly differentiated neuroendocrine carcinomas. They are extremely malignant and present with extensive local invasion and metastases at time of diagnosis [38]. These tumours are not associated with hypergastrinemia or carcinoid syndrome. The location of the tumours may be in the gastric corpus or fundus, but about a fifth of them may be seen in the antrum and are quite large, which are often ulcerated or fungating [39]. The tumours on histological examination show necrosis, significant atypia, mitosis and high proliferation index measured by Ki-67 staining. Prognosis of patients with type 4 GNETs is generally very poor.

Investigations

The mainstay of investigations in GNETs is oesophagogastroduodenoscopy (OGD). It is important to record the number and size of the lesions, with biopsies of the lesions and normal areas of the gastric mucosa from the greater and lesser curves for comparison of ECL density [37, 40]. Type 1 lesions with a size less than 1 cm do not usually require any further assessment. Assessment of *H. pylori* is important as its infection is associated with atrophic gastritis in type 1 and type 3 lesions [41]. A pH assessment using indicator strips at endoscopy or 24-h gastric pH study helps clarifying when there is uncertainty of GNETs.

Following a diagnosis of GNETs, endoscopic ultrasound (EUS) is performed to evaluate the depth of invasion of the lesions, especially in type 1 and 2 lesions more than 1 cm and all type 3 and 4 lesions [42, 43]. The added value of EUS is its ability to reveal lesions in the pancreas or duodenum in MEN1 patients and detect metastasis in the liver and regional lymph nodes [43]. Computed tomography (CT) and MRI scans are needed to delineate tumour anatomy and detect regional and distant metastasis. Scintigraphy with somatostatin analogues may reveal metastatic spread for NETs [42, 44].

Biochemical evaluation includes measuring plasma chromogranin A (CgA), plasma histamine, plasma serotonin and plasma gastrin. Elevated gastrin levels are seen in type 1 and 2 GNETs and normal in types 3 and 4. CgA is secreted by ECL cells and is elevated in chronic atrophic gastritis and ECL cell hyperplasia but may also be elevated in patients on PPI therapy, renal failure and cardiac disease. CgA is the most important tumour marker to assess response to therapy and to monitor for any recurrence [45–47].

Histological assessment of GNETs can be challenging. Type 1 and 2 tumours stain positively for argyrophil, argentaffin and CgA [37], whereas type 3 usually stains for argyrophil, CgA, neuron-specific enolase, synaptophysin and S-100 but not for argentaffin. The histological classification is based on grade and differentiation based on mitotic count and Ki-67 index. The World Health Organization 2010 classification system for neuroendocrine neoplasms is shown in Table 35.2 [48].

Treatment

Treatment of GNETs depends on the type of GNET, tumour size, location, presence of locoregional spread and metastasis.

Table 35.2 World Health Organization 2010 classification system for neuroendocrine neoplasms

WHO grading of neuroendocrine neoplasms	
Grade 1	Mitotic rate less than 2 Ki-67 index less than 3%
Grade 2	Mitotic rate of 2–20 Ki-67 index of 3%–20%
Grade 3	Mitotic rate greater than 20 Ki-67 index greater than 20%

Type 1 GNETs

The treatment of type 1 GNETs is controversial as many of these polyps behave in an indolent manner with minimal risk of invasion and metastasis [38]. Hooper et al. suggested that lesions less than 1 cm in size only require annual endoscopic surveillance, and those more than 1 cm without any features of invasion on EUS are treated with endoscopic mucosal resection or band mucosectomy [49]. A prospective study on endoscopic management of type 1 lesions reported a recurrence rate of about 63%, but repeat endoscopy and biopsy every 6–12 months demonstrated a 100% survival without any evidence of locoregional or distant spread [50]. In 2015, the National Comprehensive Cancer Network (NCCN) in its guidelines recommended that all tumours smaller than 20 mm in size without any features of invasion of the muscularis propria or metastasis should be subjected to simple surveillance or endoscopic resection (ER), regardless of the tumour number [51], while for tumours greater than 20 mm, ER or surgical resection is recommended, for single as well as multiple tumours. The European Neuroendocrine Tumor Society (ENETS) in its guidelines recommended ER as the treatment of choice for type 1 GNETs. Surgical resection is only advocated for poorly differentiated lesions, invasive tumour infiltrating beyond the submucosa, involvement of lymph nodes or distant metastasis [52].

Controversy also exists over the preferred ER technique. For a well-localized type 1 GNET, endoscopic mucosal resection (EMR) is recommended. But with better understanding of the disease pathology, it was found that type 1 GNETs commonly invade the submucosa, and hence in such cases it may be difficult to achieve complete resection by EMR or snare polypectomy. In cases where submucosal involvement is suspected, it may be better to use endoscopic submucosal dissection (ESD) techniques. In fact, multiple studies have shown that ESD is superior to EMR for achieving complete resection rates of GNETs [53, 54]. Similarly, some studies have reported no tumour-related deaths in patients with type 1 GNETs who were subjected to endoscopic surveillance alone without any treatment [55–57]. Hence, it may be reasonable to suggest endoscopic surveillance in selected patients of type 1 GNETs. Small localized tumour in elderly patients, those unfit or not willing for any active intervention and multiple comorbidities are suitable candidates for endoscopic surveillance alone taking into consideration the possibility of increased risk of local invasion or metastasis during the follow-up.

Some studies recommend surgical resection for patients with multifocal lesions, if any one of them is larger than 1 cm or in the presence of a single lesion more than 2 cm. Type 1 GNETs in association with chronic atrophic gastritis or recurrent type 1 GNETs may require an antrectomy to eliminate the source of gastrin production and thus result in tumour regression [58–60]. Antrectomy may not completely prevent recurrence or metastasis [61]. Though surgical intervention has its own complications and associated morbidity, patients with type 1 GNETs who undergo antrectomy have lower recurrence risk and require fewer follow-up endoscopies as compared to patients who undergo ER or endoscopic surveillance alone. Antrectomy removes the G-cells and hence is thought to alleviate hypergastrinemia. Improper removal of G-cells or ECL hypertrophy may result in failure to achieve desired results. This is the basis for considering subtotal gastrectomy which allows for complete removal of all the G-cells. Laparoscopy today allows us to achieve the same results as open technique with all the benefits of minimal invasive surgery. Total gastrectomy is needed in patients with substantial disease in proximal stomach. Total gastrectomy with lymph node dissection is indicated for patients with serosal involvement, extra gastric spread or recurrence [62]. Exact extent of lymph nodal dissection depends upon the patient presentation and surgeon expertise as no clear consensus is found on literature review.

Medical management should be considered in patients who are not candidates for surgical treatment (such as patient age, comorbidities, prior surgeries and compliance with medical therapy). Medical management consists of intramuscular injections of long-acting somatostatin analogues every month [63]. Thought to reduce G-cell-mediated gastrin secretion and ECL hypertrophy, discontinuation of therapy usually results in rise in gastrin levels [64]. Netazepide (YF476), an orally active and highly selective drug which is a potent human gastrin/CCK-2 receptor antagonist, has been shown to reduce gastrin secretion and serum chromogranin A levels. It also reduces the number and size of type 1 GNETs [65]. However, similar to somatostatin analogues, the CgA levels increase once therapy is discontinued [66]. Though initial results are promising, further controlled studies are needed before advocating use of netazepide.

Type 2 GNETs

All type 2 GNETs need excision due to higher risk of lymph node involvement and metastasis. Local excision is required for localized lesions with endoscopic resection [67]. Surgery is an option for those with invasive disease or metastasis [40]. Antrectomy has limited role in the management of type 2 lesions more than 1 cm, and endoscopic mucosal resection may be considered in selective cases [42, 43]. A duodenotomy for exposure of both the pancreas and duodenum may be required to remove gastrinomas and MEN1-related pancreatic lesions in some cases [68–70]. A formal gastrectomy with lymphadenectomy may be required for larger lesions [37, 42].

Type 3 GNETs

Type 3 GNETs are treated with gastrectomy (either partial or total) with lymphadenectomy as the lesions are malignant, with high risk of metastases [71, 72]. Typically, tumours more than 2 cm, atypical histology, invasion of the gastric wall and local metastasis are best dealt with by gastrectomy [71, 73]. In patients with liver metastasis, which is seen in 25–50% of patients, liver resection may be necessary to obtain a R_0 resection [31, 52, 74]. Where resection of the liver metastasis is not possible, hepatic artery embolization or chemoembolization and radiofrequency (RF) ablation may be employed [44]. Systemic chemotherapy is offered to patients with high proliferative index and may be combined with other modalities with a response rate of 20–40% [44]. In patients who present with carcinoid syndrome associated with type 3 GNET, somatostatin analogues may offer symptomatic relief, with reduction in biochemical markers and decrease in tumour size [67, 75].

Type 4 GNETs

Type 4 the poorly differentiated neuroendocrine cancers have an extremely poor prognosis, with a survival of only a few months [76]. Surgical intervention is rarely possible, and most patients are treated with chemotherapy (combination of streptozotocin plus 5-FU alternated with adriamycin) or with a combination of cisplatin plus etoposide [77, 78]. The treatment of metastatic GNET is discussed below.

Treatment of Liver Metastasis in GNETs

Metastatic GNETs usually metastasize to the liver and can present with or without symptoms. They are managed using surgery and locoregional and systemic therapies [79, 80]. Surgical resection is the gold standard with reasonably high survival at 60–80% at 5 years and morbidity around 30% [81–83]. Curative surgery is recommended for patients with operable well-differentiated metastases from GNETs, and the requirements are shown in Table 35.3. Metastasectomy is generally not recommended for poorly differentiated carcinomas.

It is important to assess the amount and quality of remnant liver prior to the resection of liver metastases. The amount of resection also depends upon whether the liver disease is unilobar or complex. The role of palliative debulking surgery mandates at least 90% of tumour volume to be resected [80]. The role of adjuvant therapy postsurgical resection is debatable. For selected patients with liver metastasis from GNETs in whom standard medical and surgical therapies have failed, liver transplantation is effective [84–86]. The criteria for liver transplantation in metastatic disease include the following [80]:

Table 35.3 Requirements for curative surgery in metastatic GNETs [80]

Requirements
Resectable G1–G2 liver disease with acceptable morbidity and less than 5% mortality
Absence of right heart insufficiency
Absence of unresectable lymph nodes and extra-abdominal metastases
Absence of diffuse or unresectable carcinomatosis peritonei

Mortality should be less than 10%.
Absence of extrahepatic disease as determined by PET/CT.
Primary tumour removed prior to transplantation.
Well-differentiated NET (NET G1, G2).

Other interventions that can be used as antitumour treatments and to relieve symptoms in patients with metastatic liver disease include radiofrequency ablation [87, 88], laser-induced thermotherapy [89] and selective transarterial embolization (TAE) or transarterial chemoembolization (TACE) [90, 91]. Similarly, medical therapies with antisecretory agents such as somatostatin analogues (octreotide, lanreotide) [92, 93], alpha interferon [94–96] and PRRT with ^{177}Lu-DOTATATE [96, 97] are used for treatment of tumours associated with hormonal hypersecretion.

Carcinoid Syndrome

Though commonly seen with midgut neuroendocrine tumour, carcinoid syndrome may rarely occur in patients with GNETs with liver metastasis. Patients present clinically with episodes of skin flushing mainly on the face, diarrhoea and abdominal cramps. Occasionally, hypotension and bronchospasm may be seen. These manifestations are a result of secretion of histamine, 5-hydroxytryptamine, bradykinins, tachykinins and prostaglandins by the cells [34]. Treatment consists of symptom control and prevention of complications and is achieved by using agents such as somatostatin analogues (octreotide or lanreotide). In refractory cases, interferon alfa can be used in low doses [98].

Prognosis and Follow Up

The prognosis of GNETs depends on size of the tumours, tumour histology, presence of metastatic disease and carcinoid syndrome. Predictors of disease recurrence include size of tumour greater than 2 cm, involvement of regional lymph nodes and high proliferative index evaluated by Ki-67. Patients should undergo follow-up with serum chromogranin A and gastrin every 6 months, imaging with CT or PET [99] every 2 years for type 1 tumours and annually for type 2 tumours [42]. Type 1 GNETs smaller than 1 cm removed by endoscopy or surgery annual endoscopic surveillance is sufficient. In patients with type 3 tumours, imaging and CgA are performed every 6-month intervals for 2 years and annually for a further 3 years [42]. In the presence of well-differentiated metastatic disease, imaging is performed every 3 months [42]. In patients with advanced, unresectable primary or metastatic disease, follow-up is every 3 months unless patients are stable in which case six monthly follow-ups may be sufficient. The 5-year survival of patients with GNETs has increased over the last few decades from nearly 50% to over 60% [100]. The 5-year survival is nearly 100% in type 1 tumours, 60–75% in type 2 and 3 tumours and 20–30% in metastatic disease.

References

1. Modlin IM, Moss SF, Oberg K, Padbury R, Hicks RJ, Gustafsson BI, et al. Gastrointestinal neuroendocrine (carcinoid) tumours: current diagnosis and management. Med J Aust. 2010;193(1):46–52.
2. Modlin IM, Shapiro MD, Kidd M. Siegfried Oberndorfer: origins and perspectives of carcinoid tumors. Hum Pathol. 2004;35(12):1440–51.
3. Modlin IM, Oberg K, Chung DC, Jensen RT, de Herder WW, Thakker RV, et al. Gastroenteropancreatic neuroendocrine tumours. Lancet Oncol. 2008;9(1):61–72.
4. Kloppel G, Couvelard A, Perren A, Komminoth P, McNicol AM, Nilsson O, et al. ENETS Consensus Guidelines for the Standards of Care in Neuroendocrine Tumors: towards a standardized approach to the diagnosis of gastroenteropancreatic neuroendocrine tumors and their prognostic stratification. Neuroendocrinology. 2009;90(2):162–6.
5. Yao JC, Hassan M, Phan A, Dagohoy C, Leary C, Mares JE, et al. One hundred years after "carcinoid": epidemiology of and prognostic factors for neuroendocrine tumors in 35,825 cases in the United States. J Clin Oncol. 2008;26(18):3063–72.
6. Akerstrom G, Hellman P. Surgery on neuroendocrine tumours. Best Pract Res Clin Endocrinol Metab. 2007;21(1):87–109.
7. Lawrence B, Gustafsson BI, Chan A, Svejda B, Kidd M, Modlin IM. The epidemiology of gastroenteropancreatic neuroendocrine tumors. Endocrinol Metab Clin N Am. 2011;40(1):1–18. vii
8. Lawrence B, Kidd M, Svejda B, Modlin I. A clinical perspective on gastric neuroendocrine neoplasia. Curr Gastroenterol Rep. 2011;13(1):101–9.
9. Hauso O, Gustafsson BI, Kidd M, Waldum HL, Drozdov I, Chan AK, et al. Neuroendocrine tumor epidemiology: contrasting Norway and North America. Cancer. 2008;113(10):2655–64.
10. Ellis L, Shale MJ, Coleman MP. Carcinoid tumors of the gastrointestinal tract: trends in incidence in England since 1971. Am J Gastroenterol. 2010;105(12):2563–9.
11. Hassan MM, Phan A, Li D, Dagohoy CG, Leary C, Yao JC. Risk factors associated with neuroendocrine tumors: a U.S.-based case-control study. Int J Cancer. 2008;123(4):867–73.
12. Lombard-Bohas C, Mitry E, O'Toole D, Louvet C, Pillon D, Cadiot G, et al. Thirteen-month registration of patients with gastroenteropancreatic endocrine tumours in France. Neuroendocrinology. 2009;89(2):217–22.
13. Niederle MB, Hackl M, Kaserer K, Niederle B. Gastroenteropancreatic neuroendocrine tumours: the current incidence and staging based on the WHO and European Neuroendocrine Tumour Society classification: an analysis based on prospectively collected parameters. Endocr Relat Cancer. 2010;17(4):909–18.
14. Jensen RT. Consequences of long-term proton pump blockade: insights from studies of patients with gastrinomas. Basic Clin Pharmacol Toxicol. 2006;98(1):4–19.
15. Abraham NS. Proton pump inhibitors: potential adverse effects. Curr Opin Gastroenterol. 2012;28(6):615–20.
16. Faggiano A, Ferolla P, Grimaldi F, Campana D, Manzoni M, Davi MV, et al. Natural history of

gastro-entero-pancreatic and thoracic neuroendocrine tumors. Data from a large prospective and retrospective Italian epidemiological study: the NET management study. J Endocrinol Investig. 2012;35(9):817–23.
17. Hemminki K, Li X. Incidence trends and risk factors of carcinoid tumors: a nationwide epidemiologic study from Sweden. Cancer. 2001;92(8):2204–10.
18. Maggard MA, O'Connell JB, Ko CY. Updated population-based review of carcinoid tumors. Ann Surg. 2004;240(1):117–22.
19. Li AF, Hsu CY, Li A, Tai LC, Liang WY, Li WY, et al. A 35-year retrospective study of carcinoid tumors in Taiwan: differences in distribution with a high probability of associated second primary malignancies. Cancer. 2008;112(2):274–83.
20. Modlin IM, Lye KD, Kidd M. A 50-year analysis of 562 gastric carcinoids: small tumor or larger problem? Am J Gastroenterol. 2004;99(1):23–32.
21. Sundler F, Ekblad E, Hakanson R. The neuroendocrine system of the gut—an update. Acta Oncol. 1991;30(4):419–27.
22. Waldum HL, Kleveland PM, Sandvik AK, Brenna E, Syversen U, Bakke I, et al. The cellular localization of the cholecystokinin 2 (gastrin) receptor in the stomach. Pharmacol Toxicol. 2002;91(6):359–62.
23. Bottcher G, Hakanson R, Nilsson G, Seensalu R, Sundler F. Effects of long-term hypergastrinaemia on the ultrastructure of enterochromaffin-like cells in the stomach of the rat, hamster and guinea pig. Cell Tissue Res. 1989;256(2):247–57.
24. Larsson H, Carlsson E, Mattsson H, Lundell L, Sundler F, Sundell G, et al. Plasma gastrin and gastric enterochromaffinlike cell activation and proliferation. Studies with omeprazole and ranitidine in intact and antrectomized rats. Gastroenterology. 1986;90(2):391–9.
25. Ryberg B, Carlsson E, Hakanson R, Lundell L, Mattsson H, Sundler F. Effects of partial resection of acid-secreting mucosa on plasma gastrin and enterochromaffin-like cells in the rat stomach. Digestion. 1990;45(2):102–8.
26. Wallmark B, Skanberg I, Mattsson H, Andersson K, Sundler F, Hakanson R, et al. Effect of 20 weeks' ranitidine treatment on plasma gastrin levels and gastric enterochromaffin-like cell density in the rat. Digestion. 1990;45(4):181–8.
27. Tielemans Y, Hakanson R, Sundler F, Willems G. Proliferation of enterochromaffinlike cells in omeprazole-treated hypergastrinemic rats. Gastroenterology. 1989;96(3):723–9.
28. Alumets J, El Munshid HA, Hakanson R, Liedberg G, Oscarson J, Rehfeld JF, et al. Effect of antrum exclusion on endocrine cells of rat stomach. J Physiol. 1979;286:145–55.
29. Solcia E, Bordi C, Creutzfeldt W, Dayal Y, Dayan AD, Falkmer S, et al. Histopathological classification of nonantral gastric endocrine growths in man. Digestion. 1988;41(4):185–200.
30. Abraham SC, Carney JA, Ooi A, Choti MA, Argani P. Achlorhydria, parietal cell hyperplasia, and multiple gastric carcinoids: a new disorder. Am J Surg Pathol. 2005;29(7):969–75.
31. Borch K, Ahren B, Ahlman H, Falkmer S, Granerus G, Grimelius L. Gastric carcinoids: biologic behavior and prognosis after differentiated treatment in relation to type. Ann Surg. 2005;242(1):64–73.
32. Bordi C. Gastric carcinoids. Ital J Gastroenterol Hepatol. 1999;31(Suppl 2):S94–7.
33. Rindi G, Bordi C, Rappel S, La Rosa S, Stolte M, Solcia E. Gastric carcinoids and neuroendocrine carcinomas: pathogenesis, pathology, and behavior. World J Surg. 1996;20(2):168–72.
34. Modlin IM, Kidd M, Latich I, Zikusoka MN, Shapiro MD. Current status of gastrointestinal carcinoids. Gastroenterology. 2005;128(6):1717–51.
35. Lehy T, Roucayrol AM, Mignon M. Histomorphological characteristics of gastric mucosa in patients with Zollinger-Ellison syndrome or autoimmune gastric atrophy: role of gastrin and atrophying gastritis. Microsc Res Tech. 2000;48(6):327–38.
36. Jensen RT. Management of the Zollinger-Ellison syndrome in patients with multiple endocrine neoplasia type 1. J Intern Med. 1998;243(6):477–88.
37. Modlin IM, Kidd M, Lye KD. Biology and management of gastric carcinoid tumours: a review. Eur J Surg. 2002;168(12):669–83.
38. Fendrich V, Bartsch DK. Surgical treatment of gastrointestinal neuroendocrine tumors. Langenbeck's Arch Surg. 2011;396(3):299–311.
39. Matsui K, Jin XM, Kitagawa M, Miwa A. Clinicopathologic features of neuroendocrine carcinomas of the stomach: appraisal of small cell and large cell variants. Arch Pathol Lab Med. 1998;122(11):1010–7.
40. Basuroy R, Srirajaskanthan R, Prachalias A, Quaglia A, Ramage JK. Review article: the investigation and management of gastric neuroendocrine tumours. Aliment Pharmacol Ther. 2014;39(10):1071–84.
41. Rappel S, Altendorf-Hofmann A, Stolte M. Prognosis of gastric carcinoid tumours. Digestion. 1995;56(6):455–62.
42. Ruszniewski P, Delle Fave G, Cadiot G, Komminoth P, Chung D, Kos-Kudla B, et al. Well-differentiated gastric tumors/carcinomas. Neuroendocrinology. 2006;84(3):158–64.
43. Yoshikane H, Tsukamoto Y, Niwa Y, Goto H, Hase S, Mizutani K, et al. Carcinoid tumors of the gastrointestinal tract: evaluation with endoscopic ultrasonography. Gastrointest Endosc. 1993;39(3):375–83.
44. Kulke MH, Anthony LB, Bushnell DL, de Herder WW, Goldsmith SJ, Klimstra DS, et al. NANETS treatment guidelines: well-differentiated neuroendo-

crine tumors of the stomach and pancreas. Pancreas. 2010;39(6):735–52.
45. Manfe AZ, Norberto L, Marchesini M, Lumachi F. Usefulness of chromogranin A, neuron-specific enolase and 5-hydroxyindolacetic acid measurements in patients with malignant carcinoids. In Vivo. 2011;25(6):1027–9.
46. Nikou GC, Lygidakis NJ, Toubanakis C, Pavlatos S, Tseleni-Balafouta S, Giannatou E, et al. Current diagnosis and treatment of gastrointestinal carcinoids in a series of 101 patients: the significance of serum chromogranin-A, somatostatin receptor scintigraphy and somatostatin analogues. Hepato-Gastroenterology. 2005;52(63):731–41.
47. Zatelli MC, Torta M, Leon A, Ambrosio MR, Gion M, Tomassetti P, et al. Chromogranin A as a marker of neuroendocrine neoplasia: an Italian Multicenter Study. Endocr Relat Cancer. 2007;14(2):473–82.
48. Bosman FT, International Agency for Research on C, World Health O. WHO classification of tumours of the digestive system. Lyon: International Agency for Research on Cancer2010. Report No.: 9789283224327;9283224329; Contract No.: Report.
49. Hopper AD, Bourke MJ, Hourigan LF, Tran K, Moss A, Swan MP. En-bloc resection of multiple type 1 gastric carcinoid tumors by endoscopic multi-band mucosectomy. J Gastroenterol Hepatol. 2009;24(9):1516–21.
50. Merola E, Sbrozzi-Vanni A, Panzuto F, D'Ambra G, Di Giulio E, Pilozzi E, et al. Type I gastric carcinoids: a prospective study on endoscopic management and recurrence rate. Neuroendocrinology. 2012;95(3):207–13.
51. Kulke MH, Shah MH, Benson AB, Bergsland E, Berlin JD, Blaszkowsky LS, Emerson L, Engstrom PF, Fanta P, Giordano T, et al. Neuroendocrine tumors, version 1.2015. J Natl Compr Cancer Netw. 2015;13:78–108.
52. Delle Fave G, Kwekkeboom DJ, Van Cutsem E, Rindi G, Kos-Kudla B, Knigge U, et al. ENETS consensus guidelines for the management of patients with gastroduodenal neoplasms. Neuroendocrinology. 2012;95(2):74–87.
53. Sato Y, Takeuchi M, Hashimoto S, Mizuno K, Kobayashi M, Iwafuchi M, Narisawa R, Aoyagi Y. Usefulness of endoscopic submucosal dissection for type I gastric carcinoid tumors compared with endoscopic mucosal resection. Hepato-Gastroenterology. 2013;60:1524–9.
54. Kim HH, Kim GH, Kim JH, Choi MG, Song GA, Kim SE. The efficacy of endoscopic submucosal dissection of type I gastric carcinoid tumors compared with conventional endoscopic mucosal resection. Gastroenterol Res Pract. 2014;2014:253860.
55. Sato Y, Imamura H, Kaizaki Y, Koizumi W, Ishido K, Kurahara K, Suzuki H, Fujisaki J, Hirakawa K, Hosokawa O, et al. Management and clinical outcomes of type I gastric carcinoid patients: retrospective, multicenter study in Japan. Dig Endosc. 2014;26:377–84.
56. Ravizza D, Fiori G, Trovato C, Fazio N, Bonomo G, Luca F, Bodei L, Pelosi G, Tamayo D, Crosta C. Long-term endoscopic and clinical follow-up of untreated type 1 gastric neuroendocrine tumours. Dig Liver Dis. 2007;39:537–43.
57. Campana D, Ravizza D, Ferolla P, Faggiano A, Grimaldi F, Albertelli M, Berretti D, Castellani D, Cacciari G, Fazio N, et al. Clinical management of patients with gastric neuroendocrine neoplasms associated with chronic atrophic gastritis: a retrospective, multicentre study. Endocrine. 2016;51:131–9.
58. Sato Y. Clinical features and management of type I gastric carcinoids. Clin J Gastroenterol. 2014;7(5):381–6.
59. Nikou GC, Angelopoulos TP. Current concepts on gastric carcinoid tumors. Gastroenterol Res Pract. 2012;2012:287825.
60. Dakin GF, Warner RR, Pomp A, Salky B, Inabnet WB. Presentation, treatment, and outcome of type 1 gastric carcinoid tumors. J Surg Oncol. 2006;93(5):368–72.
61. Gladdy RA, Strong VE, Coit D, Allen PJ, Gerdes H, Shia J, Klimstra DS, Brennan MF, Tang LH. Defining surgical indications for type I gastric carcinoid tumor. Ann Surg Oncol. 2009;16:3154–60.
62. Zhang L, Ozao J, Warner R, Divino C. Review of the pathogenesis, diagnosis, and management of type I gastric carcinoid tumor. World J Surg. 2011;35(8):1879–86.
63. Ferraro G, Annibale B, Marignani M, Azzoni C, D'Adda T, D'Ambra G, et al. Effectiveness of octreotide in controlling fasting hypergastrinemia and related enterochromaffin-like cell growth. J Clin Endocrinol Metab. 1996;81(2):677–83.
64. Jianu CS, Fossmark R, Syversen U, Hauso Ø, Fykse V, Waldum HL. Five-year follow-up of patients treated for 1 year with octreotide long-acting release for enterochromaffin-like cell carcinoids. Scand J Gastroenterol. 2011;46:456–63.
65. Fossmark R, Sørdal Ø, Jianu CS, Qvigstad G, Nordrum IS, Boyce M, Waldum HL. Treatment of gastric carcinoids type 1 with the gastrin receptor antagonist netazepide (YF476) results in regression of tumours and normalisation of serum chromogranin A. Aliment Pharmacol Ther. 2012;36:1067–75.
66. Moore AR, Boyce M, Steele IA, Campbell F, Varro A, Pritchard DM. Netazepide, a gastrin receptor antagonist, normalises tumour biomarkers and causes regression of type 1 gastric neuroendocrine tumours in a nonrandomised trial of patients with chronic atrophic gastritis. PLoS One. 2013;8:e76462.
67. Miljkovic MD, Girotra M, Abraham RR, Erlich RB. Novel medical therapies of recurrent and

metastatic gastroenteropancreatic neuroendocrine tumors. Dig Dis Sci. 2012;57(1):9–18.
68. Bordi C, Falchetti A, Azzoni C, D'Adda T, Canavese G, Guariglia A, et al. Aggressive forms of gastric neuroendocrine tumors in multiple endocrine neoplasia type I. Am J Surg Pathol. 1997;21(9):1075–82.
69. Akerstrom G, Hessman O, Skogseid B. Timing and extent of surgery in symptomatic and asymptomatic neuroendocrine tumors of the pancreas in MEN 1. Langenbeck's Arch Surg. 2002;386(8):558–69.
70. Richards ML, Gauger P, Thompson NW, Giordano TJ. Regression of type II gastric carcinoids in multiple endocrine neoplasia type 1 patients with Zollinger-Ellison syndrome after surgical excision of all gastrinomas. World J Surg. 2004;28(7):652–8.
71. Gough DB, Thompson GB, Crotty TB, Donohue JH, Kvols LK, Carney JA, et al. Diverse clinical and pathologic features of gastric carcinoid and the relevance of hypergastrinemia. World J Surg. 1994;18(4):473–9. discussion 9-80
72. Shinohara T, Ohyama S, Nagano H, Amaoka N, Ohta K, Matsubara T, et al. Minute gastric carcinoid tumor with regional lymph node metastasis. Gastric Cancer. 2003;6(4):262–6.
73. Akerstrom G. Management of carcinoid tumors of the stomach, duodenum, and pancreas. World J Surg. 1996;20(2):173–82.
74. Scherubl H, Cadiot G, Jensen RT, Rosch T, Stolzel U, Kloppel G. Neuroendocrine tumors of the stomach (gastric carcinoids) are on the rise: small tumors, small problems? Endoscopy. 2010;42(8):664–71.
75. Enzler T, Fojo T. Long-acting somatostatin analogues in the treatment of unresectable/metastatic neuroendocrine tumors. Semin Oncol. 2017;44(2):141–56.
76. Olsen IH, Langer SW, Jepsen I, Assens M, Federspiel B, Hasselby JP, et al. First-line treatment of patients with disseminated poorly differentiated neuroendocrine carcinomas with carboplatin, etoposide, and vincristine: a single institution experience. Acta Oncol. 2012;51(1):97–100.
77. Kolby L, Nilsson O, Ahlman H. Gastroduodenal endocrine tumours. Scand J Surg. 2004;93(4):317–23.
78. Nilsson O, Van Cutsem E, Delle Fave G, Yao JC, Pavel ME, McNicol AM, et al. Poorly differentiated carcinomas of the foregut (gastric, duodenal and pancreatic). Neuroendocrinology. 2006;84(3):212–5.
79. Basuroy R, Srirajaskanthan R, Ramage JK. A multimodal approach to the management of neuroendocrine tumour liver metastases. Int J Hepatol. 2012;819193(10):15.
80. Pavel M, Baudin E, Couvelard A, Krenning E, Oberg K, Steinmuller T, et al. ENETS Consensus Guidelines for the management of patients with liver and other distant metastases from neuroendocrine neoplasms of foregut, midgut, hindgut, and unknown primary. Neuroendocrinology. 2012;95(2):157–76.
81. Elias D, Lasser P, Ducreux M, Duvillard P, Ouellet JF, Dromain C, et al. Liver resection (and associated extrahepatic resections) for metastatic well-differentiated endocrine tumors: a 15-year single center prospective study. Surgery. 2003;133(4):375–82.
82. Sarmiento JM, Heywood G, Rubin J, Ilstrup DM, Nagorney DM, Que FG. Surgical treatment of neuroendocrine metastases to the liver: a plea for resection to increase survival. J Am Coll Surg. 2003;197(1):29–37.
83. Chamberlain RS, Canes D, Brown KT, Saltz L, Jarnagin W, Fong Y, et al. Hepatic neuroendocrine metastases: does intervention alter outcomes? J Am Coll Surg. 2000;190(4):432–45.
84. Moris D, Tsilimigras DI, Ntanasis-Stathopoulos I, Beal EW, Felekouras E, Vernadakis S, et al. Liver transplantation in patients with liver metastases from neuroendocrine tumors: a systematic review. Surgery. 2017;162(3):525–36.
85. Fan ST, Le Treut YP, Mazzaferro V, Burroughs AK, Olausson M, Breitenstein S, et al. Liver transplantation for neuroendocrine tumour liver metastases. HPB (Oxford). 2015;17(1):23–8.
86. Sher LS, Levi DM, Wecsler JS, Lo M, Petrovic LM, Groshen S, et al. Liver transplantation for metastatic neuroendocrine tumors: outcomes and prognostic variables. J Surg Oncol. 2015;112(2):125–32.
87. Siperstein AE, Berber E. Cryoablation, percutaneous alcohol injection, and radiofrequency ablation for treatment of neuroendocrine liver metastases. World J Surg. 2001;25(6):693–6.
88. Berber E, Flesher N, Siperstein AE. Laparoscopic radiofrequency ablation of neuroendocrine liver metastases. World J Surg. 2002;26(8):985–90.
89. Veenendaal LM, de Jager A, Stapper G, Borel Rinkes IH, van Hillegersberg R. Multiple fiber laser-induced thermotherapy for ablation of large intrahepatic tumors. Photomed Laser Surg. 2006;24(1):3–9.
90. Roche A, Girish BV, de Baere T, Baudin E, Boige V, Elias D, et al. Trans-catheter arterial chemoembolization as first-line treatment for hepatic metastases from endocrine tumors. Eur Radiol. 2003;13(1):136–40.
91. Marrache F, Vullierme MP, Roy C, El Assoued Y, Couvelard A, O'Toole D, et al. Arterial phase enhancement and body mass index are predictors of response to chemoembolisation for liver metastases of endocrine tumours. Br J Cancer. 2007;96(1):49–55.
92. Eriksson B, Kloppel G, Krenning E, Ahlman H, Plockinger U, Wiedenmann B, et al. Consensus guidelines for the management of patients with digestive neuroendocrine tumors—well-differentiated jejunal-ileal tumor/carcinoma. Neuroendocrinology. 2008;87(1):8–19.
93. Appetecchia M, Baldelli R. Somatostatin analogues in the treatment of gastroenteropancreatic neuroen-

docrine tumours, current aspects and new perspectives. J Exp Clin Cancer Res. 2010;29:19.
94. Arnold R, Rinke A, Klose KJ, Muller HH, Wied M, Zamzow K, et al. Octreotide versus octreotide plus interferon-alpha in endocrine gastroenteropancreatic tumors: a randomized trial. Clin Gastroenterol Hepatol. 2005;3(8):761–71.
95. Faiss S, Pape UF, Bohmig M, Dorffel Y, Mansmann U, Golder W, et al. Prospective, randomized, multicenter trial on the antiproliferative effect of lanreotide, interferon alfa, and their combination for therapy of metastatic neuroendocrine gastroenteropancreatic tumors—the International Lanreotide and Interferon Alfa Study Group. J Clin Oncol. 2003;21(14):2689–96.
96. Cives M, Strosberg J. Radionuclide therapy for neuroendocrine tumors. Curr Oncol Rep. 2017;19(2):9.
97. Kwekkeboom DJ, de Herder WW, van Eijck CH, Kam BL, van Essen M, Teunissen JJ, et al. Peptide receptor radionuclide therapy in patients with gastroenteropancreatic neuroendocrine tumors. Semin Nucl Med. 2010;40(2):78–88.
98. Öberg K, Knigge U, Kwekkeboom D, Perren A. ESMO Guidelines Working Group Neuroendocrine gastro-entero-pancreatic tumors ESMO Clinical Practice Guidelines for diagnosis, treatment and follow-up. Ann Oncol. 2012;23(7):vii124–30.
99. Kocha W, Maroun J, Kennecke H, Law C, Metrakos P, Ouellet JF, et al. Consensus recommendations for the diagnosis and management of well-differentiated gastroenterohepatic neuroendocrine tumours: a revised statement from a Canadian National Expert Group. Curr Oncol. 2010;17(3):49–64.
100. Modlin IM, Lye KD, Kidd M. A 5-decade analysis of 13,715 carcinoid tumors. Cancer. 2003;97(4):934–59.

36 Pancreatic Neuroendocrine Tumours

C. Chew and G. K. Bonney

Introduction

Pancreatic neuroendocrine tumours (pNETs) are relatively rare. While they comprise of only 1–2% of all pancreatic neoplasms [1], they provoke great interest amongst clinicians due to the variety of symptoms with which they present and multiple treatment options. While the overall prognosis of pNETs may be better than their exocrine counterparts, the 5-year survival rate is approximately 55% with localized disease and as low as 15% when the tumours are unresectable [2]. The incidence of pNETs has risen in the last decade, largely contributed to by the improvement of diagnostic imaging and wider use of computer tomography (CT) scanning [3, 4]. This presents clinicians with the opportunity to study the natural history of these tumours in greater detail, allowing us to further define more optimal modalities of treatment for this disease. This chapter highlights several developments and challenges regarding pNETs that have generated much debate amongst hepatobiliary surgeons about the future of treatment of this disease.

C. Chew · G. K. Bonney (✉)
Division of Hepatobiliary Surgery, National University Hospital Singapore, Singapore, Singapore
e-mail: glenn_bonney@nuhs.edu.sg

Aetiology

pNETs were initially thought to arise from the islets of Langerhans, giving rise to names such as "islet cell tumours" or "islet cell carcinomas". These terms are now deemed obsolete since Vortmeyer et al. published their findings suggesting that the origin of these neoplasms was in fact the pluripotent stem cells of the pancreatic ductules and acini [5]. The modern terminology of "pancreatic neuroendocrine tumours" is reflective of the neural and epithelial features seen in these cells.

The molecular pathogenesis of pNETs is complex and not fully understood. As with the majority of neoplasms, mutations associated with pNETs either occur sporadically or are inherited as part of a genetic syndrome. In contrast to common non-endocrine gastrointestinal tumours, such as carcinoma of the colon or stomach, alterations in common oncogenes such as ras, myc, src, or tumour-suppressor genes such as p53 and retinoblastoma1 are not seen in pNETs. Instead, alterations in genes such as the MEN1 gene, the p16/MTS1 tumour suppressor gene, DAXX/ATRX gene and the mTOR pathway have been observed to be critical in the development of pNETs [6]. Early studies of the MEN1 tumour suppressor gene in patients with multiple endocrine neoplasia (MEN) type 1 demonstrated that a germline inactivating mutation in one allele of the gene on chromosome 11q13 was followed by

R. Parameswaran, A. Agarwal (eds.), *Evidence-Based Endocrine Surgery*,
https://doi.org/10.1007/978-981-10-1124-5_36

a second somatic mutation in the other allele, which occurred by loss of heterozygosity or intragenic mutation [7, 8]. Since then, whole-exome sequencing of pNETs has detected somatic inactivating mutations in the MEN1 gene in 44% of sporadically occurring pNETs [6], a finding that has since been validated by numerous other large-volume studies [9, 10]. Determining the genetic profile in sporadic tumours may be of clinical and prognostic significance in the future as a growing number of studies show that specific molecular alterations correlate with tumour grade and spread of the disease [11, 12]. In addition to the aforementioned MEN type 1 syndrome, several other inherited syndromes such as von Hippel-Lindau disease, neurofibromatosis type 1 and tuberous sclerosis are also associated with the development of pNETs.

pNETs are classified into functional tumours and non-functional tumours. Functional tumours induce specific clinical syndromes through hormonal hypersecretion, while non-functional tumours either are void of hormonal secretion or secrete peptides that do not exhibit a distinct pattern of clinical symptoms. It was previously thought that functional tumours were of the majority; however the wider use of diagnostic imaging now suggests the inverse. Up to 90% of pNETs are non-functional tumours and are more commonly diagnosed on routine imaging [13]. Unfortunately, early diagnosis is rare with 60% of patients unfortunately presenting with metastatic disease [4]. The WHO classification for pNETs is shown in Table 36.1.

Table 36.1 WHO classification of neuroendocrine tumours and carcinomas

Well-differentiated endocrine tumour
– Benign behaviour
Confined to the pancreas
Absence of angioinvasion
Absence of perineural invasion
<2 cm in diameter
<2 mitoses/10 HPF
<2% Ki-67 activity
– Uncertain behaviour
Confined to the pancreas and ≥ 2 cm in diameter
2–10 mitoses/10 HPF
>2% Ki-67 activity
Presence of angioinvasion
Presence of perineural invasion
Well-differentiated endocrine carcinoma
– Low grade malignant
– Gross local invasion
– Metastasis
Poorly differentiated endocrine carcinoma
– High grade malignant
– >10 mitoses/10 HPF

Table 36.2 Accuracy of invasive and non-invasive investigations for insulinomas of the pancreas

Investigation	Accuracy (%)
Non-invasive	9–66
Ultrasound	50–80
Helical CT	40–70
MRI	17
Somatostatin receptor scintigraphy	
Invasive tests	25–50
Pancreatic angiogram	77–100
Intraarterial calcium stimulation	80–94
Endoscopic ultrasound	40–93
IOUS	86

Presentations, Investigations and Treatment Options

Insulinomas are the most common type of functional pNETs. They usually present as single, small benign tumours that arise almost exclusively in the pancreas, with an even distribution across the head, body and tail of the pancreas [14]. While they can be associated with MEN1, they are more often than not sporadic tumours.

The classic Whipple's triad is used in the diagnosis of insulinomas: (1) signs and symptoms of hypoglycaemia during monitored fasting or exercise (2) with blood glucose levels of <45 mg/dL during such episodes and (3) resolution of these symptoms with glucose intake [14]. Insulinomas can be reliably diagnosed by the monitoring of serum glucose, C-peptide and insulin during a 72-h fasting period. An elevated proinsulin level in combination with fasting hypoglycaemia has been shown to be the most sensitive criterion [15]. Other tests have been employed and summarized in Table 36.2.

Gastrinomas are pNETs that secrete high levels of gastrin ectopically, producing gastric acid hypersecretion otherwise known as Zollinger-Ellison syndrome. Ninety percent of gastrinomas are found within the gastrinoma triangle, bound superiorly by the cystic and common bile ducts, inferiorly by the second and third part of the duodenum and medially by the junction of the head and body of the pancreas. Within the triangle, two thirds of gastrinomas arise from the pancreas and one third from the duodenum. Sporadic gastrinomas are typically solitary, while those that develop as part of MEN1 syndrome are often multifocal [16]. Although there is no absolute level of fasting serum gastrin level that is diagnostic, a diagnosis can be made in 40–60% patients with the typical clinical syndrome of symptomatic peptic ulcer disease with a >10-fold elevation above baseline and a gastric pH ≤2, given that retained antrum syndrome (though rare) has been ruled out [16, 17]. When a >10-fold elevation is not seen, other causes such as antral G-cell hyperplasia or hyperfunction or *H. pylori* infections must be considered. A positive secretin test is useful in differentiating a gastrinoma and is demonstrated by an increase in fasting gastrin levels of >120 pg/ml above baseline following the administration of a subcutaneous secretin injection [18].

Glucagonomas are pNETs that secrete large amounts of glucagon. The clinical picture produced is best explained by considering the physiological effects of glucagon—symptoms of glucose intolerance or diabetes are seen as a result of the increased rates of gluconeogenesis stimulated by glucagonemia, and the characteristic form of dermatitis known as migratory necrolytic erythema occurs as a result of hypoaminoacidemia [19, 20]. Anaemia, diarrhoea and thromboembolism are also commonly seen. Unlike insulinomas and gastrinomas, glucagonomas tend to present as large tumours (5–10 cm), and a majority of them occur in the pancreatic tail where the mass effect of the tumour is less pronounced than tumours originating in the pancreatic head [19]. Diagnosis requires a demonstration of plasma glucagon level of >1000 pg/mL, although symptoms have been reported in patients with plasma glucagon levels <500 pg/mL [19, 20].

VIPomas are characterized by inappropriate secretion of vasoactive intestinal peptide. The syndrome observed is also known as the Verner-Morrison syndrome and comprises of symptoms of large-volume secretory diarrhoea, hypokalaemia and dehydration [21]. These tumours are usually solitary arising in the pancreatic tail and often present with hepatic metastases at diagnosis. An elevated plasma VIP level of >500 pg/mL in the presence of large-volume diarrhoea is diagnostic of a VIPoma [22].

The term "non-functional" pNET is a misnomer, as majority of such tumours in fact do secrete hormones, such as chromogranins A and B, pancreatic polypeptide and other peptides, each of which does not produce specific symptoms [22, 23]. Non-functional pancreatic tumours cause symptoms by localized mass effect of the tumour itself. They commonly originate in the pancreatic head, giving rise to symptoms of abdominal pain, jaundice and weight loss. Unfortunately, non-functional pancreatic tumours tend to present late in the course of the disease. The primary tumour is large (>5 cm) and invasive, and hepatic metastases are often already present [4, 24].

The diagnosis of non-functional pNETs is made histologically in patients without raised plasma hormones or clinical symptoms suggestive of a specific syndrome. Plasma pancreatic polypeptide is a sensitive marker for non-functional pNETs, but elevated levels are not diagnostic as plasma pancreatic polypeptide is known to be raised in several other conditions such as chronic kidney disease and diabetes [25]. With more routine imaging being done, non-functional pNETs are being diagnosed at relatively smaller sizes than before. While there are no clear treatment guidelines at present, management must balance the morbidity of pancreatic surgery with the relatively high risk of malignancy and metastasis. Historically, most clinicians would recommend surgical resection for non-functional pNETs larger than 3 cm and watchful waiting for smaller tumours [25].

The goal of imaging is to achieve localization of the primary tumour and to determine extent of disease. This knowledge is essential for reliable prognostication of the disease and to establish the goals of treatment, be it for curative or palliative intent using either surgical or systemic modalities. Conventional imaging such as triple-phase multidetector computed tomography (CT) scan is 60–83% sensitive in detecting the primary tumour [26], while magnetic resonance imaging (MRI) has a higher sensitivity of 85–100% [27]. Pancreatic neuroendocrine tumours are classically hypervascular, and the administration of intravenous contrast causes them to appear markedly enhanced during the arterial phase of CT. In MRI, these tumours exhibit a low signal intensity on T1-weighted imaging and a high signal intensity on T2-weighted imaging. However, when the tumour in question is small, they are often missed on CT, and this is where endoscopic ultrasound (EUS) has proven to be a useful tool. In fact, a large prospective study reported EUS to have an overall sensitivity of 93% for localization of pNETs [28]. pNETs tend to grow as round, homogenous and well-circumscribed lesions and hence can be easily identified using EUS. Furthermore, concurrent fine needle aspiration can be performed to obtain a tissue diagnosis, thus allowing for differentiation between pNETs and pancreatic adenocarcinomas [29].

High-affinity somatostatin receptors are frequently overexpressed in pNETs. Somatostatin radiolabelled scintigraphy employs the use of octreotide radiolabelled with 111Indium, a somatostatin analogue, to localize primary pNETs and metastases with high sensitivity. This has been shown to be particularly useful in the diagnosis of extrapancreatic glucagonomas, although it should be used with caution if an insulinoma is suspected as they do not express somatostatin receptors. Occasional false positives can occur, as high as 12% in one study, as several other diseases such as granulomas, thyroid disease and activated lymphocytes express high levels of somatostatin receptors. More recently, this principle has also been employed in positron emission tomography (PET) using 68Ga-labelled somatostatin PET (68Ga-DOTA-SSTa).

Surgical Management of Pancreatic Neuroendocrine Tumours

Surgical resection is the treatment of choice in patients with localized and resectable disease. Before proceeding with surgery, the patient's ability to tolerate a major operation must first be considered. The surgical approach is then chosen based on the size and location of the lesion. Tumours arising in the body or tail of the pancreas are resected by performing a distal pancreatectomy, whereas tumours in the pancreatic head or uncinate process require a pancreaticoduodenectomy [30]. A total pancreatectomy is often only necessary for large or multifocal tumours distributed throughout the pancreas such as MEN syndrome [31]. Apart from these standard resections, other tissue-sparing approaches have been used particularly for tumours with low malignant potential. Central pancreatectomies and enucleation allow for better preservation of pancreatic endocrine and exocrine function, but these techniques are not without disadvantages [32]. A central pancreatectomy is performed for tumours confined to the neck or body of the pancreas and allows for splenic preservation as well and the maintenance of gastrointestinal continuity [13, 32]. However, high rates of pancreatic fistulas and leaks have been reported as a pancreaticojejunostomy or pancreaticogastrostomy must be constructed for drainage of the remnant pancreatic tail [33]. Enucleation has also been described for small, superficial tumours that do not communicate or lie in close relation to the main pancreatic duct [34, 35] (Fig. 36.1). For small tumours clearly away from the main pancreatic duct, laparoscopic enucleation is a safe procedure for both functioning and non-functioning pNETs [36]. Caution should be taken that while associated with lower post-operative morbidity, the limited extent of resection provided by this technique does not allow for adequate nodal evaluation, necessitating that when a neuroendocrine carcinoma is found on pathological assessment, a formal operation must be carried out. On a practical level, these tumours are known to be vascular (Fig. 36.2c). The authors prefer energy devices

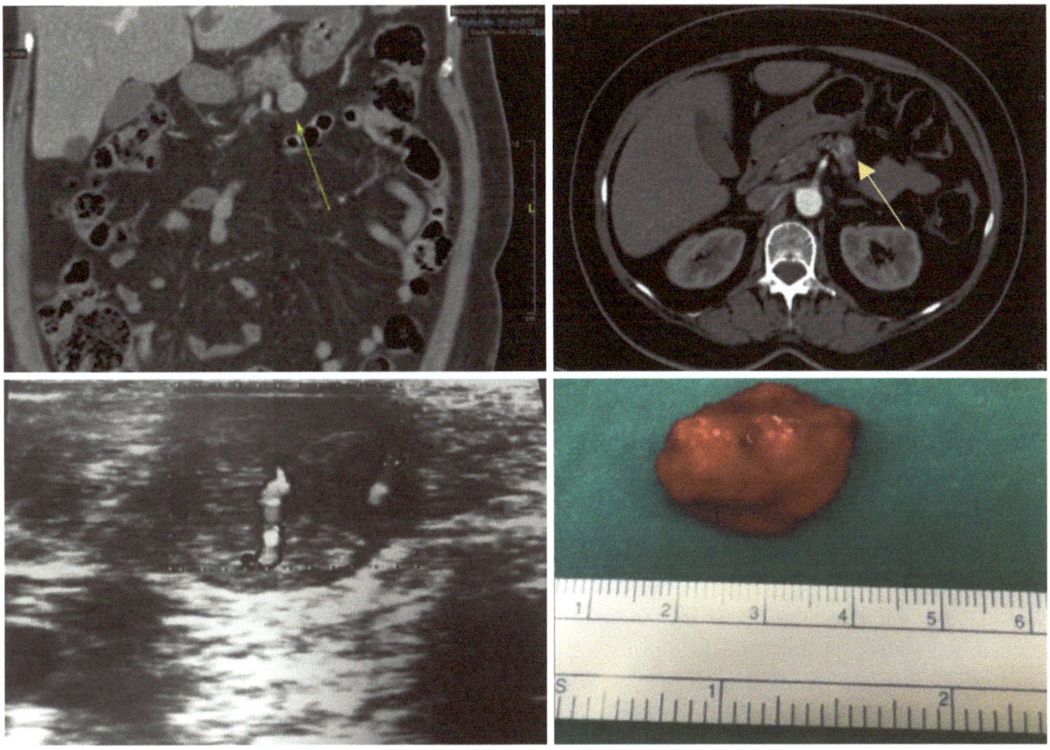

Fig. 36.1 A 2.3 cm insulinoma of the body of the pancreas that went on to have a laparoscopic enucleation. *Top left*, Coronal view of exophytic tumour on CT scanning. *Top right*, Cross-sectional view in the arterial phase. *Bottom left*, Intraoperative laparoscopic ultrasound view of hypoechoic lesion showing prominent intralesional blood vessel. *Bottom right*, Gross morphology of the laparoscopic resected specimen. Patient is now 1-year post-resection with normal blood glucose control

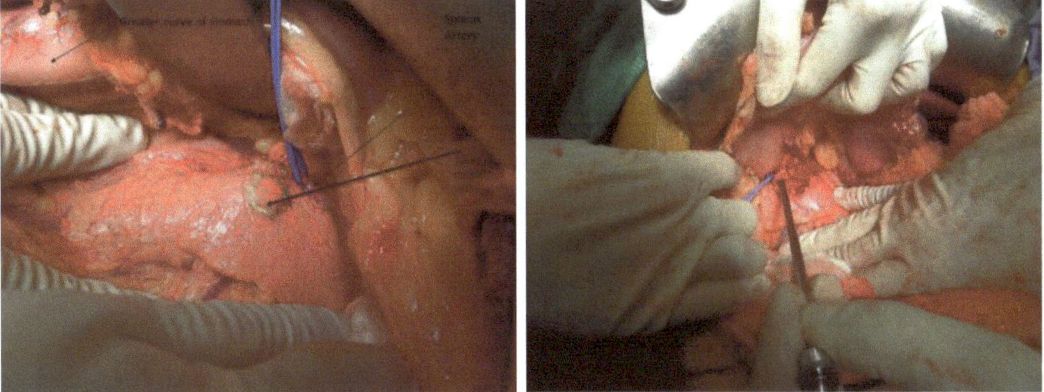

Fig. 36.2 Open enucleation of an intrapancreatic body lesion. *Left*, Lesion marked with diathermy prior to ultrasonic dissection (the splenic artery is slung). *Right*, Post-resection area

or laparoscopic ultrasonic dissectors for delimitation of small blood vessels intraoperatively. Failure to resect with adequate margin or high grade tumours may result in a higher tumour recurrence after enucleation [37].

In patients with MEN1, the role of surgery is not well established, and there is an ongoing debate regarding when and what surgical intervention should be undertaken. Patients with MEN1 present at an earlier age, with multifocal disease present in up to 80% of patients [38]. With functional non-gastrinoma pNETs, surgical resection is recommended for the management of hormonal excess. However, the approach to non-functional tumours and gastrinomas is controversial as no large scale studies or treatment guidelines exist [39]. Proponents of surgical intervention argue that early resection is beneficial in view of the fact that up to 33% of patients present with metastatic disease [40], which is a poor prognostic sign for life expectancy. On the other hand, excellent prognosis has been reported for patients with metastatic disease, with approximately 50% survival at 15 years for metastatic gastrinomas [41]. As such, metastatic disease in such pNETs may not necessarily be a reflection of the aggressiveness of the tumour [42]. Furthermore, some studies have found no survival benefit in patients undergoing surgery versus those that did not, in both small non-functioning pNETs and gastrinomas [38, 43]. Given the high morbidity and mortality associated with pancreatic surgery, the risk and benefits must be carefully considered before proceeding with surgery.

Many patients with MEN1 present with multifocal disease, and one of the challenges of surgical resection lies in determining the extent disease. In these patients, all imaging modalities are exhausted preoperatively, and additional intraoperative ultrasound of the pancreas and peripancreatic tissues is usually performed. Many surgeons also recommend duodenotomies to further evaluate the duodenal wall for tumours that may be too small to be diagnosed on imaging. The eventual surgical approach is dictated by the distribution of the tumours, and most advocate a regional peripancreatic lymphadenectomy in view of the high risk of nodal metastases [44].

pNETs most commonly metastasize to the liver, much like other gastrointestinal malignancies. In advanced metastatic disease, most consensus guidelines recommend cytoreductive therapy if greater than 90% of tumour burden can be resected [45, 46]. There are several studies that support this, demonstrating both improved survival rates compared to patients with untreated metastases, as well as improved symptom control [47, 48]. One such study found no survival difference between patients treated with curative intent and palliative intent (>90% tumour debulking) [47]. However, it must be noted that these studies were conducted retrospectively and do not take into account the high risk of eventual recurrence of disease. Given the relatively indolent course of metastatic pNETs, the survival benefit of aggressive resection is still highly debatable. On the other hand, in patients where at least 90% of tumour burden resection is unlikely to be achieved, surgical resection is not recommended as these patients would not have any survival improvement [49].

Several other treatment options exist for multifocal liver metastases that are not amenable to surgical resection. Local ablative therapy in the form of radiofrequency ablation, cryotherapy and microwave coagulation can be offered percutaneously or during surgery. It can also be offered as adjuvant therapy to patients with liver metastases that would otherwise not be suitable for resection [50]. Radiofrequency ablation is most commonly used, and good long-term outcomes have been reported with symptomatic relief achieved in 97% of patients and median disease-free survival of 1.3 years [51]. Local ablative therapy can be repeated for additional local tumour control with minimal morbidity.

In patients with extensive liver metastases, transarterial embolization can be performed. This works on the principle that hepatic metastases derive their bloody supply from the hepatic arteries instead of the portal venous circulation. This angiography-based approach also allows for embolization to be performed in conjunction with chemotherapeutic agents such as doxorubicin and cisplatin (known as transarterial chemoembolization). Response rates have been reported to be 30–85% only in retrospective studies [52–54], and to date no large scale randomized controlled trials comparing TAE and TACE are available. These procedures are relatively contraindicated in patients that have metastatic involvement of >50% of the liver. In these patients, radioembolization is a feasible alternative as it is more sparing of normal hepatic tissue hence reducing the risk of acute liver failure [55, 56]. While liver transplantation can be recommended in highly selected patients with NETs, this is not the case for pNETs that generally have a higher risk of recurrence. The author has previously described that radical resection, even when involving multiple organs, may confer a reasonable survival [57].

Systemic treatment modalities for pNETs are used in patients with advanced disease and who are not suitable candidates for surgical therapy. Until very recently, these were limited to somatostatin analogues and cytotoxic chemotherapy. Somatostatin analogues, like octreotide or lantreotide, bind to somatostatin receptors that are overexpressed on most pNETs and have been shown to be effective at regulating hormonal hypersecretion in patients with functional tumours [13]. However, somatostatin analogues are cytostatic but not cytotoxic, and while they have been shown to stabilize metastatic disease in >50% of patients with progressive disease [58], no significant survival benefit has been demonstrated with their usage.

pNETs are relatively sensitive to chemotherapy in comparison to other neuroendocrine tumours. The grade of the tumour is used to determine the chemotherapy regimen. Response to treatment is variable depending on the tumour grade. Chemotherapy drugs such as cisplatin and etoposide are used in poorly differentiated tumours and have produced response rates of up to 70% [59]. However the duration of response is relatively short, and both drugs are associated with significant toxicity that limits their usage. Most recently, a combination regime of streptomycin, 5-fluorouracil and doxorubicin has demonstrated a tumour response rate of 39% with a median response duration of 9.3 months [60].

Genomic exome sequencing has allowed us to define the most common mutations found in pNETs [13]. This has paved the way for the development of targeted molecular therapies. One such drug is everolimus, an oral inhibitor of the mammalian target of rapamycin, which inhibits cellular proliferation and angiogenesis mediated by the mTOR pathway. In a randomized controlled trial, everolimus demonstrated a significant duration of progression-free survival compared to placebo (11 months vs. 4.6 months), representing a 65% reduction in estimated risk of progression or death [61]. Sunitinib is a tyrosine kinase inhibitor that inhibits angiogenic and mitogenic proteins such as vascular endothelial growth factor receptor and platelet-derived growth factor receptors. The phase 3 clinical trial was discontinued early after the placebo group reported more serious adverse events and deaths, as well as a significant difference in progression-free survival which favoured sunitinib (11.4 months vs. 5.5 months). The objective response rate was shown to be 9.3% vs. 0% in the placebo group [62]. Both everolimus and sunitinib also have acceptable side effect profiles and have recently received US FDA approval for use in pNETs. There are ongoing studies investigating newer targeted molecular agents as well as combination therapies, such as peptide receptor radiotherapy that couples radioactive isotopes to somatostatin analogues allowing for directed delivery of radiotherapy to tumour cells [63].

Conclusion

The success in managing pNETs lies initially in early detection and treatment, where possible complete resection or near-complete (>90%) resection should be the main aim of treatment. In "low-risk tumours" located away from the main pancreatic duct, enucleation, particularly when done laparoscopically is a safe procedure with low morbidity. In "high risk" tumours, radical resection involving multiple organs where necessary results in improved survival. In disease that is unresectable, numerous oncological and radiological treatment strategies are available depending on location.

References

1. Franked M, Kim MK, Faggiano A, Valk GD. Epidemiology of gastroenteropancreatic neuroendocrine tumours. Best Pract Res Clin Gastroenterol. 2012;26(6):691–703.
2. Edge SB, Byrd DR, Compton CC, et al., editors. Exocrine and endocrine pancreas. AJCC cancer staging manual. 7th ed. New York, NY: Springer; 2010. p. 241–9.
3. Lawrence B, Gustafsson BI, Chan A, et al. The epidemiology of gastroenteropancreatic neuroendocrine tumors. Endocrinol Metab Clin North Am. 2011;40:1–18.
4. Halfdanarson TR, Rubin J, Farnell MB, et al. Pancreatic endocrine neoplasms: epidemiology and prognosis of pancreatic endocrine tumors. Endocr Relat Cancer. 2008;15:409–27.
5. Vortmeyer AO, Huang S, Lubensky I, Zhuang Z. Non-islet origin of pancreatic islet cell tumors. J Clin Endocrinol Metab. 2004;89(4):1934–8.
6. Jiao Y, Shi C, Edil BH, de Wilde RF, Klimstra DS, Maitra A, et al. DAXX/ATRX, MEN1, and mTOR pathway genes are frequently altered in pancreatic neuroendocrine tumors. Science. 2011;331(6021):1199–203.
7. Chandrasekharappa SC, et al. Positional cloning of the gene for multiple endocrine neoplasia-type 1. Science. 1997;276:404–7.
8. De Wilde RF, Edil BH, Aruban RH, Maitra A. Well-differentiated pancreatic neuroendocrine tumors: from genetics to therapy. Nat Rev Gastroenterol Hepatol. 2012;9(4):199–208.
9. Toliat MR, Berger W, Ropers HH, Neuhaus P, Wiedenmann B. Mutations in the MEN I gene in sporadic neuroendocrine tumours of gastroenteropancreatic system. Lancet. 1997;350:1223.
10. Moore PS, et al. Role of disease-causing genes in sporadic pancreatic endocrine tumors: MEN1 and VHL. Genes Chromosomes Cancer. 2001;32:177–81.
11. Dogeas E, Karagkounis G, Heathy CM, Hirose K, Pawlik TM, Wolfgang CL. Alternative lengthening of telomeres predicts site of origin in neuroendocrine tumor liver metastases. J Am Coll Surg. 2014;218(4):628–35.
12. Marinoni I, Kurrer AS, Vassella E, Deter M, Rudolph T, Banz V. Loss of DAXX and ATRX are associated with chromosome instability and reduced survival of patients with pancreatic neuroendocrine tumors. Gastroenterology. 2014;146(2):453–60.e5.
13. McKenna LR, Edil BH. Update on pancreatic neuroendocrine tumors. Gland Surg. 2014;3(4):258–75.
14. Grant CS. Insulinoma. Best Pract Res Clin Gastroenterol. 2005;19:783–98.
15. Vezzosi D, Bennet A, Fauvel J, et al. Insulin, C-peptide and proinsulin for the biochemical diagnosis of hypoglycaemia related to endogenous hyperinsulinism. Eur J Endocrinol. 2007;157:75–83.
16. Jensen RT, Niederle B, Mitry E, et al. Gastrinoma (duodenal and pancreatic). Neuroendocrinology. 2006;84:173–82.
17. Gibril F, Jensen RT. Zollinger-Ellison syndrome revisited: diagnosis, biologic markers, associated inherited disorders, and acid hypersecretion. Curr Gastroenterol Rep. 2004;6:454–63.
18. Berna MJ, Hoffmann KM, Long SH, Serrano J, Fibril F, Jensen RT. Serum gastrin in Zollinger-Ellison syndrome: II. Prospective study of gastrin provocative testing in 293 patients from the National Institutes of Health and comparison with 537 cases from the literature. Evaluation of diagnostic criteria, proposal of new criteria, and correlations with clinical and tumoral features. Medicine (Baltimore). 2006;85(6):331–64.
19. Soga J, Yakuwa Y. Glucagonomas/diabetico-dermatogenic syndrome (DDS): a statistical evaluation of 407 reported cases. J Hepatobiliary Pancreat Surg. 1998;5:312–9.
20. van Beek AP, de Haas ER, van Vloten WA, et al. The glucagonoma syndrome and necrolytic migratory erythema: a clinical review. Eur J Endocrinol. 2004;151:531–7.
21. Ghaferi AA, Chojnacki KA, Long WD, Cameron JL, Yeo CJ. Pancreatic VIPomas: subject review and one institutional experience. J Gastrointest Surg. 2008;12(2):382–93.
22. Metz DC, Jensen RT. Gastrointestinal neuroendocrine tumors: pancreatic endocrine tumors. Gastroenterology. 2008;135(5):1469–92.
23. Kloppel G. Tumour biology and histopathology of neuroendocrine tumours. Best Pract Res Clin Endocrinol Metab. 2007;21:15–31.
24. Viudez A, De Jesus-Acosta A, Carvalho FL, Vera R, Marti-Algarra S, Ramirez N. Pancreatic neuroendocrine tumors: challenges in an underestimated disease. Crit Rev Oncol Hematol. 2016;101:193–206.
25. Vinik A, Casellini C, Perry RR, Feliberti E, Vingan H. Diagnosis and management of pancreatic neuroendocrine tumors. 2015.
26. Sundin A. Radiological and nuclear medicine imaging of gastroenteropancreatic neuroendocrine tumours. Best Pract Res Clin Gastroenterol. 2012;26(6):803–18.
27. Caramel C, Domain C, De Baere T, Boulet B, Schlumberger M, Ducreux M, et al. Endocrine pancreatic tumours: which are the most useful MRI sequences? Eur Radiol. 2010;20(11):2618–27.
28. Anderson MA, Carpenter S, Thompson NW, Nostrant TT, Elta GH, Scheiman JM. Endoscopic ultrasound is highly accurate and directs management in patients with neuroendocrine tumours of the pancreas. Am J Gastroenterol. 2000;95(9):2271–7.
29. Atiq M, Bhutan MS, Bektas M, Lee JE, Gong Y, Tamm EP. EUS-FNA for pancreatic neuroendocrine tumors: a tertiary cancer center experience. Dig Dis Sci. 2012;57(3):791–800.
30. Kimura W, Tezuka K, Hirai I. Surgical management of pancreatic neuroendocrine tumors. Surg Today. 2011;41(10):1332–43.
31. Casadei R, Monari F, Buscemi S, et al. Total pancreatectomy: indications, operative technique, and

results: a single centre experience and review of literature. Updates Surg. 2010;62:41–6.
32. Falconi M, Zerbi A, Crippa S, et al. Parenchyma-preserving resections for small nonfunctioning pancreatic endocrine tumors. Ann Surg Oncol. 2010;17:1621–7.
33. Du ZY, Chen S, Han BS, et al. Middle segmental pancreatectomy: a safe and organ-preserving option for benign and low-grade malignant lesions. World J Gastroenterol. 2013;19:1458–65.
34. Hackett T, Hinz U, Fritz S, Strobel O, Schneider L, Hartwig W, et al. Enucleation in pancreatic surgery: indications, technique, and outcome compared to standard pancreatic resections. Langenbecks Arch Surg. 2011;396(8):1197–203.
35. Cauley CE, Pitt HA, Ziegler KM, Nakeeb A, Schmidt CM, Zyromski NJ, et al. Pancreatic enucleation: improved outcomes compared to resection. J Gastrointest Surg. 2012;16(7):1347–53.
36. Al-Kurd A, Chapchay K, Grozinsky-Glasberg S, Mazeh H. Laparoscopic resection of pancreatic neuroendocrine tumors. World J Gastroenterol. 2014;20(17):4908–16.
37. Jilesen AP, van Eijck CH, Busch OR, van Gulik TM, Gouma DJ, van Dijkum EJ. Postoperative outcomes of enucleation and standard resections in patients with a pancreatic neuroendocrine tumor. World J Surg. 2016;40(3):715–28.
38. Triponez F, Goudet P, Dosseh D, Cougard P, Bauters C, Murat A, et al. Is surgery beneficial for MEN1 patients with small (< = 2 cm), nonfunctioning pancreaticoduodenal endocrine tumor? An analysis of 65 patients from the GTE. World J Surg. 2006;30(5):654–62. discussion 663-4
39. Machado MC. Surgical treatment of pancreatic endocrine tumors in multiple endocrine neoplasia type 1. Clinics (Sao Paulo). 2012;67(Suppl 1):145–8.
40. Lowney JK, Frisella MM, Lairmore TC, Doherty GM, et al. Pancreatic islet cell tumor metastasis in multiple endocrine neoplasia type 1: correlation with primary tumor size. Surgery. 1998;124(6):1043–8. discussion 1048-9
41. Norton JA, Alexander HR, Fraker DL, Venzon DJ, Gibril F, Jensen RT. Comparison of surgical results in patients with advanced and limited disease with multiple endocrine neoplasia type 1 and Zollinger-Ellison syndrome. Ann Surg. 2001;234(4):495–506.
42. Gibril F, Venzon DJ, Ojeaburu JV, Bashir S, Jensen RT. Prospective study of the natural history of gastrinoma in patients with MEN1: definition of an aggressive and a nonaggressive form. J Clin Endocrinol Metab. 2001;86(11):5282–93.
43. Triponez F, Dosseh D, Goudet P, Cougard P, Bauters C, Murat A. Epidemiology data on 108 MEN 1 patients from the GTE with isolated nonfunctioning tumors of the pancreas. Ann Surg. 2006;243(2):265–72.
44. Niina Y, Fujimori N, Nakamura T, Igarashi H, Oono T, Nakamura K, et al. The current strategy for managing pancreatic neuroendocrine tumors in multiple endocrine neoplasia type 1. Gut Liver. 2012;6(3):287–94.
45. Jensen RT, Cadiot G, Brandi ML, de Herder WW, Kaltsas G, Komminoth P, et al. ENETS consensus guidelines for the management of patients with digestive neuroendocrine neoplasms: functional pancreatic endocrine tumor syndromes. Neuroendocrinology. 2012;95(2):98–119.
46. Kulke MH, Anthony LB, Bushnell DL, de Herder WW, Goldsmith SJ, Klimstra DS, et al. NANETS treatment guidelines: well-differentiated neuroendocrine tumors of the stomach and pancreas. Pancreas. 2010;39(6):735–52.
47. Cusati D, Zhang L, Harmsen WS, Hu A, Farnell MB, Nagorney DM, et al. Metastatic nonfunctioning pancreatic neuroendocrine carcinoma to liver: surgical treatment and outcomes. J Am Coll Surg. 2012;215(1):117–24; discussion 124-5.
48. Sarmiento HM, Heywood G, Rubin J, Ilstrup DM, Nargoney DM, Que FG. Surgical treatment of neuroendocrine metastases to the liver: a plea for resection to increase survival. J Am Coll Surg. 2003;197(1):29–37.
49. Bettini R, Mantovani W, Boninsegna L, Crippa S, Capelli P, Bassi C. Primary tumour resection in metastatic nonfunctioning pancreatic endocrine carcinomas. Dig Liver Dis. 2009;41(1):49–55.
50. Taner T, Atwell TD, Zhang L, Oberg TN, Harmsen WS, Slettedahl SW, et al. Adjunctive radiofrequency ablation of metastatic neuroendocrine cancer to the liver complements surgical resection. HPB (Oxford). 2013;15(3):190–5.
51. Akyildiz HY, Mitchell J, Milas M, Siperstein A, Berber E. Laparoscopic radiofrequency thermal ablation of neuroendocrine hepatic metastases: long-term follow-up. Surgery. 2010;148(6):1288–93; discussion 1293.
52. Akahori T, Sho M, Tanaka T, et al. Significant efficacy of new transcatheter arterial chemoembolization technique for hepatic metastases of pancreatic neuroendocrine tumors. Anticancer Res. 2013;33:3355–8.
53. Strosberg JR, Choi J, Cantor AB, et al. Selective hepatic artery embolization for treatment of patients with metastatic carcinoid and pancreatic endocrine tumors. Cancer Control. 2006;13:72–8.
54. Gupta S, Johnson MM, Murthy R, et al. Hepatic arterial embolization and chemoembolization for the treatment of patients with metastatic neuroendocrine tumors: variables affecting response rates and survival. Cancer. 2005;104:1590–602.
55. Ito T, Igarashi H, Jensen RT. Therapy of metastatic pancreatic neuroendocrine tumors (pNETs): recent insights and advances. J Gastroenterol. 2012;47:941–60.
56. Cao CQ, Yan TD, Bester L, et al. Radioembolization with yttrium microspheres for neuroendocrine tumour liver metastases. Br J Surg. 2010;97:537–43.
57. Bonney GK, Gomez D, Rahman SH, Verbeke CS, Prasad KR, Toogood GJ, Lodge JP, Menon KV. Results following surgical resection for malignant pancreatic neuroendocrine tumours. A single institutional experience. JOP. 2008;9(1):19–25.

58. Toumpanakis C, Caplin ME. Update on the role of somatostatin analogs for the treatment of patients with gastroenteropancreatic neuroendocrine tumors. Semin Oncol. 2013;40(1):56–68.
59. Eriksson B, Annibale B, Bajetta E, Mitry E, Pavel M, Platania M, et al. ENETS Consensus Guidelines for the Standards of Care in Neuroendocrine Tumors: chemotherapy in patients with neuroendocrine tumors. Neuroendocrinology. 2009;90(2):214–9.
60. Kouvaraki MA, Ajani JA, Hoff P, Wolff R, Evans DB, Lozano R, et al. Fluorouracil, doxorubicin, and streptozocin in the treatment of patients with locally advanced and metastatic pancreatic endocrine carcinomas. J Clin Oncol. 2004;22(23):4762–71.
61. Yao JC, Shah MH, Ito T, Bohas CL, Wolin ED, Cutsem EV, et al. Everolimus for advanced pancreatic neuroendocrine tumours. N Engl J Med. 2011;364:514–23.
62. Raymond E, Dahan L, Raoul J, Bang YJ, Borbath I, Lombard-Bohas C, et al. Sunitinib malate for the treatment of pancreatic neuroendocrine tumors. N Engl J Med. 2011;364:501–13.
63. Horsch D, Ezziddin S, Haug A, Gratz KF, Dukelmann S, Krause BJ, et al. Peptide receptor radionuclide therapy for neuroendocrine tumors in Germany: first results of a multi-institutional cancer registry. Recent Results Cancer Res. 2013;194:457–65.

Carcinoid Tumours of the Gastrointestinal System: Neuroendocrine Tumours of the Hindgut

37

Bettina Lieske

Introduction

Carcinoids are neuroendocrine tumours (NETs), small, slow-growing neoplasms, characterised by their ability to store and secrete different peptides and neuroamines [1, 2].

Langhans was the first to describe a gut carcinoid in 1867 [3, 4]. Ransom was the first to provide a comprehensive description of the classical carcinoid syndrome in 1900 [3, 5], and Oberndorfer [3, 6] first coined the term "karzinoid" in 1907 to distinguish this seemingly benign neoplasm from the typical malignant adenocarcinoma of the gastrointestinal tract. Gosset and Masson [3, 7] published a description of carcinoids of the appendix in which they recognised them as neuroendocrine tumours in 1914.

The term carcinoid represents a wide spectrum of neoplasms originating from a variety of neuroendocrine cell types. Godwin [8] published the first substantial evaluation of carcinoid tumours in 1975 and contributed significant epidemiological facts concerning incidence, distribution and survival.

His epidemiological description was only superseded in 1997, when Modlin et al. [9] revisited the analysis and added data from the NCI Surveillance Research Program, and again in 2003, when Modlin finally added SEER data and published an analysis of over 13,000 cases of carcinoid tumours [3].

B. Lieske
Division of Colorectal Surgery, University Surgical Cluster, National University Hospital, Singapore, Singapore
e-mail: bettina_lieske@nuhs.edu.sg

Background/Aetiology

Neuroendocrine tumours derive from neuroendocrine cells and are divided by anatomical location into foregut, midgut and hindgut carcinoids. They are rare and comprise less than 2% of gastrointestinal malignancies [1]. The tumours may be asymptomatic and found incidentally or can cause a variety of non-specific symptoms due to the secretion of their specific substances.

Carcinoids of the hindgut are located in the distal colon and rectum. Their incidence has increased and is currently described as 1 per 100,000 in the United States [10]. Rectal carcinoids in particular now occur at 0.86 per 100,000 (SEER database from 2004), up from 0.2 per 100,000 in 1973 [10]. This translates into 27% of all gastrointestinal NETs and 16% of NETs over all. Carcinoids of the colon are diagnosed less commonly, with an incidence of 0.2 per 100,000. True incidence of hindgut carcinoids may be higher, since many of the tumours would not have been registered in the SEER database whilst they were considered benign.

Higher rates of rectal NETs have been observed in Blacks and Asians compared with

R. Parameswaran, A. Agarwal (eds.), *Evidence-Based Endocrine Surgery*,
https://doi.org/10.1007/978-981-10-1124-5_37

Caucasians in the American population; population-corrected rates are 2.30 and 4.99, respectively [3]. There is a slight male preponderance (1.1:1), and mean age is 65 years for colonic and 56 years for rectal NETs [11].

Even though epidemiology has now been well studied [3], there is a lack of randomised prospective trial data. Management decisions are usually based on experience and expert recommendations.

The North American Neuroendocrine Tumour Society (NANETS) convened a multidisciplinary panel of leading experts from the United States, Canada and Europe and published their recommendations in 2010 [11, 12].

The American Joint Cancer Commission (AJCC) published a TNM classification system for colorectal NETs in 2010, which incorporates tumour size and depth of invasion into the T-stage classification [13] and is identical to the staging system proposed by the European Neuroendocrine Tumour Society (ENETS) in 2007 [14] (Table 37.1).

All of them divide colorectal NETs into well-differentiated and poorly differentiated categories and recommend a minimum pathological dataset to report these lesions (Table 37.2).

Even though finer aspects of nomenclature vary between the different society recommendations (Table 37.3), the distinction of well-differentiated from poorly differentiated is one of

Table 37.1 Staging of NETs of the colon and rectum

	AJCC	ENETS
Primary tumour (T)		
Tx	Primary tumour cannot be assessed	Primary tumour cannot be assessed
T0	No evidence of primary tumour	No evidence of primary tumour
T1	Tumour invades the lamina propria or submucosa and size <2 cm	Tumour invades the mucosa or submucosa
T1a	Tumour size <1 cm in greatest dimension	Size <1 cm
T1b	Tumour size 1–2 cm in greatest dimension	Size 1–2 cm
T2	Tumour invades the muscularis propria or size >2 cm with invasion of the lamina propria or submucosa	Tumour invades the muscularis propria or size >2 cm
T3	Tumour invades through the muscularis propria into subserosa or into nonperitonealized pericolic or perirectal tissue	Tumour invades subserosa/pericolic/perirectal fat
T4	Tumour invades the peritoneum or other organs	Tumour directly invades other organs/structures and/or perforates visceral peritoneum
Regional lymph nodes (N)		
Nx	Regional lymph nodes cannot be assessed	Regional lymph nodes cannot be assessed
N0	No regional lymph node metastases	No regional lymph node metastases
N1	Regional lymph node metastases	Regional lymph node metastases
Distant metastases (M)		
M0	No distant metastases	No distant metastases
M1	Distant metastases	Distant metastases

AJCC				ENETS			
Stage	T	N	M	Stage	T	N	M
I	T1	N0	M0	**IA**	T1a	N0	M0
				IB	T1b	N0	M0
IIA	T2	N0	M0	**IIA**	T2	N0	M0
IIB	T3	N0	M0	**IIB**	T3	N0	M0
IIIA	T4	N0	M0	**IIIA**	T4	N0	M0
IIIB	Any T	N1	M0	**IIIB**	Any T	N1	M0
IV	Any T	Any N	M1	**IV**	Any T	Any N	M1

Table 37.2 Minimum pathology dataset: information to be included in pathology reports on NETs of the hindgut

Details to be reported	For resection of primary tumours	For biopsy of primary tumours
Anatomic site of tumour	√	√
Diagnosis	√	√
Size (in three dimensions)	√	
Presence of unusual histologic features (oncocytic, clear cell, gland-forming and other features)	√	√
Presence of multicentric disease	√	
Immunohistochemical staining for general neuroendocrine markers: chromogranin, synaptophysin	*Optional*	*Optional*
Grade (specify grading system used)	√	√
Mitotic rate (number of mitoses per 10 high-power fields or 2 mm^2	√ count 50 high-power fields in the most active regions	√ count up to 50 high-power fields
Ki67 labelling index (count multiple regions with highest labelling density, report mean percentage; eyeballed estimate is adequate)	*Optional*	√ for biopsies in which a diagnosis of high-grade neuroendocrine carcinoma cannot be excluded
Presence of nonischaemic tumour necrosis	√	√
Presence of other pathologic components (e.g. nonneuroendocrine components)	√	√
Extent of invasion (depth of invasion into/through bowel wall)	√	
Involvement of serosal/peritoneal surfaces	√	
Invasion of adjacent organs or structures	√	
Presence of vascular invasion [perform immunohistochemical stains for endothelial markers if needed]	√ *Optional*	
Presence of perineural invasion	√	
Lymph node metastases Number of positive nodes Total number of nodes examined	√ √ √	
TNM staging (specify staging system used)	√	
Resection margins (positive/negative/close) [measure distance from margin if within 0.5 cm]	√ *Optional*	

Table 37.3 Nomenclature for NETs of the hindgut

Grade	Traditional	ENETS, WHO
Low grade	Carcinoid tumour	Neuroendocrine tumour, grade 1 (G1)
Intermediate grade	Carcinoid tumour	Neuroendocrine tumour, grade 2 (G2)
High grade	Small-cell carcinoma Large-cell neuroendocrine carcinoma	Neuroendocrine carcinoma, grade 3 (G3), small-cell carcinoma Neuroendocrine carcinoma, grade 3 (G3), large-cell neuroendocrine carcinoma

the most important pathological assessments, since the clinical course and the therapeutic interventions differ significantly between the two. The World Health Organisation (WHO) has revised its classification system in 2010 from the previous classification system in 2000 and now considers all NETs as malignant.

Presentations, Investigations and Treatment Options

Many colorectal NETs are found incidentally during routine endoscopic evaluation, and approximately 50% of patients are completely

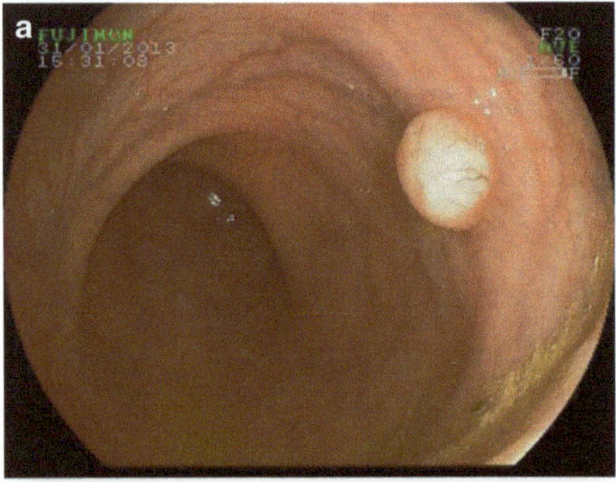

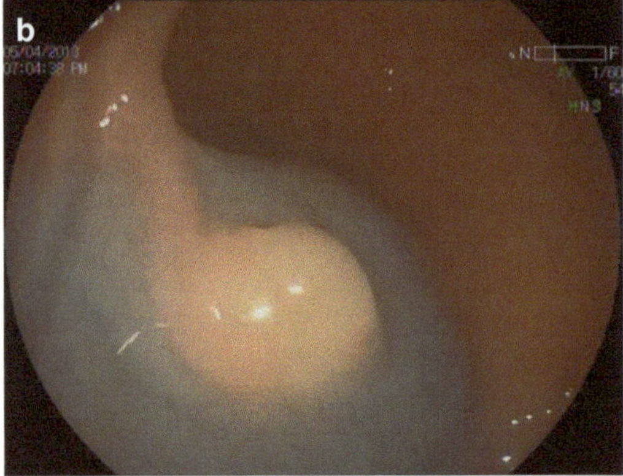

Fig. 37.1 (**a**) Neuroendocrine tumour of the rectum. (**b**) Neuroendocrine tumour of the rectum after saline lift

asymptomatic [15]. Patients who experience symptoms can present with rectal bleeding, pain and change in bowel habit [11, 15]. Unlike midgut NETs, hindgut NETs rarely exhibit hormonal syndromes such as flushing or diarrhoea, even in the metastatic stage.

Most rectal NETs arise in the mid-rectum, within 5–10 cm from the anal verge [16]. They are usually submucosal, with a typical appearance on endoscopy, which distinguishes them from adenomatous polyps arising from the mucosa (Fig. 37.1).

The risk of malignant behaviour is closely related to size and depth of invasion, and endorectal ultrasound (ERUS) is useful for evaluation of rectal NETs to assess tumour size, depth of invasion and lymph node involvement [17, 18]. NETs are usually well demarcated and either iso- or hypoechoic lesions within the hyperechoic submucosa. Kobayashi et al. [17] achieved a 100% accuracy in predicting depth of invasion in a series of 52 patients with rectal carcinoids and lesions as small as 2 mm.

ERUS can therefore be used to determine the mode of removal of the lesion and guide whether endoscopic or transanal removal versus radical surgery is appropriate.

Pathological grading as well as either mitotic index or Ki67 labelling is now recommended by WHO, ENETS and NANETS (Table 37.4). There is no data to support the use of both mitotic index and Ki67 concurrently, especially if an adequate amount of tissue is available to perform an accurate mitotic count (which requires a count of 40–50 high-power fields). Ki67 staining however provides a more accurate assessment of proliferative rate if the amount of tissue does not allow a high-quality mitotic count, e.g. in a biopsy sample. In those cases Ki67 labelling is particularly helpful to distinguish well-differentiated from poorly differentiated tumours, due to the dramatically different labelling rates [19, 20].

Routine cross-sectional imaging is only recommended for staging of rectal lesions that are bigger than 2 cm and not confined to the mucosa or submucosa on ERUS, as the risk of metastatic spread for the smaller and confined lesions is exceptionally small. Staging for the larger tumours can be performed by either computed tomography or magnetic resonance imaging [11].

The role of somatostatin receptor scintigraphy (octreoscan) for staging of localised tumours is controversial, since evidence is lacking that it improves the sensitivity of standard cross-sectional imaging techniques [11]. It can however be useful in patients with metastatic disease to ascertain the expression of somatostatin receptors, which can have therapeutic implications.

Less than 1% of hindgut NETs produce and secrete serotonin or other active hormones [21], which renders routine analysis of serum serotonin or urine 5-hydroxyindoleacetic acid (5-HIAA) unnecessary [11]. Serum chromogranin A can be a useful tumour marker to monitor patients with metastatic disease [22–24] and survey patients after resection of stage II or stage III tumours [11] or after cytoreductive surgery [25]. Chromogranin A is secreted by functional as well as less well-

Table 37.4 Grading systems for neuroendocrine tumours of the hindgut

Grade	Criteria
Low grade (G1)	<2 mitoses/10 hpf AND <3% Ki67 index
Intermediate grade (G2)	2–20 mitoses/10 hpf OR 3%–20% Ki67 index
High grade (G3)	>20 mitoses/10 hpf OR >20% Ki67 index

differentiated non-functional NETs [22]. Serum levels depend on tumour mass and grade [26], and small tumours can express normal levels. Falsely elevated chromogranin A levels however do occur in patients taking proton-pump inhibitors and have been reported in chronic gastritis, renal insufficiency and other inflammatory diseases [27]. Chromogranin B can be used as a complementary marker in such cases [27].

Carcinoid tumours appear to be associated with other non-carcinoid tumours. This has been found in 18–40% of cases, depending on the reported series [28–31] (22.4% in the SEER subset from 1992 to 99 [3]). The majority of those neoplasms occur in the gastrointestinal tract. The exact aetiology is unclear, but it is presumed that bioactive agents secreted by NETs act as mitogens and cause neoplastic transformation over time [32, 33]. It appears therefore appropriate to survey the colon, rectum, small intestine and lung, as well as the cervix and ovaries in female patients.

Surgical Technique/Rehabilitation

The main treatment goal for localised disease is removal of the primary, and modality is determined by the size and location of the lesion.

Small lesions (<1–2 cm) confined to the mucosa/submucosa can be resected endoscopically [17]. Several techniques have been described [34–38], including banding, aspiration and endoscopic submucosal dissection, to minimise the risk of positive margins. Following removal the area should be tattooed to allow identification if further resection is required and surveillance.

Intermediate lesions (1–2 cm) confined to the submucosa (T1) and small tumours (<1–2 cm) invading the muscularis propria (T2) without lymph node metastases should be considered for transanal excision, either directly [39] (distal rectum) or via transanal endoscopic microsurgery (TEMS) [40] for tumours located in the proximal rectum. TEMS can also be considered for technically challenging lesions and re-excision for positive margins after endoscopic removal [41, 42].

Larger lesions (>2 cm), tumours invading the muscularis propria (T2 and above) and tumours with loco-regional lymph nodes should be treated like a rectal adenocarcinoma and undergo a standard rectal resection [39].

Colonic lesions are usually more advanced at diagnosis and unless small should be treated with a standard segmental resection as would be appropriate for a malignant adenocarcinoma.

Postsurgical surveillance is determined by the stage of the lesion.

Stage I tumours (submucosal, <2 cm) recur rarely and do not justify long-term endoscopic or radiographic surveillance [11]. Stage II and III tumours (invasion into or beyond muscularis propria or involvement of loco-regional lymph nodes) require annual radiographic surveillance. Metastatic recurrence can occur many years after initial resection, and surveillance should therefore be extended beyond 5 years [11].

Published data on treatment outcomes for patients with metastatic colorectal NETs is scarce, and recommendations are usually extrapolated from trials for other gastrointestinal NETs. Treatment options for gastrointestinal NETs include somatostatin analogues, interferon alpha (INF-α), hepatic arterial embolization, cytotoxic chemotherapy and surgical cytoreduction. Further options are radiolabelled somatostatin analogues, angiogenesis inhibitors and mTOR inhibitors, all of which are currently undergoing evaluation in trial settings.

Since hindgut NETs are usually not associated with hormonal syndromes, the inhibitory effect of somatostatin analogues on NET growth [43, 44], which was demonstrated in human rectal NET cell lines in vitro [45], and antiproliferative effect of INF-α [46, 47] assume greater importance than their antisecretory action.

Hepatic arterial embolization can be performed for patients with diffuse, symptomatic and unresectable or progressive liver metastases. The procedure is performed in stages to reduce morbidity and with various embolic materials, including antineoplastic agents. Response can be measured radiographically, and rates have been reported to reach 50% in patients with metastatic gastrointestinal and pancreatic NETs [48–50].

Surgical cytoreduction is appropriate for patients with limited metastases and for the liver includes cryoablation and radiofrequency ablation (RFA). It is recommended if the cytoreduction can reduce the tumour burden by greater than 90%, therefore rendering the intent of the procedure curative or near-curative [51–54].

Cytotoxic chemotherapy should only be used for patients with symptomatic, advanced and aggressive tumours, who do not have other treatment options. Agents that can be used include streptozocin, 5-fluorouracil, doxorubicin, capecitabine and temozolomide. There is no published data to evaluate the outcome for hindgut NETs, and the treatment is associated with significant toxicities.

Results

In comparison with NETs in other locations, rectal NETs have favourable 5-year survival rates of 88% across stages (Table 37.5) [3, 55]. This is most likely due to the fact that the majority of lesions (82%) [3] is at a localised stage at diagnosis and on average measures 0.6cm [56]. Significant predictors of malignant behaviour in localised rectal NETs are tumour size, depth of invasion and lymph node involvement [21], as well as lymphovascular invasion and elevated mitotic rate (<2/50 hpf) [57].

There is less data available for colonic NETs. Colonic NETs have a reported poorer overall 5-year survival of 62% across stages [3]. They are usually spread more evenly across localised, regional and metastatic stage at diagnoses, leading to poorer outcomes.

Table 37.5 Five-year observed survival rates for carcinoid tumours by disease extent (from American Cancer Society, ACS [55])

Site	Localised (%)	Regional (%)	Distant (%)
Stomach	73	65	25
Duodenum	68	55	46
Jejunum/ileum	65	71	54
Cecum	68	71	54
Appendix	88	78	25
Colon	85	46	14
Rectum	90	62	24

Both rectal and colonic NETs tend to behave aggressively at the metastatic stage when compared to midgut NETs. Five-year survival is less than 30%, compared to over 50% for metastatic midgut NETs [55].

Conclusions/Personal View

Hindgut NETs are commonly found incidentally, and half of the patients are asymptomatic. Diagnosis at this early stage conveys an excellent prognosis. Primary lesions should be excised entirely and appropriately staged. Recurrences can occur years after resection, and all patients except stage I should be under follow-up for at least 7 years.

Metastatic hindgut NETs have a much worse prognosis than metastatic NETs of the midgut and are currently incurable, with survival rates similar to those of metastatic colorectal adenocarcinoma.

References

1. Vinik AI, Woltering EA, Warner RRP, et al. NANETS Consensus guidelines for the diagnosis of neuroendocrine tumours. Pancreas. 2010;39(6):713–34.
2. Massironi S, Sciola V, Peracchi M, et al. Neuroendocrine tumors of the gastro-entero-pancreatic system. World J Gastroenterol. 2008;14:5377–84.
3. Modlin IM, Lye KD, Kidd M. A 5-decade analysis of 13,715 carcinoid tumors. Cancer. 2003;97(4):934–59.
4. Langhans T. Ueber einen drusenpolyp im ileum. Virchow Arch Pathol Anat Physiol Klin Med. 1867;38:559–60.

5. Ransom WB. A case of primary carcinoma of the ileum. Lancet. 1890;2:1020–3.
6. Oberndorfer S. Karzenoide tumoren des dünndarms. Frankf Zschr Path. 1907;1:426–30.
7. Gosset A, Masson P. Tumeurs endocrines de l'appendice. Presse Med. 1914;25:237–9.
8. Godwin JD II. Carcinoid tumors, an analysis of 2837 cases. Cancer. 1975;36:560–9.
9. Modlin IM, Sandor A. An analysis of 8305 carcinoid tumors. Cancer. 1997;79:813–29.
10. Yao JC, Phan AT, Chang DZ, et al. Efficacy of RAD001 (everolimus) and octreotide LAR in advanced low- to intermediate-grade neuroendocrine tumors: results of a phase II study. [Erratum appears in J Clin Oncol. 2008; 26(34): 5660.]. J Clin Oncol. 2008;1926:4311–8.
11. Anthony LB, Strosberg JR, Klimstra DS, et al. The NANETS Consensus guidelines for the diagnosis and management of gastrointestinal neuroendocrine tumours (NETs) – well differentiated NETs of the distal colon and rectum. Pancreas. 2010;39(6):767–74.
12. Kvols LK, Brendtro KL. The North American Neuroendocrine Tumor Society (NANETS) Guidelines – mission, goals, and process. Pancreas. 2010;39(6):705–6.
13. Edge SB, Byrd DR, Compton CC. AJCC cancer staging manual. 7th ed. New York: Springer; 2010.
14. Rindi G, Kloppel G, Couvelard A, et al. TNM staging of midgut and hindgut (neuro) endocrine tumors: a consensus proposal including a grading system. Virchows Arch. 2007;451(4):757–62.
15. Wang AY, Ahmad NA. Rectal carcinoids [Review]. Curr Opin Gastroenterol. 2006;22(5):529–35.
16. Shim KN, Yang SK, Myung SJ, et al. Atypical endoscopic features of rectal carcinoids. Endoscopy. 2004;36(4):313–6.
17. Kobayashi K, Katsumata T, Yoshizawa S, et al. Indications of endoscopic polypectomy for rectal carcinoid tumors and clinical usefulness of endoscopic ultrasonography. Dis Colon Rectum. 2005;48(2):285–91.
18. Fujishima H, Misawa T, Maruoka A, et al. Rectal carcinoid tumor: endoscopic ultrasonographic detection and endoscopic removal. Eur J Radiol. 1993;16(3):198–200.
19. Lin O, Olgac S, Green I, et al. Immunohistochemical staining of cytologic smears with MIB-1 helps distinguish low-grade from high-grade neuroendocrine neoplasms. Am J Clin Pathol. 2003;120(2):209–16.
20. Pelosi G, Rodriguez J, Viale G, et al. Typical and atypical pulmonary carcinoid tumor overdiagnosed as small-cell carcinoma on biopsy specimens: a major pitfall in the management of lung cancer patients. Am J Surg Pathol. 2005;29(2):179–87.
21. Mani S, Modlin IM, Ballantyne G, et al. Carcinoids of the rectum [Review]. J Am Coll Surg. 1994;179(2):231–48.
22. Eriksson B, Oberg K, Stridsberg M, et al. Tumor markers in neuroendocrine tumors [Review]. Digestion. 2000;62(suppl 1):33–8.
23. O'Connor DT, Deftos LJ. Secretion of chromogranin A by peptide-producing endocrine neoplasms. New Engl J Med. 1986;314(18):1145–51.
24. Nobels FR, Kwekkeboom DJ, Bouillon R, et al. Chromogranin A: its clinical value as marker of neuroendocrine tumours. Eur J Clin Invest. 1998;28:431–40.
25. Jensen EH, Kvols L, McLoughlin JM, et al. Biomarkers predict outcomes following cytoreductive surgery for hepatic metastases from functional carcinoid tumors. Ann Surg Oncol. 2007;14:780–5.
26. Nobels FR, Kwekkeboom DJ, Coopmans W, et al. Chromogranin A as serum marker for neuroendocrine neoplasia: comparison with neuron-specific enolase and the alpha-subunit of glycoprotein hormones. J Clin Endocrinol Metab. 1997;82:2622–8.
27. Stridsberg M, Eriksson B, Fellstrom B, et al. Measurements of chromogranin B can serve as a complement to chromogranin A. Regul Pept. 2007;139:80–3.
28. Berge T, Linell F. Carcinoid tumors. Frequency in a defined population during a 12-year-period. Acta Pathol Microbiol Scand. 1976;84:322–30.
29. Saha S, Hoda S, Godfrey R, Sutherland C, Raybon K. Carcinoid tumors of the gastrointestinal tract: a 44-year experience. South Med J. 1989;82:1501–5.
30. Marshall JB, Bodnarchuk G. Carcinoid tumors of the gut. J Clin Gastroenterol. 1993;16:123–9.
31. Olney JR, Urdaneta LF, Al-Jurf AS, Jochimsen PR, Shirazi SS. Carcinoid tumors of the gastrointestinal tract. Am Surg. 1985;51:37–41.
32. Oberg K. Expression of growth factors and their receptors in neuroendocrine gut and pancreatic tumors, and prognostic factors for survival. Ann N Y Acad Sci. 1994;733:46–55.
33. Modlin IM, Goldenring JR, Lawton GP, Hunt R. Aspects of the theoretical basis and clinical relevance of low acid states. Am J Gastroenterol. 1994;89:308–18.
34. Berkelhammer C, Jasper I, Kirvaitis E, et al. "Band-snare" resection of small rectal carcinoid tumors. Gastrointest Endosc. 1999;50(4):582–5.
35. Fujishiro M, Yahagi N, Nakamura M, et al. Successful outcomes of a novel endoscopic treatment for GI tumors: endoscopic submucosal dissection with a mixture of high-molecular-weight hyaluronic acid, glycerin, and sugar. Gastrointest Endosc. 2006;63(2):243–9.
36. Ono A, Fujii T, Saito Y, et al. Endoscopic submucosal resection of rectal carcinoid tumors with a ligation device. Gastrointest Endosc. 2003;57(4):583–7.
37. Okamoto Y, Fujii M, Tateiwa S, et al. Treatment of multiple rectal carcinoids by endoscopic mucosal resection using a device for esophageal variceal ligation. Endoscopy. 2004;36(5):469–70.
38. Imada-Shirakata Y, Sakai M, Kajiyama T, et al. Endoscopic resection of rectal carcinoid tumors using aspiration lumpectomy. Endoscopy. 1997;29(1):34–8.
39. Schindl M, Niederle B, Hafner M, et al. Stage-dependent therapy of rectal carcinoid tumors. World J Surg. 1998;22(6):628–33.

40. Buess G, Hutterer F, Theiss J, et al. A system for a transanal endoscopic rectum operation. [in German]. Chirurg. 1984;55(10):677–80.
41. Kinoshita T, Kanehira E, Omura K, et al. Transanal endoscopic microsurgery in the treatment of rectal carcinoid tumor. Surg Endosc. 2007;21(6):970–4.
42. Tsai BM, Finne CO, Nordenstam JF, et al. Transanal endoscopic microsurgery resection of rectal tumors: outcomes and recommendations. Dis Colon Rectum. 2010;53(1):16–23.
43. Arnold R, Trautmann ME, Creutzfeldt W, et al. Somatostatin analogue octreotide and inhibition of tumour growth in metastatic endocrine gastroentero-pancreatic tumours. Gut. 1996;38(3):430–8.
44. Ducreux M, Ruszniewski P, Chayvialle JA, et al. The antitumoral effect of the long-acting somatostatin analog lanreotide in neuroendocrine tumors. Am J Gastroenterol. 2000;95(11):3276–81.
45. Koizumi M, Onda M, Tanaka N, et al. Antiangiogenic effect of octreotide inhibits the growth of human rectal neuroendocrine carcinoma. Digestion. 2002;1965:200–6.
46. Arnold R, Rinke A, Klose KJ, et al. Octreotide versus octreotide plus interferon-alpha in endocrine gastroenteropancreatic tumors: a randomized trial. Clin Gastroenterol Hepatol. 2005;3(8):761–71.
47. Kolby L, Persson G, Franzen S, et al. Randomized clinical trial of the effect of interferon alpha on survival in patients with disseminated midgut carcinoid tumours. Br J Surg. 2003;1990:687–93.
48. Eriksson BK, Larsson EG, Skogseid BM, et al. Liver embolizations of patients with malignant neuroendocrine gastrointestinal tumors. Cancer. 1998;83(11):2293–301.
49. Gupta S, Yao JC, Ahrar K, et al. Hepatic artery embolization and chemoembolization for treatment of patients with metastatic carcinoid tumors: the M.D. Anderson experience. Cancer J. 2003;9(4):261–7.
50. Strosberg JR, Choi J, Cantor AB, et al. Selective hepatic artery embolization for treatment of patients with metastatic carcinoid and pancreatic endocrine tumors. Cancer Control. 2006;13(1):72–8.
51. Norton JA, Warren RS, Kelly MG, et al. Aggressive surgery for metastatic liver neuroendocrine tumors. Surgery. 2003;134(6):1057–63.
52. Osborne DA, Zervos EE, Strosberg J, et al. Improved outcome with cytoreduction versus embolization for symptomatic hepatic metastases of carcinoid and neuroendocrine tumors. [erratum appears in Ann Surg Oncol. 2006;13(8):1162. Note: Strosberg, Jonathon [corrected to Strosberg, Jonathan]]. Ann Surg Oncol. 2006;13(4):572–81.
53. Sarmiento JM, Que FG, Sarmiento JM, et al. Hepatic surgery for metastases from neuroendocrine tumors. Surg Oncol Clin N Am. 2003;12(1):231–42.
54. Boudreaux JP, Putty B, Frey DJ, et al. Surgical treatment of advanced-stage carcinoid tumors: lessons learned. Ann Surg. 2005;241:839–45.
55. http://www.cancer.org/acs/groups/cid/documents/webcontent/003102-pdf.pdf.
56. Landry CS, Brock G, Scoggins CR, et al. A proposed staging system for rectal carcinoid tumors based on an analysis of 4701 patients. Surgery. 2008;144(3):460–6.
57. Fahy BN, Tang LH, Klimstra D, et al. Carcinoid of the rectum risk stratification (CaRRS): a strategy for preoperative outcome assessment. Ann Surg Oncol. 2007;14(2):396–404.